Exit 199
N. Service Rd.
50's Cafe

Mosby's Q&A for NCLEX-PN

EDITOR

Mary Yannes-Eyles, *RN, MA*

Director, Education Department
Kessler Institute for Rehabilitation, Inc.
West Orange, New Jersey

Instructor, LPN Review Course
Rockland Community College
Suffern, New York

(formerly) Director of Continuing Education
National Association for Practical Nurse Education and Service, Inc. (N.A.P.N.E.S.)

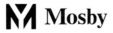 **Mosby**

St. Louis Baltimore Boston Chicago London Madrid Philadelphia Sydney Toronto

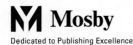

Editor: Susan Epstein
Developmental Editor: Beverly Copland
Project Manager: Gayle May Morris
Production Editor: Mary Cusick Drone
Manufacturing Supervisor: Betty Richmond
Designer: Susan Lane

Printed in the United States of America

Composition by Graphic World, Inc.
Printing/binding by Maple-Vail Book Mfg. Group

Mosby–Year Book, Inc.
11830 Westline Industrial Drive
St. Louis, Missouri 63146

International Standard Book Number 0-8016-6952-9

93 94 95 96 97 / 9 8 7 6 5 4 3 2 1

To
my mother, *Mary E. Yannes*
and to the memory of my father, *William P. Yannes*
without whom I would not be,
and who, more importantly,
offered the encouragement and support
necessary for me to believe in myself
as they did in me.

Associate Editor

Martha Phillips, RN, MA

Associate Professor of Nursing, Iona College, New Rochelle, New York

Contributors

Persephone C. Agrafiotis, RN, PhD, BSN, MEd

Management Consultant, Manchester, New Hampshire.

Lora Jean Miller Alley, RN

Former Instructor of Practical Nursing, Jacksboro Vocational-Technical School, Jacksboro, Tennessee.

Cynthia Amerson, RN, BSN, MS

Director, Nursing Science, Northeast Texas Community College, Mount Pleasant, Texas.

Gwendolyn Price Berry, RN, MS, MEd

Instructor, Level I and II, Vocational Nursing Program, Houston Community College System, Southeast College, Houston, Texas.

Gloria Depole-Coschigano, RN, MSN, CS

Assistant Professor, Iona College, New Rochelle, New York.

Nancy M. Daniels, RN, MN, CS

Lieutenant Colonel, Army Nurse Corps, Department of Nursing, Brooke Army Medical Center, Fort Sam Houston, Texas.

Karen Hill, RN, MN

Assistant Professor, School of Nursing, Southeastern Louisiana University, Hammond, Louisiana.

Larita Norris Kaspar, MSN, RN

Assistant Professor, Division of Allied Health and Nursing, Lorain County Community College, Elyria, Ohio.

Frances Jean Kelley, PhD, RN

Assistant Professor of Clinical Nursing, The University of Texas Houston Health Science Center, School of Nursing, Houston, Texas.

Lucy Longoria Miller, RN, BSN, MS

Nursing Instructor, Del Mar College, Corpus Christi, Texas.

Sally L. Persons-Beck, RN, MS, CPC

Occupational Health Coordinator, Midwest Power Systems, Des Moines, Iowa.

Judith L. Pulito, RN, MSN

Instructor, Lorain County Community College, Elyria, Ohio.

Rita Harrison Raymond, RN, MSN, CS

School of Nursing, Duquesne University, Pittsburgh, Pennsylvania.

Virginia Ann Smith, PhD, RN

Grayson County College, Sherman, Texas; University of Texas, Arlington, Texas.

REVIEWER PANEL

Catherine Burke, BSN, MS

Pat Castaldi, RN, BSN, MSN

Linda Clark-Cutchen, MSN

Mary Ann Cosgarea, RN, BA, BSN

Cathy Franklin, RN, BSN, MA

Joyce Hamlin, BSN, MSN

Wendy F. Higden, BN

Patricia Jacobson, RN, MSN

Marjorie Knox, BSN, MA, MPA

Dorothy Thomas, RN, MSN

Wendy Wilson-Weslowski, RN, BSN, MSN, NHA

Beverly Yeshion, RN, BSN, ACCE

Preface

This new review tool from Mosby was developed to help you prepare for the NCLEX-PN examination in the United States and the Practical Nurse/Nursing Assistant Registration/Licensure examination in Canada. More than 1600 questions provide ample experience in answering questions. The broad scope of content covered enables you to evaluate your knowledge of nursing and your readiness for the NCLEX-PN. Answers with rationales promote understanding and help you learn from your mistakes.

The questions in this text were developed by experienced educators and practitioners. All questions follow the stand-alone, multiple choice format used in the new, computerized NCLEX examination. The content covered by the questions was selected from the areas identified in the Test Plan for the NCLEX-PN.

Chapter 1 discusses the NCLEX examination—what it will test and how. Study techniques and test-taking tips are provided to help you make the best use of your time and abilities.

Chapters 2, 3, and 4 include 1150 questions covering medical-surgical, psychiatric/mental health, and maternal/child nursing. Questions in each of these chapters are grouped by subtopic to enable you to review and evaluate specific content areas.

Chapter 5 provides two comprehensive practice examinations that reflect the scope of the NCLEX examination. Use these practice tests to evaluate your overall knowledge and to help learn to pace yourself for the actual examination.

Chapters 6 and 7 include the answers and rationales for all questions, and are tabbed and perforated for easy location and removal. Rationales explain why the correct answers are right and why each of the other options is wrong. Rationales also indicate the cognitive level, step of the nursing process, client needs category, and level of difficulty for each question. Use this information to determine your specific areas of strengths and weakness.

This text is a logical companion to *Mosby's PN AssessTest* and *Mosby's Comprehensive Review of Practical Nursing.* These three components make up a complete review and study package for any student preparing for the NCLEX-PN.

• • •

I would like to take this opportunity to thank my colleagues for their efforts, which has culminated in the development of this text. My appreciation also extends to the professionals who have served on the editorial review panel. In addition, I would like to thank those at Mosby for assisting in the development of this review book, especially Susan Epstein, Beverly Copland, Mary Drone, and Susan Lane. And of course, thanks and gratitude to Martha Phillips, Associate Editor, and to my family, especially my husband Robert, who have been extremely supportive throughout the duration of the entire project.

To all who are about to become LP/VNs, our best wishes for a successful examination and a rewarding career.

Mary Yannes–Eyles

Contents

Chapters list question numbers by subject.

3 Maternal/Child Health Nursing Questions 50

CHAPTER 1

Preparing for the NCLEX-PN Examination

The practice of nursing is regulated by law for the principal purpose of public protection. The respective State Boards of Nursing are charged with the responsibility of upholding the regulation of such law. The National Council Licensure Examination for Practical Nurses (NCLEX-PN) covers all areas of the practical/vocational nursing curriculum and has been further designed to test nursing knowledge, including the ability to apply principles of that knowledge to individual clinical situations in a safe and effective manner.

NCLEX-PN

THE NCLEX-PN was developed by the National Council of State Boards of Nursing (NCSBN). The examination is based on a test plan that is designed to evaluate entry-level performance while incorporating the nursing process and identified client needs. As stated in the actual test plan, "the Practical Nurse Test Plan is distinguished from the Registered Nurse Test Plan by the scope of practice as defined by member jurisdictions, by the practical nurse job analyses, and by the tested levels of cognitive abilities."

As of April 1994 the NCLEX-PN examination will be administered via computerized adaptive testing (CAT), a change from the traditional paper-and-pencil method of testing. The number of questions per individual will vary on the CAT and will be based on the candidate's performance, which measures knowledge, skills, and abilities. All successful candidates will answer no fewer than 75 questions and a maximum of approximately 195 questions within a 5-hour time frame. Rest periods (one mandatory after the first 2 hours of testing and one optional following the next 90 minutes of testing) and a computer tutorial are included within the 5-hour testing session. Tests are scored to determine the number of correct answers (raw score). The raw score is then measured against the set standard, which is the minimum score set to guarantee that the test taker is competent in the nursing knowledge and skills being tested. Scores reflect the "pass" or "fail" status of the candidate with the majority of the boards using the same pass/fail score as determined by the Angoff method, a criterion-referenced, standard-setting technique commonly used by the NCSBN.

A candidate who fails the examination will receive a diagnostic profile that will assist in focusing further study efforts for retaking the examination.

The examination has been developed with the basic knowledge necessary for the practice of practical/vocational nursing, and contains test items reflecting the cognitive levels of knowledge, comprehension, and application.

The two major components of the test plan are (1) the phases of the nursing process and (2) client needs.* Keep in mind that the elements of accountability, nutrition, anatomy and physiology, growth and development, documen-

tation, communication, fundamentals, and patient education are found throughout the examination.

Percentage of test items on the examination relative to the *phases of the nursing process* as set forth in the test plan are as follows:*

1. Data collection (assessment) 30%: the collection of data in clients with predictable outcomes, which contributes to a data base and assists in the formulation of a nursing diagnosis.
   * Observes total needs of client—physiologic, psychosocial, health, and saftey
   * Collects information from various sources—client, family, records, team members
   * Determines needs for additional information
   * Communicates findings of collected data
2. Planning 20%: contributes to the nursing care plan by assisting in setting goals, identifying client needs (some of which may require a change in the plan of care), and communicating with all those involved in the client's care.
   * Contributes to development of nursing care plans for clients with health needs
   * Assists in goal formulation
   * Participates in identifying client needs and those nursing measures that will aid in achieving set goals
   * Communicates needs that may indicate a change in the care plan
   * Communicates with client, family, and team members when planning nursing care
3. Implementation 30%: performing basic therapeutic and preventive nursing measures in a safe and effective environment. The measures follow a prescribed plan to achieve established goals, including appropriate data reporting and documenting and assistance to the client, family, and other members of the health team in understanding the plan of care.
   * Provides a safe and effective care environment
   * Assists all concerned in understanding the care plan
   * Records information and reports it to other members of the health team

*Adapted from NCLEX-PN Test Plan for National Council Licensure Examination for Practical Nurses, 1989.

4. Evaluation 20%: participates in evaluating effectiveness of care, observing and documenting client response to care, and how/if identified outcomes have been realized.
   * Participates in evaluating effectiveness of nursing care
   * Assists in evaluating client response to nursing care and in making necessary changes
   * Evaluates extent to which specific outcomes of the care plan are achieved
   * Records/describes client response to therapy and nursing care

Percentage of items on the examination relative to *client needs* as set forth in the test plan are as follows:

1. Safe, effective care environment 24% to 30%: includes coordinated care; standards of care; goal-oriented care; environmental safety; preparation for treatments and procedures; safe and effective treatments and procedures.
   Examples of the knowledge, skills, and abilities for this category of client need are as follows:
   * Data gathering techniques; communication skills, preparation for prescribed treatments and procedures; environmental and client safety; infection control; clients' rights; confidentiality; individualized care relative to religious, cultural, and developmental influences; team participation in care planning and evaluation; and general knowledge of community agencies

2. Physiologic integrity 42% to 48%: includes physiologic adaptation; reduction of risk potential; mobility; comfort provisions of basic care.
   Examples of the knowledge, skills, and abilities for this category of client need are as follows:
   * Therapeutic and life-saving techniques; specialized equipment; principles of administering medications; maintenance of optimal body functioning and prevention of complications; principles of body mechanics and assistive devices; comfort measures; routine nursing measures; and reporting changes in condition

3. Psychosocial integrity 7% to 13%: includes psychosocial adaptation and coping skills.
   Examples of the knowledge, skills, and abilities for this category of client need are as follows:
   * Obvious signs of emotional and mental health problems; self-concept; life crisis; chemical dependency; adaptive and maladaptive behavior; sensory deprivation and overload; abusive and self-destructive behavior; therapeutic communication; common therapies; and general knowledge of community resources

4. Health promotion/maintenance 15% to 21%: includes continued growth and development; self-care; integrity of support system; prevention and early treatment of disease.
   Examples of the knowledge, skills, and abilities for this category of client need are as follows:
   * Family interactions; concepts of wellness; adaptation to altered health states; reproduction and human sexuality; birthing and parenting; growth and development, including death and dying; immunization; health teaching that is appropriate to the scope of practice; and general knowledge of community resources

Please note that the NCLEX-PN examination contains several test items that are being validated for use in future NCLEX-PN examinations. These questions are not identifiable and whether answered correctly or not, the test taker neither gains nor loses points.

REVIEW AND PREPARATION FOR NCLEX-PN

The key to effective review and preparation for the examination lies solely with YOU and the goals you have set for yourself. Review is necessary in order to become familiar with the extent of your nursing knowledge, allowing you to identify your areas of strength as well as those areas in which you need additional study. Review texts, such as *Mosby's Comprehensive Review of Practical Nursing* and *Mosby's PN Assess Test,* will give you the added benefit of increasing your familiarity with and ability to respond to test questions similar to those presented in the NCLEX-PN examination.

How, what, when, and where you study are entirely up to you; however, being practical and using common sense are vital to the study process. The following suggestions will be helpful to you when devising a study plan that is right for *you*:

* Begin with a *positive attitude!*
* Establish the priority of the study plan as a means of accomplishing the ultimate goal—passing the NCLEX-PN examination.
* Develop a realistic study-time schedule that is somewhat flexible to accommodate what needs to be done within the time available; follow the schedule as closely as possible, revising the schedule if necessary; pinpoint a study time that is convenient for you rather than someone else; specify the amount of time you will need for study; be prepared for the unexpected; provide for free time in the overall schedule.
* Improve your organizational ability by developing a checklist for the study plan and schedule you have designed for yourself.
* Improve your ability to remember through repetition, visualization, associating facts and concepts with use of the senses (touch, smell, hearing), and creating a cue system that will serve to jog your memory on difficult/complicated concepts.
* Choose a quiet study environment where interruptions will be minimal or eliminated.
* Plan to study in an upright position by sitting in a chair at a desk or a table; refrain from using the comfortable overstuffed chair or studying in bed.
* Include a few quick stretch breaks in each block of study time.

What and how to study must be included in the study plan. Most nursing professionals would agree that whether you decide to study by yourself, with a friend, or as part of a group, you will need to allow a good 6 to 8 weeks or more of study prior to sitting for NCLEX-PN. Cramming is *not* recommended. You may also wish to consider taking a review course that provides for more study structure and in most cases incorporates a review book such as *Mosby's Comprehensive Review of Practical Nursing.* Use of a review text is recommended because the most important and vital areas of the practical/vocational nursing curriculum are usually presented in an outline format that allows for a much quicker yet thorough review of the topic. Also included are questions and comprehensive examinations similar to NCLEX-PN. The review text thus increases students' familiarity and self-confidence with multiple-choice questions and the format of NCLEX-PN.

Review of material and exposure to questions relevant to that material provide a means to identify strengths and weaknesses, thus allowing for quality study time on weaker areas of comprehension. Once weaker areas have been identified, it may be necessary to refer to nursing school texts, handouts, class notes, or nursing journals for further study in that particular area of content.

In whichever way you decide to study, do not simply read through the material looking only for facts and hoping you will be able to recall what you've read. It will be necessary to think in-depth as you read, looking for main and associated ideas. Review what you've read, repeating important information in context of larger ideas as a means of retaining what you've just learned.

This text contains two examinations, each having two parts. Each part contains 120 questions with a recommended completion time of 2 hours. Although time may no longer be a major concern during the actual examination, which in a way decreases the anxiety of taking a timed test, becoming more proficient in time-management skills will only be to your advantage during the actual examination.

TEST-TAKING SKILLS: STRATEGIES FOR SUCCESS

No matter how many tests you have taken, preparation for a licensing examination creates a bit more anxiety than usual. Being prepared and becoming more comfortable and familiar with the testing format will help decrease your anxiety level. A certain amount of anxiety will always be present, however, serving to sharpen your senses and make you more alert to the realities of the testing procedure and content.

While in school, you were most likely exposed to several methods of testing. The NCLEX-PN examination deals only with the objective method and more specifically with the objective multiple-choice form of testing. Each question contains a stem (the main intent of the question), followed by four possible options/answers that either complete a statement or answer the question presented. Only *one* of the four choices is the best or most appropriate answer; the remaining three options are known as *distractors,* so named because they are written in such a way that they *could* be correct and so distract you to a certain degree. Knowing that your nursing knowledge is being subtly tested, your strength in that knowledge will lead you to the correct response.

Although this form of testing may be familiar to you, consider the following in an attempt to avoid some of the more common test-taking errors:

- **Answer the question that is being asked.** To do so you need to read, not scan, the situation and the question carefully, looking for key words or phrases. Do not read anything into the question or apply what you did in a similar situation during one of your clinical experiences. Instead, think about what the question is really asking. Reflect back on your nursing knowledge, asking yourself how you would handle the situation in an ideal setting. Then choose what you feel to be the best or most appropriate response.
- **Identify key words or phrases.** Key words or phrases in the stem of the question, such as *first, only, primary, early, best,* or *most appropriate* are essential when determining the intent of the question. Words such as *only, always, never* and *all* in the options will frequently be evidence of an incorrect response. There are no absolutes in nursing, as there are none in life. Of course, there are exceptions to every rule, so answer with care.
- **Identify option parts (components) as being correct or incorrect.** If for instance each option contained three supposed side effects of a given drug, you would be wise to consider each side effect individually as being correct or not for the drug in question. If even one of the three in any given option is incorrect, then the option itself is not the correct answer.
- **Identify and eliminate options that you know are definitely incorrect.** By doing so you will have increased your chances of selecting the correct answer, in addition to having more time to focus on the true nature of the question.
- **Identify options that are similar in nature.** If three of the options all share a direct relationship to one another, then the fourth option (not necessarily in that order) will most likely be the correct answer, as it is this option that will either include the other three or totally exclude them from the situation. If neither is the case, then the question is not written properly.
- **Identify words in options that are identical, similar in nature, or closely related to those in the stem.** Such similarities can provide clues to the correct response.
- **Be alert to grammatical inconsistencies.** If the response, which is intended to complete the stem (presented as an incomplete sentence), makes no grammatical sense, it can be considered to be a distractor rather than the correct answer. Likewise, if the stem phrase indicates a singular in the response and several of the options provide responses that are plural in nature, one can safely eliminate those as the correct answer.
- **Answering questions.** You have at least a 25% chance of selecting the correct answer. Wild guesses should be avoided at all costs. Should you feel insecure about a question, try to eliminate the options you feel are definitely incorrect by calling on your nursing knowledge and one or more of the methods listed. This will increase your chances of making an educated guess at the correct answer. *Remember,* although there is no penalty for guessing on the examination, the subsequent question will, to an extent, be based on the respone to a given question. That is, if you answer incorrectly, the computer will formulate the next question accordingly based on your knowledge/skill performance on the examination up to that point.
- **At times, the correct answer may be the longest option given.** Although the longest answer option may be correct in some cases, don't consider it foolproof. Test developers are very much aware of this technique and may include wordy options that are incorrect as a way of testing your knowledge.
- **Avoid looking for an answer pattern or code.** Often four or five consecutive questions will have the same letter or number for the correct answer.
- **Have confidence in your initial response.** It will probably be the correct answer. Serious consideration should be given before recording a response, because once a response has been entered, another question will appear on the screen. On the CAT test, skipping questions or going back to review and/or change responses is not possible.
- **Budget your time wisely.** Remember, although time is not a factor, don't spend too much time on any one question. One minute is the recommended time that should be allotted to a single question. Not all questions will consume a full minute; some may take only 15 or 20 seconds to read and answer.
- **Answer those questions that you know first.** *During practice study sessions* in which the more traditional pa-

per-and-pencil method of testing is used, it is recommended that you answer those questions that you know first, returning to the more difficult questions at a later time, as this is an excellent way to build confidence in preparation for the actual examination. As already noted, skipping and/or returning to change a response is not possible on the CAT test.

The night before the examination you may wish to review some material; but then relax and get a good night's sleep. Make sure to set your alarm or arrange to have someone call you. In the morning allow yourself plenty of time to dress, have breakfast, and arrive at the testing site at least 15 to 30 minutes before the start of the test. Be sure you know where to park and where the test will be given (room location). In addition, remember to take eyeglasses (if needed), your admission card, and a second proof of identity. Once seated in

the testing center, listen to the examiner carefully. All candidates will be given a short training session that includes a keyboard tutorial complete with a practice session. No prior computer experience is necessary. Failure to listen to the directions thoroughly may lead to an error that could cost considerable points. Should you have any question about these instructions, ask the examiner for further explanation. By doing so, you will be able to control your stress level and proceed confidently.

One final note: no two candidates will be given the same questions to answer, because the examination is individualized according to the candidate's knowledge and skills while meeting test plan requirements.

Above all, approach the examination with a *positive attitude* about yourself, your nursing knowledge, and your test-taking abilities.

CHAPTER 2

Medical-Surgical Nursing Review Questions

1. Carmella Bennitto, age 52, is seen in the clinic with bilateral pain and swelling in her knees and fingers. Her diagnosis is rheumatoid arthritis. Additional assessment data would most likely reveal the following:
   1. Pain more severe in the late evening, less severe in the morning
   2. Low-grade fever only during the night
   3. Pain and stiffness more severe in the morning
   4. Constant bone pain, with a history of fractures

2. For a patient with rheumatoid arthritis, instructions to best decrease pain and stiffness would include:
   1. Taking a cool bath or shower on arising
   2. Active exercises to all joints using weights
   3. Taking aspirin 20 minutes before arising
   4. Aerobic exercise for 30 minutes three times a week

3. To prevent flexion deformities in a patient with rheumatoid arthritis, the nurse should include which of the following positions in the turning schedule?
   1. High Fowler's
   2. Prone
   3. Sims'
   4. Trendelenburg's

4. A patient with rheumatoid arthritis asks if she can substitute acetaminophen (Tylenol) for her aspirin because it is on sale. The nurse's response will be based on the understanding that:
   1. Both can be used interchangeably
   2. Both are analgesic drugs
   3. Acetaminophen (Tylenol) increases gastric secretions
   4. Aspirin is an antiinflammatory drug

5. Mrs. Polter suffers from severe arthritis. The nurse is aware that the term *arthritis* refers to:
   1. Chronic inflammatory disease of the diarthrodial joints
   2. Acute joint problems
   3. Infectious condition of the joints
   4. Infection of synarthrodial joints

6. A patient asks the nurse if there are different forms of arthritis. The nurse explains that rheumatoid arthritis is differentiated from osteoarthritis because it is characterized by:
   1. Degeneration of the joint
   2. Chronic inflammatory reaction in the synovial membrane
   3. Porous and brittle bones
   4. Inflammation of the bone

7. Carrie Lynn has been in a nursing home for several years because of increasing disability from rheumatoid arthritis. The main nursing measure in Carrie's treatment is:
   1. Ensuring complete bed rest with range-of-motion exercises
   2. Limiting activities because they tire her
   3. Keeping the joints immobilized
   4. Preventing contractures and maintaining range of motion in all joints

8. In treating a patient who has rheumatoid arthritis that was diagnosed several years ago, a major goal is relieving her pain and inflammation through antiinflammatory agents. The nurse should administer this medication:
   1. Between meals
   2. With meals
   3. At bedtime
   4. On a limited basis

9. Rehabilitation for a patient with rheumatoid arthritis is directed toward:
   1. Bed rest
   2. Feeding her meals
   3. Total care
   4. Adaptation to physical limitations

10. A patient tells the nurse that she has heard of a new cure for her condition, rheumatoid arthritis, and is seeking information on it. The nurse's response should be:
    1. "That's great! You should be happy that this is really happening."
    2. "You should talk to your physician about this."
    3. "Tell me about it, and we can let your physician know."
    4. "You have to be careful about these cures. They are just a lot of empty promises that are quite costly."

11. Mr. Wilson is a 35-year-old electrician who has been admitted to the hospital with gouty arthritis (gout). Mr. Wilson questions the nurse about his condition. The nurse explains that gout is a disorder:
    1. That is metabolic and results in decreased bone mass
    2. In which excessive amounts of uric acid accumulate in the blood
    3. That is a chronic inflammatory process involving connective tissue
    4. Affects local weight-bearing joints and results in disintegration of cartilage

12. When planning nursing care for a patient with gout, the nurse remembers that the pathologic cause of gout is the body's inability to metabolize:
    ① Purines
    ② Fats
    ③ Carbohydrates
    ④ Calcium

13. When assessing a patient with a diagnosis of gouty arthritis, the nurse is aware that the most common subjective complaint is:
    ① Limited range of motion of all joints
    ② Sweating of hands and feet
    ③ Acute pain in the great toe
    ④ Morning stiffness

14. The dietitian and patient have already discussed the dietary restrictions related to gout. Later the patient, Mr. T, tells the nurse that he forgot which foods to avoid. The nurse should instruct Mr. T to avoid:
    ① Cheese, milk, and dairy products
    ② Marbled hamburger, lean steaks, and pork
    ③ Potatoes, breads, and sugar
    ④ Liver, kidney, and sardines

15. For a patient with gout, which of the following drugs would most likely be on the drug profile?
    ① Allopurinol
    ② Corticosteroids
    ③ Acetaminophen
    ④ Estrogen replacement

16. Mr. Henderson, a 43-year-old construction worker, had been working on a housing project when he felt a sudden, sharp pain in his lower back. He is brought to the emergency room for evaluation, and the initial diagnosis is a herniated intervertebral disk at L5-S1. What signs and symptoms would you most expect Mr. Henderson to exhibit?
    ① Acute pain in the lower back, pain radiating across his buttock, and sciatic leg pain
    ② Pain aggravated by motion, edema, and crepitus
    ③ Subjective pain, limited motion, and localized swelling
    ④ Bone pain, progressive weakness, and anemia

17. Mr. Higgins, a 50-year-old printer, had been working in his print shop when he felt something snap in his back. He is brought to the emergency department for evaluation, and his initial diagnosis is a herniated intervertebral disk at L5-S1. For a confirmation of this diagnosis, which tests would the nurse anticipate?
    ① Health history, blood chemistries, and x-ray examination
    ② Computed tomography, magnetic resonance imaging, and physical examination
    ③ Bone scan, x-ray examination, and bone biopsy
    ④ Bone scan, arthroscopy, and x-ray examination

18. Mr. Smith, a 46-year-old railroad worker, had been laying new track when he felt something snap in his back. He is brought to the emergency room for evaluation, and his initial diagnosis a herniated intervertebral disk at L5-S1. Conservative treatment that the nurse could expect in planning Mr. Smith's care would include:
    ① The maintenance of spinal cord alignment, log rolling, and frequent observations of respiratory and neurologic functioning
    ② The administration of analgesics, antiinflammatories as ordered, application of heat and cold, and provision of range-of-motion exercises
    ③ The administration of antiinflammatory and uriocosuric agents as prescribed, weight loss if indicated, and provision of patient education
    ④ Application of heat, administration of analgesics as ordered, back brace, and bed rest

19. Mr. Ross, a 53-year-old electrical lineman, had been installing new electrical lines and felt a sudden pain in his back. Diagnostic tests reveal that Mr. Ross has a herniated lumbar disk with spinal nerve impingement. He is scheduled for a laminectomy. The nurse explains to Mr. Ross that this surgical procedure involves:
    ① Removing only the extruding disk material
    ② Usually fusing several disks together to stabilize the spine
    ③ Removing the arch of the vertebrae and then removing the disk
    ④ Guiding a needle into the nucleus pulposus to inject chymopapain, performed under a local anesthetic agent

20. Mr. Lee, a 45-year-old gas installation worker, has a herniated intervertebral disk at L4-5 and is scheduled for a laminectomy. Postoperative laminectomy care involves:
    ① Maintaining bed rest, providing complete care, anticipating needs by leaving call bell within reach, and establishing means of communication
    ② Frequent observation of respiratory and neurologic functioning, maintaining spinal alignment at all times, and instituting active and passive range-of-motion exercises as soon as prescribed
    ③ Not turning patient on side, observing for signs of hemorrhage, observing for swelling, notifying physician if necessary, and administering analgesics judiciously
    ④ Assessing incision for signs of infection, monitoring intake and output, encouraging sitting in a straight-back chair for a limited period, and monitoring for respiratory distress

21. Mr. Scott, a 53-year-old carpenter, had a back injury that required a lumbar laminectomy. On discharge, Mr. Scott should be instructed:
    1. Not to drive until permitted by surgeon, to avoid twisting motions of trunk, and not to lift weights over 5 lb
    2. To practice environmental safety, including use of grab bars in the bathroom, rubber mats in the shower or tub, and a side rail on the bed
    3. To carefully monitor intake and output, to wear thigh-high antiembolism stockings, and to do isometric exercises
    4. To eat only a soft diet, to work toward independence in hygiene and dressing, and to exercise daily as tolerated

22. John Curtis, a 26-year-old male, was admitted to the emergency department with a fracture of the tibia following a skiing accident. While preparing to care for John, the nurse is aware that the tibia is:
    1. The main weight-bearing bone of the leg
    2. Located at the upper aspect of the leg
    3. Surrounded by little muscular tissue
    4. Connected to the lateral malleolus

23. Mark, 27 years old, was admitted to the emergency deparment with a fractured tibia following a biking accident. X-ray examination of the leg shows a complete fracture, which means:
    1. It is a torsion fracture
    2. The bone is splintered into three or more fragments
    3. It is a telescoped fracture
    4. The fracture line extends entirely through the bone

24. A young man was admitted to the emergency department with a fracture of the tibia and a full leg cast was applied. Primary nursing care for a patient in a cast is to:
    1. Turn the patient frequently
    2. Keep the patient dry and clean
    3. Observe closely for circulatory impairment
    4. Check the drying time of the cast

25. A patient who recently suffered a fractured leg during a skiing accident asks the nurse if he will be able to ski again. The nurse's most appropriate response is:
    1. "Of course. You'll be on skis again in no time!"
    2. "A fractured bone never heals completely, and it leaves the bone weak. You should hang up your skis."
    3. "It is a bit early to determine this, but it usually doesn't affect future skiing. What kinds of concerns do you have?"
    4. "You should ask your physician when he comes in."

26. When caring for a patient in a full leg cast, the nurse's main goal is:
    1. Application of support to prevent further injury
    2. Immobilization of the leg to promote healing
    3. Ensuring comfort and pain relief
    4. Prevention of hemorrhage and shock

27. When placing a patient with a full leg cast on a bedpan, the nurse should:
    1. Support the cast with pillows
    2. Protect the edge of cast with plastic
    3. Elevate the head of the bed
    4. Ask the patient to lift himself

28. Mr. Cardenas, age 69, is admitted to the hospital with an open wound on his right forearm and a fractured right leg that he sustained in an automobile accident. The physician ordered the wound to be cleansed with povidone-iodine and a sterile dressing to be applied. What is the best technique to clean debris and drainage from the wound?
    1. Using a sterile 4 × 4 pad, move from outer edge of wound to center
    2. Using a sterile 4 × 4 pad, move from center of wound outward
    3. Using a sterile 4 × 4 pad, move from center of wound outward in a circular motion
    4. Using a new sterile 4 × 4 pad for each area cleaned, move from center of wound outward

29. In planning for a patient's wound care, what important nursing measures should the nurse consider *first?*
    1. Preparing supplies
    2. Checking drainage tubes
    3. Giving assistance to patient's needs
    4. Reducing the transfer of microorganisms

30. The nurse is to apply a roller bandage to a patient's arm. The arm should be wrapped starting at:
    1. The wrist, wrapping toward the hand
    2. The wrist, wrapping toward the elbow
    3. The elbow, wrapping toward the wrist
    4. The fingers, wrapping toward the wrist

31. The physician writes an order concerning the frequency of observing a patient's cast. How often should the casted area be inspected for signs of possible complications during the first 24 hours after it is applied?
    1. Every 15 minutes
    2. Every hour
    3. Every 3 hours
    4. Every 4 hours

32. The nurse prepares to petal a patient's cast. The primary purpose of petaling a cast is to help prevent:
    1. The cast from becoming wet
    2. The cast from becoming too tight
    3. Debris from getting under the cast
    4. The cast from irritating the patient's skin

33. Mr. Thompson, a 76-year-old man, is admitted to the hospital with a fracture of the left femur. Surgical reduction of the fracture and insertion of an Austin-Moore prosthesis is done. In planning nursing care for Mr. Thompson, it is important that the leg with the hip prosthesis be kept slightly:
    1. Abducted
    2. Adducted
    3. Flexed
    4. Prone

34. When turning a patient with a hip prosthesis, the nurse should know to:
    1. Place the patient on the affected side
    2. Place the patient on the unaffected side
    3. Maintain the patient's head at a 90-degree angle
    4. Maintain the patient's head at a 45-degree angle

35. Mr. Jackson, who has a hip prosthesis, tells you he does not like lying in bed all the time. He thinks he is well enough to walk with assistance. The nurse explains to him that a patient with a hip prosthesis:
    1. Will be getting up the next day after surgery
    2. Is not allowed to have full weight bearing until 3 days after surgery
    3. Will be allowed partial weight bearing in 7 to 10 days and can use crutches in 3 to 6 months
    4. Will be allowed partial weight bearing in 10 to 14 days and full weight bearing in about 4 weeks

36. Mr. Corbin, who has a hip prosthesis, becomes depressed and says, "I'm never going to walk right again, am I?" The nurse's best response would be:
    1. "What makes you think you will never walk right again?"
    2. "Of course you will, it is just going to take time!"
    3. "You will be up and walking before you know it."
    4. "Why don't we see if there is something good on television?"

37. Mr. Jeff Hoffa, age 66, is admitted to the hospital for a below-the-knee amputation. Following surgery, his orders include meperidine (Demerol) 50 mg intramuscularly for relief of pain and intravenous fluids. Mr. Hoffa tells the nurse, "It hurts so much." Before administering Mr. Hoffa's medication for pain relief, the nurse should make which initial assessment?
    1. Where is his discomfort?
    2. Does he have a pulse deficit?
    3. Is his urine output adequate?
    4. Does he have active bowel sounds?

38. A patient with a below-the-knee amputation has a compression bandage applied. The compression bandage would be achieving the desired effect on his residual limb if which of these observations were made?
    1. The incision is well approximated
    2. The wound is free of drainage
    3. There is no evidence of edema
    4. The skin edges are pink

39. Following his below-the-knee amputation, Mr. Malloy received instructions about care of his residual limb. Which of these comments by him indicates the need for further teaching?
    1. "I'll rub my residual limb with alcohol twice a day."
    2. "I'll press my residual limb against a pillow when the wound is healed."
    3. "I'll bathe my residual limb with soap and water every day."
    4. "I'll be sure to exercise the joints above and below my residual limb every day."

40. A patient with a below-the-knee amputation is being taught to walk with crutches. Which basic principle of crutch walking should the nurse emphasize for this patient?
    1. When ascending stairs, the crutch and the residual limb should go up first
    2. The major part of the body weight is maintained by the patient's axilla
    3. The patient should continually check his foot position when walking with crutches
    4. Before starting to walk, the patient begins the gait in the tripod position

41. Juan Thomas, a 68-year-old man with severe arteriosclerosis, is scheduled for a left midthigh amputation. Preoperative teaching for Mr. Thomas should include making him aware:
    1. Of the adjustment period needed when using an artificial limb
    2. Of the need to turn frequently
    3. That he will not experience phantom limb pain
    4. Of the need to lie on his back without too much movement

42. Preoperative care for a patient scheduled in surgery for a left midthigh amputation should include:
    1. Elevation of the affected leg to decrease the need for blood to circulate to the area
    2. Repeated blood work to determine the amount of blood flow to the lower extremity
    3. Bed rest to decrease movement of the affected leg
    4. Palpation of bilateral pedal pulses

43. In caring for a patient immediately following a left midthigh amputation and for the first 48 hours following surgery, the nurse should:
    1. Keep the residual limb lowered in the bed to promote circulation to the operative site
    2. Elevate the residual limb on pillows
    3. Observe for signs of bleeding under the dressing
    4. Place bed boards under the mattress for firm support under the residual limb

44. The most common postoperative complication that the nurse should watch for following a midthigh amputation is:
    1. Contractions of hip flexors and abductor muscles
    2. Hemorrhage at the operative site
    3. Infection at the operative site
    4. Embolism caused by decreased mobility

45. Following a midthigh amputation, application of elastic wraps to the residual limb is necessary primarily to:
    1. Decrease the chance of hemorrhage at the operative site
    2. Shrink and reshape the residual limb
    3. Decrease the chance of edema at the operative site
    4. Decrease the chance of infection at the operative site

46. After an above-the-knee amputation (AKA), Mr. Kent will be fitted for his prosthesis when his physical exercise has:
    1. Strengthened the normal leg so it can bear the weight of the body
    2. Strengthened the muscle tone in both legs
    3. Prevented flexion of both hips
    4. Strengthened the muscle power in the residual limb to equal that of the normal leg

47. A patient is brought to the emergency department with profuse epistaxis. As the nurse on duty, your immediate action would be to:
    1. Obtain the patient's medical history and available insurance
    2. Decrease the patient's level of anxiety, if present
    3. Apply pressure on the bridge of the nose
    4. Assess patient's vital signs every 15 minutes

48. When caring for a patient with an epistaxis, the nurse should place the patient in:
    1. Supine position with the head tilted backward
    2. Supine position with the head leaning forward
    3. Fowler's position with the head leaning forward
    4. Fowler's position with the head tilted backward

49. A 65-year-old man is admitted to the hospital with cancer of the larynx. An early sign of laryngeal cancer is:
    1. Pain
    2. Hoarseness
    3. Weight loss
    4. Difficulty swallowing

50. A total laryngectomy and radical neck dissection is planned for a patient with cancer of the larynx. The patient asks the nurse about the effect the surgery will have on his breathing. The nurse's response is based on the fact that the patient will breathe through:
    1. His nose
    2. His mouth
    3. A temporary tracheostomy
    4. A permanent tracheostomy

51. When suctioning secretions of a patient with a tracheostomy, suction is turned off as the catheter is inserted to prevent:
    1. Irritation of the lining of the trachea and loss of additional oxygen
    2. Blocking of the catheter with mucus
    3. Infection of the oral cavity
    4. "Kinking" of the catheter

52. Following a total laryngectomy, which of the following findings during the nurse's assessment indicates a need to suction the patient's laryngectomy tube?
    1. Decreased pulse, and decreased respiratory rate
    2. Moisture on the neck dressing and increased swallowing
    3. Increasing respirations and use of accessory muscles
    4. Chest pain and a dry, hacking cough

53. Nursing actions during suctioning of a laryngectomy tube would include:
    1. Continuous suctioning while withdrawing the catheter
    2. Suctioning limited to no more than 10 seconds
    3. Applying suction while inserting the catheter
    4. Positioning patient in the supine position

54. When a patient is first admitted to the postanesthesia unit (recovery room) following a laryngectomy, he or she should be positioned:
    1. On his or her back
    2. On his or her side
    3. With his or her head down
    4. In a sitting position

55. As part of discharge planning for the patient who has a total laryngectomy, the nurse would include teaching about which of the following daily activities that would require modification?
    1. Bathing
    2. Walking
    3. Sleeping
    4. Exercising

56. Mrs. Brown, a 90-year-old alert, homebound woman, was admitted to the hospital with pneumonia. She has a painful, productive cough with thick sputum, chest pain, and chills. Her vital signs are temperature 103° F, pulse rate 110, and respirations 58. The physician ordered acetaminophen (Tylenol) 500 mg PO q4h for discomfort, oxygen at 3 L, and penicillin liquid 500 mg PO tid. In planning care for Mrs. Brown, the nurse knows that elderly persons are primarily susceptible to pneumonia because of:
    1. Limited activity
    2. Poor diet
    3. Age
    4. Limited expansion of rib cage

57. Chest pain is a common symptom in a patient with pneumonia, usually occurring on the affected side. When it does occur, the nurse should encourage the patient to:
    1. Breathe deeply to relieve the pain
    2. Lie on the affected side to cough
    3. Cough frequently
    4. Lie on the unaffected side to cough

58. When planning care for a 90-year-old patient who is ill, the nurse is aware that dehydration can occur when:
    1. The body is unable to excrete sufficient amounts of sodium
    2. There is inadequate food or fluid intake
    3. The kidneys are unable to excrete wastes normally
    4. The bladder is unable to hold urine

59. Mrs. Sandler, age 95, was admitted to the hospital with pneumonia. The orders written for the patient include forcing fluids by mouth. In planning care for this patient, the nurse is aware that the main purpose of this order is to:
    1. Help rid the body of waste products
    2. Maintain proper nutrition
    3. Dilute the toxins in the body
    4. Lower the body temperature

60. Treatment protocol and overall prognosis for a patient with pneumonia depend on the causative organism, which is determined by which of the following diagnostic tests?
    1. X-ray examination
    2. Gastric lavage
    3. Blood/sputum tests
    4. Bronchoscopy

61. The physician ordered acetaminophen (Tylenol) 500 mg PO q4h for a patient with diagnosed pneumonia. When evaluating patient response to the drug, the nurse is aware that acetaminophen is used specifically to aid in:
    1. Kidney function
    2. Sputum reduction
    3. Fever reduction
    4. Fluid retention

62. Mrs. Samson, age 60, is admitted to the unit with a diagnosis of pneumonia. Admitting vital signs are temperature 103° F, pulse rate 116, and respirations 58. The predominant indication that oxygen shortage is occurring is evidenced by:
    1. Cyanosis
    2. Dyspnea
    3. Increased respiratory rate
    4. Increased pulse rate

63. Mr. England, age 20, is brought to the emergency room. His diagnosis is spontaneous right pneumothorax. On Mr. England's admission, which of these signs and symptoms should the nurse expect to find?
    1. Breathing that is not symmetric
    2. Harsh productive cough
    3. Pain that is increased by sitting up
    4. Audible wheezing or rhonchi

64. A patient has a chest tube connected to an underwater-seal drainage system. He has been given instructions about the chest drainage system. Which of these comments by the patient would indicate that he has accurate knowledge about the system?
    1. "I'll empty the drainage container and record the results."
    2. "I'll lie on my right side while the drainage system is in place."
    3. "I'll keep the drainage system below the level of my chest."
    4. "I will remain in bed until the drainage system is removed."

65. While bathing a patient with a chest tube connected to an underwater-seal drainage system, the nurse observes that the chest tube has fallen out. Which of these actions should the nurse perform *first?*
    1. Seal off the wound
    2. Call the team leader
    3. Prepare for CPR
    4. Reinsert the tube

66. When planning the nursing care for a patient in general, the nurse should remember that:
    1. All patients require constant attention
    2. The diagnosis determines the patient's needs, more than maintaining the patient's independence
    3. Patients are admitted to a hospital when they cannot care for themselves
    4. A patient is an individual with unique needs and problems; therefore, nursing care should be planned according to needs and problems

67. A man is brought to the emergency room with multiple knife wounds to the chest. His diagnosis is a sucking chest wound. In preparing this patient's care plan, the nurse should be aware that this condition is commonly known as:
    1. Pneumothorax
    2. Pneumonia
    3. Epistaxis
    4. Hemathorax

68. Which of the following observations by the nurse would most likely indicate that a lung has been punctured?
    1. White, frothy sputum from the mouth
    2. Bright red, frothy sputum from the mouth
    3. Thick, purulent drainage from the mouth
    4. Copious, dark red drainage from the mouth

69. A patient has returned from surgery with underwater-seal drainage. In assisting the patient to understand more about his postoperative care, the nurse explains that the chest tubes are inserted into:
    1. Thoracic cavity
    2. Punctured lung
    3. Pleural space
    4. Visceral space

70. In planning nursing care for a patient with underwater-seal drainage, the nurse should remember that the primary goal for using this procedure is to:
    1. Allow expansions of the affected lung by draining secretions and air by gravitation
    2. Restore the negative pressure within the thoracic cavity
    3. Restore the atmospheric pressure within the thoracic cavity
    4. Equalize the pressure within the thoracic cavity by allowing expansion of both lungs

71. When caring for a patient with an underwater-seal drainage system, the nurse must know that the bottle closest to the patient:
    1. Provides drainage of secretions by suction
    2. Provides drainage of secretions via gravity
    3. Measures the patient's inspiration
    4. Measures the patient's expiration

72. When caring for a patient with an underwater-seal drainage system, the nurse should make sure the bottles remain:
    1. Higher than the patient
    2. Lower than the patient
    3. At the same level of the patient's chest
    4. The level of the bottles is not important

73. The nurse's prime responsibility when caring for a patient with underwater-seal drainage is to:
    1. Keep the drainage system at eye level
    2. Monitor the patient's weight daily
    3. Empty the drainage bottles every hour
    4. Observe the patient and drainage system every hour

74. If a bottle in the underwater-seal drainage system breaks, which action should the nurse carry out *first?*
    1. Call for help
    2. Observe for respiratory distress
    3. Raise the head of the bed and check vital signs
    4. Clamp the chest tubes immediately

75. A 30-year-old mechanic was injured in an automobile accident and is brought to the hospital for observations of possible pneumothorax and the insertion of a chest tube. Assessment is *most* likely to reveal:
    1. Shortness of breath and sharp pain on affected side
    2. Sharp pain that is relieved by leaning forward
    3. Increased breath sounds on the affected side
    4. Absence of breath sounds on the unaffected side

76. A chest x-ray examination confirms a pneumothorax, and the physician inserts a pleural tube in the anterior chest. The nurse tells the patient that the purpose of the chest tube is to:
    1. Instill antibiotics
    2. Drain secretions
    3. Remove blood
    4. Remove air

77. A patient who has had a chest tube inserted for a pneumothorax is transferred to the nursing unit. After he is moved from the stretcher to the bed, the *most* appropriate action is to:
    1. "Strip" the tube to enhance drainage
    2. Mark the time of measurement and the fluid level
    3. Raise the bottle to chest height to check for air bubbles
    4. Place the drainage system at the foot of the bed

78. Following insertion, a pleural tube is connected to a drainage system with low suction. The nurse assesses the water-seal chamber of the drainage system. Which finding indicates that the system is working effectively?
    1. No fluctuation is observed in the water-seal chamber
    2. Continuous and constant bubbling is noted in the water seal
    3. Fluctuations are observed rising with inspirations and falling with expirations
    4. The fluctuation of the fluid in the water-seal chamber increases the first 24 hours

79. The physician is preparing to remove a chest tube. The nurse should instruct the patient to:
    1. Take several rapid, shallow breaths
    2. Inhale deeply and hold the breath
    3. Perform a Valsalva's maneuver
    4. Do pursed-lip breathing

80. A nursing colleague had a Mantoux test performed after being notified that her patient has an active case of tuberculosis. The nurse is aware that this test is read after:
    1. 24 hours
    2. 36 hours
    3. 48 hours
    4. 96 hours

81. Mary Ellen has a diagnosis of tuberculosis and is seen in the respiratory clinic. Signs and symptoms Mary Ellen would be expected to report:
    1. Thick, rusty-colored sputum
    2. Consistent high fever
    3. Development of dependent edema
    4. Generalized skin rash

82. A patient with tuberculosis requires a sputum specimen for acid-fast bacillus. The most appropriate nursing intervention for sputum collection is:
    1. Encourage her to do abdominal breathing while coughing
    2. Cleanse her mouth with hydrogen peroxide before taking the specimen
    3. Instruct her to take a deep breath and cough from the diaphragm
    4. Keep her in a semi-Fowler's position while obtaining the specimen

83. A patient with tuberculosis is placed on isoniazid (INH) and pyrazinamide (Tebrazid). A realistic goal for this patient would be that he or she will have:
    1. Negative sputum tests in 1 week
    2. A return of energy in 2 to 3 days
    3. Absence of a cough in 1 week
    4. A normal temperature in 3 weeks

84. When teaching a patient with tuberculosis who is taking rifampin on an outpatient basis, the nurse should instruct her to:
    1. Double the next dose if a dose is missed
    2. Weigh herself once a week
    3. Expect urine color to be dark orange
    4. Decrease the dose if anorexia and nausea develops

85. Mr. Adams, a 32-year-old unemployed laborer, has been admitted with fever, weight loss, weakness, a productive cough, bloody sputum, and night sweats. Because these symptoms suggest tuberculosis (TB), the physician's orders include a Mantoux test, three sputum specimens to be sent to the laboratory, and a chest x-ray examination. A positive reading of the Mantoux test indicates that Mr. Adams has:
    1. Been exposed to the disease but does not necessarily have it
    2. An active case of TB
    3. No active case of TB at this time
    4. Been exposed to the disease and has it

86. Alex, a 21-year-old college student, has a diagnosis of tuberculosis. The nurse knows that sputum specimens must be obtained in the early morning because:
    1. It is easier for the night nurse to collect the specimen
    2. Coughing up sputum does not occur during the day hours
    3. An arbitrary assignment of time has been given
    4. Secretions pool overnight and are less likely to be contaminated

87. Mr. Abrams, a 32-year-old unemployed laborer, is admitted with a diagnosis of tuberculosis. The nurse has identified that the primary patient teaching for Mr. Abrams should include:
    1. Strict isolation technique, avoiding family and friends
    2. Proper disposal and handwashing techniques related to coughing and sneezing
    3. Proper diet to gain weight
    4. Rest to regain his strength

88. The main pharmacologic treatment for tuberculosis (TB) includes isoniazid (INH) and *para*-aminosalicylate sodium (PAS). In planning care for a patient receiving these medications, the nurse is aware that they are used:
    1. To prevent the TB organisms from multiplying
    2. For 6 to 8 weeks
    3. To destroy the TB organisms
    4. For the rest of his life

89. A patient with a diagnosis of tuberculosis (TB) asks the nurse the main purpose of drug therapy. The nurse's best response is that drug therapy is used:
    1. To cure him of the disease
    2. To prevent recurrence of the disease
    3. To arrest the disease
    4. To develop immunity to the TB organism

90. Mr. Brown is seen in the physician's office with complaints of chest pain, hemoptysis, anorexia, and weight loss. The physician admits Mr. Brown to the hospital to rule out tuberculosis. In addition to Mr. Brown's signs and symptoms of tuberculosis, the nurse would expect Mr. Brown to have:
    ① Expiratory wheeze
    ② Confusion
    ③ Night sweats
    ④ Hemothorax

91. To confirm a patient's diagnosis of tuberculosis, further diagnostic testing is necessary, and the physician orders a sputum test for AFB. The nurse knows this test is done to identify the causative organism known as:
    ① Shigella bacillus
    ② Gas bacillus
    ③ Koch's bacillus
    ④ Epstein-Barr virus

92. The family of a recently admitted patient with a diagnosis of tuberculosis has been advised by the physician that each family member should receive a tuberculin test. When administering the test, which method of injection would the nurse use for the skin test?
    ① Intramuscular
    ② Subcutaneous
    ③ Intradermal
    ④ Z-track method

93. When administering a tuberculin skin test, the nurse would insert the needle at an angle of:
    ① 15 degrees
    ② 25 degrees
    ③ 45 degrees
    ④ 90 degrees

94. After administering a tuberculin skin test, it is important for the nurse to:
    ① Massage the area with firm strokes
    ② Massage the area with gentle strokes
    ③ Refrain from massaging the site of injection
    ④ Rub the site with an alcohol swab

95. Mr. Barnes has a diagnosis of tuberculosis (TB). Mr. Barnes' wife expresses her concern about her own positive result to the tuberculin skin test. The nurse should explain to her that a positive skin test indicates that:
    ① She is infected and needs to be admitted to the hospital
    ② Exposure to the TB organism; further tests may be required
    ③ She has an immunity to the TB organism and does not need to worry
    ④ She has had an allergic reaction to the skin test and should not take it again

96. Marilee Ann, age 43, has a diagnosis of asthma. When planning care for this patient, the nurse should know that asthma is defined as:
    ① A chronic, progressive condition that involves destruction of the elastic tissues of the alveolar walls
    ② A chronic dilation of a bronchus or bronchi, with secretions of large amounts of purulent sputum
    ③ A respiratory disorder characterized by recurring episodes of labored breathing with wheezing on expiration
    ④ An infectious disease caused by a tubercle bacillus

97. Mr. Tom, age 58, has chronic emphysema. His condition has deteriorated in the past several months, and he is admitted to the hospital. While obtaining a patient history, which of the following risk factors should the nurse identify as the primary cause of Mr. Tom's emphysema?
    ① History of pneumonia last month
    ② Smoking two packs of cigarettes a day
    ③ Living in an industrial area
    ④ High-fat and high-cholesterol diet

98. Theophylline (Theo-Dur) therapy was started for a patient with emphysema. The main pharmacologic action of this drug is:
    ① Relaxation of bronchial smooth muscle
    ② Bronchial constriction
    ③ Liquefying and thinning secretions
    ④ Vasoconstriction of major vessels

99. A patient with emphysema is receiving aminophylline intravenously. The most common side effect that the nurse must observe for is:
    ① Bradycardia
    ② Hypotension
    ③ Lethargy
    ④ Weight gain

100. Mr. Thomas has emphysema. Which of the following characteristics would the nurse expect him to exhibit?
    ① Thin body build and a pigeon chest
    ② Cyanotic skin color and dry, sparse hair
    ③ Peripheral edema and moist, shiny skin
    ④ Barreled chest and clubbing of the fingers

101. Mr. Thomas requires a tracheotomy. Which of the following procedures should be carried out by the nurse when suctioning secretions in Mr. Thomas?
    ① Oxygenate, suction for 30 seconds, oxygenate
    ② Oxygenate, suction for 15 seconds, cough and deep-breath
    ③ Oxygenate, suction for 10 seconds, oxygenate
    ④ Oxygenate, suction for 25 seconds, allow to rest

102. A patient is admitted to the hospital with a history of weakness, a productive cough, and a 15-pound weight loss over the last month. The physician suspects lung cancer. A bronchoscopy is performed, and the patient has returned to the nursing unit. Which postprocedural order would *most likely* be included in the plan of care?
    ① Save all sputum
    ② Observe the neck dressing for drainage
    ③ Keep NPO until the gag reflex has returned
    ④ Whisper rather than talk for at least 1 week

103. A localized lesion was observed during a bronchoscopy, and the patient is scheduled for a pneumonectomy. In this surgical procedure:
    ① The localized, diseased portion is removed
    ② Segments of diseased lung are removed
    ③ One lobe of the lung is removed
    ④ An entire lung is removed

104. Nursing interventions during the postoperative period following a pneumonectomy will *most likely* include:
    ① Monitoring closed chest drainage
    ② Placing the patient in semi-Fowler's position
    ③ Administering anticoagulant medications
    ④ Positioning the patient in the supine position for the first 24 hours

105. Niki Neals, age 68, is admitted with dyspnea and pitting edema of both ankles. Physician's orders include bed rest, oxygen at 4 L, morphine sulfate 5 mg subcutaneously q4h, Lasix 40 mg PO stat, and a chest x-ray examination. The preliminary diagnosis is pulmonary edema. The chest x-ray examination report, which confirmed the diagnosis of pulmonary edema, showed:
① Thickened bronchial margins
② Widened intercostal spaces
③ Enlarged main pulmonary artery
④ Increased fluid in the pleural space and an enlarged heart

106. Pulmonary edema is caused by the:
① Increase of fluid in the circulating blood
② Decrease of fluid in the bronchi
③ Increase of fluid in the bronchi
④ Decrease of fluid in the circulating blood

107. Rebecca Morris, age 68, is admitted with dyspnea and pitting edema of both ankles. Physician's orders include Lasix 40 mg PO stat. What measures would the nurse take to evaluate the effects of Lasix?
① Monitor intake and output and check for facial edema
② Record daily weights and monitor intake and output
③ Limit fluid intake and check for pedal edema
④ Check for pedal and facial edema

108. A patient with pulmonary edema tells the nurse she is frightened by her difficult breathing. She says she feels she is suffocating. The nurse's response would be to:
① Have her take some deep breaths to relax, and report the condition to the charge nurse
② Tell her that there is medication she can have that will help her breathing
③ Tell her that she is too anxious over this and that the anxiety is making her worse
④ Report this condition to the charge nurse

109. At a discharge planning meeting, the need for oxygen administration is discussed for Ms. Robinson, a patient with pulmonary edema. Which device for administering oxygen should be recommended for Ms. Robinson?
① Face mask
② Oxygen tent
③ Nasal catheter
④ Nasal cannula

110. Chlorothiazide is given to expel fluid from the body and prevent pulmonary edema. When evaluating patient response to the drug, the nurse should also observe for:
① Hematuria
② Nausea and vomiting
③ Diarrhea
④ Muscular weakness and cramping

111. Venous blood is pumped from the right atrium into the right ventricle through the:
① Tricuspid valve
② Biscuspid valve
③ Aortic valve
④ Mitral valve

112. The sinoatrial node is located in the:
① Left atrium
② Right atrium
③ Left ventricle
④ Right ventricle

113. A patient complains of pain in the lower extremities, tingling and numbness of the toes, and cramping of the calf muscles. The nurse knows that this is commonly called intermittent claudication and is caused by:
① Poor circulation
② Tight clothing
③ Poor diet
④ Inadequate rest

114. Michael Sands, a 65-year-old laborer, is admitted to the hospital complaining of pain in the lower extremities, tingling and numbness of the toes, cramplike pain in the calf muscles at night, and angina. Nursing care for Mr. Sands should include:
① Keeping extremities uncovered to relieve undue pressure on the legs
② Instructing him to lie still in bed to prevent the possibility of thrombi forming
③ Keeping him warm
④ Instructing him to bathe infrequently to decrease the risk of dislodging emboli

115. A patient is admitted to the hospital complaining of pain in the lower extremities; tingling and numbness of the toes; and cramplike pain in the calf muscles at night. When planning care, the nurse should discourage this patient from:
① Drinking alcoholic beverages
② Smoking
③ Drinking coffee
④ Drinking tea

116. A patient states that he is afraid he will lose his job as a laborer because of his pending surgery. The nurse's response should be:
① "Don't worry about that now; there's time later to think about it."
② "Being a laborer is stressful. You'll have to get another job."
③ "You're surely eligible for unemployment benefits. Why not sit back and collect what is due you?"
④ "You seem concerned about your job. Do you want to talk about it?"

117. When planning the nursing care for a patient with angina pectoris, the nurse understands that this condition results from:
① Arteries that harden, thicken, and lose their elasticity
② Obstruction of a coronary artery or one of its branches
③ Failure of the heart to pump sufficient blood through the body
④ Insufficient oxygenated blood to the myocardial tissue

118. To appropriately assess a patient's symptoms related to angina pectoris, the nurse understands that the factor distinguishing angina pectoris from myocardial infarction is that the pain:
    ① Usually lasts longer than 15 minutes
    ② Usually occurs during periods of exertion
    ③ Is accompanied by diaphoresis and tachycardia
    ④ Does not radiate to the upper extremities

119. When a patient complains of anginal pain, the nurse would expect him or her to describe it in which of the following ways?
    ① Mild midepigastric pain
    ② Sharp, burning, substernal pain
    ③ Severe, crushing chest pain
    ④ Dull, ache-like pain in the arm

120. Which of these statements made by a patient would indicate that teaching about a low-sodium diet was effective?
    ① "Canned vegetables have the same sodium content as fresh."
    ② "I will read all labels on packaged foods."
    ③ "Beef has the same sodium content as cheese."
    ④ "Canned fruits are high in sodium."

121. Which of these statements made by a patient with angina would indicate the need for further teaching about nitroglycerin therapy?
    ① "I will take one nitroglycerin tablet before engaging in strenuous activity."
    ② "I will store the nitroglycerin tablets in a dark container."
    ③ "I will discard nitroglycerin tablets that cause a burning sensation under my tongue."
    ④ "I can take three nitroglycerin tablets 5 minutes apart to control chest pain."

122. Mr. Kelly, age 60, has been experiencing intermittent chest pain for the last 6 months. He seems to be more aware of the pain during exertion. He takes nitroglycerin sublingual and rests, and his pain seems to subside. The outstanding symptom of angina pectoris is:
    ① Acute pain that is often mistaken for indigestion
    ② Severe cyanosis
    ③ Elevation of blood pressure
    ④ Chest pain that radiates down the left arm

123. A patient who has angina pectoris is receiving nitroglycerin and wants to know how the drug works in the body. The nurse would explain that the drug:
    ① Constricts the coronary vessels
    ② Dilates the coronary arteries
    ③ Relieves pain by depressing the nervous system
    ④ Relaxes the muscles of the heart

124. If the nurse leaves a supply of nitroglycerin tablets at the patient's bedside, she should:
    ① Check on the number of tablets left in the bottle and record the amount taken by the patient each time
    ② Check the patient's blood pressure q6h and record
    ③ Discourage the patient from taking too many pills, which could lead to drug dependency
    ④ Realize that she has no responsibility for the patient regarding nitroglycerin

125. When planning nursing care for a patient with angina pectoris, which of the following should be considered a primary goal?
    ① Administering vasodilating drugs promptly
    ② Restricting dietary fat and cholesterol
    ③ Relieving the patient's anxiety
    ④ Monitoring the patient's weight daily

126. If a patient has an angina attack, the nurse should record:
    ① Onset, duration, and intensity of the pain
    ② Activity, vital signs, and intensity of the pain
    ③ Onset, duration of pain, vital signs, and activity
    ④ Duration, intensity of the pain, and activity

127. When planning care for a patient with angina, the nurse would expect the physician to order an agent that would provide immediate relief for anginal pain. The medication most likely ordered would be:
    ① Propranolol hydrochloride (Inderal)
    ② Nitroglycerin
    ③ Digoxin (Lanoxin)
    ④ Isoproterenol hydrochloride (Isuprel)

128. Mrs. C, admitted to the hospital with angina pectoris, is being discharged to go home. Nursing instructions for the patient and family members regarding continuity of care would include:
    ① Diet, activity, drug therapy, and avoiding risk factors
    ② Avoiding emotions of anxiety and avoiding exercise
    ③ Exercise, eating heavy meals, and extreme temperature changes
    ④ Diagnostic tests, exercise, and dietary modifications

129. Mr. Wayne has a diagnosis of angina pectoris. This condition is best described by which of the following?
    ① An area of necrosis of the myocardium
    ② Rubbing of an enlarged epicardium against the pericardial sac
    ③ Inability of the coronary arteries to meet the oxygen needs of the myocardium
    ④ Generalized vasospasm throughout the endocardium and surrounding structures

130. Findings on an adult's voided urine are described below. The finding that should be considered *abnormal* unless proved otherwise is that the urine:
    ① Contains protein
    ② Is acidic in reaction
    ③ Is light yellow
    ④ Amounts to 1200 ml collected in a 24-hour period

131. In teaching Mr. Jones about nitroglycerin, the nurse knows that the main function of this drug is to:
    ① Cause venous pooling throughout the body
    ② Constrict arterioles to lessen peripheral resistance
    ③ Dilate the coronary arteries to increase oxygen supply
    ④ Lower the systemic blood pressure

132. Mrs. Duke is a 45-year-old teacher who is admitted to the hospital for essential hypertension. Which of the following is the most significant factor predisposing Mrs. Duke to hypertension?
    ① She has two small children
    ② She has been losing weight lately
    ③ She has lost both parents because of the disease
    ④ She has a cousin with the disease

133. Mrs. Miller worries about her diagnosis of essential hypertension. She exhibits signs of anxiety and apprehension. The best nursing intervention is to:
① Teach her about hypertension
② Let the patient express her feelings
③ Explain that everybody has the same feelings
④ Avoid the subject of her disease

134. A patient with essential hypertension is to receive 1 g of methyldopa (Aldomet) daily. Because each dose is 250 mg, the nurse will give her:
① 1 tablet daily
② 3 tablets daily
③ 4 tablets daily
④ 8 tablets daily

135. The nurse knows that it is not unusual for the patient with hypertension to stop taking the prescribed medication. The usual reason for this is:
① The medications are too expensive
② All the symptoms of hypertension disappear
③ The patient did not receive adequate instructions
④ The patient finds the side effects too bothersome

136. The dietitian has instructed a patient with essential hypertension to moderate caffeine intake. The nurse understands the reason for this is that caffeine acts in the body to:
① Constrict blood vessels
② Increase cholesterol in the blood levels
③ Harden the blood vessels
④ Dilate the blood vessels

137. Mr. Clover's blood pressure is 140/88. He exercises very little and smokes at least one pack of cigarettes a day. The nurse would recommend which of the following as a priority in Mr. Clover's health teaching?
① Mr. Clover should get 10 to 12 hours of sleep
② Mr. Clover should give up smoking
③ Mr. Clover should consider early retirement
④ Additional exercise is not appropriate for the patient at this time

138. In assessing a patient with hypertension, the nurse is aware that a sign of primary hypertension, as opposed to other types of hypertension, is an elevation of:
① Atrioventricular pressure
② Diastolic pressure
③ Systolic pressure
④ Pulse pressure

139. While caring for a patient being treated for hypertension, the nurse can increase patient compliance to treatment by explaining that hypertension is a disease that:
① Can be cured
② Disappears without treatment
③ Can be controlled with treatment
④ Is usually fatal

140. The nurse is discussing the appropriate diet with Mrs. Wilson, a patient with hypertension. She enjoys the following snacks but should try to avoid:
① Carrots
② Pretzels
③ Oranges
④ Jello

141. In planning care for patients with hypertension, the nurse knows that the treatment is usually directed toward:
① Preventing further damage to the blood vessels
② Increasing the urine output
③ Lowering the blood pressure below normal level
④ Repairing the damaged blood vessels

142. The diet for a patient with a diagnosis of hypertension would most likely be:
① Bland
② Low sodium
③ High fat
④ High cholesterol

143. Which of the following health care suggestions made by the nurse would be most helpful to a patient who has a history of hypertension, weighs 250 pounds, and is 5 feet, 8 inches tall?
① Enroll in a quick weight-loss program
② A gradual weight loss is best
③ Use a vegetarian diet
④ Count calories but do not exceed 1000 calories per day

144. Mr. Jones rushes into the physician's office, very anxious and agitated because he is late for his appointment. Suddenly he grabs his chest and tells the nurse that he is having chest pain, as well as pain radiating down both arms. His lips are cyanotic, and he is perspiring heavily. Mr. Jones' symptoms most likely indicate:
① Angina pectoris
② Myocardial infarction
③ Anxiety attack
④ Indigestion

145. Nursing assessment for a patient with a myocardial infarction includes collecting subjective and objective data. Subjective data includes noting the patient's:
① Dyspnea, vertigo, and weakness
② Behavior and pulse abnormalities
③ Vital signs and skin color
④ Dyspnea, pallor, and diaphoresis

146. A primary nursing goal in caring for a patient with a myocardial infarction is to:
① Reduce stress and anxiety level
② Allow gradual increase in activities
③ Provide diversional activities
④ Provide complete bed rest

147. The *most important* aspect of the nursing care for a patient with chest pain should be to:
① Elevate legs and note degree of pitting edema
② Note color, character, and amount of sputum
③ Monitor intake and output and weigh daily
④ Evaluate/record onset, duration, and intensity of chest pain

148. Mr. Garcia is admitted to the cardiac unit with a diagnosis of acute anterior myocardial infarction. He remains in the cardiac intensive care unit for a week and then is transferred to the intermediate care unit. The nurse realizes that this is an appropriate time to provide health teaching. With which of the following would the nurse begin her teaching?
    ① Nutritional counseling, because it is the easiest for the patient to understand
    ② Assessing the patient's knowledge about coronary artery disease and myocardial infarctions
    ③ Medication therapy, because it is the most essential
    ④ Asking the patient what he would like to know about his illness

149. A patient's serum cholesterol level is 260 mg/dl. Which of the following recommendations by the nurse is the best nutritional counseling for this patient?
    ① Eat only foods low in cholesterol
    ② Eat a soft, high-protein diet
    ③ Maintain a low-fat diet
    ④ Eat only easily digestible foods

150. Mr. Garcia is ordered to take nitroglycerin tablets as needed. The nurse knows that the correct method of administering this medication is to:
    ① Place the tablet under the tongue
    ② Drink with plenty of water or juice
    ③ Always take with meals
    ④ Always take before bedtime

151. The pain associated with a myocardial infarction differs from that of angina in that the pain is:
    ① Relieved with rest
    ② Not relieved by rest
    ③ Considerably less severe
    ④ Quickly relieved with nitroglycerin

152. A patient who has been admitted with an acute myocardial infarction becomes restless and experiences a rapid drop in blood pressure. He develops sudden dyspnea; productive coughing of pink-tinged, frothy sputum; and orthopnea. Crackles in the lungs and a respiratory rate of 32 are noted. These symptoms *most likely* indicate:
    ① Pulmonary edema
    ② Cardiogenic shock
    ③ Pulmonary embolus
    ④ Right-sided failure

153. Appropriate nursing measures to promote oxygenation for the patient with dyspnea include positioning the patient:
    ① Upright to decrease venous return
    ② In the supine position to encourage rest
    ③ With the legs elevated to promote venous return
    ④ With the head down to facilitate drainage of the upper respiratory tract

154. The diagnostic test *most* often ordered to evaluate the presence and scope of valvular heart disease is:
    ① Chest x-ray examination
    ② Electrocardiogram (ECG)
    ③ Serial blood cultures
    ④ Echocardiogram

155. Martin enters the emergency room with rapid, shallow, dyspneic respirations. His diagnosis is congestive heart failure (CHF). In planning Martin's nursing care, the nurse would consider which of the following nursing interventions?
    ① Encourage interaction with others; get patient out of bed and room; and have the patient do short, focused activities
    ② Limit activities while providing and maintaining periods of rest; instruct patient to avoid smoking or use of nicotine products; and induce analgesia and sedation as ordered
    ③ Avoid having the patient sit for prolonged periods of time; ascultate abdomen for bowel sounds; and assess skin and mucous membranes
    ④ Reinforce the importance of daily planning activities to conserve energy; encourage self-care as tolerated; and provide small, frequent feedings

156. Mrs. Wilson is being seen by her physician for congestive heart failure. She complains of being short of breath. This is primarily caused by:
    ① Increased anxiety and feelings of helplessness
    ② Pulmonary embolism
    ③ Acute bronchitis
    ④ Decreased cardiac output

157. John, age 68, enters the emergency room with rapid, shallow, dyspneic respirations. His diagnosis is congestive heart failure. The admitting nurse would assess for *early* signs of congestive heart failure, which are:
    ① Shallow, rapid, dyspneic respirations
    ② Paroxysmal nocturnal dyspnea and dyspnea on exertion
    ③ Dyspnea on exertion, cerebral anoxia, and chronic cough
    ④ Malaise, elevation of temperature, and night sweats

158. In planning care for a patient with congestive heart failure, the nurse should know that the condition is:
    ① An occlusion of a major coronary artery or one its branches
    ② An infection or inflammation of the inner membranous lining of the heart, particularly the valves
    ③ A decrease of blood flow through the heart and great vessels
    ④ An enlargement or ballooning of an artery

159. When auscultating respirations of a patient with congestive heart failure, the types of sounds the nurse would expect to hear are:
    ① Diminished or absent breath sounds
    ② Crackling
    ③ Expiratory wheezing
    ④ Inspiratory sounds louder than expiratory sounds

160. A patient has fallen and bruised his right lower leg. In assessing the injury, the nurse must distinguish the body's response. The process of the body's reaction to injury or irritation is called:
    ① Inflammation
    ② Allergy
    ③ Infection
    ④ Immunity

161. Mild exercises of the legs and wearing antiembolitic stockings are prescribed for Mr. Jones, a patient with congestive heart failure. When applying the stockings, the nurse explains that the purpose for these orders are to:
    ① Reduce circulation to the legs and ease the workload of the heart
    ② Prevent abdominal edema
    ③ Prevent clot formation in the lower extremities
    ④ Reduce edema of the extremities

162. For a patient with cardiac disease, a low-salt diet is prescribed. Which of the following foods contain the least amount of sodium?
    ① Baking soda
    ② Citrus fruits
    ③ Milk and cheese
    ④ Canned meats

163. The nurse is to administer digitalis to a patient. This drug is classified as a(n):
    ① Antianxiety agent
    ② Coagulant
    ③ Respiratory stimulant
    ④ Cardiotonic

164. A major complication of congestive heart failure is pulmonary edema. Some of the findings that suggest a patient has pulmonary edema are:
    ① Dyspnea on exertion, nausea and vomiting
    ② Orthopnea and angina
    ③ Thick, tenacious sputum and anxiety
    ④ Dyspnea and frothy, pink-tinged sputum

165. The nurse is to weigh a patient with congestive heart failure daily. The purpose of daily weigh-ins is to determine loss of:
    ① Blood volume
    ② Tissue fluid
    ③ Body fat
    ④ Appetite

166. Mr. Lincoln, age 62, was admitted to the hospital with a diagnosis of congestive heart failure. This disease occurs most often because of:
    ① Incomplete emptying of the left ventricle
    ② Incomplete emptying of the right ventricle
    ③ Rapid emptying of the left ventricle
    ④ Rapid emptying of the right ventricle

167. In planning care for a 60-year-old patient with congestive heart failure, the nurse should observe for which of the following signs and symptoms?
    ① Fatigue
    ② Restlessness
    ③ Excessive thirst
    ④ Respiratory difficulty

168. When developing the nursing care plan for a patient with a diagnosis of congestive heart failure, which of the following should be an important consideration?
    ① Prevention of infection
    ② Early ambulation
    ③ Skin integrity
    ④ Increased fluid intake

169. Fluid and electrolyte balance need to be maintained for patients with congestive heart failure by which of the following?
    ① Maintaining strict input and output and daily levels
    ② Limiting fluid intake and maintaining daily levels
    ③ Limiting activity and maintaining a salt-free diet
    ④ Limiting activity and maintaining a low-sodium diet

170. A 44-year-old patient with valvular heart disease was treated for endocarditis. Discharge teaching will focus on:
    ① The need for a sedentary life-style
    ② Forcing fluids to prevent dehydration
    ③ Prophylactic antibiotic therapy for dental procedures
    ④ The need for wearing a mask in crowds to prevent upper respiratory tract infections

171. Melissa Morris has an apical systolic murmur and a history of rheumatic fever. A diagnosis of rheumatic heart disease was made after the physician received the results of her electrocardiogram and cardiac catheterization. Her blood pressure is to be taken q4h. In setting up the care plan for Melissa, the nurse is aware that rheumatic fever is:
    ① A disease of adults
    ② More prevalent in males
    ③ More prevalent in females
    ④ More prevalent in children

172. In preparing a patient for a cardiac catheterization the nurse should explain that the patient will:
    ① Experience a great deal of pain
    ② Be able to see the catheter pass through the superior vena cava on the monitor
    ③ Have her meals held for 24 hours before the examination
    ④ Not have blood samples taken

173. It is important that the nurse understands the purpose of diagnostic testing. In an electrocardiogram the P wave is:
    ① The impulse from the sinoatrial node
    ② The ventricular contractions
    ③ Helpful in diagnosing myocardial infarction
    ④ Helpful in diagnosing valvular lesions

174. When taking a blood pressure, the nurse is aware that the period of relaxation of the heart muscle is called:
    ① Refractory period
    ② Systole
    ③ Diastole
    ④ Atrial systole

175. Chronic valvular disorders develop when healing occurs in rheumatic fever. The heart valves frequently affected are the:
    ① Mitral and aortic
    ② Tricuspid and mitral
    ③ Aortic and pulmonary
    ④ Pulmonary and semilunar

176. The nurse caring for a patient with arteriosclerotic heart disease knows that delayed treatment of the disease may result in:
    ① Myocardial infarction
    ② Pulmonary edema
    ③ Congestive heart failure
    ④ Endocarditis

177. A patient with rheumatic heart disease has orders that blood pressure be checked q4h. When taking blood pressure, the nurse is aware that the best site to use is the:
    ① Radial artery
    ② Popliteal artery
    ③ Femoral artery
    ④ Brachial artery

178. In caring for a patient with rheumatic heart disease, the primary nursing intervention that the nurse will implement includes:
    ① A low-sodium diet
    ② Bed rest
    ③ Steroid therapy
    ④ Sublingual nitroglycerin

179. The physician has diagnosed a coronary occlusion in Mrs. Zale. When planning this patient's nursing care, the nurse knows this diagnosis means the patient has:
    ① A seizure
    ② A spasm of the muscles
    ③ A stationary blood clot
    ④ An obstruction or cutting-off

180. A coronary artery bypass graft is performed on a patient with a diagnosis of coronary artery disease. In planning postoperative care for this patient, the nurse is aware that this procedure is done:
    ① In the heart catheterization laboratory
    ② To bypass occluded vessels
    ③ To insert a pacemaker
    ④ To remove the lining of the artery

181. The most common use of cardiac catheterization is to determine the:
    ① Amount of blood entering the right atrium
    ② Degree of blockage of the coronary arteries
    ③ Pressure in the left ventricle
    ④ Strength of ventricular contraction

182. Patients requiring cardiac diagnostic studies that involve the use of a contrast medium are questioned before the study about their:
    ① Dietary intake of foods high in fat
    ② Use of an antihistamine in the past week
    ③ Recent gain or loss of weight
    ④ Allergies, especially to seafood and iodine

183. A patient has a cardiac catheterization. Which of the following nursing interventions is *most* important during the first 4 to 6 hours after the procedure?
    ① Assess circulation to extremity used for catheter insertion
    ② Maintain extremity used for the procedure in a flexed position
    ③ Keep the extremity elevated on at least two pillows
    ④ Limit the intake of fluids

184. Mr. Meer receives regular treatment for arteriosclerosis of his lower extremities. He is concerned about his condition and wonders why his physician has asked him to stop smoking. The nurse's best response to Mr. Meer is:
    ① "There is no connection between smoking and your condition."
    ② "Smoking dulls your appetite and prevents healing of your legs."
    ③ "The physician is afraid your condition might spread to your lungs."
    ④ "Nicotine is a drug present in cigarettes that narrows the blood vessels and makes your condition worse."

185. Mr. Shield, age 60, was admitted to the hospital because of an ischemic left foot. The admission diagnosis is arterial insufficiency of the left foot related to generalized arteriosclerosis. Other information that the nurse might obtain during an assessment would most likely include:
    ① Loss of hair on the extremity
    ② Enlarged blood vessels in his leg
    ③ Warm, moist skin on the affected extremity
    ④ Swelling of the feet at the end of the day

186. A patient with peripheral vascular disease suddenly develops pain in his left foot. Which of these assessments of the patient's foot would the nurse report immediately to the team leader?
    ① Numbness and tingling
    ② Warm to the touch
    ③ Brisk capillary refill
    ④ Absent pedal pulse

187. A femoral/popliteal bypass is performed on Mr. Shane's left extremity. In the immediate postoperative period, which of these measures would be the most important indication that blood supply to the leg was improving?
    ① Obtaining his vital signs q4h
    ② Checking the temperature of his leg
    ③ Monitoring his urine output q1h
    ④ Encouraging a high fluid intake

188. The nurse would assess a patient for signs of thrombophlebitis in a lower extremity by noting:
    ① An elevated platelet count
    ② A positive Chvostek's sign
    ③ A positive Homans' sign
    ④ Decreased hemoglobin level

189. The nurse must recognize that the primary symptoms of superficial thrombophlebitis include:
    ① Fever, nausea, and vomiting
    ② Pain, heat, and redness
    ③ Diarrhea or constipation, and abdominal discomfort
    ④ Anorexia, and pain when walking

190. Mrs. Adams has developed thrombophlebitis after being confined to bed for several weeks. To explain the diagnosis to Mrs. Adams, the nurse's best statement would be that thrombophlebitis is:
    ① An ulcer that becomes infected
    ② A traumatic inflammation of blood vessels
    ③ An inflammation of the vein with clot formation
    ④ An inflammation of an artery with clot formation

191. The nurse should observe the patient with deep vein thrombosis for the possibility of an embolism, as indicated by:
   ① Pain at the site
   ② Warm affected areas
   ③ Bradycardia
   ④ Decreased respirations

192. While caring for a patient with deep vein thrombosis, the nurse is aware of the possibility of an embolism, which is defined as:
   ① A stationary blood clot
   ② A blood clot in the arteries
   ③ A blood clot that lodges in the brain only
   ④ A clot circulating in the blood

193. The nurse is caring for a patient on the first postoperative day. Knowing that immobility is one of the causes of thrombophlebitis, the nurse is aware that this complication is best prevented by:
   ① Taking vitamin C daily
   ② Early ambulation to increase circulation
   ③ Massaging the extremities
   ④ Restricting activity, even in bed

194. The nurse is bathing a patient. She knows that which of the following is contraindicated with a diagnosis of thrombophlebitis?
   ① Massaging the legs
   ② Rubbing the neck
   ③ Turning in bed as necessary
   ④ Elevating the head of the bed

195. The nurse is instructing Mr. Myer, a patient with arteriosclerosis of his lower extremities, on proper care of his feet and legs. Which of the following would the nurse include in her teaching program?
   ① To be careful applying heat to feet and legs
   ② To wear snug shoes
   ③ To allow legs to hang/dangle independently at all times
   ④ That it's okay to go out in extremely cold weather

196. Mr. Casey, age 76, has been hospitalized with bed rest prescribed for a week. The nurse assists Mr. Casey out of bed for the first time. As he begins to walk, he complains of pain in his right leg. To establish the basis of this patient's complaint, which of these assessments should the nurse carry out *first?*
   ① Ask him to describe the pain
   ② Inspect his leg for evidence of trauma
   ③ Test for Homans' sign
   ④ Check his pedal pulses

197. If a patient's diagnosis is thrombophlebitis, what other signs or symptoms might the nurse expect to find?
   ① Decreased pedal pulses on the affected leg
   ② Ecchymosis on the area that has pain
   ③ Dry, flaky skin particularly on the foot
   ④ Redness, edema of the affected leg

198. Nursing interventions on the care plan of a patient with thrombophlebitis would most likely include:
   ① Increasing foods containing vitamin C
   ② Range-of-motion exercises to all extremities
   ③ Bed cradle and cold compresses to the extremities
   ④ Continual use of elastic stockings

199. A patient is discharged on a regimen of warfarin sodium (Coumadin). Which food, if avoided by the patient, would indicate that he understands his teaching plan about vitamin K?
   ① Milk
   ② Oranges
   ③ Spinach
   ④ Bran cereal

200. A condition that makes a person more susceptible to the development of varicose veins is:
   ① Repeated bacterial infection in the veins
   ② Improper functioning of the valves that control the flow of blood through the veins
   ③ Congenital malformation of the lower extremities in which there is improper circulation
   ④ Deposits of material along the wall of the veins

201. Mrs. Jones, age 56, has developed varicose veins of both lower extremities. In planning care for Mrs. Jones, the nurse knows that varicose veins are those that have become:
   ① Enlarged and engorged with blood
   ② Hardened, with narrowed openings
   ③ Atrophied because of blood vessel constriction
   ④ Infected by invasion of bacteria

202. In preparing to administer a drug used to treat a patient with an embolism, the nurse understands that the classification of the drug should be:
   ① Antibiotics
   ② Vitamins
   ③ Thrombolytic agents
   ④ Antineoplastic agents

203. A 28-year-old patient has pallor of the mucous membranes and nailbeds. She has a history of fatigue and exertional dyspnea. Her hemoglobin level is 8 g/dl. A diagnosis of iron deficiency anemia is made. What is the *most* likely physiologic reason for the assessment findings?
   ① Impaired production of red blood cells
   ② Decreased production of white blood cells
   ③ Platelet destruction and internal bleeding
   ④ Oxygen-carrying capacity of hemoglobin is reduced

204. Which nursing assessment is *most* appropriate for the patient with iron deficiency anemia?
   ① Pain
   ② Anxiety
   ③ Fluid volume deficit
   ④ Activity intolerance

205. A specific nursing intervention for the patient with iron deficiency anemia would be:
   ① Absolute bed rest
   ② Increased use of vitamins
   ③ Increased periods of exercise
   ④ Short work sessions with rest periods

206. Mrs. Benson's diagnosis is anemia. Which statement by Mrs. Benson would indicate that she understands the dietary plan related to the treatment of anemia?
   ① "I won't drink tea or coffee with my meals."
   ② "I will include eggs in my diet daily."
   ③ "I'll drink a quart of milk every day."
   ④ "I'll include green, leafy vegetables every day."

207. To provide appropriate nursing care for a patient in sickle cell crisis, the nurse is aware that sickle cell anemia is caused by:
① The herpes virus
② *Staphylococcus* bacteria
③ Repeated blood transfusions
④ An abnormal heredity trait

208. A 50-year-old patient has recently been told that he has leukemia. A bone marrow biopsy helped confirm the diagnosis. What would the nurse expect the laboratory reports to indicate?
① Large numbers of immature white blood cells
② Decreased number of T-lymphocytes
③ Marked increase in hematocrit
④ Low level of hemoglobin

209. An intensive course of chemotherapy is started for a patient with recently diagnosed leukemia. After the first week of therapy, the patient develops thrombocytopenia and therefore should be cautioned against which of the following?
① Keeping flowers in his room
② Using a disposable razor
③ Engaging in activity
④ Having visitors

210. A patient receiving an intensive course of chemotherapy for acute leukemia has developed leukopenia. His temperature, taken orally, is 99.8° F (37.67° C). What nursing action is *most* warranted?
① Take future temperatures rectally
② Look for a source of infection
③ Monitor for bleeding
④ Force fluids

211. While caring for a patient with leukemia, the nurse is concerned about controlling possible complications. An example of good medical asepsis to follow in *all* situations is:
① Changing a dressing with nonsterile gloves
② Slowing the IV when the site is red and warm to touch
③ Cleansing the rubber stopper on the penicillin before drawing up the medication
④ Wearing the same isolation gown for each day of the patient's care

212. Bob Burke is a 25-year-old sales clerk who has been admitted for a diagnostic work-up because of symptoms of fever, chills, itchy rash, headache, myalgia, sore throat, vomiting, diarrhea, and swollen lymph nodes. He has had these symptoms for the last 3 months. His physician thinks that he may have the acquired immune deficiency syndrome (AIDS) virus. The admitting nurse knows that AIDS is a disease caused by:
① Mononeucleosis
② Herpes simplex
③ Human immunodeficiency virus (HIV)
④ Hepatitis B virus

213. Universal precautions used in caring for a patient with AIDS include:
① Blood and body fluid precautions
② Private room with door closed
③ Use of disposable utensils, dishes, and trays
④ Full isolation technique

214. Once the diagnosis of AIDS is confirmed, the nurse should focus patient teaching on:
① Changing his or her life-style, friends, and relationships
② Balance of diet, rest, and activity with health-care follow-ups as needed
③ Isolation from family and society in general
④ The legal implications around his or her rights to working, living arrangements, and anonymity

215. Social isolation among patients with AIDS is common. Establishing a therapeutic relationship with these patients is achieved when they:
① Share feelings about their condition
② Talk about AIDS in general terms
③ Talk freely on all subjects excluding their condition, which they feel is private
④ Introduce the nurse to close friends

216. Karra, age 22, visits a clinic and appears quite anxious. Her best friend has been diagnosed as HIV positive. The three major routes of transmission of AIDS are:
① Breast milk, sexual intercourse, and lacrimal secretions
② Cerebrospinal fluid, sexual intercourse, and blood
③ Saliva, lacrimal secretions, and urine
④ Sexual intercourse, blood, and transplacenta (perinatal)

217. The diagnostic test enzyme-linked immunosorbent assay (ELISA) is used for diagnosis of which of the following?
① Kaposi's sarcoma
② AIDS
③ Cytomegalovarus
④ Herpes simplex virus type II

218. Melissa, age 17, comes to a clinic in an agitated state. She reports that her best friend's diagnosis is HIV positive. The nurse's most appropriate response would be:
① Tell Melissa there is no cause for concern as long as there has been no sexual contact
② Tell her to avoid all contact with her friend
③ Listen carefully, then educate Melissa on symptoms, protective measures, mode of spread; provide list of potential support groups
④ Request an immediate blood test for HIV or human T-cell leukemia virus III, CT scan, and lumbar puncture

219. A 32-year-old male is admitted to the hospital with a diagnosis of AIDS. Findings in the nursing assessment would most likely reveal:
① A history of constipation
② A red, itchy rash on his legs
③ A subnormal temperature in the late afternoon
④ The presence of purplish lesions on his trunk

220. A patient with AIDS also has candidiasis. Which information given on the assessment would most likely indicate this condition?
① "I have pain in my legs at night."
② "My skin is very dry."
③ "My throat is sore."
④ "I have difficulty digesting fats."

221. When caring for a patient with AIDS, the nurse would include which of following in the treatment plan?
     ① Have visitors and staff wear cap, mask, and gown
     ② Isolate blood pressure equipment and thermometer
     ③ Be sure the patient has his or her own bathroom
     ④ Wash spilled body fluid with chlorine bleach

222. Which of the following would be considered a secondary organ to the GI system?
     ① Liver
     ② Ileum
     ③ Stomach
     ④ Sigmoid colon

223. A hernia in which the blood supply has been cut off is termed:
     ① Incarcerated
     ② Incisional
     ③ Strangulated
     ④ Umbilical

224. A patient is scheduled to have an upper GI series. While instructing the patient on the procedure, the nurse explains that it aids in the identification of:
     ① Oropharyngeal pathology
     ② Esophageal and stomach pathology
     ③ Stomach and duodenal pathology
     ④ Pharyngeal and esophageal pathology

225. A patient is scheduled for an upper GI Series and barium enema. The nurse explains that because of the procedure for a barium enema, the patient can expect to:
     ① Have coffee and toast the morning of the tests
     ② Take radiographic dye tablets
     ③ Have a needle inserted in the liver area
     ④ Be NPO after midnight and receive enemas until clear

226. When preparing a patient for an endoscopy procedure, the nurse should:
     ① Administer radiographic dye tablets as prescribed
     ② Monitor the patient for bleeding or bile leakage
     ③ Obtain a signed consent form
     ④ Know there are no specific preparations

227. After a patient returns from having an endoscopy, he asks for a drink of water and something to eat. The appropriate nursing action would be to:
     ① Offer a drink of water and order the prescribed diet
     ② Explain that the patient needs to wait until his gag reflex is functional
     ③ Explain to the patient that solid food or drink is not allowed for 24 hours
     ④ Instruct the patient to take small sips of water until the meal trays are served

228. Mrs. Jane Farrett, age 65, is admitted to the hospital for a gastric ulcer work-up. While obtaining the admission history, which of the following complaints would suggest to the nurse that the patient has a gastric ulcer?
     ① Pain experienced 3 hours after meals, relieved by food
     ② Pain experienced before meals, not relieved by vomiting
     ③ Pain 1 hour after eating, increased by food
     ④ Pain experienced only during the night

229. A patient is admitted to the hospital with a diagnosis of perforated gastric ulcer. Which of the following signs and symptoms would most probably alert the nurse to the perforation?
     ① Gradual decrease in body temperature
     ② Epigastric fullness and regurgitation
     ③ Blood-tinged drainage in the vomitus
     ④ Persistent and intense abdominal pain

230. Mrs. Jarrett has a subtotal gastrectomy. She returns to the unit with a nasogastric tube in place. Which of the following is a priority nursing action at this time?
     ① Start clear fluids as soon as bowel sounds are heard
     ② Irrigate the nasogastric tube per order with sterile water
     ③ Connect the nasogastric tube to low, intermittent suction
     ④ Advance the tube hourly as ordered by the physician

231. The nurse is teaching a postgastrectomy patient about dumping syndrome. The patient would indicate the need for further instruction if she made which of the following statements?
     ① "I will lie down after eating a meal."
     ② "I will eat smaller portions of food, more frequently."
     ③ "I will not drink liquids when I eat."
     ④ "I will avoid fats and increase carbohydrates."

232. After returning from lunch the nurse notices that a patient's urine specimen collected for culture and sensitivity has not been delivered to the laboratory. The nurse would be concerned because the specimen:
     ① Should be warm when it arrives in the laboratory
     ② May accidentally spill and require another collection
     ③ Sitting on the counter for a long period could result in growth of microorganisms
     ④ Sitting on the counter for a long period could result in the microorganisms dying and producing a false report

233. To confirm a diagnosis of duodenal ulcers, a fiberoptic endoscopy was one of the diagnostic procedures performed. In preparing the patient for this procedure, the nurse should instruct him to:
     ① Not take anything by mouth after midnight
     ② Take a cleansing enema the night before
     ③ Take a cleansing enema the morning of the examination
     ④ Take a laxative the night before the examination

234. The primary medical treatment for a patient with duodenal ulcers is:
     ① Promote healing by diet therapy
     ② Reduce the signs and symptoms with drug therapy
     ③ A diet low in fat and carbohydrates
     ④ A diet high in protein and milk products

235. After a trial of medical management for duodenal ulcers, John's vomiting and abdominal distention became worse. He was admitted for a vagotomy. In planning postoperative care for John, the nurse knows that this type of surgery is performed to remove:
     ① The gastric-producing portion of the lower stomach
     ② The scar tissue lining the stomach
     ③ The vagal innervation to the fundus of the stomach
     ④ The entire stomach

236. The complication known as dumping syndrome occurs after gastroenterostomy surgery. In planning care for this type of patient, the nurse knows that this syndrome is caused by:
    ① Decreased intestinal mobility
    ② Increased hydrochloride acid in the stomach
    ③ Decreased hydrochloride acid in the stomach
    ④ A rapid gastric emptying

237. The nurse would instruct a patient with dumping syndrome to:
    ① Recline for 1 hour after meals
    ② Recline for 1 hour before meals
    ③ Drink a lot of fluid during meals
    ④ Increase the intake of carbohydrate foods

238. Mrs. Susan Mack, age 31, is admitted to the hospital with ulcerative colitis. She is scheduled to have an ileostomy because she has not responded to conservative treatment. When interviewing Mrs. Mack, which of the following symptoms would the nurse expect her to report?
    ① Anorexia and constipation
    ② Liquid, tarry stools
    ③ Epigastric pain after meals
    ④ Frequent bloody diarrhea

239. Mrs. Jones, a patient with ulcerative colitis, has been instructed to follow a low-residue diet. Which breakfast food selected by her would indicate that she needs further instruction?
    ① Oatmeal, orange slices, and milk
    ② Soft-cooked egg, toast, and herb tea
    ③ Apple juice, English muffin, and jelly
    ④ Cream of rice cereal, white toast, and marmalade

240. Mrs. Mack has a total colectomy and ileostomy. She has an ileostomy appliance in place when she is brought to her room. The nurse should expect the drainage from Mrs. Mack's ileostomy to have which of these characteristics?
    ① Semiliquid consistency with mucus
    ② Semiformed consistency with blood
    ③ Formed stool, brown in color
    ④ Tarry and soft consistency

241. Twenty-four hours after ileostomy surgery, the nurse should expect the stoma to have which of the following appearances?
    ① Light pink and edematous
    ② Retracted below the skin surface
    ③ Edematous and red
    ④ Small and purplish

242. Mrs. Gingras, a 42-year-old executive, has been undergoing diagnostic testing in the outpatient clinic because of nausea, vomiting, diarrhea, and multiple stomach problems. After reviewing the results of her tests, the physician has diagnosed ulcerative colitis. One of the diagnostic tests performed on Mrs. Gingras was a gastric analysis to determine the:
    ① Amount of blood in the stool
    ② Presence of pus in the stomach
    ③ Amount of free hydrochloride in the stomach
    ④ Functioning of the lower GI tract

243. In preparing a patient for a gastric analysis, the nurse must know that the drug used to stimulate the flow of gastric juices is:
    ① Histamine
    ② Belladonna
    ③ Atropine
    ④ Opium tincture (Paregoric)

244. At a team conference, the nurse would contribute which of the following toward the development of a care plan for a patient with ulcerative colitis?
    ① Bed rest with bedside commode privileges
    ② No restriction of visitors or phone calls
    ③ Attention given to the patient's emotional state, rest, and a private room with a bathroom
    ④ Semiprivate room, bedside commode, and restriction of visitors

245. An expected outcome of treatment for a patient with ulcerative colitis would be:
    ① Fewer stools, better formed with no mucus, blood, or pus in them
    ② A softening of the hard and constipated stools
    ③ No change in the formed, soft, brown stools
    ④ A decrease in the watery, brown stools

246. Ms. Potter, a 51-year-old housewife, has a diagnosis of ulcerative colitis. While teaching the patient about the condition, the nurse informs her that the principal cause of ulcerative colitis is:
    ① Poor dietary habits
    ② Hypermotility of the large intestine
    ③ Bacterial infection of the intestines
    ④ Emotional stress

247. It is important for the nurse to expect the stools of a patient with ulcerative colitis to be:
    ① Loose, containing mucus and blood
    ② Hard and constipated
    ③ Formed, soft, and brown
    ④ Watery and brown

248. Mr. Lou Green has had a colon resection with the creation of a permanent colostomy to treat a medical diagnosis of primary sigmoid colon cancer. Mr. Green has a transverse loop colostomy, leaving one stoma. What would the nurse expect the first bowel movements to be like?
    ① Mostly bloody, with small clots mixed with liquid stool
    ② Liquid, light-brown stool
    ③ Semisolid, brown stool
    ④ Solid brown stool, with a small amount of blood

249. Following a transverse loop colostomy, the nurse inspects Mr. Green's stoma. The stoma appears mostly pink with some purple discoloration at the lower border. Which of the following is an appropriate action by the nurse?
    ① Clean the area around the stoma and record the observation in the nurses' notes
    ② Carefully place a clean pouch over the stoma to prevent any further bruising
    ③ Cover the stoma with a petroleum gauze dressing to prevent any further irritation to the stoma
    ④ Apply a clean dressing and pouch, and notify the physician about the discoloration

250. Mrs. Carmen is recovering from colon surgery. She has a nasogastric tube in place, and the nurse is to instill liquids into the tube. Before instillation the most prudent nursing action should include:
① Checking the tube for patency
② Ascertaining that the tube is in the stomach
③ Firmly securing the tube to the nose
④ Clamping the tube for 5 minutes before instillation of liquid

251. Irene Todd, a 52-year-old woman, was admitted to the hospital complaining of increased weight loss over the last 3 months, a change in her bowel habits, and constant nausea and vomiting. A diagnosis of cancer of the colon was made. Symptoms of a partial intestinal obstruction with the passage of "pencil-shaped" stools are characteristic of cancer of the:
① Sigmoid
② Cecum
③ Transverse colon
④ Descending colon

252. A 50-year-old woman has symptoms suggestive of cancer of the colon. One of the diagnostic procedures performed to confirm cancer of the colon is a sigmoidoscopy. To prepare the patient for this procedure, the nurse will:
① Administer a cathartic the evening before the procedure
② Administer an enema the morning before the procedure
③ Explain to her that she will drink a chalk-like fluid
④ Administer a cathartic and enema the evening before the procedure and an enema the morning of the procedure

253. While being prepared for a sigmoidoscopy because of suspected cancer of the colon, a patient asks, "Am I going to die?" The nurse's response should be:
① "It is too early to tell."
② "Do *you feel* you're going to die . . . ?"
③ "Oh, don't say things like that."
④ "Have you discussed this with your family?"

254. A patient received a diagnosis of cancer of the colon. Following a sigmoidoscopy, the diagnosis was stated as cancer of the descending colon with rectal involvement. In planning care for this patient, the nurse knows that the surgical procedure most likely to be done would be a:
① Sigmoid colostomy
② Ileostomy
③ Colectomy
④ Right hemicoloctomy

255. If a patient complains of cramping during a colostomy irrigation, the nurse should:
① Lower the container containing the fluid
② Discontinue the irrigation
③ Advance the catheter 2 more inches
④ Stop the flow until the cramping subsides

256. During a recent team conference that was held to discuss immediate postoperative care for a patient with a sigmoid colostomy, the nurse's main concern would have included problems related to:
① Identifying specific type of colostomy pouch needed
② Teaching the patient to change her own colostomy
③ Monitoring of urinary elimination
④ Identifying foods that the patient can eat

257. A colostomy irrigation was ordered for a patient with a sigmoid colostomy. When doing an irrigation, the cone should be inserted into the stoma opening no more than:
① 2 inches
② 4 inches
③ 10 inches
④ 12 inches

258. Which of the following behaviors exhibited by a patient with a colostomy just before discharge should be of concern to the nurse and reported to the charge nurse?
① Not eating the food sent at each meal
② Refusing to care for the colostomy
③ Wearing loose-fitting clothing
④ Having periods of anger over why this happened

259. Patient education is an important aspect of patient care, and the nurse must remember to:
① Have answers to anticipated questions written out so you can read them to the patient
② Involve the patient in decision making concerning his or her care
③ Identify community resources available to the patient
④ Encourage involvement of family and significant others

260. Mrs. G, a 40-year-old obese housewife, has been admitted with the diagnosis of cholelithiasis. To plan appropriate nursing care, the nurse must understand that cholelithiasis is the medical term for:
① Presence of gallstones in the gallbladder or biliary tree
② An inflammation of the gallbladder
③ Presence of renal calculi in one or both kidneys
④ An inflammation of the nephrons of the kidneys

261. In caring for a patient with cholelithiasis, the nurse should observe for which of the two following characteristic symptoms:
① Jaundice and liver tenderness
② Abdominal rigidity and paralytic ileus
③ Liver enlargement and bleeding disorders
④ Indigestion after a high-fat meal and jaundice

262. A patient with cholelithiasis has been scheduled for surgery. To plan appropriate postoperative nursing care, the nurse understands that the surgical procedure for this condition is a:
① Colonectomy
② Cholecystectomy
③ Gastrectomy
④ Nephrectomy

263. A patient is scheduled for surgery with a common bile duct exploration. The nurse would expect the patient to return from surgery with:
① An underwater-seal drainage
② A T-tube
③ A penrose drain
④ A tracheotomy

264. A low-fat diet has been ordered for a patient with cholelithiasis. Which of the following food sources would be most appropriate?
① Ground sausage, vegetables, and fruits
② Ground turkey, avocados, and fruits
③ Marbled hamburger, lean steak, and vegetables
④ Skinless chicken, vegetables, and fruits

265. A patient is admitted to the emergency room with a primary diagnosis of cholecystitis. The nurse should carefully observe for which of the following symptoms?
① Voiding large amounts of light yellow urine
② Sensation of nausea and bloating after eating fried food
③ Stool becomes dark, may evidence blood
④ Abdominal pain after eating a diet high in carbohydrates

266. Ms. Jenson is scheduled for a gallbladder series. She is to receive an oral contrast media the evening before the test. What additional preparation should be completed before this test?
① An IV should be started the evening before the test
② The upper abdominal area should be prepped and shaved
③ The patient should be NPO after the evening meal
④ A low-fat, high-carbohydrate breakfast should be given before the test

267. Following a cholecystectomy, Ms. Taylor has a nasogastric tube in place. What nursing measure should be implemented when Ms. Taylor returns to her room?
① Irrigate the nasogastric tube with normal saline every 6 hours
② Wrap the open end of the tube with sterile gauze
③ Obtain a clear-liquid diet for her
④ Attach the nasogastric tube to low, intermittent suction

268. Because Ms. Smith has a common bile duct exploration with a cholecystectomy, she also has a T-tube in place. Which of the following postoperative nursing measures would be most correct?
① Complete a sterile dressing change as necessary
② Reinforce the dressing as often as needed
③ Encourage the patient to lie as still as possible
④ Keep the patient sedated as long as the T-tube is in place

269. Ms. Johnson is to be discharged with the T-tube and drainage system in place. Which of the following discharge instructions are correctly given by the nurse?
① Wear snug clothing, or a binder, to prevent any movement of the T-tube
② Soak in the bathtub for 20 minutes twice a day to clean the incision site
③ Tape the drainage tubing to the abdomen below the level of the T-tube
④ Expect a certain amount of redness and tenderness around the incision site

270. Thomas Sparks, a 19-year-old college student, was admitted with jaundice, back pain, high temperature, and a diagnosis of hepatitis A. The admitting nurse knows that jaundice is caused by:
① A poorly functioning pancreas
② Intestinal obstruction
③ Large amounts of bile pigment in the blood
④ An unknown factor

271. John Thomas, a 16-year-old student, was admitted with a diagnosis of hepatitis A. In developing his care plan, the nurse should include:
① Universal precautions and disinfection of body fluids and secretions
② Monitoring antibiotic intravenous administration
③ Bed rest with bathroom privileges
④ Restrictive fluid intake

272. Changes in the liver caused by the viral hepatitis affects certain laboratory test results. In planning care for these patients, the nurse is aware that the laboratory results would most likely show:
① Elevated hemoglobin and hematocrit levels
② Elevated direct bilirubin and SGOT levels
③ Increased serum albumin and SGOT levels
④ Decreased serum albumin and elevated hemoglobin levels

273. Daniel Glass, age 36, has a diagnosis of hepatitis B. In planning care for this patient, the nurse knows that treatment considerations include:
① A high-fat diet
② Bed rest for several weeks
③ No specific dietary regimen
④ A moderate exercise regimen

274. Monitoring stools of a patient with hepatitis A is important. As the nurse caring for such a patient, you would expect that the stools will be:
① Dark brown
② Black
③ Clay-colored
④ Green

275. Janet, age 53, is admitted to the hospital for treatment of cirrhosis of the liver. Sam, Janet's husband, has frequently called her employer to say she was sick when she was actually intoxicated. Sam has exhibited what type of behavior?
① Caring
② Codependent
③ Confrontational
④ Realistic

276. George Jensen, age 46, has been experiencing epigastric pain and episodes of vomiting. On admission his pulse rate is 120, respirations 22, blood pressure 90/60, and temperature 101.6° F (38.67° C). His diagnosis is acute pancreatitis. Other signs or symptoms of acute pancreatitis most likely include:
① Soft abdomen
② Bloody urine
③ Elevated serum amylase level
④ Elevated serum creatinine level

277. Discharge teaching for a patient with pancreatitis included information about a low-fat diet. Which of the following meals selected by the patient would best indicate an understanding of patient teaching?
① A tuna salad sandwich and tea
② Hamburger, roll, and decaffeinated coffee
③ Steamed vegetables and skimmed milk
④ Grilled cheese sandwich and ginger ale

278. As part of the diagnostic work-up for a patient exhibiting symptoms of a ruptured appendix, a complete blood count (CBC) is ordered. What laboratory results would the nurse expect that would confirm the diagnosis of appendicitis?
① Agranulocytosis
② Leukopenia
③ Leukocytosis
④ Aplastic anemia

279. If surgery is not performed on a patient with appendicitis and the appendix ruptures, the nurse would watch closely for signs and symptoms of which of the following complications?
① Peritonitis
② Ileitus
③ Colitis
④ Diverticulitis

280. Before surgery, until laboratory results are returned, the nurse can expect the physician to order which of the following for a patient exhibiting symptoms of appendicitis?
① Narcotics for pain relief
② Heat applied to the abdomen
③ Cleansing enema
④ Ice bag applied to the abdomen

281. Scott, a 19-year-old college student, was admitted with sharp lower-right quadrant pain, nausea, vomiting, and an elevated temperature. The pain stopped suddenly after admission, with further elevation in his temperature. After a diagnosis of a ruptured appendix, he is being prepared for an appendectomy. In planning postoperative care for Scott, the nurse knows that the cause of acute appendicitis is:
① Unknown
② Overeating
③ Infection
④ Overexertion

282. Immediate postoperative teaching that is imperative for a patient who has undergone an appendectomy includes:
① The fact that he or she will be able to play sports again
② The fact that he or she will no longer have pain
③ What he or she is to expect and why it is done
④ That he or she doesn't need his appendix for any specific body function

283. Nancy Martin, age 22, is admitted with a head injury and to rule out a subdural hematoma from being hit in the head with a baseball bat and then falling down 10 stairs. When assessing for the earliest sign of increased intracranial pressure, the nurse observes for changes in which of the following?
① Level of responsiveness
② Intensity of a headache
③ Pupillary status
④ Vital signs

284. When assessing vital-sign changes in a patient with increased intracranial pressure, the nurse observes for which of the following?
① Bradycardia, hypertension, and subnormal temperature
② Fever and hypertension
③ Bradycardia, hypertension, and fever
④ Tachycardia and normal temperature

285. Which of the following is the position of choice when caring for a patient with increased intracranial pressure (ICP)?
① Supine, with the bed flat
② Prone, with the head of the bed flat
③ Sims' position, with foot of the bed elevated 30 degrees

286. The Glasgow Coma Scale is used to determine a patient's level of consciousness. The nurse has completed her assessment and finds the numerical value totals 14. This means the patient is:
① Neurologically impaired
② Not neurologically impaired
③ Comatose
④ Disoriented

287. When the nurse collects subjective data from a patient with a head injury, which of the following would apply?
① Vertigo, diplopia, and headache
② Results of diagnostic tests such as brain scan
③ Pupillary reaction to light
④ Cerebrospinal drainage from the ears and/or nose

288. While observing a patient for signs of increased intracranial pressure, the nurse notes that the blood pressure changes from 110/70 to 130/60, and pulse rate is now 120. What would be the appropriate nursing action?
① Report the vital-sign changes to the physician when he makes rounds
② Recheck vital signs and report immediately to the charge nurse
③ Wait 1 hour, recheck vital signs, and document immediately
④ These changes are not necessary to report because they are insignificant

289. When caring for a patient with increased intracranial pressure, the nurse knows to *avoid* which of the following positions?
① Semi Fowler's
② Lateral
③ Supine
④ Trendelenburg's

290. Mr. Mann is scheduled for a craniotomy. The nurse explains preoperative and postoperative routines to him. This is done primarily to reduce fear of:
① Increased intracranial pressure
② Hair loss
③ Loss of self-esteem
④ The unknown

291. Mr. James has had a craniotomy. Following surgery, the nurse assesses Mr. James for signs of increased intracranial pressure. Which of the following signs would be most critical?
① Dilated and fixed pupils
② Decreasing pulse pressure
③ Motor response is flaccid
④ Vital signs are blood pressure 140/82, pulse rate 72, and respirations 20

292. Following Mrs. Warren's craniotomy, which of the following signs indicates that she is at risk for developing a complication common to this type of surgery?
① Glucose in the urine
② Clear discharge from the nose
③ Ecchymotic areas around the eyes
④ Abdominal pain and diarrhea

293. A patient has a grand mal seizure. A priority nursing intervention for the patient during a seizure is to:
① Loosen constrictive clothing and monitor vital signs
② Open the patient's jaw and insert a seizure stick
③ Position the patient on his or her side and suction mouth
④ Provide for privacy and a safe environment

294. After receiving patient teaching about phenytoin (Dilantin), a patient with epilepsy would indicate understanding of the teaching plan if he or she made which of the following statements?
① "I will expect to gain weight on Dilantin."
② "I will notify my physician if my gums bleed."
③ "I will stop the Dilantin if my urine turns pink."
④ "I will drive a car now that I'm on Dilantin."

295. The nurse observes her co-worker, Mary, arriving to her shift apparently intoxicated. The nurse sees that Mary behaves as if she were partially conscious, aimlessly picking at her clothing. The nurse is aware Mary has a seizure disorder and has symptoms of which characteristic seizure activity?
① Psychomotor
② Akinetic
③ Jacksonian
④ Myoclonic

296. Barbara, a 25-year-old bookkeeper, is admitted to the emergency room with a history of two seizures a day for the last 3 days. What nursing assessment is considered most valuable in establishing Barbara's medical diagnosis?
① A complete skull series of examinations
② A neurologic examination
③ Developmental health history
④ Complete blood count

297. Rachel, a 43-year-old epileptic patient, reports her seizure activity has doubled in the last few days. While in the office, she demonstrates recurrent, generalized seizure activity. In assessing the patient, the nurse is aware that this type of seizure is called:
① Grand mal
② Psychomotor
③ Petit mal
④ Status epilepticus

298. Mrs. Jones, a 78-year-old with a diagnosis of myocardial infarction, is admitted to the unit and placed on a heart monitor. She complains of constipation, and an order is obtained to give her an enema as needed. In planning care for this patient, the nurse knows that the physician will most likely order:
① Fleet enema
② Saline solution
③ Oil retention enema
④ 1500 ml soap solution

299. Jane, a 34-year-old patient with a history of epilepsy, comes to the clinic reporting increased seizure activity for the past 4 days. While in the clinic, Jane has several seizures and does not regain consciousness between seizures. A primary nursing goal would be prevention of:
① Toxic disturbances
② Metabolic problems
③ Hypertension
④ Brain damage

300. Christine, a 34-year-old vocational rehabilitation evaluator, places a call to the clinic and requests to be seen today. She reports increased epileptic seizure activities the last 3 days. Christine is concerned about driving a car. The nurse's responsibility is to inform her that driving will depend on local laws; however, most laws require:
① Driving only during daylight hours
② Evidence that seizures occur no more frequently than every 6 months
③ Evidence that seizures are under medical control
④ That carry a medical identification card at all times

301. While leading a self-help group of individuals with seizure disorders, the nurse informs them that not everyone has an aura before a seizure. The nurse should describe an aura as a:
① Postseizure amnesia state
② Generalized feeling of relaxation
③ Hallucination during a seizure
④ Warning of impending seizure

302. Rick seeks medical care at an outpatient clinic. He reports an increase in epileptic seizure activity over the last week. The clinic nurse knows that a typical postictal phenomenon would include:
① Status epilepticus
② Headache
③ Reduced blood pressure
④ Kidney failure

303. Anticonvulsants are used in treating seizure disorders and are considered:
① Cholinergic blocking agents
② Central nervous system (CNS) stimulants
③ Antispasmodics
④ CNS depressants

304. Which of the following individuals is at greatest risk for a cerebrovascular accident (CVA)?
① 40-year-old male schoolteacher
② 35-year-old sedentary male manager
③ 55-year-old female with hypertension
④ 80-year-old female with renal disease

305. Mrs. Parks, a 33-year-old teacher, is admitted with the diagnosis of multiple sclerosis. To provide appropriate nursing care, the nurse should understand that this disease is characterized by:
① Seizures that last longer than 15 minutes
② Progressive degeneration of nerve cells caused by insufficient dopamine
③ Progressive degeneration of the myelin sheath of the brain and spinal cord
④ Attacks of vertigo and tinnitus with progressive hearing loss

306. When observing a patient with interference of motor nerve impulses, the nurse would note:
① Premonition or sign (aura) and a seizure lasting 1 to 2 minutes
② Loss of muscle tone, slurred speech, and paresthesia
③ Disorientation and drainage of cerebrospinal fluid from ears and nose
④ Tremor and fingers having a "pill-rolling" movement

307. In planning the nursing care for a patient with multiple sclerosis, the nurse should encourage the patient to:
① Remain as active as possible without becoming fatigued
② Exercise all joints several times a day
③ Adapt to complete bed rest and antibiotic therapy
④ Maintain a low-calorie, low-protein, and low-fat diet

308. Nursing interventions for a patient hospitalized with multiple sclerosis should be directed toward:
① Assisting the patient with social and occupational activities
② Encouraging the patient to seek treatment that promises a cure
③ Preventing decubitus ulcers and contractures by use of proper supports
④ Providing complete bed rest and breathing exercises twice a day

309. When teaching the patient and family members about multiple sclerosis, the nurse should include all of the following *except*:
① Drugs that stop the degenerative process
② Facts about the disease process
③ Ways to conserve energy and avoid fatigue
④ How to contact the National Multiple Sclerosis Society

310. Kelly, age 67, has had Parkinson's disease for 8 years. To promote Kelly's optimal functions, which activity could the nurse recommend as being most beneficial?
① Discussing current events with neighbors
② Building model airplanes
③ Playing bridge
④ Planting a vegetable garden

311. Mr. Gray, age 64, has a 7-year history of Parkinson's disease. Which of the following goals are most appropriate and realistic in planning his nursing care?
① Preparing for terminal care
② Stopping progression of disease
③ Maintaining optimal body functioning
④ Curing the disease

312. Ken, age 60, has a 5-year history of Parkinson's disease. Nursing diagnosis would include all of the following *except*:
① Alteration in comfort, resulting from the disease process
② Impaired physical mobility related to neuromuscular deterioration
③ Alteration in self-care ability: feeding, hygiene, and toileting
④ Knowledge deficit regarding the disease process

313. While reading Mr. Jones' medical record, a nurse notices he has hypersecretion of the growth hormone. The medical term for this condition in adults is:
① Simmonds' disease
② Graves' disease
③ Gigantism
④ Acromegaly

314. When caring for a patient with hypersecretion of the growth hormone, the nurse should observe for which of the following?
① Coarse facial features; broad hands, fingers, and feet
② Headache, weakness, and visual disturbances
③ Symmetric overgrowth of the long bones of the body
④ Increased height (8 to 9 feet tall)

315. The primary nursing intervention in treating adult patients who have increased growth hormone is to:
① Observe for tetany: tingling of hands and feet, facial muscle spasms, and muscle twitching
② Explain the need for a diet high in calcium, but low in phosphorus; instruct to avoid milk, cheese, and egg yolks
③ Observe for adrenal crisis: falling blood pressure, tachycardia, elevated temperature, convulsions, and coma
④ Assist the patient to accept altered body image by emphasizing the person's value as an individual

316. Mrs. Susan Thomas, age 45, is admitted to the hospital with a diagnosis of hyperthyroidism. During the initial assessment of Mrs. Thomas, the nurse should expect her to exhibit which of these signs?
① Excitability
② Lethargy
③ Intolerance to cold
④ Anorexia

317. A patient has a subtotal thyroidectomy. In the immediate postoperative period, the patient should be kept in which of these positions?
① Flat in bed, without a pillow
② Side-lying, with the head of the bed elevated 15 degrees
③ Semi-Fowler's, with the head on a small pillow
④ Prone, with a small pillow under the head

318. In the postoperative room of the thyroidectomy patient, the most important thing the nurse should be sure to have at the bedside is a:
① Warmed blanket
② Padded tongue blade
③ Foley catheter setup
④ Tracheostomy set

319. In the early postoperative period, Mrs. Roland, a thyroidectomy patient should be given which of these instructions?
① "Expectorate your saliva until you are able to swallow."
② "Range-of-motion exercises will prevent contractures."
③ "Do not turn your head from side to side."
④ "Deep-breathe and cough every hour to avoid respiratory complications."

320. A patient has had a thyroidectomy. The nurse caring for this patient must remember that postoperatively the patient is:
① Restricted to fluid intake
② Cautioned not to cough
③ Placed in a prone position
④ Administered morphine frequently

321. After a thyroidectomy, a patient should be carefully observed for decreases in calcium levels. A sign of this would be:
① Muscle pain
② Dependent edema
③ Cold intolerance
④ Involuntary tremors

322. When caring for a patient with hyperthyroidism, the nurse is aware that the principal action of the iodine preparation just administered is to:
① Reduce the activity of the thyroid gland
② Increase production of thyroxin
③ Increase the activity of the thyroid gland
④ Increase the activity of the pancreas

323. In teaching a patient about hyperthyroidism, the nurse should also inform the patient that the condition is also known as:
① Myxedema
② Cretinism
③ Colloid goiter
④ Graves' disease

324. After the diagnosis of hyperthyroidism is confirmed by a basal metabolic rate (BMR), a patient was placed on an iodine preparation by mouth. In caring for this patient, the nurse must know that the diagnostic test, a BMR, measures the functioning of which of the following glands?
① Parotid
② Parathyroid
③ Thyroid
④ Pituitary

325. Ms. Jordan, a 35-year-old lawyer, has a diagnosis of hyperthyroidism. After her basal metabolic rate was measured, she was placed on an iodine preparation by mouth. In planning care for this patient, the nurse must know that hyperthyroidism exists when the:
① Basal metabolic rate is low
② Thyroxin blood level is high
③ Thyroxin blood level is low
④ Amount of thyroid hormone is unchanged

326. When caring for a thyroidectomy patient, the nurse should observe for which major complication associated with this type of surgery?
① Urinary retention
② Tetany
③ Shrill voice
④ Dehydration

327. When preparing an iodine preparation for oral administration, to a thyroidectomy patient, the nurse should:
① Dilute it well
② Give it at bedtime
③ Give it whenever necessary
④ Give it the first thing in the morning

328. One of the major complications for the thyroidectomy patient is thyroid crisis. A major nursing priority would be to observe for:
① Increased pulse rate
② Decreased pulse rate
③ Slowed respirations
④ Subnormal temperature

329. Jack Moriarity, a 21-year-old college student, was admitted to the hospital. The physician has ordered capillary blood glucose monitoring four times a day with insulin coverage. He is to receive 20 U NPH insulin plus 5 U regular insulin in the morning. When giving regular insulin which of the following is it important to remember?
① Food must be taken at least 2 to 3 hours after the injection
② Regular insulin must be taken at least 1 hour after meals
③ Food must be taken approximately a ½ hour after the injection
④ Regular insulin peaks in 8 hours, food must be taken at that time

330. A patient's diagnosis is diabetes ketoacidosis. The nurse should carefully assess this patient for:
① Profuse diaphoresis
② Lethargy
③ Tremors
④ Tachycardia

331. Mr. Dixon is to be taught to monitor his blood glucose level using the capillary glucose test (Dextrostix). Because of his insulin prescription, it would be most important to teach Mr. Dixon to check his blood glucose level:
① After strenuous activity
② Two hours after meals
③ Before his lunch
④ Before strenuous activity

332. The nurse should teach a patient with diabetes that early symptoms of hypoglycemia include:
① Flushed face
② Diploplia
③ Slurred speech
④ Hunger

333. A patient would understand how to use the diabetic food exchange list if he or she selected which of these foods as an appropriate substitute for a serving of peanut butter?
① Fruit salad
② Hamburger
③ Tomato soup
④ Corn muffin

334. The nurse is teaching a patient the relationship between exercise and insulin requirements. Which of these statements made by the patient would indicate correct understanding of this relationship?
① "When I exercise, I may need less insulin."
② "When I exercise more, I need more insulin."
③ "There is no change in the insulin requirement when exercise is increased."
④ "If I eat enough, I don't need to exercise or adjust my insulin".

335. A patient will be taking NPH insulin in the morning before breakfast and another smaller dose of NPH insulin at bedtime. The nurse should teach this patient that on this regimen, the most common times for a hypoglycemic reaction would be:
① Before breakfast and 1 hour after lunch
② Between 4 to 5 PM and during the night
③ 1 hour after breakfast and 1 hour after dinner
④ 1 hour after lunch and during the night

336. Mrs. Moriarity, age 48, has adult onset diabetes mellitus. She tells the nurse that she is surprised she developed diabetes at 48 years of age, and she asks the nurse to review what she should know about diabetes mellitus. The development of type II diabetes mellitus in middle-aged people is most directly related to which of these risk factors?
① A history of obesity
② Eating many sweets
③ An infection that doesn't heal
④ A history of polyria

337. Because Mrs. Jones, who has type II diabetes, takes glyburide (Micronase) 2.5 mg daily, which of these instructions should she be given?
① To adjust glyburide according to her capillary blood glucose levels
② Exercise immediately following the ingestion of glyburide
③ Take glyburide in the morning after breakfast
④ Avoid drinking alcohol with the drug

338. The nurse is teaching a type II diabetic patient about the mechanism of action of oral hypoglycemic agents. Which of the following statements made by the patient would indicate understanding of the teaching plan?
① "The medication will replace my insulin."
② "The medication will help me digest glucose better."
③ "The medication will help me lose weight."
④ "The medication will help my pancreas produce more insulin."

339. To control type II diabetes, the patient's priority goal would be to:
① Participate in a trial of insulin injections
② Achieve and maintain ideal body weight
③ Avoid carbohydrate-containing foods
④ Test her capillary blood sugar four times a day

340. When planning care for a patient with diabetes mellitus, the nurse knows that this condition:
① Interferes with the absorption of minerals
② Interferes with the absorption of vitamins
③ Involves a disorder in carbohydrate metabolism
④ Involves the pituitary gland

341. Allen, a newly diagnosed diabetic patient, asks the nurse about the excess glucose in his bloodstream and how it is measured. The nurse tells him that a fasting blood test is done to determine the amount and that the normal blood glucose level is:
① 50 to 75 mg/100 ml of blood
② 70 to 160 mg/100 ml of blood
③ 100 to 200 mg/100 ml of blood
④ 60 to 110 mg/100 ml of blood

342. The physician has ordered tolbutamide (Orinase) for Steve, a newly diagnosed diabetic patient. In preparing to teach Steve about the drug, the nurse knows that tolbutamide is:
① An oral insulin
② A drug that does not have to be taken regularly
③ A hypoglycemic agent that lowers the blood sugar
④ A drug that can be given to all diabetic patients

343. While caring for a diabetic patient, the nurse observes that the patient appears to be in a diabetic coma. Signs and symptoms of diabetic coma include:
① Cool, moist skin
② Rapid, shallow respirations
③ Increased blood pressure
④ Fruity odor to breath

344. A 52-year-old patient with diabetes wants to know how he can lower his blood sugar level if his body is not producing enough insulin on its own. The nurse explains to him that:
① Diet, exercise, and oral hypoglycemic agents are indicated in adult onset diabetes
② Diet, exercise, and insulin injections are needed
③ Insulin injections replace what the body doesn't produce
④ Major weight loss is necessary

345. It is imperative that John, a diabetic patient, understands the signs and symptoms of complications that may occur as a result of having diabetes. Acidosis is one of the complications and is caused by:
① Too much insulin
② Too little insulin
③ The absence of ketone bodies
④ Overeating

346. The nurse should know that the two outstanding characteristic symptoms of diabetes mellitus are:
① Hypoglycemia and glycosuria
② Hyperglycemia and glycosuria
③ Hypoglycemia and hypokalemia
④ Hyperglycemia and glycogen

347. When a patient is diagnosed with diabetes mellitus, the nurse should observe for symptoms of impending diabetic coma. These symptoms include:
① Skin moist and pale, and extreme thirst
② Skin dry and pale, and extreme hunger
③ Skin dry and flushed, and extreme thirst
④ Skin flushed and moist, and anorexia

348. The nurse should understand that diabetic acidosis may occur as a complication of diabetes mellitus. This is caused by:
① Increased amounts of glucose in the blood
② Decreased amounts of glucose in the blood
③ The pancreas producing an excessive amount of insulin
④ The pancreas producing an excessive amount of pancreatic juices

349. If diabetic acidosis is left untreated, the nurse should expect which of the following symptoms to occur?
① Trembling sensation and profuse perspiration
② Decreased blood pressure and a fruity odor to the breath
③ Generalized muscle weakness and blurred vision
④ Tingling sensation of the lips or tongue, and headaches

350. The nurse is caring for a patient who refuses to adhere to the appropriate insulin and diet prescribed for diabetes mellitus. The nurse should know that increased metabolism of fats and proteins caused by accumulated glucose and waste products would most likely manifest itself in the condition known as:
① Insulin reaction
② Hypoglycemia
③ Diabetic retinopathy
④ Ketoacidosis

351. Mr. Wilson is a 51-year-old accountant with a history of allergy-related asthma for which he has taken corticosteroid medications. He now is admitted with Cushing's syndrome. Assessment of Mr. Wilson for the signs and symptoms of Cushing's syndrome should include:
① Weight loss
② Skin breakdown
③ Low blood pressure
④ Hypoglycemia

352. One of the primary goals of nursing care of a patient with Cushing's syndrome should be that the patient:
① Consume a high-carbohydrate, low-fat diet
② Increase fluids to 3 liters per day
③ Experience increased mental stability
④ Gains weight of 2 pounds within 1 week

353. Discharge teaching for a patient with Cushing's syndrome includes:
① Avoiding foods with a high sodium content
② Maintaining a high-protein, low-calcium diet
③ Frequently shaving skin to prevent infection
④ Frequently monitoring urine and blood glucose levels

354. Mrs. Gray, a 60-year-old woman with Cushing's syndrome, is admitted for an adrenalectomy. In planning care for Mrs. Gray, the nurse is aware that Cushing's syndrome is a condition involving:
① Hyperplasia of the adrenal gland
② Hypoplasia of the adrenal gland
③ Diminished secretions of the adrenal gland
④ Increased secretions of the adrenal gland

355. Mrs. White, age 56, has a diagnosis of Cushing's syndrome. The admitting nurse should expect Mrs. White's symptoms to include:
① Hypotension and weight loss
② Anorexia and muscle weakness
③ Muscle weakness and osteoporosis
④ Moon face and hypotension

356. Mrs. Brown recently received a diagnosis of Cushing's syndrome. In planning her care, the nurse's primary concern should be to:
① Accurately record intake and output
② Protect her from infection
③ Test urine for sugar
④ Prepare her for surgery

357. A patient with Cushing's syndrome is admitted for an adrenalectomy. In planning postoperative care for this patient, the nurse knows that the adrenocorticotropic hormone (ACTH):
① Is secreted by the adrenal glands
② Is a factor that influences growth
③ Influences the activity of the cortex of the adrenal glands
④ Diminishes the function of the medulla of the adrenal glands

358. The priority postoperative nursing measure for a patient with an adrenalectomy is to:
① Observe for hemorrhage
② Prevent hypertension
③ Encourage fluid intake
④ Accurately record intake and output

359. In caring for a patient with an adrenalectomy, the nurse knows that an unavoidable sequela after surgery is:
① Addison's disease
② Hypoparathyroidism
③ Hyperparathyroidism
④ Simple goiter condition

360. For a patient with an adrenalectomy, discharge planning should include the recommendation to:
① Increase salt intake
② Avoid stress
③ Restrict activity
④ Administer insulin

361. The physician has scheduled a cystoscopic examination for Mr. James. When preparing him for his procedure, the nurse explains to Mr. James that the purpose of the examination is to:
① Determine the size, shape, and location of the kidneys
② Visualize the prostate gland
③ Visualize the size of the ureters
④ Visualize the inside of the bladder

362. A patient has been admitted to the medical unit from the emergency room with a diagnosis of renal calculi. The nurse anticipates that the physician will order which of the following diagnostic examinations to confirm that renal calculi is lodged in a ureter?
① KUB
② Cystourethrogram
③ Cystometry
④ Proctoscopy

363. Mr. Richard Lander, age 46, is seen by the physician for recurrent symptoms of cystitis. He is to have a urine culture and sensitivity determination and a 24-hour urine collection for laboratory analysis. Mr. Lander should be informed that the urine culture and sensitivity studies are required to:
① Analyze the elements present in the urine
② Determine if the urine contains evidence of malignant cells
③ Identify the organism causing the infection in the urinary tract
④ Localize the site of the inflammatory process in the urinary tract

364. To obtain a 24-hour urine specimen, a patient should be given which of these instructions?
① Collect each voiding in separate containers for the next 24 hours
② For the next 24 hours, retain a 30-ml specimen of each voiding after recording the amount voided
③ Keep a record of the time and amount of each voiding for 24 hours
④ Discard the first voided specimen and then collect the total volume of each voiding for 24 hours

365. The most common x-ray examination procedure used to visualize the kidney and related structures is a(n):
① Cholecystography
② Cystography
③ Intravenous pyelogram
④ Retrograde pyelography

366. When caring for a patient with symptoms suggestive of renal calculi, the nurse should know the clinical manifestations of renal calculi, which include:
① Dribbling at the end of urination; and pyuria
② Severe, flank pain; and hematuria
③ Frequency of urination; and dysuria
④ Urgent, uncontrollable urination; and polyuria

367. If a patient is admitted with a diagnosis of renal calculi, which of the following should the nurse assess for during the admission procedure?
① Flank pain radiating to the testes
② Polyuria and thirst
③ Burning and frequency of urination
④ Painless hematuria

368. Jessie Grant, age 50, was admitted to the medical unit from the emergency room with a diagnosis of renal calculi. His symptoms are flank pain, difficulty with urination, voiding small amounts, nausea, and vomiting. He was given hydromorphone (Dilaudid) 5 mg intramuscularly stat and then q4h prn for the pain. The renal calculi are lodged in Jessie's ureter. In planning his care the nurse knows the pain he is having is referred to as:
① Floating kidney
② Nephrosclerosis
③ Hydronephrosis
④ Renal colic

369. When a patient is admitted with renal calculi, the nursing care plan should include:
① Limiting fluid intake
② Straining the urine
③ Limiting food intake
④ Maintaining bed rest

370. The physician orders hydromorphone (Dilaudid) 5 mg intramuscularly for pain for a patient with renal calculi. The nurse is preparing the medication and finds a multiple-dose vial that indicates hydromorphone 2 mg/ml for intramuscular use. How much hydromorphone should the nurse administer to the patient?
① 1.5 ml
② 2 ml
③ 2.5 ml
④ 5 ml

371. When caring for a postoperative patient, the nurse knows that the determining factor for advancing a diet from clear liquids to solid foods is:
① Recovering from the anesthesia
② Return of peristalsis
③ Discontinuing the IV
④ Absence of abdominal pain

372. When initiating dietary teaching for the patient with kidney stones, the nurse should advise limiting intake of which of the following foods?
① Meat, fish, and poultry
② Eggs, cheese, and milk
③ Plums, prunes, and cranberries
④ Vegetables, fruits, and carbohydrates

373. A patient must restrict calcium in his diet because of the development of calcium stones. He would demonstrate understanding of his dietary plan if he selected which of the following foods for lunch?
① Macaroni and cheese, green salad, and tea
② Broiled hamburger, roll, and steamed carrots
③ Yogurt, mixed fruit, and broccoli
④ Baked fish, spinach, and skimmed milk

374. The most common early symptom of a malignant bladder tumor is:
① Suprapubic pain
② Elevation of temperature
③ Painless hematuria
④ Dysuria

375. Mr. Mansfield, age 76, has a benign hypertrophy of the prostate gland. The nurse would expect him to have which of these symptoms?
① Hematuria with associated pain
② A persistent low-grade temperature
③ Perineal tenderness during a bowel movement
④ Complaints of inability to void

376. Mr. Jones had a transurethral resection of the prostate gland. He is returned to his room with a three-way urethral catheter attached to a continuous bladder irrigation system. At the end of the shift, the nurse is calculating his urine output. His intake is as follows: IV fluids 800 ml, irrigating solution 2000 ml, and amount of drainage in the Foley bag 3800 ml. His urine output should be documented as:
    1. 3800 ml
    2. 1800 ml
    3. 1000 ml
    4. 800 ml

377. A patient has had a transurethral prostatic resection (TURP). During a continuous bladder irrigation, the patient states that he feels like he has to void. The nurse's *first action* should be to:
    1. Explain to him that this is a normal sensation
    2. Manually irrigate the Foley catheter with 100 ml of irrigant
    3. Palpate the bladder above the symphysis pubis
    4. Report this to the team leader immediately

378. Mr. Mann had a TURP. Several days later, his urethral catheter is removed. To help Mr. Mann regain bladder control, which of these measures would be part of his care plan?
    1. Drinking 1500 ml of fluid daily
    2. Taking a sitz bath twice a day
    3. Doing leg-raising exercises three times a day
    4. Tensing and relaxing the perineal muscles

379. Mr. Garcia, age 72, was admitted from the nursing home with a neoplasm of the prostate, and his symptoms have progressively worsened. The major problem he has been experiencing is:
    1. Urgency
    2. Frequency
    3. Difficulty in urinating
    4. Burning on urination

380. Mr. Jenson is a 60-year-old man with a neoplasm of the prostate. In planning his care, the nurse knows that this condition occurs most often in men who:
    1. Have a high incidence of infection
    2. Are over 55 years of age
    3. Have sedentary jobs
    4. Are sexually inactive

381. A patient has had a suprapubic prostatectomy. In planning postoperative care for this patient, the nurse knows that the incision is made:
    1. Through the perineum
    2. In the urethra
    3. Under the bladder
    4. Over the bladder

382. Following a patient's surgery for a suprapubic prostatectomy, the nurse notes a suprapubic catheter was left in place. The nurse's *major* responsibility in caring for this patient is:
    1. Administering analgesics because this procedure is painful
    2. Limiting fluid intake to decrease output and facilitate healing
    3. Frequently checking the amount, color, and consistency of urine from the catheter
    4. Administering antibiotics

383. The physician left an order to irrigate a patient's suprapubic catheter prn. The nurse should plan on irrigating the catheter when:
    1. The flow of urine decreases and there are blood clots in the tubing
    2. There are a few blood clots flowing through the tubing
    3. Her judgment, with no specific times or indications, deems it to be appropriate
    4. The patient asks for pain medication, which indicates problems with the catheter

384. Mr. Joseph has undergone a suprapubic prostatectomy. The dressing must be changed frequently, because it becomes saturated with urine during a bladder spasm and the urine doesn't flow through the catheter. Because there is urine in the wound, the nurse should:
    1. Change the dressing without following clean technique
    2. Change the dressing following sterile technique
    3. Leave the wound open and put an emesis basin by his side to catch the urine
    4. Give him analgesics frequently to stop the spasm and flow of urine onto the abdomen

385. Mr. Sam Bell, age 62, is admitted to the surgical unit for a repeat bilateral inguinal herniorrhaphy with a mesh graft reinforcement. During the late afternoon after surgery, Mr. Bell complains that he is hungry and wants to know when he can have something to eat. What is the *best response* by the nurse?
    1. "When you are able to 'pass gas.'"
    2. "The day after surgery."
    3. "When bowel sounds are present in all four quadrants of your abdomen."
    4. "When the IV fluids the physician ordered are finished."

386. At dinnertime following surgery, Mr. Clyde is to be given a clear-liquid diet. Which of the following *would not* be included in this diet?
    1. Tea and coffee
    2. Popsicles and gelatin
    3. Ice cream
    4. Chicken or beef broth

387. Mr. Small has not been able to void for 8 hours after his surgery. What is the *best* nursing intervention for Mr. Small?
    1. Help Mr. Small stand beside the bed to void
    2. Apply pressure over the bladder area (Credé's maneuver)
    3. Catheterize Mr. Small with a straight catheter
    4. Notify the physician

388. Mr. James is to be discharged 48 hours after his surgery for repair of a bilateral inguinal hernias. Which of the following instructions should the nurse include in the discharge teaching?
    1. Return to work after a 4- to 6-week recuperation period
    2. Remain on a soft diet, low in roughage, for 2 weeks
    3. Avoid lifting objects heavier than a book for 4 to 6 weeks
    4. Avoid bathing or showering until seeing the physician for a checkup

389. Mr. Billy Lane, age 54, develops acute renal failure. He is admitted to the hospital. When taking Mr. Lane's vital signs, the nurse should expect to obtain which of these results?
    ① A weak, thready pulse
    ② A low body temperature
    ③ Shallow respirations
    ④ An elevated blood pressure

390. A patient tells the nurse that he is having trouble breathing. The nurse should take which of these actions *first?*
    ① Determine the pulse rate
    ② Report this to the team leader
    ③ Elevate the head of the bed to high-Fowler's position
    ④ Instruct to breathe deeply

391. Mr. Tate is scheduled to have hemodialysis. An external shunt is inserted into his left forearm. The nurse should assess the patient for which of the following to ensure proper functioning of the external shunt?
    ① There is no bleeding at the site
    ② The arm is not edematous
    ③ A radial pulse is palpable
    ④ A bruit is audible

392. The nurse teaches a patient with renal failure about his low-protein diet. The patient would demonstrate an understanding of the protein content of food if he selected which of these desserts?
    ① Baked custard with caramel sugar
    ② Yogurt with fruit
    ③ Applesauce with raisins
    ④ Gelatin with whipped cream

393. Mr. Lassiter, age 36, appears in the clinic complaining of dysuria and a purulent discharge from the penis. The patient states he has had these symptoms for the past 2 weeks. Because the symptoms are suggestive of gonorrhea, the physician plans to begin treatment on a presumptive basis. To establish a diagnosis, the physician advises the nurse to prepare this patient for which of the following tests?
    ① Blood test
    ② Anal culture
    ③ Throat culture
    ④ Culture of penal discharge

394. The physician asks for the nurse's assistance during a routine gynecologic examination on Ms. Kinney. The nurse assists the patient onto the examination table and explains the procedure to her. Which of the following is the position of choice for a pelvic examination?
    ① Sims'
    ② Lithotomy
    ③ Trendelenburg's
    ④ Dorsal recumbent

395. The physician asks the nurse to assist in performing a Pap test on 24-year-old Mrs. Zikiel. When Mrs. Zikiel asks the nurse how often a Pap test should be done, the nurse's response should be:
    ① "Whenever you have irregular menstrual periods."
    ② "Annually for someone your age."
    ③ "Every 5 years until you are 40 years old."
    ④ "Every 3 years until you are 40 years old."

396. When preparing a patient for a gynecologic examination, the nurse should:
    ① Have the patient empty her bladder
    ② Withhold meals before the examination
    ③ Restrict fluid intake for 24 hours before the examination
    ④ Encourage the patient to drink 500 to 1000 ml of fluid before the examination

397. A nurse is preparing to assist the physician in a gynecologic examination. The patient is 29 years old and has been taking birth control pills since she was 18. It is important for the nurse to know that a Pap test is done to:
    ① Determine ovarian functioning
    ② Measure the length of the cervix
    ③ Test the acidity level of vaginal secretions
    ④ Detect the presence of cervical cancer early

398. Ms. Sams comes to the clinic complaining of extremely heavy bleeding during her menstrual period. Which of the following symptoms should the nurse document as part of an initial patient assessment?
    ① Amenorrhea
    ② Menorrhagia
    ③ Metrorrhagia
    ④ Dysmenorrhea

399. Ms. Pearl, age 36, has had a hysterectomy for uterine cancer and will soon begin chemotherapy. Five days following surgery the patient appears anxious and asks, "How will my husband feel about me now that I am half a woman and will soon have no hair?" Which of the following responses by the nurse is the *most appropriate?*
    ① "I wouldn't really worry about it. He's your husband, and I'm sure he loves you very much."
    ② "Would you like to discuss this matter with your physician?"
    ③ "Would you like me to sit for a while so that we could talk about how you feel?"
    ④ "I can recommend a fine store that will design a wig for you."

400. Ms. Jay is being discharged following a radical hysterectomy for uterine cancer. Which of the following would the nurse include in her teaching plan for Ms. Jay?
    ① It is okay to resume normal sexual activity within 2 weeks
    ② It is recommended to resume all previous activities, even jogging
    ③ Physical activity should be limited to that which avoids strain
    ④ Heavy lifting is to be avoided for at least 12 months

401. Mrs. Peters, age 24, comes to OB-GYN clinic with symptoms of metrorrhagia and dyspareunia. Closer examination by the physician indicates endometrial-like cells growing elsewhere in the pelvic cavity. When planning care for this patient, the nurse must be aware that this condition is called:
    ① Endometritis
    ② Endometriosis
    ③ Endophthalmitis
    ④ Endamoebiasis

402. Ms. Willard is admitted to the surgical unit for repair of a rectocele. The patient's symptoms include a history of pain and constipation, and a pelvic examination revealed structural changes. Early postoperative nursing care for a patient who has had a posterior colporrhaphy includes:
① Low-Fowler's position
② A regular diet
③ A stool softener
④ Enemas

403. Mrs. James, age 45, came to OB-GYN clinic complaining of bleeding between periods. A Pap smear was done and revealed cancer of the cervix, stage I. Mrs. James returns to the clinic for a follow-up appointment, and the physician tells her of his findings and recommended treatment. After the physician leaves the room, Mrs. James asks the nurse what the physician really said. The nurse's best explanation of cervical cancer, stage I would be:
① The cancer extends beyond the cervix, but not the pelvic wall
② The cancer is confined to the epithelium of the cervix
③ The cancer is completely confined to the cervix
④ The cancer involves the bladder and the rectum

404. Sally Jones, age 22, was admitted to the unit with a temperature of 102° F, hypotension, diarrhea, impaired renal function, and hyperemia of the conjunctivae. Following a history, physical examination, and several diagnostic tests, a diagnosis of toxic shock syndrome (TSS) was made. Which of the following expected patient outcomes should the nurse consider a *priority* in planning care for this patient?
① Activity tolerance with a pulse rate increase of no more than 60
② Describes methods of practicing safe sex
③ Urine output returns to normal limits
④ Demonstrates increased knowledge of condition

405. Amy, age 24, visits her physician complaining of severe itching of the vulva and a vaginal discharge. Her symptoms suggest candidiasis, and the physician requests the nurse to more closely assess the patient's symptoms. Which of the following descriptions of the vaginal discharge is the nurse most likely to document for the possible diagnosis of candidiasis?
① White
② Grayish white
③ Thick, white, curdlike
④ Copious, frothy, greenish yellow

406. Jennifer, age 18, comes to the clinic complaining of difficulty voiding, vaginal bleeding, and dyspareunia. The initial diagnosis is *Chlamydia trachomatis* infection, which is later confirmed by a culture. The patient is ordered to receive tetracycline and sees the nurse for counseling. While counseling Jennifer, the nurse should:
① Discuss infertility with the patient
② Suggest she share her medication with her partner
③ Explain the life-threatening aspects of the condition
④ Include prevention of recurrence of the infection

407. Prognosis of breast cancer is dependent on a variety of factors, one of which is early detection. The nurse plays a vital role in teaching patients the significance of early diagnosis relative to cancer of the breast. Which of the following recommendations by the nurse is vital in early detection of the disease?
① Ultrasonography
② Yearly mammogram
③ Breast self-examinations
④ Annual examinations by the physician

408. Ms. Kuster, age 54, returns to her room following a radical mastectomy. The most comfortable position for the patient appears to be on her back with the head of the bed elevated. The affected arm is elevated to facilitate circulation and prevent edema. When preparing the patient's environment, it is vital the nurse:
① Ensure complete privacy
② Maintain a dimly lighted room
③ Place the telephone on the side of the unaffected arm
④ Indicate that no injections or blood tests be done on affected arm

409. Mrs. Williams has just returned from surgery. She has had a modified radical mastectomy for treatment of a malignant tumor of the left breast. Mrs. Williams has a dressing over the surgical area. When checking the dressing for hemhorrhage it will be necessary for the nurse to:
① Remove the uppermost layers of the dressing and observe for drainage
② Turn the patient q4h to check the dressing
③ Remove the entire dressing to observe the operative site
④ Feel with the hand under the patient's side and turn the patient to check for drainage

410. Mrs. Kahn has a modified radical mastectomy. To facilitate proper positioning of the patient's arm the nurse should take which of these actions?
① Flex her left arm across her chest while she is in a semi-Fowler's position
② Abduct her left arm at least 8 inches and suspend it from trapeze or IV pole.
③ Place her left arm on pillows with her elbow higher than her shoulders and her wrist higher than her elbow
④ Keep her in high-Fowler's position with her hand on one pillow

411. As the nurse prepares to change a mastectomy patient's dressing for the first time, the patient begins to cry and says, "I can't bear to look at my ugly body." The nurse's *best* response should be:
① "Even though you feel disfigured now, you can always have reconstruction surgery."
② Say nothing, and change the dressing
③ "Everyone feels that way after a mastectomy. You'll get used to it."
④ "You're having a difficult time right now."

412. Discharge teaching is begun for a postmastectomy patient. Which of these instructions is important to include?
① Eat a diet that is high in carbohydrates and vitamin C
② Exercise the affected arm once a day
③ Avoid having blood pressure taken in the affected arm
④ Take frequest rest periods throughout the day

413. A nurse is teaching a patient how to do a self-breast examination. On return demonstration, which action by the patient would indicate understanding of the instructions?
① Raising her arms above her head and inspecting her breast
② Putting a small pillow under her left shoulder when she examines her right breast
③ Lying on her side while she examines the breast
④ Keeping her right arm at her side while examining her right breast

414. Cecil Gagnon, age 60, was admitted to the medical/surgical unit from the emergency room with severe burns. Most of her chest is burned, as well as her hands and upper, inner parts of her arms. On the basis of the rule of nines, what percentage of her body surface is involved?
① 26%
② 27%
③ 45%
④ 54%

415. Jan Jones, age 59, was admitted to the medical/surgical unit from the emergency department with severe burns. An IV of 1000 ml Ringer's Lactate was started by the physician. The amount of Ringer's Lactate solution that she should receive is based on:
① The percentage of body surface area that is burned relative to her body weight
② The total amount of fluid she usually drinks in a 24-hour period
③ A standard amount of 4000 ml, which is given to all burn patients
④ The percentage of body surface that is burned

416. Janie Nelson, age 61, was admitted to the medical/surgical unit from the emergency room with severe burns. On admission to the unit, the nurse noted that a Foley catheter was in place. The primary reason for inserting a Foley catheter is to:
① Avoid using the bedpan
② Avoid urinary incontinence
③ Measure the amount of urine in the bladder
④ Measure urine output hourly

417. A burn patient was placed on "reverse precautions." When the patient asks the nurse why this is necessary, the nurse's *most appropriate* response should be:
① "To prevent the spread of microorganisms to other patients"
② "To prevent potential exposure of microorganisms to hospital personnel"
③ "To protect visitors from exposure to microorganisms"
④ "To protect you from the transmission of microorganisms that may be present in the hospital"

418. Marian Williams, age 19, was badly burned when her clothing caught on fire while cooking. She has partial-thickness (second degree) and full-thickness (third degree) burns over her abdomen and down the front of both upper legs. Marian is placed in isolation. Which of the following isolation techniques should the nurse be prepared to observe in Marian's hospital environment?
① Enteric precaution
② Drainage precaution
③ Protective isolation
④ Respiratory isolation

419. The nurse notes that a patient is to have a homograft. This type of skin graft is used primarily to help:
① Decrease pain at the burn sites
② Improve circulation at the burn sites
③ Prevent fluid loss from the burn sites
④ Stimulate growth of tissue at the burn sites

420. Meperidine hydrochloride (Demerol) was prescribed for a patient with second-degree burns. The nurse should know that the primary reason for this drug is to:
① Reduce anxiety
② Prevent nausea
③ Promote sleep
④ Relieve discomfort

421. The nurse is asked to assist in the selection of a between-meal snack for a patient with second- and third-degree burns. The patient is ordered a diet high in protein. Of the following combinations of foods, which have the highest protein content?
① Cheese cubes and peanuts
② Cheese spread and potato chips
③ Jello with cream, and glass of milk
④ Popcorn with butter, and pretzels

422. The most common complication and cause of death in burn patients after the first 72 hours is:
① Heart failure
② Infection
③ Renal failure
④ Contractures

423. A team conference is held to discuss a burn patient's readiness for discharge. Major considerations for the patient should include:
① The degree of healing and scarring of the burns, as well as emotional and physical well-being
② The fact that the patient has pledged not to smoke in bed
③ The degree of return demonstration the patient exhibits changing the dressing
④ The degree of family involvement in patient care

424. While assisting Dr. Mell with a patient's examination, the nurse is asked to prepare the instrument for examining the patient's ears. Which of the following instruments would the nurse prepare?
① Ophthalmoscope
② Laryngeal mirror
③ Otoscope
④ Pomeroy syringe

425. As the physician prepares to examine the patient's throat, the nurse should have which of the following instruments ready for use?
    ① Schioetz tonometer
    ② Laryngeal mirror
    ③ Ophthalmoscope
    ④ Otoscope

426. Mrs. I, a 35-year-old computer technician, is talking with her neighbor, a nurse. Mrs. I mentions that her vision has been blurry in the left eye and it seems to be getting progressively worse. She says, "It's like a film over my eye that I've had for 3 months, and I can't wipe it away." The nurse realizes this could be indicative of:
    ① Refractive errors
    ② Glaucoma
    ③ Retinal detachment
    ④ Cataracts

427. The nurse should recommend that patients having eye problems make an appointment to have their eyes examined. The most appropriate eye care professional should be a(n):
    ① Ophthalmologist
    ② Optometrist
    ③ Optician
    ④ Neurologist

428. When a patient under the age of 40 develops a cataract, the most probable causative factor is:
    ① Trauma
    ② Age
    ③ Weight
    ④ Job related

429. Which of the following should the nurse observe as signs and symptoms of an impending complication of cataract extraction?
    ① Nausea and vomiting
    ② Blurred vision and diplopia
    ③ Myopia and purulent drainage
    ④ Spots (floaters) and flashes of light

430. Mrs. Kent, age 73, was admitted to the one-day surgical unit for cataract surgery in her right eye. The admitting nurse is aware that Mrs. Kent has difficulty seeing because the cataract is caused by:
    ① Increased intraocular pressure
    ② An opacity and clouding of the lens
    ③ A contagious infection of the eye
    ④ Retinal detachment

431. Mrs. Jason, age 67, was admitted to the one-day surgical unit for cataract surgery. In postoperative teaching, the nurse should:
    ① Explain to her the need for bed rest for 3 months
    ② Explain to her the need to wear dark glasses at all times
    ③ Demonstrate how to instill eye drops
    ④ Demonstrate how to apply warm, wet compresses

432. Mrs. Clark, age 75, is scheduled for cataract surgery. She tells the nurse that she is too old to go through a surgical procedure and hesitates to learn about her postoperative care. The nurse's response should be:
    ① "Oh, you're not too old! There's not that much to learn."
    ② "You'll be surprised how well you will do!"
    ③ "The physician and nursing staff will assist you!"
    ④ "You seem concerned about your surgery and your postoperative care. Do you want to talk about it?"

433. During cataract surgery for a 72-year-old woman, the surgeon implanted an intraocular lens in her right eye. The nurse should caution the patient to notify her or the physician of any complications such as:
    ① Sudden pain, erythema, drainage, or sudden visual change
    ② Flash of light, increase in "floaters," or blurred vision
    ③ A drooping eyelid
    ④ Blurred vision

434. During the admission process for a patient scheduled for cataract surgery, which of the following interventions is *not* necessary?
    ① Orient the patient to the room
    ② Speak in a louder voice than normal
    ③ Ask the patient what assistance he or she will need
    ④ Place the call light where the patient can find it

435. Mr. Charles had cataract surgery with a local anesthetic and sedation. Which of the following is an appropriate postoperative nursing action?
    ① Encourage coughing and deep-breathing exercises
    ② Do not move Mr. Charles in bed. This patient should have complete bed rest
    ③ Administer medication promptly if nausea occurs
    ④ Do not allow visitors in the room because they may disturb the patient's rest

436. How can the nurse best help Mr. Thompson at mealtime following his return to the unit after cataract surgery?
    ① Feed him his meal
    ② Chop his food into small pieces
    ③ Allow him to manage the meal by himself
    ④ Orient him to where the food is on the plate

437. Which of the following *best* describes a glaucoma screening program?
    ① Color blindness evaluation
    ② Acuity testing with a Snellen chart
    ③ Tonometer used to detect increasing intraocular pressure
    ④ Obtaining a specimen for culture and sensitivity studies

438. The nurse is to prepare Mr. G for a glaucoma test. The instrument used to test for glaucoma is the:
    ① Ophthalmoscope
    ② Snellen chart
    ③ Otoscope
    ④ Tonometer

439. The nurse should identify glaucoma as the physiologic result of a(n):
    ① Increase in the vitreous humor fluid
    ② Increase in the intraocular pressure
    ③ Decrease in the aqueous fluid
    ④ Decrease in the intraocular pressure

440. Mr. C, a 52-year-old male, was admitted with a diagnosis of closed-angle glaucoma. The nurse prepares to meet Mr. C's needs by knowing that another name for closed-angle glaucoma is:
① "The sneak thief" glaucoma
② Preglaucoma
③ Acute glaucoma
④ Chronic glaucoma

441. Mr. Shepherd is a 54-year-old man with closed-angle glaucoma. Mr. Shepherd tells the nurse that he thinks he caused his condition by reading a lot. The nurse should explain that the occurrence of glaucoma is most often related to:
① Height
② Weight
③ Race
④ Age

442. Mr. William Bailey, age 54, goes to a clinic for an eye examination. The results of the examination reveal that he has open-angle (chronic) glaucoma. His orders include timolol maleate (Timoptic) eyedrops and acetazolamide (Diamox). Which of these statements made by Mr. Bailey would indicate a symptom of open-angle glaucoma?
① "I have a greenish discharge from my eye."
② "I bump into people I don't see walking alongside of me."
③ "Sometimes I have pain in my eyes."
④ "My eyes have a reddened appearance sometimes."

443. Mr. Rogers, a patient with glaucoma, asks the nurse why he has to take the timolol maleate (Timoptic) eyedrops. The nurse should inform him that the medicine acts by:
① Dilating the pupil
② Promoting production of aqueous humor
③ Reducing muscle contractions of the eye
④ Decreasing the formation of aqueous humor

444. A glaucoma patient is taking timolol maleate (Timoptic) eyedrops and acetazolamide (Diamox). The two *most important* assessments for this patient would be:
① Blood pressure and electrolyte readings
② Apical pulse and serum drug levels
③ Urinalysis and blood pressure readings
④ Hemoglobin and hematocrit readings

445. A glaucoma patient indicates an understanding of discharge instructions if he or she makes which of the following statements?
① "I will avoid antihistamines for the treatment of a cold."
② "I will keep the affected eye patched at night."
③ "I will keep the lights dim so that I won't hurt my eyes."
④ "I will discontinue my medication if I feel well."

446. Jane Sheely, age 50, is admitted to the hospital with the diagnosis of detached retina of the right eye. She was bending over and lifting up her clothes basket when she saw "floating spots" with her right eye. What additional signs and symptoms would the nurse expect Mrs. Sheely to report?
① Periorbital pain
② Flashes of light
③ Blurred vision
④ Rainbows around lights

447. The preoperative nursing care plan for a patient with a detached retina includes:
① Maintaining the patient on bed rest
② Having the patient cough every 2 hours
③ Irrigating the affected eye
④ Keep one eye patched

448. A patient is admitted with a diagnosis of Ménière's disease, which is:
① Characterized by recurrent episodes of vertigo, progressive unilateral nerve deafness, and tinnitus
② Acute disease of the inner ear
③ Most common in men who are 30 to 40 years of age
④ Diagnosed through specific blood tests

449. Jodi is brought to the local clinic with symptoms of heatstroke, which the nurse would expect to include:
① Double vision; nausea and vomiting; muscle incoordination; and dyspnea
② Muscle cramps; cool, pale, damp skin; tachycardia; and marked diaphoresis
③ Edema; discoloration of skin; blister formation; complaints of numbness, tingling, and burning of the skin
④ Hot, flushed, dry skin; hypotention; tachycardia; and hyperpyrexia

450. Sal is brought to the first aid tent at the local fair because he is exhibiting symptoms of heatstroke. Nursing interventions for a heatstroke should include:
① Removing constrictive clothing; providing warm soaks; and if conscious, giving warm liquids
② Ensuring adequate airway and ventilation, administering quick-acting carbohydrates, and recording vital signs
③ Maintaining adequate airway, breathing, and circulation; providing rapid cooling; and administering oxygen, if prescribed by physician
④ Making sure the patient is in a cool area, giving salt water if the patient is conscious and not vomiting, and relieving muscle cramps

451. The physician has ordered an antihistamine to be given immediately to treat a patient's allergic reaction to an insect bite. In this situation, the emergency room nurse should expect which of the following drugs to be administered?
① Ephedrine
② Epinephrine
③ Neosynephrine
④ Hydroxyzine (Vistaril)

452. Emergency room nurses are always vigilant for a severe, allergic, systemic reaction to a foreign substance, which could cause a condition known as:
① Psychogenic shock
② Neurogenic shock
③ Cardiogenic shock
④ Anaphylactic shock

453. Julie Green was stung by a bee. Within the next 45 minutes she developed an itchy rash, began to wheeze, and felt her lips and tongue begin to thicken. On admission to the emergency room, where she was treated for an allergic reaction to an insect bite, Julia presented additional symptoms. The nurse on duty should have noted which of the following?
    ① Increased pulse rate and drop in blood pressure
    ② Decreased pulse rate and increase in blood pressure
    ③ Sensation of being hot and feverish
    ④ Increased respiratory rate

454. Mr. Raphael Garcia, age 70, has been in good health since his retirement. While mowing his lawn on a summer morning, he suddenly experienced a sharp pain in his midsternal area that radiated down his left arm. At this time he also suddenly experienced nausea. What is the most common patient response to chest pain?
    ① Dialing 9-1-1 immediately
    ② Lying down and delaying calling for help
    ③ Calling the physician
    ④ Ignoring the pain and continuing to work

455. The nurse knows that the immediate rescuer response to a patient experiencing chest pain should be which of the following?
    ① Walk with the patient to help him or her remain conscious
    ② Start CPR before the patient's heart stops beating completely
    ③ Put the patient in the car and drive to the hospital immediately
    ④ Keep the patient at rest and call 9-1-1

456. The nurse's first consideration when a patient has a cardiac arrest is:
    ① Airway
    ② Breathing
    ③ Circulation
    ④ Definitive therapy

457. A patient's heart rate is 100 to 160 beats/min, rhythm is regular, the P waves are normal, the P-R interval is normal, the QRS is normal. The nurse in the emergency room should interpret this rhythm as:
    ① Complete heart block
    ② Atrial fibrillation
    ③ Sinus tachycardia
    ④ Sinus bradycardia

458. Concerning emergency procedures, the nurse must know that elective cardioversion is a procedure performed by the physician to:
    ① Restore ventricular function
    ② Decrease the work of the right ventricle
    ③ Terminate heart block
    ④ Terminate rapid dysrhythmias

459. The first choice of treatment for ventricular fibrillation is:
    ① Emergency administration of IV atropine
    ② Immediate defibrillation
    ③ Endotracheal intubation
    ④ Cardioversion

460. An electrocardiogram was done for Mrs. Palmer immediately after her admission for severe chest pain. In planning care for Mrs. Palmer, the nurse should understand that this test:
    ① Records the flow of blood through the heart
    ② Measures the strength of the heartbeats
    ③ Records the activity of the heart muscle
    ④ Measures the rate at which oxygen is used

461. On learning of her diagnosis of a coronary occlusion, Mrs. Zale became very apprehensive and expressed fear she was going to die. Her husband was frightened by her behavior and asked the nurse why his wife was feeling this way. The nurse's *best* response should be:
    ① Your wife realizes she had a heart attack and that it is probably serious
    ② This reaction is not unusual for patients with a heart attack, and she needs reassurance
    ③ So many people die when they have this condition. It's typical
    ④ Your wife's heart attack probably affected her mind, so don't worry

462. In providing appropriate nursing care to patients with cardiac disease, it is helpful for the nurse to understand that arteries supplying heart muscle tissue receive their oxygenated blood from the:
    ① Ascending aorta
    ② Left subclavian artery
    ③ Carotid arteries
    ④ Intercostal arteries

463. During a team conference, patient data is reviewed as a means of planning care. Of the following data, which indicates myocardial damage?
    ① Decrease in heart rate
    ② Elevated cardiac enzyme levels
    ③ Severe cyanosis
    ④ Decreased cardiac enzyme levels

464. Connie, a rape victim, is brought to the emergency room for treatment. To protect the patient legally, what is the most important measure the nursing staff should follow?
    ① Personally take evidence to the laboratory
    ② Obtain an account of what happened in Connie's own words
    ③ Do not allow people around her
    ④ Arrange for Connie to be escorted home by someone she trusts

465. Amy, a rape victim, is brought to the emergency department for treatment. A physical examination is recommended for early detection of:
    ① Dysuria
    ② Dysmenorrhea
    ③ Pregnancy
    ④ Venereal disease

466. The nurse informed the physician that she forgot to give Mrs. Stark's 10:00 AM blood pressure medication. This is an example of which of the following professional characteristics?
    ① Responsibility
    ② Accountability
    ③ Autonomy
    ④ Advocacy

467. When the nurse takes the initiative for making an independent decision about her patient's care, it is known in nursing practice as:
① Independence
② Accountability
③ Responsibility
④ Autonomy

468. Peer assistance programs are present in most states to assist nurses who are impaired by either alcohol or drugs. The goals of the peer assistance program include all the following *except:*
① To assist the nurse who is impaired to receive treatment
② To protect the public from the untreated nurse
③ To assist the nurse in pursuing other vocational options
④ To assist the nurse in monitoring continued recovery for a period of time

469. When providing nursing care for elderly people in institutions, which of the following is a major consideration?
① Providing personal hygiene
② Eliminating all patient responsibilities
③ Fostering social privacy
④ Making decisions for the patient

470. One of the most common myths associated with aging is that:
① The majority of elderly reside in their own home
② Most elderly people have at least one chronic condition
③ All people become senile when they become old
④ Most elderly are isolated and alone, averaging one weekly contact with family

471. Which of the following is *not* a common myth associated with aging?
① All people become senile when they become old
② Most older people are not isolated and alone
③ Most elderly are in nursing homes or care facilities
④ Old people are ill and disabled

472. The Health Care Financing Administration (HCFA) mandates comprehensive assessment as a basis for developing a plan of care to assist nursing home residents in attaining the highest physical, mental, and psychosocial functioning possible. To meet this requirement, nursing homes throughout the country have developed the Minimum Data Set (MDS) for Nursing Home Resident Assessment and Care Screening, and 18 Resident Assessment Protocols (RAPs) for problem identification. The MDS is a tool regarding resident care that:
① Has added a great deal of paperwork to caring for the elderly
② Provides a simple list of problems that a nurse uses to assess each resident
③ Is a functionally based assessment tool identifying pertinent information needed to develop a comprehensive care plan
④ Is the same for all states

473. Nursing home administrations developed 18 Resident Assessment Protocols (RAPs) for problem identification. The RAPs specify "trigger" definitions that:
① Have added a great deal of paperwork to caring for the elderly
② Provide a simple listing of problems that a nurse uses to assess each resident
③ Are the same as the MDS
④ Explicitly suggest specific care that requires implementation

474. HCFA received a federal mandate through the Omnibus Budget Reconciliation Act (OBRA) to ensure that the MDS and RAPs systems are implemented. These requirements are for:
① All long-term care facilities participating in Medicare or Medicaid programs
② All long-term care facilities participating in Medicare programs
③ All long-term care facilities participating in Medicaid programs
④ For everyone covered by Medicare, Medicaid, and private insurance plans

475. OBRA requires that each assessment be conducted or coordinated by:
① Any staff members directly caring for the resident
② Any licensed persons
③ Only registered nurses
④ Any staff members caring indirectly for the resident

476. After completing the initial history and assessment on Mr. Hall, a newly admitted 56-year-old patient, the nurse documents the following:

"Speaks frequently of his children being 'all grown up' and being at home all alone with his wife. States he has always cared for his wife, has never been sick for any length of time, and is concerned about loss of his job because of illness."

From this statement the nurse should conclude that Mr. Hall is:
① Having trouble adjusting to the hospital and will need help from a social worker
② Too concerned about his wife and should be more concerned about himself
③ Demonstrating the normal characteristics of middle adulthood and the demands of illness
④ Demonstrating pity for himself and does not want to admit that he is getting older

477. Of the following methods of charting, which one *best* describes the recording of events as they occur throughout the day?
① Narrative charting
② SOAP charting
③ Focus charting
④ PIE charting

478. In SOAP charting, the *S* is best represented by which of the following entries?
    1. WBC count is elevated
    2. Patient says, "I feel better today."
    3. Temperature is 102.8° F (39.3° C)
    4. Incisional line is well approximated

479. In most agencies, the use of a pencil to record patient information is acceptable on which of the following documents?
    1. Flow sheet
    2. Discharge summary
    3. Medication record
    4. Kardex

480. Which of the following documentation provides the *most* objective information about the patient's neuromuscular status?
    1. Limited response to painful stimuli
    2. Decreased strength of the lower extremities
    3. Confused at intervals; lethargic most of the time
    4. Not able to grip nurse's hand with right hand, but strong grip with left hand

481. Which of the following barriers to communication is being demonstrated by a nurse who says to a patient, "There, there . . . don't worry. Everything will turn out for the best."
    1. Disagreeing with the patient
    2. Offering a cliché as an expression of reassurance
    3. Belittling the patient's feelings
    4. Giving approval

482. Which of the following is an example of a communication technique that *best* expresses the nurse's interest in what the patient has to say?
    1. Maintaining direct eye contact with the patient during the interaction
    2. Sharing several personal experiences with the patient
    3. Smiling throughout the interaction
    4. Providing privacy so that the patient's concerns will not be overheard

483. Mrs. Todd, age 58, is brought to the emergency room because she is experiencing chest pain. It is determined that she is to be admitted to the coronary care unit. She states to the emergency department nurse, "I don't know what all the fuss is about. I'm sure this is just a bad case of indigestion." Which coping mechanism is this patient demonstrating?
    1. Rationalization
    2. Regression
    3. Denial
    4. Compensation

484. The nurse notes that a male patient who has had a stroke has expressive aphasia. A plan is developed to help him communicate his needs more effectively. Which nursing intervention is *most* appropriate?
    1. Associate words with physical objects
    2. Inform the family that he cannot communicate
    3. Immediately correct any of his mispronounced words
    4. Anticipate his needs to minimize efforts at talking

485. Which of the following diagnostic tests would be *excluded* in establishing a diagnosis for a patient who exhibits symptoms of stomach cancer?
    1. Cholecystogram
    2. Gastroscopy
    3. Fluoroscopy
    4. Gastric analysis

486. Mr. P has been admitted to the urology unit for diagnostic testing. Included in the laboratory work was an order for a serum BUN test. The nurse knows the value of the test because blood urea nitrogen (BUN) is:
    1. Elevated in renal failure
    2. Lowered in renal failure
    3. Not related to kidney disease
    4. Not a very significant test to measure kidney function

487. Which of the following enzyme studies are *most* specific for measuring cardiac damage?
    1. SGOT, SGPT
    2. CPK, SGPT
    3. CK-MB, isoenzymes LDH_1 and LDH_2
    4. CH, CPT

488. The nurse's aid reports to the nurse that Mr. Meeker's bedpan was accidentally emptied and the urine was not saved in the 24-hour collection container. Since the 24-hour collection was started 6 hours earlier, the nurse should:
    1. Continue with the specimen collection, making note in the chart
    2. Start the collection over, obtaining a new container and making a note in the chart
    3. Start the collection over, using the same container and adding to the urine already collected
    4. Stop the collection and wait to start a new specimen the next morning

489. Bill Johnson is a 42-year-old high school teacher who complains about a burning and gnawing sensation in his stomach after eating. He is frequently nauseated, has eructations, abdominal distention, and melena. After diagnostic studies were performed at the outpatient clinic, a diagnosis of duodenal ulcers was made. In planning care for Mr. Johnson, the nurse knows that the burning and gnawing sensation in the stomach associated with duodenal ulcers is known to:
    1. Be constant
    2. Be more severe when eating
    3. Occur 2 hours before meals
    4. Occur 2 hours after meals

490. Mrs. V needs to be catheterized for residual urine. During the procedure, the nurse notes resistence to the catheter at the external urinary meatus. Which of the following actions is the *most* appropriate for the nurse to implement?
    1. Ask the patient to cough several times
    2. Remove the catheter, then try again
    3. Have the patient take several deep breaths
    4. Pull back the catheter, then push forward again

491. Urine that remains in the bladder after a person voids is called:
    1. Reflex incontinence
    2. Residual urine
    3. Urge incontinence
    4. Retention urine

492. Which of the following procedures would be appropriate for the nurse in obtaining and measuring a patient's residual urine?
① Empty the collection receptacle and record the amount q8h
② Remove the retention catheter and measure the amount the patient voids
③ Have the patient void and then catheterize immediately, measuring the amount obtained from the catheterization
④ Instruct the patient to void, and then wait 2 hours and have her void again

493. When collecting a routine urine sample, the nurse should instruct the patient to:
① Completely fill the container
② Void 50 to 100 ml of urine
③ Add a few drops of water to the empty container
④ Use a sterile container

494. Mr. Hill had an appendectomy 2 days ago. During his morning care, he complains of nausea, shortness of breath, and light-headedness. The nurse's *first* action should be to:
① Notify the nurse in charge
② Take his vital signs and report them along with his symptoms
③ Wait a short time to see if he is feeling better
④ Inspect the abdominal dressing

495. Mr. Harry Bell, age 46, has a diagnosis of benign adenoma of the descending colon. He undergoes a colon resection with an end-to-end anastomosis. During the procedure, he receives a general anesthetic. In the recovery room, Mr. Bell is given oxygen to promote tissue perfusion. What is the best method of oxygen administration for Mr. Bell?
① Nasal canula with the O_2 flow rate set at 1 to 4 L/min
② Face mask with the O_2 flow rate set at 6 to 12 L/min
③ Oxygen tubing held by his face with the O_2 flow rate set at 6 to 12 L/min
④ Deep breathing exercises with a paper bag

496. Mr. Bates has been transferred from the recovery room to the unit. The physician's postoperative orders include use of the incentive spirometer to avoid respiratory complications. To help Mr. Bates correctly use the incentive spirometer, the nurse should:
① Encourage the patient to cough to remove as much mucus as possible before the treatment
② Have the patient breathe as rapidly as possible during the treatment
③ Have the patient lie flat in the side-lying position to use the spirometer
④ Ask the patient to use the spirometer only when he thinks he is able

497. During surgery, Mr. Thompson had a penrose drain inserted near the incision site. On the third postoperative day the dressing inadvertently becomes wet during the patient's bath, and the physician orders a sterile dressing change. What is the *best* method for the nurse to use during the dressing change?
① With sterile gloves, remove the dressing layers all at once to avoid contaminating the wound
② With clean, nonsterile gloves, remove the dressing one layer at a time
③ With sterile gloves, remove only the outer dressing and apply additional gauze pads
④ Gloves are not needed as long as the gauze for the dressing change is not touched

498. During a dressing change, the nurse observes the patient and the incision site for any signs of infection. Which of the following signs should the nurse report to the surgeon?
① An oral temperature of 99.2° F on the first postoperative day
② A small amount of clear, yellow exudate at the edges of the incision
③ Redness and swelling around the incision
④ A sudden drop in blood pressure on the day of surgery

499. Which of the following postoperative nursing measures will best help the nurse assess a patient for postoperative complications?
① Allowing bed rest for as long as the patient feels the need
② Removing the elastic stockings during the morning bath and reapplying them at bedtime
③ Dorsiflexing the patient's foot and evaluating the patient for lower leg pain
④ Rubbing the patient's lower leg as a response to any complaints of leg cramps

500. The nurse is providing a sitz bath for Mrs. Pauling. The nurse knows to establish the temperature of the water at:
① 75° to 80° F (23.8° to 26.6° C)
② 85° to 90° F (29.4° to 32.2° C)
③ 100° to 105° F (37.7° to 40.5° C)
④ 120° to 125° F (48.8° to 51.6° C)

501. The nurse must turn a patient from his left side to his right side. What is the *most important* safety measure to use when moving the patient?
① Maintain the bed in a low position
② Keep the opposite side rail up
③ Remove the pillow from under the patient's head
④ Ensure that the bed is in a locked position

502. The nurse's aide reports a patient's blood pressure is 80/50. The nurse rechecks the blood pressure and obtains the same reading. The patient states that he feels fine; however, the nurse would:
① Call the physician immediately
② Check the blood pressure in the other arm
③ Ask another nurse to check the blood pressure
④ Document the blood pressure and retake it in 10 min

503. The nurse is preparing to give Mr. Haltom a bath and assess his skin. He notices that the nurse uses gloves and questions why. He feels that the gloves imply that he is dirty or contaminated. The nurse's *best response* is:
  1. "I'm sorry it offends you, but it is hospital policy."
  2. "I never said that you are contaminated; you are assuming that I feel this way."
  3. "I would wear these gloves whether you were contaminated or not."
  4. "It is hospital policy for gloves to be worn for all patients to protect them as well as staff."

504. While transferring a patient with an indwelling catheter from the bed to the chair, the nurse should:
  1. Place the Foley bag on the overbed table
  2. Place the Foley bag in the patient's lap
  3. Disconnect the Foley bag and clamp the tubing
  4. Hang the bag on the side of the chair, below the bladder

505. When making rounds at 11 AM, the nurse notices that her patient's catheter bag is empty and has had no drainage since 7 AM. After checking to see that no one emptied the bag, the nurse should:
  1. Check for kinks in the tubing
  2. Notify the physician immediately
  3. Question the patient about how he feels
  4. Increase the patient's IV from keep vein open (TKO) rate to 50 ml/h

506. The amount of fluid used in the irrigation of a ureteral catheter is:
  1. 1 to 2 ml
  2. 5 ml
  3. 15 to 30 ml
  4. 20 to 50 ml

507. Kidney stones most often occur in persons who:
  1. Drink large amounts of fluids
  2. Eat foods high in fats and proteins
  3. Are not following a regular exercise schedule
  4. Are on long-term bed rest

508. Mr. L has a long history of angina attacks. A drug used to relieve attacks of angina is:
  1. Meperidinet (Demerol)
  2. Aspirin
  3. Nitroglycerin
  4. Morphine

509. Perineal exercises are most often used to help:
  1. Reduce residual urine
  2. Relieve urinary retention
  3. Overcome painful urination
  4. Control urinary incontinence

510. When the nurse discovers a reddened area on the coccyx, an appropriate nursing intervention is to:
  1. Rub the area with alcohol
  2. Keep the patient in a semi-Fowler's position
  3. Massage the surrounding area gently with lotion
  4. Apply warm compresses four times a day

511. Which of the following *best* indicates a risk factor in a patient's state of health?
  1. A health behavior that decreases the risk of disease or injury
  2. A health behavior that promotes physiologic health
  3. A life-style practice that increases a patient's susceptibility to a disease or accident
  4. A health behavior that promotes spiritual and emotional well-being

512. Mrs. Smith, age 40, was admitted to the surgical unit for complaints of abdominal pain, nausea, and vomiting. Her temperature was 100.4° F (38° C), blood pressure 140/76, pulse rate 80, and respirations 24 and slightly shallow. When planning care for Mrs. Smith, which of the following actions should the nurse implement *first*?
  1. Nursing actions necessary for achieving a goal
  2. Revising the plan of care
  3. Collecting data
  4. Formulating a nursing diagnosis

513. While collecting data for further assessment of a patient, the nurse notes a decrease in the number of red blood cells and in the hemoglobin level. This information is vital in planning nursing care because it could indicate that the patient has:
  1. Leukemia
  2. Anemia
  3. Hemolysis
  4. Leukocytosis

514. If a patient has the following symptoms, the one *most* indicative of a fluid imbalance is:
  1. Heartburn
  2. A skin rash
  3. Swollen fingers
  4. Excessive tearing

515. When you are assigned to care for a patient who is ill because of an invasion of microorganisms, you would know that the most appropriate term to use for this condition would be:
  1. Inflammation
  2. Allergy
  3. Infection
  4. Immunity

516. Mrs. Stevens, age 64, has congestive heart failure (CHF), which the nurse knows is best described as:
  1. A sudden spasm of the heart muscle caused by a decreased blood supply
  2. A formed clot within one of the heart chambers
  3. Failure of the pumping mechanism of the heart resulting in decreased blood flow to the heart
  4. An abnormality in the structure of the heart

517. A patient is admitted to the hospital with the diagnosis of nephrosis. This condition is characterized by a group of symptoms, which are proteinuria, hypoalbuminemia, and edema. The nurse knows that a patient who has a disorder characterized by a group of symptoms is said to have a(n):
  1. Subjective symptom
  2. Objective symptom
  3. Sign
  4. Syndrome

518. The nurse is assisting the physician with a physical examination. In using a sphygmomanometer to check the patient's blood pressure, the nurse helps to determine any significant changes. A symptom that is detected through special examination and is observed is termed a(n):
① Subjective symptom
② Objective symptom
③ Sign
④ Syndrome

519. Mrs. Samson, age 55, was admitted to the surgical unit after complaints of abdominal pain, nausea, and vomiting. Her temperature was 100.4° F (38° C), blood pressure 140/76, pulse rate 80, and respirations 24 and slightly shallow. What information about Mrs. Samson is an example of subjective data?
① Temperature elevation
② Complaints of nausea
③ Blood pressure measurement
④ Rapid, shallow respirations

520. Ms. Tam, age 25, was admitted to the surgical unit after complaints of abdominal pain, nausea, and vomiting. Her temperature was 100.4° F (38° C), blood pressure 140/76, pulse rate 80, and respirations 24 and slightly shallow. Which of the following best describes objective data?
① Anorexia
② Pain
③ Nausea
④ Temperature

521. In evaluating the proper functioning of a chest tube connected to an underwater-seal drainage system, the nurse should assess for:
① Pleural drainage above 100 ml/hr
② Constant bubbling in the water-seal chamber
③ No bubbling in the suction chamber
④ Fluctuation of water in the water-seal chamber

522. Jill St. Clair is an emergency medical technician (EMT) who has been careful to wear gloves, goggles, or masks whenever there was a lot of blood present at the scene of an accident. She recently had a cold with runny nose and itchy eyes. She was constantly blowing her nose and rubbing her eyes. Today, she is admitted to the unit with fatigue, swollen joints, dark urine, yellow skin and sclera. A diagnosis of hepatitis B was made. Jill cannot understand how she contracted hepatitis. The nurse knows that a major reason for contamination was:
① Being on an ambulance run with a patient infected with the hepatitis B virus
② Being exposed to a person with hepatitis in the hospital
③ Rubbing her eyes after touching sheets contaminated with blood, vomitus, and urine
④ Being in contact with other EMTs who have been exposed to patients with hepatitis

523. In maintaining safe practice procedures, which of the following is the *best* nursing method for preventing an accidental puncture from a contaminated needle?
① Remove the needle from the syringe and discard in special container
② Recover the needle with its cap and discard in regular containers
③ Leave the needle uncapped after use and discard entire syringe in a special container
④ Bend or break the needle from the syringe and discard in regular container

524. The Occupational Safety and Health Administration (OSHA) recommends that high-risk public safety workers be given hepatitis B vaccine. The nurse in a public health clinic knows this vaccine is:
① A cure for the disease, once a person is infected
② Made from human blood plasma and can spread the disease
③ A method of controlling the virus
④ Good for both HBV and HAV viruses

525. Which of the following juices should the nurse recommend to the patient to help keep the urine acid?
① Apple juice
② Tomato juice
③ Pineapple juice
④ Cranberry juice

526. Mrs. Adams has a physician's order that reads, "Restrict fluids." The nurse would understand that the patient's general fluid intake should probably be limited to:
① 200 to 400 ml/24 hr
② 800 to 1000 ml/24 hr
③ 2000 ml/24 hr
④ 3000 ml/24 hr

527. A patient is NPO and has a nasogastric tube in place with low intermittent suction. He complains that he is thirsty. An appropriate nursing intervention is to:
① Offer sips of water by mouth
② Increase the flow of IV fluids
③ Offer him mouth care
④ Decrease the force of the suction

528. Which of the following diets is usually prescribed for patients with constipation?
① Low-fiber
② Low-fat
③ High-fiber
④ High-fat

529. Mrs. Stevens does not like to drink milk. To supply food of equal nutrient value, the nurse would encourage her to eat:
① Fresh pineapple
② Fish
③ Potatoes
④ Puddings

530. Mr. Cohen is placed on a clear-liquid diet. Which of these foods may be included in his diet plan?
① Lime sherbet
② Cream of celery soup
③ Oatmeal
④ Weak tea with skim milk

531. A patient is to have dressings changed on burned areas of his body. The procedure is extremely painful. To promote the patient's comfort, which of the following actions should the nurse take?
① Have the patient take a nap immediately before and after the procedure
② Assist the patient to use relaxation exercises immediately before the procedure
③ Arrange to have the patient's favorite television or radio program on during the procedure
④ Administer to the patient a prescribed pain medication 15 to 30 minutes before the procedure

532. Which of the following nursing techniques has been found *most* helpful when caring for the patient in pain?
① Leaving the patient to rest in a quiet, darkened room
② Asking the patient why he or she thinks there is pain
③ Asking family members to remain with the patient
④ Allowing the patient to describe the nature of the pain

533. To promote measures directed at reversing inappropriate health behaviors in the patient, the nurse should:
① Inform the patient that unhealthy behaviors can harm other people
② Ask the patient to explain why he or she still engages in this unhealthy practice
③ Supply the patient with educational materials aimed at reducing the unhealthy practice
④ Realize that the patient may resist changing a behavior that has become a habit

534. Mr. Dunn's history indicates that he is 40 pounds overweight, smokes two packs of cigarettes a day, and drinks 8 to 10 cups of coffee a day. In developing a teaching plan, the nurse should take which of these actions first?
① Explain to him the effects of smoking on the cardiovascular system
② Give him a pamphlet that explains the benefits of exercise in reducing stress
③ Talk with his wife regarding his intake of calories and cholesterol
④ Determine his understanding of the relationship between his behavior and his condition

535. Which of the following nursing behaviors *best indicates* that the nurse is meeting a patient's need for emotional support?
① The nurse spends time listening to the concerns of a patient scheduled for surgery
② The nurse assists an elderly patient in eating a meal
③ The nurse accompanies a patient to have a x-ray examination
④ The nurse avoids disturbing a patient who is praying

536. Hospice nurses often provide narcotic analgesics for patients in pain. One of the most common side effects of narcotic analgesics is:
① Constipation
② Anorexia
③ Nausea
④ Muscle weakness

537. The licensed practical nurse/vocational nurse (LPN/VN) is a secondary nurse in a primary hospice team. The LPN/VN's functions and responsibilities include:
① Providing physical assistance for the patient, and emotional and spiritual support for the patient and family
② Providing instruction to the patient and family about health care management and the effects of medication and illness
③ Providing companionship, respite care for family relief, and emotional support
④ Providing opportunities for spiritual reconciliation and healing, and prayer

538. A hospice nurse provides palliative care, which is defined as:
① Support care
② Curative care
③ Holistic care
④ Symptom-control care

539. Mr. Gehringer, age 87, has been living in his son's home for 6 years. He has been admitted to the hospital for incontinence and burning on urination. He is alert and oriented but occasionally has difficulty communicating his needs because of his heavy German accent. Who should make the decisions regarding his care?
① Mr. Gehringer
② The physician
③ The primary care giver
④ Mr. Gehringer's son

540. On admission to nursing homes, residents designate a person as having durable power of attorney. This means that the resident legally appoints a person on his behalf to:
① Make decisions regarding his finances
② Make health care decisions for him even when he is able
③ Make decisions as to how he will spend his money for health care
④ Make health care decisions for him when he is unable to do so

541. The status of durable power of attorney that nursing home residents give to a person shall include but is not limited to:
① Selling his home, property, and other possessions that he has while he is alive, whether mentally competent or not
② Obtaining, inspecting, receiving, and disclosing medical records and information related to his physical/mental health history and medications
③ Giving the nursing home all his finances once he has passed away
④ Taking care of all his property, finances, and other responsibilities upon his death

542. Mrs. Smith is a 1-day postoperative patient complaining of severe pain. The physician has ordered hydromorphone (Dilaudid) q4h prn for pain. In planning for the pain management of Mrs. Smith, the nurse should instruct the patient to inform her of the need for medication:
① Every time she is able to have a dose of medication, even if it is before she is aware of much pain
② As she begins to have the sensation of pain
③ When the pain has risen to 7 or 8 on a 10-point scale
④ When she has pain, but only if the 4-hour period is up

543. Before intramuscular injection of medication, the nurse should aspirate for blood. If blood returns in the syringe, the nurse should:
① Proceed with the injection of medication
② Withdraw needle and prepare a new syringe
③ Slowly inject medication and massage the site
④ Withdraw the needle and give the injection in another site

544. When preparing to administer medications to geriatric patients, the nurse knows that as a general rule, medications for elderly patients should be given in:
① Smaller doses, closer together
② Larger doses, closer together
③ Smaller doses, farther apart
④ Larger doses, farther apart

545. Which of the following actions that the nurse performs is most likely to decrease discomfort from an intramuscular gluteal injection?
① Rub skin firmly with antiseptic swab
② Pull the skin tissue taut
③ Aspirate for blood
④ Inject medication rapidly but consistently

546. The nurse is preparing furosemide (Lasix) 40 mg PO for administration. The most important time the label should be checked is:
① When checking the medication record with the physician's orders
② Immediately before pouring the medication
③ After pouring the medication
④ After administering the medication

547. While on duty, the nurse notices that the medication refrigerator is very warm, registering 80° F (26.6° C), and that the vaccines stored inside are all warm. The nurse should:
① Notify the pharmacy and adjust the thermometer
② Close the door and report it later to the supervisor
③ Adjust the temperature and recheck in an hour to be sure the temperature has dropped
④ Remove all of the medication and return it to the pharmacy

548. A nurse on the unit has a critically ill patient who is being transferred to the intensive care unit. Being very busy, she obtains a scheduled drug from the narcotics cabinet and prepares to administer it as ordered. No one has seen her prepare the drug. She asks a co-worker to sign the record that the excess was wasted. The nurse's correct response should be to:
① Sign the record because she trusts her co-worker
② Refuse to sign the record, and inform the co-worker of this decision when she returns
③ Refuse to sign the record and hope the co-worker will not ask about it on her return
④ Sign the co-worker's name with her own initials next to the signature, indicating that the excess was wasted

549. An air lock should be used with a subcutaneous injection of insulin for a hospitalized patient if:
① The nurse prefers to use an air lock with insulin
② The patient is obese and needs a longer needle for administration
③ A pediatric patient were receiving insulin twice a day
④ The patient has been using an air lock during self-administration of insulin at home

550. Which of these sites is preferred for the subcutaneous administration of heparin?
① In the deltoid muscle
② On the top of the thigh
③ In the buttocks at a 45-degree angle
④ Below the ribs to the iliac crest

551. To ensure that the right patient is receiving a prescribed medication, it is *essential* that the nurse take which of these actions?
① Check the name on the patient's wristband
② Call the patient by name
③ Read the name of the patient on the bed card
④ Check the medication record for the patient's room number

552. The physician orders penicillin 250,000 U IM. The label on the vial reads 100,000 U/ml. How much medication should the nurse prepare to administer to the patient?
① 1 ml
② 1.5 ml
③ 2 ml
④ 2.5 ml

553. The physician orders penicillin liquid 500 mg PO tid. The bottle of penicillin that comes from the pharmacy is labeled 125 mg/tsp. Which of the following would be the appropriate dose for the nurse to administer to the patient?
① 15 ml
② 16 ml
③ 20 ml
④ 25 ml

554. Heparin 5000 U is to be give subcutaneously. In stock is heparin 10,000 U/ml. The nurse should administer:
① 0.5 ml
② 1 ml
③ 1.25 ml
④ 1.5 ml

555. Mrs. G has codeine, 1.5 gr, ordered. On hand are scored tablets labeled 60 mg. The nurse should give:
① ½ tablet
② 1 tablet
③ 1½ tablets
④ 2 tablets

556. The order for penicillin 150,000 U IM is written on the medication record sheet. The drug label reads penicillin 1,000,000 U/6 ml. How many ml should the nurse give?
① 0.01 ml
② 0.5 ml
③ 0.9 ml
④ 1.5 ml

557. The nurse is to administer pain medication. The physician ordered Demerol 75 mg. The ampule reads Demerol 100 mg/2 ml. What quantity does the nurse administer?
① 0.6 ml
② 1 ml
③ 1.2 ml
④ 1.5 ml

558. Mrs. Neetle has an order for her IV to infuse at 1000 ml q8h. The drop factor is 10 gtt/ml. How many gtt/min will be needed for the IV to infuse?
① 12 gtt
② 13 gtt
③ 20 gtt
④ 21 gtt

559. Ms. G refuses her stool softener because she states that she does not need it. The nurse's *best* response is:
① "Ms. G, the physician has ordered this medication; you really need it."
② "Ms. G, you have the right to refuse this. I will respect your right."
③ "Ms. G, let me give you this medicine now and in a while I will call your physician to see if we can hold it in the future."
④ "Ms. G, you do not have to take this medicine, but let me explain what this medication is for."

560. Besides an adequate diet with sufficient fluid intake, which of the following nursing interventions should be ordered to relieve a patient's constipation?
① Oil retention enema every other day
② Strong laxative every third day
③ Stool softeners once a day
④ Saline enema as needed

561. The physician discontinues a patient's use of topical nitroglycerin and orders nitroglycerin as a sublingual tablet. Normally, this form of nitroglycerin:
① Is only given three to four times a day
② Cannot be used more frequently than every ½ hour
③ Takes approximately ½ hour to relieve anginal pain
④ May be used for a maximum of 3 to 5 doses

562. A nurse helps in transcribing some physician's orders on the medication record. The nurse notices that the patient is taking digitalis every morning and Maalox 1 hour before meals and at bedtime. If breakfast comes at 8 AM, which schedule would be *most* effective for the patient?
① Maalox and digitalis at 9 AM
② Maalox at 8 AM and the digitalis at 9 AM
③ Maalox at 9 AM and the digitalis at 10 AM
④ Maalox at 8:30 AM and the digitalis at 9 AM

563. On reviewing a patient's medication record, the nurse notices that there is an order for warfarin (Coumadin) 5 mg PO qd and an order for Fiorinal tablets PO q4h prn. The nurse's concern should result in which?
① Leave the prn order on the medication administration record, but note that the patient is on warfarin
② Inform the patient that he will not be able to receive any pain medication for awhile
③ Call the physician and request an order for a different pain medication
④ Call the physician and request an order for heparin instead of warfarin

564. A patient is receiving warfarin (Coumadin) every day at 9 AM. Her laboratory work comes back with her prothrombin time four times the control. The nurse discovers that the patient's laboratory work was within normal limits the day before. The nurse's *first* action should be to:
① Call the physician immediately and then report to the charge nurse
② Check the time the laboratory work was drawn and report to the charge nurse
③ Prepare an injection of vitamin K while the charge nurse calls the physician
④ Prepare to administer protamine sulfate while the charge nurse calls the physician

565. Mr. Bills was in the emergency room with chest pain. He admitted to drinking heavily during the day and indicated that he is voiding large amounts. The nurse explained that he was voiding large amounts because alcohol causes diuresis by:
① Increasing cardiac output
② Increasing renal blood flow
③ Inhibiting secretion of the pituitary antidiuretic hormone
④ Stimulating the posterior pituitary gland

566. Before administering digoxin (Lanoxin) to a patient with congestive heart failure, the nurse will hold giving the medication and report to the charge nurse if the patient:
① Complains of nausea and vomiting and has a pulse rate of 52
② Complains of nausea and vomiting and has a pulse rate of 80
③ Has a regular and strong pulse
④ Complains of nausea and vomiting

567. The following order is transcribed onto a patient's medication record sheet: "Acetaminophen (tylenol) tablets prn for pain or temperature of 102° F (38.7° C)." The nurse should:
① Assume that two tablets are to be given every 4 hours
② Give the acetaminophen if pain or fever occurs and note the reason in the nurses' notes
③ Call the physician to clarify the dosage and frequency of the medication before giving it
④ Call the physician to clarify the dosage and frequency of the medication after giving a dose for pain

568. Which of the following symptoms should concern the nurse if observed in a patient after receiving a bronchodilator?
① Fremitus
② Wheezing
③ Rales (crackles)
④ Yellow, thick sputum

569. Ms. Putman has been placed on birth control pills. She should notify her physician of birth control pill use before beginning which of the following medication?
① Propylthyracil (Propylthiouracil)
② Ranitidine hydrochloride (Zantac)
③ Tetracycline hydrochloride (Achromycin V)
④ Gelusil (aluminum hydroxide, magnesium hydroxide, simethicone)

570. When Ms. Moates asks about the rhythm method of birth control, the nurse should teach Ms. Moates that the most effective way to use this method is to keep careful records of her:
① Weight
② Pulse rate
③ Body temperature
④ Blood pressure

571. Mrs. G had enteric-coated salicylates ordered, before having a nasogastric (NG) tube inserted. When preparing to administer the medication, the nurse should:
① Check with the physician regarding the status of this drug
② Hold the medication, because it cannot be administered at this time
③ Crush the medicine and mix it in water; administer it down the NG tube and clamp the tube
④ Have the patient swallow the tablet with sips of water

572. Mrs. R has an order to begin receiving penicillin VK. Which of the following questions should the nurse ask the patient before administering this medication?
① "Do you understand how often you will be taking this medicine?"
② "Do you have any medication allergies?"
③ "Have you eaten recently?"
④ "Do you know what this medication is for?"

573. A neighbor confides in you, because you are a nurse, that she has been chronically using tetrahydrocannibinol (THC) for the past several years. She asks, "What will happen to me if I suddenly quit?" The nurse could tell her that she may experience any of the following symptoms *except:*
① Tremors
② Increased perspiration
③ Increased appetite
④ Nausea

574. Which of the following is an accurate statement about diuretics?
① Diuretics act by increasing sodium reabsorption
② Osmotics are often used before eye surgery to increase intraocular pressure
③ Diuretics should be scheduled early in the morning or no later than 5 PM if possible
④ Carbonic anhydrase inhibitors are strong and frequently used to lower blood pressure

575. Mr. Amero has been given instructions about the effects of oral anticoagulants. Which of these comments by the patient indicates he understood the instructions?
① "I will brush my teeth with a soft toothbrush."
② "I will eat plenty of green, leafy vegetables each day."
③ "I will use aspirin if I get a headache."
④ "I will stop driving now that I'm on Coumadin."

576. In planning nursing care for a patient receiving warfarin (Coumadin), the nurse must be aware that the antidote for warfarin is:
① Protamine sulfate
② Vitamin K
③ Folic acid
④ Calcium gluconate

577. The drug trimethobenzamide hydrochloride (Tigan) is used to control nausea and vomiting and is classified as a(n):
① Antispasmodic
② Anticholinergic
③ Antiemetic
④ Cathartic

578. Miss DeMarco's temperature was 103.8° F (39° C), and the physician ordered a drug to lower her body fever. Drugs of this kind are classified as:
① Antibiotics
② Antipyretics
③ Antiemetics
④ Antihistamines

579. Mrs. Andrews has a diuretic ordered for congestive heart failure (CHF). It would be best to administer the diuretic at:
① 6 PM
② 1 PM
③ 9 AM
④ 4 PM

580. A potassium-sparing (retaining) diuretic used to reduce hypertension and/or edema is:
① furosemide (Lasix)
② spironolactone (Aldactone)
③ sulfisoxazole (Gantrisin)
④ methenamine (Mandelamine)

581. A patient receiving heparin must be observed for:
① Bleeding
② Numbness
③ Convulsions
④ Muscle twitching

582. Cimetidine (Tagamet) is prescribed for Ms. Jones during her hospitalization. Cimetidine's primary action is to:
① Directly promote healing of an ulcer
② Neutralize gastric acidity
③ Inhibit the secretion of hydrochloric acid
④ Decrease gastric motility

583. What signs and symptoms should a nurse be alert for in detecting a patient's recent use of cocaine?
① Clear, constricted pupils
② White, patchy areas of the tongue
③ Red, excoriated nostrils
④ Seizure activity

584. Mr. Franklin is a patient in the nursing home. While taking his medication, amitriptyline hydrochloride (Elavil), he reports that his mouth feels dry. An appropriate nursing intervention should be to:
① Tell him that this is just his imagination and to ignore it
② Tell him to suck on hard candies
③ Recommend chewing sugarless gum or drinking plenty of fluids
④ Instruct to rinse his mouth with salt water

585. Frequently used medications for myocardial infarctions are:
① Salicylates, antiinflammatory agents, and gold salts
② Antidysrhythmics, analgesics, and anticoagulants
③ Cardial glycosides, diuretics, and nitrates
④ Anticoagulants, vasodilators, and fibronolytics

586. The physician orders promethazine (Phenergan) for a patient with nausea. The charting method for an injection of promethazine intramuscularly, Z-track would be which of the following?
① "Phenergan 50 mg IM given Z-track for complaint of nausea"
② "Phenergan 50 mg IM in the right dorsogluteal for complaint of nausea"
③ "Phenergan 50 mg IM given in the dorsogluteal Z-track for complaint of nausea"
④ "Phenergan 50 mg IM, Z-track in the right dorsogluteal for complaint of nausea"

587. The following medications are all ordered prn by the physician. Which should be administered when the patient complains of anxiety and inability to sleep?
① nalbuphine hydrochloride (Nubain)
② Magaltrate Hydroxymagnesium aluminate (Magaltrate)
③ Indomethacin (Indameth)
④ Flurazepam hydrochloride (Dalmane)

588. Mr. Brandon is receiving acetazolamide (Diamox) for his glaucoma. In planning his care the nurse should include instructions on:
① The photosensitivity effect of this drug
② The hypoglycemic effects of this drug
③ The diuretic effect of this drug
④ The cardiac effects of this drug

589. Mrs. J has had a Hickman catheter inserted and is scheduled to begin antineoplastic chemotherapy. The nurse would plan to:
① Place her in strict isolation
② Offer frequent skin care of the site to promote comfort
③ Use strict infection-control procedures
④ Serve only bland foods

590. Mrs. Leftwich is ordered to receive corticosteroids. Which information would be appropriate for the nurse to assess as baseline data?
① Bone length and calcium levels
② Sleep patterns and understanding of disease
③ Abdominal girth and leg circumference
④ Weight and blood pressure

591. Mr. Jones is being prepared for surgery this morning. The physician has ordered a preoperative injection including atropine. Mr. Jones asks the nurse the purpose of his needing a "shot" before surgery. The nurse should explain to him that the medication will:
① Help to decrease secretions in the digestive tract, thus lessening the chance of complications with surgery
② Promote the cardiac response to stress
③ Help control anxiety and pain
④ Help him sleep and potentiate the anesthesia

592. Dr. K orders lenoxin (Digoxin) 5 mg for his patients. Recognizing this to be a high dose for the patient, the nurse's *most* appropriate action should be to:
① Transcribe the order as Digoxin 0.5 mg, because this is a normal dose for your patient
② Transcribe the order as written
③ Seek clarification now from the physician regarding the required dose
④ Hold the medication until the physician next makes rounds

593. The following three medications are to be given to different patients at the same time:
Mr. D receives Demerol 100 mg intramuscularly, which he has just requested for pain he describes as "pretty strong"
Mr. L receives nitroglycerin sublingual stat
Ms. J receives ampicillin IVPB q6h, and it was time for her dose 10 minutes ago
In which order should the medications be administered?
① Ampicillin IVPB, nitroglycerin SC, Demerol IM
② Nitroglycerin, Demerol, ampicillin
③ Demerol, nitroglycerin, ampicillin
④ Demerol, ampicillin, nitroglycerin

594. Mrs. Sams was brought to the emergency room because she was experiencing sudden, severe, sharp chest pain. She exhibited shortness of breath, profuse perspiration, and nausea. The nurse administered morphine sulfate ¼ gr (15 mg) intravenously. The morphine was given primarily to:
① Relieve the severe chest pain
② Relieve the nausea
③ Relieve the vomiting
④ Relieve shortness of breath

595. A patient has a daily prothrombin time level ordered. The nurse gives the anticoagulant, warfarin (Coumadin). The main action of this drug is to:
① Prevent hemorrhage
② Prevent infection in the blood
③ Interfere with clotting mechanisms
④ Stimulate the heart action

596. Chloral hydrate was ordered for Mrs. Zeff, an 83-year-old resident in a nursing home. In planning care for Mrs. Zeff, the nurse must know that chloral hydrate is a(n):
① Sedative
② Antiepileptic
③ Antidepressant
④ Tranquilizer

597. Mr. Dale was admitted complaining of chest pain. He admitted to drinking heavily during the day, later becoming quite anxious at the prospect of having a heart attack. He was given a tranquilizer. The minor tranquilizers are useful mainly for the symptomatic treatment of:
① Common psychoneuroses
② Acute psychoses
③ Chronic psychoses
④ Epilepsy

598. Shortly after her admission to the emergency room, Mrs. Nelson has a seizure. The nurse's *initial* intervention is to:
① Control the seizure
② Restrain the patient
③ Protect the patient
④ Increase circulation to the brain

599. Ms. Solita, age 46, has been admitted for a total hip replacement. The evening before surgery, the patient is anxious and is unable to fall asleep. Her physician left an order for pentobarbital (Nembutal). The nurse would expect the patient to fall asleep once the medication was given because the action of this drug is to:
① Depress the cough center of the brain
② Relieve moderate-to-severe pain
③ Allay apprehension
④ Increase blood pressure

600. The nurse is about to give meperidine hydrochloride to her patient for pain. When preparing to administer this medication, the nurse must know that the brand name for this medication is:
① Dilaudid
② Demerol
③ Dilantin
④ Dicumarol

CHAPTER 3

Maternal-Child Health Nursing Questions

1. The nurse should be aware of and prepared to counsel prospective parents on which of the following trends in maternal-child nursing that has benefited all expectant families:
   ① Improved quality and availability of prenatal care
   ② Having the father present in labor and delivery
   ③ The use of birthing rooms in most hospitals
   ④ The increased knowledge and use of antibiotics

2. In planning health care for pregnant women, newborns, and children from preschool to adolescence, a nurse should know that new United States government—sponsored health programs have:
   ① Ceased to be created after 1976
   ② Continued to be created after 1976
   ③ Had to be dismantled because of budgetary cuts
   ④ Been relegated to individual states and local communities

3. To implement the best possible patient care and to counsel effectively in patient teaching, the nurse must understand the normal anatomy and physiology of pregnancy as well as the complications that may occur. During a training session for childbirth educators, the following question was asked: "Which type of pelvis can be classified as the 'true' female pelvis?" Participants, demonstrating their readiness for their new role, would answer:
   ① Android
   ② Anthropoid
   ③ Gynecoid
   ④ Platypelloid

4. During childbirth classes, the nurse teaches the patients and their significant others that the fetus is fully developed in the:
   ① Third month
   ② Fourth month
   ③ Fifth month
   ④ Sixth month

5. When working in a prenatal clinic, the nurse must be aware that during pregnancy there are definite changes that occur in all the major body systems, including the hematologic system. Which of the following is a major change within this system?
   ① Decreased red blood cell count
   ② Increased hemoglobin level
   ③ Decreased white blood cell count
   ④ Increased coagulation factors

6. As the nurse explains fetal circulation to the expectant parents, she notes their fascination with the fact that, during fetal circulation, blood flowing through the heart actually bypasses the:
   ① Liver
   ② Lungs
   ③ Brain
   ④ Kidneys

7. During prenatal class, Ms. Guys asks the nurse just how the fetus receives nutrients from the mother. The nurse explains that the link between mother and fetus is the umbilical cord, which contains:
   ① One artery and one vein
   ② One artery and two veins
   ③ Two arteries and one vein
   ④ Two arteries and two veins

8. A patient asks how oxygen gets to her baby in utero. The nurse's most appropriate response would be to:
   ① Show the patient a picture of the umbilical cord
   ② Show the patient a picture of the fetal circulation
   ③ Use a chart, explaining that the umbilical vein carries oxygen
   ④ Use a chart, explaining that the umbilical artery carries oxygen

9. When teaching patients about the processes of fertilization and implantation, the nurse must know that fertilization normally occurs in the:
   ① Ovary
   ② Fundus of the uterus
   ③ Upper third of the cervix
   ④ Distal end of the fallopian tube

10. Ms. Tippen is pregnant for the first time and asks the nurse questions on basic anatomy and physiology of pregnancy, such as "How much amniotic fluid will be in the bag of waters when I reach term?" The nurse responds:
    ① "300 ml, which is replaced on a continual basis"
    ② "500 ml, which is replaced at the rate of 250 ml/hr"
    ③ "1000 ml,ml, which is replaced every 3 hours"
    ④ "2000 ml, which is replaced every 3 hours"

11. A patient complains that she hates milk, but because she is pregnant she will drink a lot of it anyway. Which of the following could the nurse recommend as a milk substitute that supplies adequate amounts of calcium for the expectant mother?
    ① Liver and organ meats
    ② Cheddar-type cheeses
    ③ Dark yellow vegetables
    ④ Enriched macaroni products

12. Which of the following sources of milk might the nurse suggest to a patient who is 6 months' pregnant and on a tight budget?
    ① Fortified skim milk
    ② Condensed milk
    ③ Evaporated milk
    ④ Powdered milk

13. During a routine prenatal examination, a patient complains of being constipated. Which of the following could the nurse suggest to minimize this discomfort?
    ① Increase her intake of milk and dairy products
    ② Increase her intake of refined cereals
    ③ Increase her intake of raw fruits and vegetables
    ④ Increase her intake of ground meats

14. A nurse's neighbor is pregnant for the first time and asks the nurse what she should and shouldn't eat during her pregnancy. The nurse advises her that her diet should include a(n):
    ① Increase of sodium and potassium
    ② Decrease in calories and sodium
    ③ Decrease in carbohydrates and protein
    ④ Increase in protein and calcium

15. Ms. Mendle is a recently divorced, working mother with two small children at home. She is 8 months' pregnant with her third child and is having trouble making ends meet. She asks the nurse at the prenatal clinic if she knows of any organization that might provide food after the baby arrives. Which of the following responses by the nurse is the most appropriate?
    ① "The food stamp program will provide adequate food for your family; the social worker will help you to apply."
    ② "If you are eligible, there is a federal supplementary program that provides nutritionally good food for you and your children."
    ③ "The Women, Infants, and Children (WIC) program will provide plenty of food for you, your infant and children under 5 years of age."
    ④ "You should apply for welfare immediately."

16. Ms. Paul is a 16-year-old pregnant high school student who attends prenatal clinic on a regular basis. During counseling sessions, the nurse emphasizes the patient's need for extra calcium because of her age. Which of the following statements correctly explains this need?
    ① During pregnancy, the calcium need is higher for this age group than it is for an expectant mother who is age 21 or older
    ② During pregnancy, the calcium need is lower for this age group than it is for an expectant mother who is age 21 or older
    ③ During pregnancy, the calcium need is the same as it is for an expectant mother who is age 21 or older
    ④ During pregnancy, the calcium need is always met naturally in persons of this age group

17. Because nutrition is an important component of prenatal care, the nurse includes in her patient education classes the teaching that the primary need for the growing and developing fetus is:
    ① Iron
    ② Proteins
    ③ Vitamin K
    ④ Calcium supplements

18. Ms. Sheridan, age 23, is 2 months' pregnant with her first child and is visiting her physician for the first time. The office nurse prepares to counsel the new mother about proper nutrition. It is important that the nurse include the need for sufficient iron in the patient's diet because in the last trimester the fetus stores iron that will be needed for the first:
    ① 3 Months of life
    ② 6 Months of life
    ③ 9 Months of life
    ④ Year of life

19. Which of the following available snack foods should the nurse suggest to a pregnant patient as the best source of complete protein?
    ① Cereal
    ② Peanuts
    ③ Cheese on crackers
    ④ Peanut butter on apple wedges

20. Marilyn is 4 months' pregnant and asks the nurse to recommend economical sources of protein. Which of the following foods would be most appropriate for the nurse to recommend to Marilyn?
    ① Red meats and fish
    ② In-season fruits and vegetables
    ③ Breads and macaroni
    ④ Dried beans and lentils

21. The nurse would plan for all of the following tests to be routinely done on all expectant mothers during their initial prenatal visit *except:*
    ① Hemoglobin and hematocrit levels
    ② Abdominal ultrasound
    ③ Maternal blood type and Rh factor
    ④ Urinalysis

22. Ms. Blue, a 30-year-old gravida 1 para 0, attends prenatal clinic on a regular basis. The physician has ordered an ultrasound to confirm a multiple pregnancy. Ms. Blue appears anxious about this procedure and asks the nurse what she might expect. The best explanation the nurse can give is that:
    ① Radiopaque dye will be injected into the uterus and an x-ray will be taken
    ② A jelly like substance will be applied to your abdomen, then a small device will be moved back and forth over the abdominal area
    ③ During the test you will be placed in several different positions so that the uterus can be viewed from different angles
    ④ A small area on your abdomen will be numbed; then a needle will be inserted and a small amount of fluid will be removed

23. Ms. Paul, age 30, is 6 months' pregnant with her second child. Because she was exposed to rubella during her fourth month, the physician orders a rubella titer drawn. The patient exhibits anxiety over the prospect of this new test. In preparing to counsel the patient, the nurse must know that the test actually:
    ① Indicates active disease during this pregnancy
    ② Measures the level of maternal antibodies
    ③ Indicates teratogenic effects on the fetus
    ④ Protects the patient from getting active disease

24. Ms. Charles, age 38, is pregnant for the first time and schedules an appointment with her obstetrician. During the initial visit, she appears healthy and gives an unimpressive medical history. The nurse explains to the patient that because of her age special tests will be done. Which of the following tests would be indicated because of the patient's age?
    ① Test for gestational diabetes
    ② Alpha-fetoprotein level
    ③ Heterozygote testing
    ④ Estriol levels
25. Nursing assessment during routine prenatal visits includes a urinalysis, a blood pressure check, and a weight check to:
    ① Prevent pregnancy-induced hypertension
    ② Ensure good prenatal care
    ③ Detect diabetes
    ④ Detect anomalies
26. The clinic nurse can inform patients that a pregnancy can be positively confirmed by:
    ① A palpable enlargement in uterine size, and shape
    ② A positive gravindex test
    ③ Fetal heart tones heard by the examiner
    ④ Amenorrhea for past 2 months
27. Ms. Charles attends the prenatal clinic exhibiting presumptive signs of pregnancy. The clinic nurse knows that these signs would most likely include:
    ① Urinary frequency, Chadwick's sign, and quickening
    ② Fatigue, positive gravindex, nausea, and vomiting
    ③ Amenorrhea, fatigue, and urinary frequency
    ④ Chadwick's sign, breast enlargement, and fetal movement felt by examiner
28. During the first trimester of Ms. Tallman's pregnancy, the nurse can expect that the patient's complaints of nausea and vomiting can be controlled by:
    ① Antiemetics and rest
    ② Plenty of fluids and a well-fitting girdle
    ③ Increasing bulk in her diet and restricting salt
    ④ Rest periods and a high-carbohydrate diet
29. When caring for the prenatal patient, the nurse should include which of the following in her teaching plan?
    ① No sexual intercourse during the first trimester
    ② Weight gain of over 25 pounds by due date
    ③ Need to report epigastric/abdominal pain
    ④ Need to participate in childbirth classes
30. Mrs. Bissell, gravida 2 para 1, asks if it is really beneficial to attend natural childbirth education classes. The clinic nurse caring for Mrs. Bissell explains that the primary benefit of such classes is that:
    ① Labor and delivery will be more rapid and less painful
    ② Most likely no pain medication will have to be administered
    ③ She will deliver the baby in a natural and quiet environment
    ④ Preparation will allow her to more fully assist in the birth

31. Ms. Newbarry tells the nurse that her EDC is January 5. When planning the essentials of prenatal care for this patient, the nurse knows that this means:
    ① Her expected delivery date
    ② The day her labor will begin
    ③ The first day of last menstrual period
    ④ The date her pregnancy was confirmed
32. The nurse at the clinic explains to her patient that a woman who is pregnant for the first time is called a:
    ① Primigravida
    ② Multipara
    ③ Primipara
    ④ Multigravida
33. A woman who thinks that she is pregnant asks when she should consult the physician. The nurse's best reply would be:
    ① "As soon as lightening occurs"
    ② "As soon as you miss one or two menstrual periods"
    ③ "As soon as morning sickness stops"
    ④ "As soon as you feel movement"
34. During a routine prenatal visit to her physician's office, Mrs. Todd asks if a thin watery secretion that she has noted from her breasts was normal in the third trimester of pregnancy. The nurse reassures her that this is a fairly common symptom at this time and that the proper term for this secretion is:
    ① Lochia
    ② Colostrum
    ③ Chloasma
    ④ Chorion
35. The nurse working in a physician's office should know that the communicable disease that can cause severe deformities in the fetus if contracted early in pregnancy is:
    ① Scarlet fever
    ② German measles
    ③ Chicken pox
    ③ Gonorrhea
36. Ms. Jones, age 23, is pregnant for the second time. Her first pregnancy was a difficult one, resulting in a miscarriage at 4 months. She is concerned that this will happen again and asks the nurse why this may have occurred. Although unable to give her a definite answer, the nurse can tell the patient that the major hormone necessary for maintaining a pregnancy is:
    ① Estrogen
    ② Progesterone
    ③ Luteinizing hormone
    ④ Follicle-stimulating hormone
37. Ms. Dell is approaching her estimated date of confinement (EDC). Because this is her first pregnancy, she is quite anxious and reports that although she has been able to breathe more easily for the past 2 days, she now has to void more frequently. The office nurse would:
    ① Explain that this is normal since lightening has occurred
    ② Obtain a urine sample for culture and sensitivity
    ③ Recommend that she restrict fluid intake
    ④ Report to physician immediately

38. Ms. Marcus asks the clinic nurse when she will most likely feel the baby move. The nurse responds that the fetus is most likely to move during which of the following months of pregnancy?
    1. Fifth
    2. Sixth
    3. Third
    4. Fourth

39. During pregnancy a patient's weight is carefully monitored. The nurse knows that the maximum weight gain usually recommended for an entire pregnancy is:
    1. 10 to 15 pounds
    2. 15 to 18 pounds
    3. 20 to 25 pounds
    4. 28 to 30 pounds

40. During the initial visit of a patient in a prenatal clinic, for which of the following assessments would the nurse be responsible?
    1. Enlargement of the uterus
    2. Examining for goodell's sign
    3. Enlargement of the breasts
    4. Fetal heart tones

41. Camille is now in her seventh month of pregnancy, and the nurse notes that she is wearing high-heel shoes. The nurse should advise her to:
    1. Continue wearing the shoes she is now wearing
    2. Wear heels of a moderate height to prevent varicose veins
    3. Wear low-heel shoes to avoid additional strain on her back
    4. Wear athletic shoes for walking

42. Mrs. Simpson is 35 weeks' pregnant and has ankle edema in the afternoon and evening but *not* when she arises in the morning. The nurse should inform Mrs. Simpson that:
    1. Edema with this pattern requires complete bed rest
    2. She is in the beginning stages of pregnancy-induced hypertension
    3. She must restrict her sodium intake
    4. This dependent edema that disappears after a night of sleep is not unusual during pregnancy

43. Maria Thomas is 6 months' pregnant with her second child. During her prenatal visit, she tells the nurse that Seth, her 5-year-old son, is asking a lot of questions about the baby, particularly its sex. Which of the following suggestions by the nurse is the most appropriate approach to this situation?
    1. Divert Seth's attention to his toys, telling him that there is time after the baby is born to answer his questions
    2. Tell Seth that the stork will decide whether the baby will be a boy or a girl
    3. Tell Seth that she honestly doesn't know at this time and will not know until the baby is born
    4. Refer Seth to his father for answers on a "man-to-man" level

44. Sally Wood is 8 months' pregnant with her second child. She tells the nurse that Peter, her 6-year-old son, has been asking her why she is getting so fat. Which of the following responses should the nurse suggest?
    1. "I've been eating for two people, for me and the baby, so I'm gaining a lot of weight."
    2. "The baby is growing inside mommy's uterus, which is a special place where babies grow."
    3. "The baby is growing inside mommy's stomach, so I am getting fat."
    4. "The baby is getting so big that he is using up all my energy and I have to eat a lot more, which is making me fat."

45. Marilyn Green is 6 months' pregnant. She tells the nurse that her 5-year-old son, Jonas, who has been toilet trained for a while, is now wetting and soiling his pants like a new baby. The best guidance the nurse can give Marilyn is:
    1. That this will pass, it is just a phase he is going through
    2. To sit down and have a heart-to-heart talk with him, explaining that big boys don't do this
    3. To scold him so he knows this is wrong
    4. To include him when going to prenatal visits and in getting the baby's room ready

46. Mrs. Parsons, gravida 1 para 0, is a class B insulin-treated diabetic patient. She wants to know why she has to take more insulin during the second half of her pregnancy. The nurse tells her that:
    1. Hormonal activity tends to counteract the effects of insulin in the second half of pregnancy
    2. Because her activity level will increase, her insulin needs will also increase
    3. Taking more insulin tends to prevent urinary tract infections
    4. The baby is growing and needs extra insulin

47. During her pregnancy, Darlene has developed a urinary tract infection. The nurse teaches Darlene that it is important to:
    1. Drink four to six 8-oz glasses of fluids per day
    2. Eat extra carbohydrates and sugar
    3. Void before and after sexual intercourse
    4. Wear only nylon underwear

48. Ms. Page is 20 weeks' pregnant and has had persistent nausea and vomiting for the past 2 days. Her physician decides to admit her to the obstetric unit. In planning care for this patient, the nurse should know that the diagnosis for Ms. Page is most likely to be:
    1. Pregnancy-induced hypertension
    2. Morning sickness
    3. Hyperemesis gravidarum
    4. Preeclampsia

49. The nurse caring for a patient with a diagnosis of hyperemesis gravidarum knows that, if left untreated, this condition could result in:
    1. A low-birth-weight infant
    2. Anorexia nervosa
    3. Premature delivery
    4. Maternal and/or fetal death

50. Ms. Masters, 38 weeks' pregnant, is admitted to the labor room following a seizure at home. The patient is extremely anxious and is complaining of epigastric pain. Her blood pressure is 190/112. The physician orders 4 g magnesium sulfate to be given intravenously in 250 ml D₅W. When planning care for this patient, the nurse knows that this medication will:
    ① Reduce the pulse rate
    ② Stimulate labor
    ③ Reduce edema
    ④ Increase peristalsis

51. Mrs. Godfrey is being evaluated for preeclampsia. Which of the following assessments would the nurse make first?
    ① Fundal height
    ② Blood pressure
    ③ Urine for sugar/acetone
    ④ Fetal heart tone

52. Mrs. Ferguson is gravida 3 para 0, having miscarried as a result of two preterm labors. To reduce the risk of preterm labor, the nurse teaches this patient to:
    ① Avoid salt in her diet
    ② Comply with prescribed amount of bed rest
    ③ Reduce calorie intake
    ④ Reduce fluid intake

53. Mrs. Harold is having her full-term baby. She is admitted to the hospital in the first stage of labor. True labor is best described as having started when Mrs. Harold's:
    ① Mucus plug is expelled from the cervical canal
    ② Membranes rupture spontaneously
    ③ Uterine contractions are regular
    ④ Fetus drops into the brim of the pelvis

54. The nurse is administering an enema to a woman in early labor. An important reason for giving an enema at this time is to:
    ① Prevent constipation during labor
    ② Relieve pressure in case of an episiotomy
    ③ Ease the contractions
    ④ Provide for a clean delivery

55. Mrs. Harold is to have a vaginal examination to determine how much the cervix has dilated. To prepare for the procedure, the nurse should include:
    ① Having a sterile speculum
    ② Cleaning the patient's vulva
    ③ Placing the patient in lithotomy position
    ④ Telling the patient to bear down

56. The nurse is caring for a patient in the latent phase of the first stage of labor. Which of the following situations would necessitate immediate notification of the physician?
    ① Meconium in the amniotic fluid
    ② No palpable movement of the fetus
    ③ Spontaneous rupture of the membranes
    ④ Fetal heart rate of 90 beats/min

57. The physician has just completed his examination of a newly admitted patient in labor and requests that the nurse recheck the fetal heart tones. The nurse knows that the best location on the abdomen to hear the fetal heart tones is:
    ① Above the umbilicus
    ② Below the umbilicus
    ③ The upper right quadrant
    ③ The upper left quadrant

58. Mr. Bauer has been coaching his wife during labor. The patient now informs her husband and her nurse that she feels like pushing. The physician examines the patient and informs the nurse that she is completely dilated and ready to begin pushing. Which of the following instructions would the nurse be correct in giving the patient?
    ① Head back, arms forward, hips back, lips closed, and push down
    ② Inhale, head on chest, elbows out, push down toward anus and count to 10; pelvic tilt helps
    ③ Spread legs apart, take deep breath, and bear down while exhaling
    ④ Pant and blow until the fetus is completely delivered

59. Mrs. Hempstead's physician informs the nurse that the patient is 3 cm dilated and that the fetus is in cephalic presentation. In planning care for the patient, the nurse knows that this means the:
    ① Cervix is 3 cm thick, and the head of the fetus is high in the pelvis
    ② Fetal head is against the cervix, and the cervix is thinning
    ③ Cervix has opened 3 cm, and the fetal head is presenting
    ④ Fetal head is 3 cm above the ischial spines of the pelvis

60. Mrs. Sullivan is admitted in active labor. Fetal heart rate is determined to be 150 beats/min. The nurse caring for Mrs. Sullivan knows that this rate is:
    ① High; oxygen should be administered
    ② Within normal limits
    ③ High; physician should be notified
    ④ Expected during contractions; should decrease afterward

61. Mr. Chaucer tells the nurse that he has learned how to count fetal heart tones in childbirth classes and that he will record them for her on the labor record because she is so busy. The most appropriate action/response by the nurse would be to:
    ① Provide him with paper to record fetal heart tones and check his accuracy at intervals
    ② Tell him that this is the nurse's job and doing this would only increase his anxiety about the infant's condition
    ③ Explain that the nurse must monitor the fetal heart tones and ask him to assist in timing contractions
    ④ Explain that childbirth classes don't teach students everything they need to know about monitoring fetal heart tones

62. Mrs. Smith has been in labor for 6 hours. Her membranes have just ruptured. The nurse's priority now is to assess:
① Amniotic fluid with nitrazine
② Duration of contractions
③ Fetal heart rate
④ Maternal vital signs

63. Mrs. Hoover, a primipara, has been in labor for some time and has been using the Lamaze method. The physician has just completed a vaginal examination, which revealed the cervix to be 7 cm dilated and 100% effaced. The presenting part is at 0 station. Contractions are every 3 to 4 minutes, lasting 35 to 45 seconds. While attending to this patient in the labor room, the nurse would expect the patient to:
① Have an irresistible urge to push
② Ask many questions about the impending delivery
③ Be more preoccupied with proper breathing techniques
④ Fall asleep during contractions

64. Ms. Black, a 25-year-old gravida 2 para 1, is admitted to the labor room having contractions every 5 to 7 mintues, each lasting 30 to 35 seconds. She states that her contractions started about 2 hours ago and that her bag of waters (bow) is intact. Vaginal examination reveals a cervix that is 2 cm dilated and 25% effaced. When planning care for Ms. Black, the nurse knows that this patient is in:
① False labor; Braxton-Hicks contractions
② Early labor; latent phase
③ True labor; transitional phase
④ Active labor; third stage

65. Mrs. Black's labor intensifies, with the cervix fully dilated and 100% effaced. The physician administers a pudendal block. When caring for a patient with a pudendal block, the nurse can expect which of the following to occur?
① A decrease in discomfort from contractions
② An absence of sensation in the perineal area
③ An absence of sensation in the lower extremities
④ A decrease in the strength of contractions

66. Mrs. Proctor, gravida 12 para 10, is admitted to the labor and delivery suite in active labor. Contractions are approximately every 2 to 3 minutes, strong, lasting 45 to 50 seconds. She states that her membranes are still intact and that she has very fast labors. During her admission, which one of the following nursing actions would be contraindicated for this patient?
① Application of an external fetal monitor
② Requesting a urine specimen from the patient
③ Administering a small-volume enema
④ Requesting stat blood work

67. Ms. Jopo, a newly admitted labor patient, appears anxious and states, "I wish that my husband could be here. He's at work, and if he leaves, he'll lose his job." Which of the following interventions indicate caring and understanding on the part of the nurse?
① Ask the patient if there is another person she would like to have with her at this time
② Follow through with routine procedures according to hospital policy and procedure
③ Explain that many women go through labor and delivery without their husbands
④ Listen empathetically, but say nothing in anticipation of being with her most of the time

68. Ms. Charles is admitted to the labor room in what appears to be very early labor. She is anxious but excited because this is her first pregnancy. When planning care for this patient, the nurse knows that, once active labor begins, Ms. Charles can expect to give birth to her infant in approximately:
① 14 to 16 hours
② 18 to 20 hours
③ 22 to 24 hours
④ 26 to 28 hours

69. The patient plans to have a saddle block anesthetic for the delivery of her baby. The nurse knows that the anesthetic would be injected into the:
① Pudendal nerves
② Perineum
③ Spinal canal
④ Cervix

70. The nurse is timing Mrs. Tao's contractions. To document correctly the nurse must know that the term used to describe the length of the contraction from beginning to end is called the:
① Duration
② Intensity
③ Frequency
④ Interval

71. The nurse is palpating a patient's contractions. She should place her hand:
① Just above the patient's pubis
② Just above the patient's umbilicus
③ On either side of the patient's abdomen
④ Between the pubis and the perineum

72. Mrs. Harold will need support and encouragement during labor, especially during the:
① Second stage
② Third stage
③ The early part of the first stage
④ The transition phase of the first stage

73. The physician delivers the baby, and the nurse gives an oxytocic drug to the new mother soon after the delivery of the placenta. This is done primarily to help:
① Decrease the likelihood of uterine spasms
② Strengthen contractions of the uterus
③ Hasten the process of involution
④ Prevent uterine inversion

74. The delivery room nurse in caring for Ms. Sams knows that this patient's labor is truly complete when the:
    ① Infant is delivered
    ② Cord is cut
    ③ Placenta is delivered
    ④ Uterus becomes inverted

75. The nurse in the delivery room writes the notation "VBAC" on the patient's delivery room record. A student nurse who had observed the delivery asks what "VBAC" means. Which of the following nurse's responses correctly answers the student's question?
    ① "It's a new organization for mothers called *Volunteers for Baby's Active Care.*
    ② "It indicates a specific type of aortic valve correction that the infant will need to have done."
    ③ "It stands for the latest type of carrier, especially for vaginally delivered babies."
    ④ "It means that the mother is having a vaginal delivery after having had a cesarean section for the last pregnancy."

76. Mrs. Gray delivers a healthy, 7 lb 7 oz (3375 g) baby girl. Soon after delivery the patient begins to shiver, and her teeth start chattering. Which of the following nursing interventions is appropriate?
    ① Check her temperature immediately
    ② Cover her with several warmed blankets
    ③ Administer oxygen via nasal canula
    ④ Administer acetaminophen

77. The infant is taken to the nursery, and the patient's legs are removed from the stirrups. The physician had performed a midline episiotomy to facilitate a safe delivery; the perineum is cleansed, and a pad is applied. While checking the patient's fundus, the nurse notes that it is soft (boggy); the nurse's first clinical priority is to:
    ① Immediately notify the charge nurse
    ② Check the perineum for vaginal bleeding
    ③ Check the patient's blood pressure and pulse rate
    ④ Massage the fundus immediately

78. When Julie is admitted to the obstetric unit with a diagnosis of preeclampsia, the physician orders IV magnesium sulfate. In planning care for Julie, the nurse knows that this drug is administered to:
    ① Prevent convulsions
    ② Relieve pain
    ③ Increase blood pressure
    ④ Induce labor

79. Julie, gravida 1 para 0, has a diagnosis of preeclampsia and is receiving magnesium sulfate during early labor. The nurse observes that Julie's respirations are 9 and that her patellar reflexes (DTRs) have decreased. This information should be:
    ① Recorded and monitored
    ② Immediately brought to the physician's attention
    ③ Considered an indication for increasing the dose
    ④ Considered to be a normal result

80. Julie's labor progresses without incident. She delivers a healthy baby boy and is taken to the recovery room. Because Julie was diagnosed as having preeclampsia, the nurse knows that Julie must still be observed for impending eclampsia for at least:
    ① 3 hours
    ② 24 hours
    ③ 36 hours
    ④ 72 hours

81. Mrs. Omni has just been admitted to the recovery room following a cesarean section for which she had received spinal anesthesia. Which of the following actions by the recovery room nurse is appropriate in caring for this patient?
    ① Avoid palpating the uterine fundus
    ② Restrict oral fluids until the gag reflex returns
    ③ Catheterize the patient every 4 hours following surgery
    ④ Keep the patient lying flat for 8 to 12 hours following surgery

82. The patient is going to surgery for an emergency cesarean section. Which of the following anesthetics would the nurse recognize as being the best choice for both mother and infant?
    ① An epidural block
    ② A general anesthetic
    ③ A pudendal block
    ④ A Bier's block

83. The patient asks if she will be able to breast-feed her baby after a cesarean delivery. The nurse's best reply would be:
    ① "You'd better bottle-feed, because you will probably be in a lot of pain."
    ② "You can still breast-feed, and we will help you."
    ③ "It's best that you ask your doctor."
    ④ "You don't have to decide now."

84. At 36 weeks' gestation, Mrs. Hanson has had no contractions, but amniotic fluid has been slowly leaking from her vagina. Priority nursing assessment includes:
    ① Nutritional history
    ② Onset of contractions
    ③ Urinalysis
    ④ Vital signs

85. Nursing assessment of a patient with placenta previa often reveals:
    ① Pain with no bleeding
    ② Pain with passage of clots
    ③ Painless bleeding with a hard uterus
    ④ Painless bleeding with a soft uterus

86. While working in the labor and delivery area, the nurse must be aware of the signs and symptoms of premature separation of the placenta from the uterine wall. This is known as a (an):
    ① Ectopic pregnancy
    ② Placenta previa
    ③ Abruptio placentae
    ④ Complete abortion

87. Mrs. Johnson enters the hospital with third-trimester bleeding. She is crying and very nervous. The appropriate nursing action is to:
   ① Ask the chaplain to talk to the Johnsons
   ② Explain possible causes for the bleeding
   ③ Leave Mr. and Mrs. Johnson alone after the initial assessment
   ④ Reassure the Johnsons that everything will probably be all right

88. Ms. Ketzler, gravida 2 para 1, has been in labor for the past 8 hours. During the last 2 hours, contractions have become progressively weaker, with no noticeable effect on cervical dilation or effacement. The physician orders an IV drip with oxytocin (Pitocin). Which of the following nursing interventions is of prime importance when observing a patient with an oxytocin drip?
   ① Time contractions; report to physician at frequent intervals
   ② Monitor the intervals during and after contractions; report if longer than 5 minutes apart
   ③ Monitor the blood pressure and patient reactions to IV drip
   ④ Monitor intervals carefully; if less than 1 minute or absent, stop IV and notify physician immediately

89. When planning care for cocaine-addicted mothers in labor, the nurse must know that they will experience:
   ① Fewer labor contractions than do nonaddicted mothers
   ② Stronger labor contractions than do nonaddicted mothers
   ③ No more or less discomfort than that experienced by nonaddicted mothers
   ④ Less need for sedation than do nonaddicted mothers, because of their cocaine addiction

90. Julie is a 14-year-old single primigravida. Her membranes have ruptured spontaneously; she has slight, bloody show; and her contractions are 10 to 12 minutes apart, lasting about 20 seconds. She reveals that she was seen by a physician for the first time 3 weeks ago. The nurse finds that Julie's blood pressure is 150/98, her face is edematous, and her urine shows 2 + protein. The nurse would know that these are symptoms of:
   ① Normal delivery progress
   ② Impending delivery
   ③ Preeclampsia
   ④ Gestational diabetes

91. Ms. Torry, a 15-year-old pregnant patient, has just been admitted to the labor and delivery suite. She has had no prenatal care and on examination by the physician is noted to have an advanced case of herpes genitalis. In developing a plan of care for this patient, the nurse must:
   ① Suggest that the patient be placed in complete isolation
   ② Use extreme caution when preparing the patient for delivery
   ③ Implement universal precautions for blood and body fluids
   ④ Use strict handwashing procedures

92. Because she is breast-feeding, Ms. John's nutritional requirements will increase. In planning care for Ms. John, the nurse knows that this increase includes:
   ① An additional 1000 ml of fluids daily and increased protein
   ② An additional 3000 ml of fluids and an additional 640 calories daily
   ③ Additional vitamin supplements and protein every other day
   ④ An additional half-quart of milk and vitamin supplements daily

93. On the second day after delivery, Ms. Taylor, who is breast feeding, complains that her breasts feel tight and are tender. The correct nursing action in response to the patient's complaint is to:
   ① Offer to bottle-feed her baby in the nursery for the next several feedings
   ② Notify the physician, because this may be a sign of mastitis
   ③ Apply a breast binder and ice packs to the breasts
   ④ Tell her that nursing her baby will offer relief

94. Mrs. Sims is breast-feeding her infant daughter and using the demand feeding method. In planning care for baby Sims, the nursery nurse understands that this method allows baby Sims to be fed:
   ① Whenever she cries
   ② Approximately every 4 hours
   ③ At the time and in the amount the newborn wishes
   ④ Whenever Mrs. Sims feels her breasts to be full

95. Sally wants to know how soon it will be before she can start to breast-feed and is anxious to know when her milk will begin to flow. Which of the following statements by the nurse is the most appropriate in answering this patient's questions?
   ① "I really can't answer that; perhaps you should ask your physician."
   ② "Your baby will be brought to you for the next feeding; your milk will probably start right after that."
   ③ "We encourage you to nurse as soon as you can; your milk will probably start in about 3 days."
   ④ "The baby can nurse anytime after birth."

96. Mrs. Johnson has decided to try "rooming in" with her first baby. In helping the patient prepare, the nursery nurse should inform her that rooming in means that:
   ① Mr. Johnson will be allowed to stay in the room and assist in caring for his new baby
   ② A private duty nurse will care for Mrs. Johnson for the first few days
   ③ Mrs. Johnson will be sharing her room with another mother who is more experienced in infant care
   ④ Mrs. Johnson's infant will be at her bedside so that she may care for her as long as she feels up to it

97. In addition to using an anesthetic ointment, another common measure the nurse could suggest to relieve discomfort from an episiotomy is to have the patient:
   ① Ambulate frequently
   ② Take sitz baths
   ③ Elevate her hips while in bed
   ④ Apply cortisone ointment to the perineal area

98. When caring for a postpartum patient, the nurse may best facilitate the return of normal bowel and bladder function by which of the following nursing interventions?
    ① Providing perineal care and administering sitz baths as ordered
    ② Encouraging ambulation and eating of a well-balanced diet
    ③ Obtaining orders for simple catheterization and a cathartic
    ④ Recording intake and output, and instructing the patient in perineal care

99. Ellen says, "I haven't had a bowel movement since delivery." This patient is 2 days postpartum. The most appropriate nursing intervention would be to:
    ① Obtain an order for a Fleet enema; encourage ambulation
    ② Check for fecal impaction; suggest additional fluids
    ③ Encourage fluids and bulk-forming foods
    ④ Check for fecal impaction; administer a laxative

100. The patient is planning to bottle-feed. Which of the following medications would the nurse expect the physician to order to suppress lactation?
    ① Ibuprofen (Motrin)
    ② Docusate sodium (Colace)
    ③ Oxytocin (Pitocin)
    ④ Bromocriptine mesylate (Parlodel)

101. Theresa has decided not to breast-feed her newborn son because of recurrent mastitis. She asks the nurse how much formula she should give the infant, and how often. Which of the following suggestions offered by the nurse is in line with the general guidelines for formula feedings?
    ① Allow the infant as much as he likes as often as he likes
    ② 30 ml every 1 to 2 hours for the first 2 months
    ③ 60 to 120 ml every 3 to 4 hours for the first 2 months
    ④ 180 to 280 ml every 3 hours for the first 2 months

102. It is essential that the nurse observe the postpartum patient closely for hemorrhage after delivery, because excessive bleeding is most likely to occur:
    ① During the first hour after delivery
    ② About 8 to 10 hours after delivery
    ③ About 10 to 24 hours after delivery
    ④ About 24 to 72 hours after delivery

103. A new postpartum patient's lochia has several clots and has saturated the perineal pad. When documenting, the nurse would describe this amount of lochia as:
    ① Moderate
    ② Gross
    ③ Scant
    ④ Heavy

104. The nurse is giving postpartum instructions to her patient. She explains that for the first 2 to 3 days her lochia will be:
    ① Pale pink or brownish
    ② Yellowish, creamy discharge
    ③ Excessive and bright red
    ④ Dark red to bright red

105. On doing a routine third postpartum day check, the nurse notes that Mrs. Cole's lochia is red and moderate and charts it as:
    ① Lochia rubra
    ② Lochia serosa
    ③ Lochia alba
    ④ Lochia puerpera

106. Several hours after delivery, Julie's uterus lies to the right side of her abdomen. The nurse knows that the most likely reason for this position is that Julie's:
    ① Stomach is distended
    ② Urinary bladder is full
    ③ Uterus has returned to normal position
    ④ Uterus is filling with blood

107. A variety of nursing interventions are implemented to help the patient void after delivery. An overdistended bladder is likely to predispose the patient to development of:
    ① A hematoma
    ② Phlebitis
    ③ An infection
    ④ A tumor

108. The Greys are concerned that their 5-year-old daughter, Betsy, will have difficulty adjusting to the new baby. When counseling the Greys, the nurse knows that it is important for them to:
    ① Buy presents for Betsy, equal to the number they feel the new baby will receive
    ② Allow Betsy to kiss and hold the new baby so she will begin to love the new baby
    ③ Tell Betsy that she is a big girl and can help mommy with some chores around the house
    ④ Plan to spend time alone with Betsy, doing the things that Betsy wants to do

109. Theresa Green, gravida 5 para 3ab2, is being discharged from the maternity unit after delivering a 9 lb 2 oz (413 g) baby boy 2 days earlier. How many live births did Theresa have?
    ① Three
    ② Five
    ③ Eight
    ④ Ten

110. Theresa is concerned that her other children have not shown any interest in the new baby when they have come to visit her in the hospital. The nurse responds to this concern with:
    ① "It's just as well, because babies need their rest. They can stay away until he's older."
    ② "It's just as well, because they may hurt him if they get too close to him."
    ③ "Time will take care of things; just wait, they will come around."
    ④ "Include them in the care and attention you give the baby."

111. Mrs. Tillman has just delivered twin sons via a normal vaginal delivery. The nurse is aware that she is now at increased risk for:
    ① Early postpartum hemorrhage
    ② Mastitis
    ③ Postpartum infection
    ④ Thrombophlebitis

112. On the second postpartum day, the nurse finds Ellen crying and complaining of feeling "down in the dumps." When caring for this patient, the nurse should:
    ① Leave her alone to work through her feelings
    ② Tell her to cheer up because she has a fine healthy baby
    ③ Explain that this is a normal response that many women experience
    ④ Consult the psychiatric clinical nurse specialist for guidance

113. Kim's family is very supportive, but she expresses concern about how to financially support herself and the baby. She is only 14 years old. The best response by the nurse should be:
    ① "Why didn't you think about that before you got pregnant?"
    ② "Ask the baby's father to help; it's his responsibility too."
    ③ "Tell me some things you have considered so we can research some possibilities."
    ④ "Welfare seems to be the only answer."

114. Baby Jane has just been delivered. The nurse knows that before the newborn takes her first breath, the physician will most likely:
    ① Clamp and cut the cord
    ② Evaluate the Apgar score
    ③ Clear the infant's airway of mucus
    ④ Repair the episiotomy

115. The nurse is to give the infant an injection of vitamin K. The best site to use for an intramuscular injection on an infant is:
    ① Biceps femoris
    ② Gluteus maximus
    ③ Vastus lateralis
    ④ Biceps brachii

116. Baby Jane is given vitamin K soon after birth. The nurse knows this is done primarily to help:
    ① Start peristalsis
    ② Increase calcium level
    ③ Stimulate respirations
    ④ Improve blood coagulation

117. When evaluating a newborn's heart rate, respiratory rate, muscle activity, reflex irritability, and color, the best possible score the team can obtain when using the Apgar scoring system is:
    ① 4
    ② 10
    ③ 14
    ④ 18

118. The nurse, in cooperation with the physician, is using the Apgar scoring system. She has scored the infant's color, respiratory effort, reflex response, and heart rate. The next item to score is the:
    ① Weight
    ② Blood pressure
    ③ Length
    ④ Muscle tone

119. Newborns have many needs. When planning for immediate care of a newborn, the nurse knows that the highest priority for the newborn following delivery is the need to be:
    ① Weighed
    ② Kept warm
    ③ Bathed
    ④ Circumcised

120. Routine newborn care following delivery includes administration of silver nitrate eyedrops or an antibiotic ointment for the eyes. It is important that this be included in the nursing care plan for all infants, because these medications prevent blindness as a result of:
    ① Herpes
    ② Syphilis
    ③ Gonorrhea
    ④ Retrolental fibroplasia

121. Capillary blood is often used to determine blood glucose levels and test for specific conditions such as phenylketonuria in the newborn. The site used to obtain the specimen is the heel. To increase blood flow to the area, the nurse should:
    ① Do nothing specific
    ② Elevate the foot of the crib
    ③ Wrap the foot in a warm wet cloth
    ④ Soak both feet in a saline solution

122. Accompanied to the delivery room by her husband, Mrs. Sands gives birth to a female infant with an Apgar rating of 9 at 1 minute after birth. According to most states, the nurse legally identifies the infant by:
    ① Placing identification bracelets on mother and infant
    ② Attaching laboratory slips of the mother to the infant's chart to verify blood type
    ③ Obtaining the signature of the physician on the identification sheet
    ④ Obtaining the infant's footprints and the mother's fingerprint on the delivery record

123. Ms. White is unsure as to whether she should have her newborn baby boy circumcised. Which of the following comments by the nurse is most appropriate in responding to the patient's uncertainty?
    ① "Circumcision is necessary for good hygiene."
    ② "Circumcision reduces the incidence of disease."
    ③ "Circumcision decreases the risk of sexually transmitted diseases (STDs)."
    ④ "Circumcision is a matter of the parents' personal choice."

124. Sarah's baby was circumcised the morning of discharge. The nurse's discharge teaching should include the fact that:
    ① Frequent checking for bleeding and keeping the incision well-lubricated is important
    ② Complications frequently occur after the procedure
    ③ Voiding is frequently affected, causing the baby's abdomen to become distended
    ④ Healing takes a long time because circulation to the site is poor

125. Greta Swift, a primipara who just delivered a baby girl, states, "My baby is breathing so fast. I count around 58 breaths. Is something wrong with her?" The nurse's most appropriate response would be:
    1. "A newborn's respirations vary, going up to 58 at times and as low as 30."
    2. "We should watch her closely. That seems high to me, too!"
    3. "Why don't you let us check her vital signs for accurate information?"
    4. "You don't need to worry; her color is okay."

126. The nursery nurse meets all new mothers on a daily basis. During a recent encounter, a patient asked, "Why does she have such black, sticky stuff in her diaper? It looks awful and it's so hard to clean. Is she bleeding internally? I know something is wrong with her!" The nurse's response should be:
    1. "You should know that it is meconium. Didn't they cover that in your prenatal classes?"
    2. "That is meconium. It's baby's first bowel movement until the normal yellow stool comes through."
    3. "Oh, that's nothing to worry about. It's normal."
    4. "She's not bleeding. You're worrying needlessly."

127. Greta, a new mother, examines her baby. She says, "Look, my baby's hands and feet are purple! She must have a heart condition. I know there is something wrong with her!" The nurse's response to this should be:
    1. "Bluish discoloration of hands and feet occurs with newborns and usually lasts for a few days."
    2. "Your baby is cold because you've kept her undressed for so long."
    3. "Your baby worked hard during delivery by kicking and pushing. She has bruised herself."
    4. "Your baby probably does have problems. We will have to call the doctor."

128. Three days after birth, Baby Collins appears to be slightly jaundiced. In caring for this newborn, the nursery nurse is aware that this condition is most likely the result of:
    1. Rh incompatability
    2. ABO incompatability
    3. Normal destruction of red blood cells
    4. A liver malfunction

129. When Baby Murray's cheek is stroked, she turns her head in the direction of the stroked cheek. The nurse caring for Baby Murray knows that this reflex, present at birth, is known as the:
    1. Rooting reflex
    2. Moro reflex
    3. Tonic neck reflex
    4. Sucking reflex

130. During a routine check on the newest addition to the nursery, the nurse notes that Baby Tomby has acrocyanosis. She knows that this means:
    1. The skin is reddish-blue in color
    2. Extremities are bluish in color
    3. The skin has a mottled appearance
    4. Extremities are covered with a bluish-white substance

131. Baby Boy Rodnik is admitted to the newborn nursery in good condition. On assessment, the nurse knows that the respirations of the normal neonate will be:
    1. Regular, 24 to 36 per minute
    2. Irregular, 40 to 58 per minute
    3. Regular, 30 to 44 per minute
    4. Irregular, 32 to 48 per minute

132. When planning care, the nurse should be aware that all newborns should be burped (bubbled) during and after each feeding to prevent:
    1. Regurgitation of the feeding
    2. Gas pains/colic
    3. Pneumonia
    4. Pneumaturia

133. In observing Baby Girl Newby the first 12 hours after delivery, the nurse notes that the infant's eyelids are puffy and red. The most appropriate nursing action is to:
    1. Notify the pediatrician immediately
    2. Culture any exudate noted at the inner canthus
    3. Gently clean any exudate with warm sterile water
    4. Review the labor record to see if any trauma to the head or eyes was noted

134. Which of the following descriptions would the nurse be correct in using to chart the newborn's first stool?
    1. Sticky, dark brown
    2. Blackish green and tarry
    3. Soft, greenish brown
    4. Sticky, reddish brown

135. The nurse has just admitted a newborn baby girl from the delivery room. While reviewing the chart, the nurse notes the weight to be 8 lb (3600 g). In planning care for this infant, the nurse can expect that she will lose up to 10% of her birth weight. The nurse would be correct in estimating the newborn's weight to drop to:
    1. 7 lb 8 oz (3400 g)
    2. 7 lb 3 oz (3200 g)
    3. 7 lb (3100 g)
    4. 7 lb 5 oz (3300 g)

136. The newest addition to the nursery, a baby girl, is noted to have an enlarged breast. Which of the following instructions would the nurse give the parents on how to care for this condition?
    1. Squeeze it daily
    2. Bind the breasts
    3. Apply hot packs
    4. Do nothing

137. The nursery nurse notes that a newborn baby girl has a small amount of pink vaginal discharge. The nurse knows that this is:
    1. Normal because of maternal hormones
    2. Normal because of birth trauma
    3. Abnormal because of excessive hormones
    4. Baby's first menses

138. In caring for a normal newborn, it is important that the nurse know that physiologic jaundice appears:
    1. Within the first 24 hours of life
    2. Before 48 hours
    3. Within 72 hours
    4. 5 Days after birth

139. The nurse is preparing to give Baby Luke his first bath following delivery. It would be appropriate for the nurse to:
    1. Hold the bath until he has begun taking PO fluids
    2. Initially clean only face and torso
    3. Provide cord care first
    4. Use gloves throughout the entire procedure

140. Baby Sue, a newborn, is being given a PO elixir. The best technique for the nurse to use would be to:
    1. Mix the medication with 1 mg of formula
    2. Place small amount in a spoon and give slowly
    3. Mix with a small amount of rice cereal and give slowly
    4. Give through a 1-ml syringe placed against the buccal wall

141. In caring for a newborn, it is important for the nurse to know that a pulse rate of 160 in the newborn who had just been crying probably indicates:
    1. Normalcy
    2. Infarction
    3. Heart disease
    4. Respiratory distress syndrome

142. Which of the following would the nurse recognize as a normal respiratory rate for a newborn infant?
    1. 20 to 25 per minute, regular
    2. 35 to 50 per minute, slightly irregular
    3. 130 to 140 per minute, regular
    4. Hard to determine because they are shallow

143. Greta, a new mother, puts her baby on the bed and begins to walk away, stating that she has to go to the bathroom down the hall. The appropriate nursing action would be to:
    1. Watch and say nothing
    2. Pick up the baby and put her in the crib
    3. Sit on the edge of the bed next to the baby
    4. Caution the new mother never to leave the baby unattended

144. One minute Greta shows concern for her new baby by asking a lot of questions. The next minute she appears not to care as she leaves the baby unattended. Observation of the patient leads the nurse to assume which of the following?
    1. She has answered all of Greta's questions satisfactorily and doesn't need to do anything else
    2. She has taken care of all of Greta's concerns, this patient is all right
    3. Greta's questions are the kind usually asked by new mothers, and there is no need for concern
    4. The changes in Greta's behavior are of concern and should be reported to the charge nurse immediately

145. Baby Jeffrey has been undergoing phototherapy for high bilirubin levels because of ABO incompatability. In caring for this infant, the nurse might expect baby Jeffrey's stools to be:
    1. Watery and green
    2. Golden yellow and loose
    3. Greenish black and sticky
    4. Pale yellow and soft

146. Mrs. Thomas is a gravida 2, para 1. Her blood type is O positive, and her husband's is A negative. During the first day after delivery, the nurse observes slight yellowing of the sclera in baby Thomas. By the second day, the jaundice is more obvious and is noted over the infant's entire body. Laboratory studies indicate the unconjugated bilirubin level to be 9 mg/dl. When planning further care for this infant, the nurse must consider that the jaundice is most likely related to:
    1. Normal physiology of the newborn
    2. Rh incompatibility
    3. Hepatitis B
    4. ABO incompatibility

147. The physician orders phototherapy for Baby Seth, who is 2 days old and has a bilirubin level of 13 mg/dl. Which of the following nursing interventions is of prime importance in caring for an infant undergoing phototherapy?
    1. Cover the eyes loosely with cotton balls
    2. Restrict fluids to enhance effects of therapy
    3. Remove all clothing, including the diaper
    4. Monitor skin temperature

148. In caring for the newborn with hyperbilirubinemia, it is important for the nurse to know that this is a hemolytic disease caused by a(n):
    1. Rh-negative father and Rh-negative mother giving birth to an Rh-positive baby
    2. Rh-negative mother giving birth to Rh-positive baby fathered by Rh-positive father
    3. Rh-positive mother giving birth to Rh-positive baby fathered by Rh-positive father
    4. Rh-positive mother giving birth to Rh-negative baby fathered by Rh-positive father

149. Baby Boy Sims has been diagnosed with ophthalmia neonatorum. It is important for the nurse to know that ophthalmia neonatorum refers to:
    1. Congenital cataracts
    2. Congenital syphilis
    3. Gonorrheal infection of the conjunctiva
    4. Congenital deformities

150. Baby Zio was admitted to the newborn nursery at 5:01 AM. Ms. Zio, age 16, had an active case of syphilis diagnosed during her pregnancy, but she did not comply with treatment protocol for the disease. In caring for a newborn possibly infected with syphilis, the nurse must observe for which of the following signs and symptoms?
    1. Rash and nasal discharge
    2. Vomiting and diarrhea
    3. Central nervous system instability and seizures
    4. Conjunctivitis and septicemia

151. In planning care for a newborn who has tested HIV positive, it is most important for the nurse to:
    1. Wash hands frequently
    2. Notify the Centers for Disease Control
    3. Implement universal precaution protocol
    4. Wear mask, gown and gloves at all times

152. In caring for a newborn addicted to cocaine, the nurse must know that the infant reacts to the drug because:
① Of the inability of the infant's immature liver to excrete the drug rapidly
② Of use of the drug by the mother just before conception
③ When taken by the mother in combination with other drugs, cocaine is doubly addictive
④ It impairs uterine growth and fosters respiratory distress syndrome problems following birth

153. Knowledge of child growth and development principles is essential when planning care for a pediatric patient. Therefore the nurse knows that punishment is most effective when:
① The child knows that his mother loves him
② It is a logical consequence of wrong-doing
③ It enables the parent to constructively channel his or her anger
④ The child has been disobedient

154. Parent education classes are being offered by the Health Maintenance Organization (HMO) clinic. Because the nurse is an important part of these classes, it is essential that the principles of child growth and development be understood. In regard to diet, the basic factor in forming good eating habits in a child is:
① Not insisting that toddlers eat everything
② Serving attractive, nutritious foods
③ Allowing the child choices at mealtime
④ Making mealtime a pleasant social situation

155. In caring for pediatric patients, it is important that the nurse understand normal growth and development periods. A sense of trust is developed at a definite period in the life of the child. This period is primary during:
① Adolescence
② Preschool
③ School age
④ Infancy

156. Mrs. Green brings 1-month-old Billy to the pediatric clinic. The nurse recognizes which of the following developmental achievements as normal for Billy?
① He rolls from his back to his right side
② He smiles and laughs aloud when talked to
③ He holds a rattle for a brief period
④ He turns his head from side to side while on his abdomen

157. Mrs. Allen brings Paula to the pediatric clinic. The nurse observes Paula to be competent in various developmental skills, including holding her head erect when in a sitting position, staring at an object when it is placed in her hand and putting it in her mouth, cooing and gurgling when talked to, and sustaining part of her own weight when held in a standing position. The nurse is correct when she assesses Paula's age to be approximately:
① 2 months
② 4 months
③ 6 months
④ 8 months

158. A mother states, "The soft spot near the front of my child's head is still big. When will it close?" The nurse's response should be guided by knowledge that most often the anterior fontanel closes when the infant is between the ages of:
① 2 and 4 months
② 4 and 8 months
③ 8 and 12 months
④ 15 and 18 months

159. Knowledge of the principles of child growth and development is essential in planning care for a pediatric patient. The nurse knows that language and speech development is promoted by speaking to the 18 month old:
① Clearly and simply
② With a rich vocabulary
③ "In baby talk"
④ As if he or she were an adult

160. In caring for a toddler, the nurse must know that a physiologic task that would be unrealistic for most toddlers between 12 and 14 months of age to achieve is:
① Helping to feed self
② Walking with assistance
③ Manipulating building blocks
④ Controlling the anal sphincter

161. Knowledge of the principles of child growth and development is essential in planning the care of a pediatric patient. The nurse knows that to facilitate readiness for toilet training, the child should wear:
① Diapers
② Rubber pants
③ Training pants
④ Overalls

162. Knowledge of child growth and development principles is essential in planning care for a pediatric patient. The nurse knows that for toddlers, temper tantrums can be avoided or decreased in number and severity by:
① Letting the toddler have his own way
② Providing regular periods of active physical exercise
③ Giving him what he wants to quiet him down
④ Making him understand that this is unacceptable behavior

163. Knowledge of child growth and development principles is essential in planning care for the pediatric patient. The nurse knows that toddlers often ingest or aspirate foreign bodies because they:
① Want to frighten their mothers
② Want to get attention
③ Have easy access to them
④ Learn through exploring

164. Jimmy's mother expressed concern that Jimmy, age 2, does not play with other children or share his toys. The nurse's appropriate response to the mother would be:
① "You'd better take him to counseling sessions."
② "He has probably inherited his father's behavior."
③ "You should strongly encourage him to share toys."
④ "He is demonstrating normal behavior for his age."

165. Two-year-old Tommy's mother states that her son's favorite word lately has been "no!" The nurse can explain that according to Erickson's developmental stage, Tommy is in a stage of:
① Industry vs. inferiority
② Autonomy vs. doubt
③ Trust vs. mistrust
④ Initiative vs. guilt

166. In observing a pediatric patient, the nurse knows that gross motor coordination is demonstrated by:
① Running
② Tying shoelaces
③ Writing
④ Sewing

167. In caring for a 5 year old, the nurse knows that the normal pulse rate for a child of this age is:
① 76 to 90 beats/min
② 90 to 110 beats/min
③ 110 to 140 beats/min
④ 120 to 150 beats/min

168. Knowledge of child growth and development principles is important in caring for a pediatric patient. The nurse knows that a major benefit a preschool child receives from attending nursery school is:
① Lessening of sibling rivalry
② Improvement in eating and sleeping habits
③ An opportunity to learn to play with peers
④ Decreased tension and anxiety for his age

169. The nurse knows that according to Erikson, when a child starts engaging in tasks in the real world (learning to win recognition by producing things), this change is a sign of the emergence of the child's sense of:
① Autonomy
② Industry
③ Initiative
④ Intimacy

170. The nurse knows that an important aspect of development of the child during the middle childhood years is his or her ability to engage in:
① Abstract thinking
② Logical thinking
③ Perceptual thinking
④ Preconceptual thinking

171. Which of the following statements would be *best* for the nurse to use when describing findings in relation to the onset of puberty in males and females?
① "Males and females experience the onset of puberty at about the same age."
② "Males experience the onset of puberty about 1 to 2 years earlier than females."
③ "Females experience the onset of puberty about 1 to 2 years earlier than males."
④ "Males and females experience the onset of puberty at the same age, but females decline in development 1 year after males."

172. In caring for the adolescent, the nurse must understand adolescent characteristics. Which statement regarding adolescence is *least true?*
① Sexual experiences have repercussions on budding identity
② Adolescent rebellion is inevitable in our society
③ A major problem for adolescents today is pregnancy
④ Current sexual attitudes and behaviors are more liberal than in the past

173. Richard is 13 years old. Which of the following behaviors would the nurse expect to be characteristic of this age group?
① Predictability
② Seclusive and moody
③ Acceptance of parents' ideals
④ Move from autonomy to dependency

174. In caring for the adolescent patient, the nurse must know that Erikson's theory of development states that adolescents are in the stage of:
① Industry vs. inferiority
② Trust vs. mistrust
③ Initiative vs. guilt
④ Identity vs. role confusion

175. The nurse working on an adolescent unit knows that, in planning care for patients, consideration should be given to the developmental tasks of the adolescent. These include all of the following except:
① Development of body image
② Being dependent on their parents
③ Achieving proper social roles
④ Establishment of career goals

176. It is important for the nurse working in the local well-baby clinic to know that the total number of deciduous teeth is:
① 18
② 20
③ 22
④ 24

177. The U. S. Department of Health and Human Services publishes an immunization schedule for children. Which of the following schedules do they recommend?
① 1 month: DPT, OPV
  3 months: DPT, OPV
  5 months: DPT
  10 months: DPT, OPV, MMR
② 2 months: DPT, OPV
  4 months: DPT, OPV
  6 months: DPT
  15 months: DPT, OPV, MMR
③ 4 months: DPT, OPV
  8 months: DPT, OPV
  12 months: DPT
  16 months: DPT, OPV, MMR
④ 3 months: DPT, OPV
  6 months: DPT, OPV
  9 months: DPT
  12 months: DPT, OPV, MMR

178. A preschool child's mother asks the nurse about immunizations and communicable diseases. Which of the following statements best describes the incidence of communicable diseases in children?
    ① Communicable diseases have been eradicated by immunizations
    ② Immunizations have reduced the incidence of communicable disease; however, communicable diseases are still a major cause of illness in children
    ③ Communicable diseases are absolutely necessary in a child's life
    ④ Communicable diseases are never severe

179. A mother has just been instructed by the nurse that the first immunization her child will be given, at the age of 2 months, is:
    ① Diphtheria, pertussis, and tetanus (DPT) and rubella
    ② DPT
    ③ DPT and trivalent oral polio virus
    ④ Measles and mumps

180. It is important for the nurse working in the local well-baby clinic to know that the age when a child should receive a measles-mumps-rubella (MMR) immunization is:
    ① 4 months
    ② 6 months
    ③ 12 months
    ④ 15 months

181. A school-age child is receiving a low-sodium diet. She has requested an evening snack. In planning her diet, which of the following foods would the nurse consider?
    ① Banana
    ② Candy bar
    ③ Ham sandwich
    ④ Tuna salad

182. When explaining an infant's diet and feeding schedule to a new mother, the nurse must include the following principles. Which is *the most* important for the nurse to emphasize?
    ① New foods are introduced one at a time to observe for allergies
    ② Pureed fruits and cereals are added when formula no longer satisfies the infant
    ③ Solid foods are added when the infant begins to chew
    ④ Formula feedings are supplemental, along with plenty of water

183. The schedule for introduction of semisolid foods depends on the infant and the physician's recommendation. The nurse would instruct the mother to introduce cereal at:
    ① 1 to 2 months
    ② 2 to 3 months
    ③ 5 to 6 months
    ④ 7 to 8 months

184. Penny, age 5, does not like to drink milk. Which of the following foods would the nurse suggest to Penny's mother to meet the need for essential amino acids provided by milk?
    ① Cereals
    ② Eggs
    ③ Lentils
    ④ Legumes

185. A urinalysis performed on Susie, age 5, shows a high bacteria count. Which of the following instructions should be included in teaching Susie's mother?
    ① Bathe Susie daily in a tub, using soap and water
    ② Discontinue antibiotics as soon as symptoms disappear
    ③ Drink only cranberry juice
    ③ Wipe perineum from front to back after voiding

186. Documentation that the nurse would make immediately after a child returns from a cardiac catheterization includes:
    ① Assessing insertion site
    ② Monitoring vital signs q2h
    ③ Frequent turning of patient
    ④ Recording preoperative medications

187. Following a cardiac catheterization, a child has an intravenous infusion running at 20 ml/hr. The infusion set delivers 60 drops (gtt)/ml. The nurse regulates the drops per minute at:
    ① 2 gtt/min
    ② 5 gtt/min
    ③ 10 gtt/min
    ④ 20 gtt/min

188. Brian, age 2 months, has been in the neonatal ICU since birth. The nursing staff observes Brian closely because he exhibits symptoms such as a large pulse pressure, dyspnea on exertion, and growth retardation. These symptoms could be indicative of:
    ① Aortic stenosis
    ② Pulmonary stenosis
    ③ Coarctation of the aorta
    ④ Patent ductus arteriosus

189. Baby George, age 6 weeks, has been diagnosed with patent ductus arteriosus. In caring for this infant, the nurse knows that cyanoisis is *not* present because of the connection between the:
    ① Right and left atria
    ② Right and left ventricles
    ③ Pulmonary artery and aorta
    ④ Pulmonary vein and right atrium

190. Brittany, 4-year-old girl admitted to the hospital for diagnostic tests, is suspected of having leukemia. The nurse anticipates that the test most likely to be ordered to determine whether Brittany has leukemia is:
    ① Bone marrow aspiration
    ② Gastric analysis
    ③ Arterial blood gases
    ④ Cardiac echogram

191. Bed rest is ordered for Brittany, a 4-year-old with leukemia. The reason bed rest is ordered is to relieve:
    ① Cyanosis
    ② Palpitations
    ③ Painful joints
    ④ Blurred vision

192. Brittany, a 4-year-old leukemia patient, is not responding to treatment. Which of the following signs would indicate to the nurse that the disease is progressing?
    ① Edema
    ② Cyanosis
    ③ Rectal bleeding
    ④ Clubbed fingers

193. Prednisone (Meticorten) and vincristine sulfate (Oncovin) are prescribed for Brittany, a 4-year-old leukemia patient. The nurse knows that this combination of drugs in the body acts to:
    1. Reduce symptoms of pain
    2. Induce prolonged remissions
    3. Prevent infections
    4. Promote white cell production

194. Lisa, a 6-year-old leukemia patient, asks the nurse, "Am I going to die?" The nurse wants to help relieve Lisa's anxieties. Her best response would be:
    1. "Do you really feel that bad today?"
    2. "We are all going to die someday. Tell me more about how you feel."
    3. "Let's talk about something else."
    4. "Don't worry about that; let's watch televison."

195. Johnny, age 6, has been diagnosed with acute leukemia. In planning care for this patient, it is important for the nurse to be aware of the signs and symptoms of this disease, which include:
    1. Decreased white blood cell (WBC) count, decreased hemoglobin, petechiae, and anorexia
    2. Decreased WBC count, pallor, lethargy, and fever
    3. Increased WBC count, increased hemoglobin, petechiae, and pallor
    4. Increased WBC count, pallor, anemia, and petechiae

196. Sara Jane is a 16-year-old high school student who has not been feeling well. On the basis of her presenting symptoms, she is being given a diagnostic workup for leukemia. During the admission procedure, the nurse would closely observe the patient for symptoms of leukemia that include:
    1. Epistaxis, easy bruising, and malaise
    2. Gastrointestinal bleeding, nausea, and vomiting
    3. Pruitis, rash, and fever
    4. Petechiae, gastrointestinal bleeding, and rash

197. In planning care for a patient with leukemia, the nurse must understand that the disease is characterized by:
    1. An increase in the number of red blood cells (RBCs)
    2. Severe weight gain from edema
    3. Increase in the number of white blood cells
    4. Immature RBCs in circulating blood

198. Discharge planning for a patient with leukemia will most likely include a treatment plan for:
    1. A diet high in vitamins
    2. Loss of weight by controlling edema
    3. Home care as soon as possible
    4. Antibiotics and blood transfusions

199. A major nursing goal in caring for a teenager diagnosed with leukemia includes assisting her to:
    1. Cope with the diagnosis/prognosis
    2. Deal with her body image
    3. Continue with school
    4. Go home as soon as possible

200. George is a 9-year-old boy who is being admitted to the hospital for further testing. He has been having low-grade fever, weight loss, and pain in his arms and legs. He recently had a sore throat and was diagnosed as having rheumatic fever. In planning care for this patient, the nurse knows that the organism most likely responsible for the sore throat is:
    1. A virus
    2. *Pneumococcus*
    3. *Staphylococcus*
    4. *Streptococcus*

201. George, age 9, has a diagnosis of rheumatic fever. During the acute stage of his illness, the nursing care should include:
    1. Assisting him to the shower
    2. Walking him to the bathroom
    3. Protecting him from sunlight
    4. Turning him in bed

202. The physician orders aspirin for George, a 9-year-old with rheumatic fever. The nurse knows that the most probable reason for this medication is to relieve:
    1. Carditis
    2. Cardiac enlargement
    3. Joint pain
    4. Nausea

203. In caring for a child with rheumatic fever, the nurse must know that the most potentially serious complication from it is:
    1. Disintegration of the joints
    2. Cardiac involvement
    3. Cerebral involvement
    4. Paralysis of limbs

204. Jimmy, a newly diagnosed diabetic patient, plays soccer on the school team. What is the best advice that the nurse can give Jimmy about diabetes and playing sports?
    1. Administer an extra dose of insulin before playing
    2. Skip the meal before playing
    3. Consider not playing until his diabetes is stabilized
    4. Eat an extra high-carbohydrate snack before playing

205. Which of the following would be an acceptable nutritional practice for Jimmy, a boy with newly diagnosed diabetes, who wants to eat at a fast food restaurant with his friends?
    1. Order only lettuce and tomato salads without dressing
    2. Order foods as desired, later adjusting the insulin dose based on the blood glucose check
    3. When ordering, use a dietary exchange list specific to fast-food restaurants
    4. Order whatever is desired; all adolescents need time away from restrictions

206. Jimmy, a newly diagnosed diabetic patient, would like to take driver's education and obtain his driver's license. What advice should the nurse give Jimmy about driving a car?
    ① Jimmy should not drive until he is older and is sure that he will not have problems with his diabetes
    ② Jimmy should carry a snack with him in the car in case he begins to feel hypoglycemic
    ③ Jimmy will need to have another driver with him at all times
    ④ The Department of Public Safety will not issue him a driver's license

207. A 15-year-old patient tells the nurse he wants to be on the basketball team next year, but he has been told he is too short. He asks what can be done to make him grow taller. The nurse explains that growth occurs as a result of the growth hormone produced by the:
    ① Thyroid gland
    ② Anterior pituitary gland
    ③ Posterior pituitary gland
    ④ Adrenal medulla

208. In planning postoperative care for a young patient following surgical intervention for removal of the structure that produces the growth hormone, the nurse plans care for which of the following?
    ① Hypophysectomy
    ② Thyroidectomy
    ③ Parathyroidectomy
    ④ Adrenalectomy

209. The nurse should observe for potential complications following surgical intervention in the structure that produces the growth hormone. This will include assessing for:
    ① Adrenal insufficiency, diabetes insipidus, and hypothyroidism
    ② Thyroid storm, tetany, and respiratory obstruction
    ③ Ketoacidosis, hypoglycemia, and coma
    ④ Adrenal crisis; hypotension, tachycardia, convulsions, and coma

210. In counseling the parents of a child with celiac syndrome, the nurse would strongly recommend which of the following foods to be eliminated from the child's diet?
    ① Rye bread
    ② Lean meats
    ③ Green beans
    ④ Strawberries

211. Nursing management of the patient with Crohn's disease includes monitoring the patient's diet. Which of the following diets would the physician most likely order for this patient?
    ① Full liquid diet
    ② Clear liquid with potassium
    ③ Soft diet, no foods high in fiber
    ④ Soft diet with bulk-containing foods

212. James is a 4 year old admitted to the hospital with the diagnosis of nephrosis. During the admission process, the nurse knows that the prime presenting symptom of the child would be:
    ① Edema
    ② Hematuria
    ③ Petechial rash
    ④ Dehydration

213. In caring for a 4-year-old with nephrosis, the nurse would expect that the urinalysis would reveal:
    ① Gross hematuria
    ② Gross albuminuria
    ③ Glycosuria
    ④ No abnormalities

214. In planning care for a patient with nephrosis, the nurse knows that the proper diet for the condition would most likely contain:
    ① Decreased sodium and increased fluids
    ② Decreased protein and sodium
    ③ Increased fiber and vitamins
    ④ Increased protein and decreased sodium

215. Ms. Sam brings her 6-week-old newborn to the clinic because of an apparent red rash on the infant's arms. The earliest indication of an allergic response in an infant is:
    ① Impetigo
    ② Acne vulgaris
    ③ Eczema
    ④ Dysplasia

216. Janine, age 5, has been admitted to the pediatric unit with a diagnosis of eczema. Nursing care for Janine should include which of the following nursing interventions?
    ① Maintaining the child in one position
    ② Keeping the child fully clothed
    ③ Maintaining skin integrity
    ④ Applying moist dressings

217. Sally Foster, a recent nursing graduate, has taken a summer job as a nurse for the local childrens' camp. As the camp nurse, Sally must know that a common fungal infection of the skin on the scalp, body, and feet is:
    ① Ringworm
    ② Pediculosis
    ③ Herpes
    ④ Urticaria

218. In caring for a child with tinea capitis, it is important for the nurse to know that the organism responsible for causing the condition is a:
    ① Virus
    ② Bacillus
    ③ Bacterium
    ④ Fungus

219. Will sustained second- and third-degree burns over 43% of his body. Before the burn dressing is changed, Will is to receive 20 mg of Demerol elixir. The elixir has 50 mg of Demerol per teaspoon. How many milliliters of the elixir would the nurse administer to Will?
    ① 1 ml
    ② 2 ml
    ③ 4 ml
    ④ 6 ml

220. Will's burned areas have healed enough so that Will can receive skin grafts. After skin grafting, the most important nursing action to promote acceptance of the graft is to:
    1. Debride the outer edge of the recipient site to facilitate healing
    2. Restrict movement of graft site to prevent dislodging of graft
    3. Apply a heat light to decrease drainage
    4. Change the petroleum gauze dressings daily
221. In caring for a burn victim who has just received skin grafts, the nurse must encourage the patient to drink fluids to prevent:
    1. Renal calculi
    2. Dehydration
    3. Electrolyte imbalance
    4. Weight loss
222. Sally, age 12, is brought to the pediatric clinic by her mother, who states the child appears to be "walking funny." On further examination, the physician discovers that Sally has a lateral S-shaped curvature of the spine. In planning home care for this patient, it is important for the nurse to know that this condition is called:
    1. Scoliosis
    2. Nephrosis
    3. Lordosis
    4. Kyphosis
223. In caring for a child with scoliosis over a period of time, the nurse knows that which of the following statements regarding the condition is true?
    1. Pain is a common presenting symptom
    2. Disability is confined only to the spine
    3. Detection is difficult and requires radiography
    4. A compensatory curve usually results in an effort to maintain an erect posture
224. Jeff, age 10, was admitted to the emergency room with a suspected fracture of the right wrist. Following confirmation of the diagnosis by x-ray examination, the physician applied a cast. The nurse in the emergency room shows Jeff's mother the correct way to check for tightness of the cast. Which of the following statements made by the nurse is an appropriate teaching statement?
    1. "After the cast has dried, insert your fingers between the skin and the cast."
    2. "Pull the cast up and down to determine movement."
    3. "Insert a gauze dressing as far down the cast as possible."
    4. "Insert a rigid object as far down inside the cast as possible."

225. Willy, age 3, has been admitted to the pediatric unit with a fractured left femur. He was placed in Russell traction and is having a difficult time adjusting to being immobilized. His grandmother is concerned about his wetting the bed at night. The most appropriate response by the nurse in answer to the woman's concern would be:
    1. "Willy may need to be toilet trained again after his discharge from the hospital."
    2. "Don't worry about his wetting the bed at night. We change his sheets frequently."
    3. "Willy has had a traumatic experience. When he gets used to being in the hospital he will stop wetting the bed."
    4. "Wetting the bed is not unusual for a child Willy's age. Children often regress in some behaviors in the hospital."
226. Jimmy is a 2-year-old boy who is in the hospital with a fractured right femur. The physician has ordered Bryant's traction. In planning care for a child in Bryant's traction, the nurse must know:
    1. The type/purpose of traction
    2. The function of the traction only
    3. The method used to order the traction
    4. That she need not be concerned with the age of the child
227. In caring for a child in traction, it is important to maintain proper use of the traction. Therefore, the nurse should check:
    1. That the weights rest on the floor
    2. The pulleys and correct weights
    3. The splints, and reposition them as necessary
    3. The position of the bed
228. While bathing Jimmy, a 2-year-old in traction with a fractured right femur, the nurse carefully assesses him. It is important that the nurse check the child's:
    1. Skin condition
    2. Circulation to the left lower extremity
    3. Immobility in bed only
    4. Mother's reaction to the situation
229. The nurse develops a plan of care for Jimmy, a 2-year-old in Bryant's traction. Because bed rest is ordered, the plan should include which of the following?
    1. Promote as little activity in bed as possible
    2. Change the weights on the traction daily
    3. Administer pain medication q2h
    4. Change position, still maintaining proper traction
230. In planning care for a child in traction as a result of a fracture, the nurse must understand that the purpose of the traction is to:
    1. Cure the fracture immediately
    2. Keep the patient in bed
    3. Promote comfort in bed
    4. Align/immobilize the limb

231. Dennis Edwards is a 7-year-old boy who has cerebral palsy. He is cared for at home by his parents with the assistance of home-care nurses. He has a gastrostomy tube in place for his feedings. In planning care for this patient, it is important for the nurse to know that cerebral palsy may be caused by:
    ① Premature birth
    ② Injury to the brain
    ③ A genetic disorder
    ④ Erythroblastosis fetalis

232. A major nursing consideration that the nurse must deal with during the early years of a cerebral palsy patient's life is:
    ① Seizure activity
    ② Increased muscle tone
    ③ Decreased muscle tone
    ④ Sensory impairment

233. Tommy, age 5, is a cerebral palsy patient who has a gastrostomy tube in place for his feedings. When giving Tommy his gastrostomy feeding, the nurse would:
    ① Push the formula in with a 50 ml syringe to ensure that the feeding gets into the stomach
    ② Aspirate formula in the stomach and discard it
    ③ Allow the formula to flow in by gravity and flush with 10 ml of water
    ④ Reinsert the gastrostomy tube each feeding

234. Sammy, age 10, has cerebral palsy and is cared for at home by his parents with the assistance of home-care nurses. Nursing management of his care should include:
    ① Educational and social programs
    ② Long-term planning and care
    ③ Patience and tolerance
    ④ Knowledge of the general disease processes

235. Developing family relationships is important for a child with cerebral palsy. The nurse knows this goal has been achieved when:
    ① Ritualization management is accepted
    ② There is acceptance of his growing independence
    ③ A study is completed to determine how much help the parents need in caring for him
    ④ There is acceptance of him as he is now

236. Baby Paul is admitted to the newborn nursery with a confirmed diagnosis of Down's syndrome. In preparing to care for the infant and to respond to questions the mother may have, it is important for the nursery nurse to know that this condition is:
    ① A congenital abnormality
    ② Caused by a bacterial infection
    ③ Caused by a viral infection
    ④ A result of oxygen deprivation

237. In caring for a child admitted with recurrent seizures that are a result of uncontrolled epilepsy, the nurse is aware that an anticonvulsant drug commonly used to control such seizures is:
    ① Cimetidine (Tagamet)
    ② Hydroxyzine pamoate (Vistaril)
    ③ Prochlorperazine (Compazine)
    ④ Phenytoin (Dilantin)

238. The Stemples anxiously awaited the birth of their first child. Baby girl Stemple was born with a myelomeningocele. As the delivery room nurse cares for the infant, the new father suddenly leaves the delivery room. The best way for the nurse to approach Mr. Stemple is to:
    ① Offer him a cup of coffee and leave him alone
    ② Sit down beside him and ask if he needs help
    ③ Tell him that, although deformed, the baby can live a normal life
    ④ Ask him several questions about the delivery to start conversation

239. An infant was born with a myelomeningocele. Seeing his new son for the first time, the father asks, "What is that horrible thing on my baby's back?" An appropriate first response from the nurse would include:
    ① The term "myelomeningocele" and a simple description of the anomaly
    ② A description of the long-term care the infant will need
    ③ A full description of the condition, including complications
    ④ Conversation that would direct his attention away from the situation

240. In caring for a newborn with a myelomeningocele, it is important that the nurse observe closely for:
    ① Bowel elimination
    ② Moro's reflex
    ③ Relationship with mother
    ④ Hemoglobin levels

241. The nurse can assist the physician in determining the extent of neuromuscular damage in an infant with spina bifida by:
    ① Observing movement of extremities
    ② Testing response to deep pain
    ③ Checking tendon reflexes
    ④ Recording type of cry heard

242. Baby girl Sims was born with a myelomeningocele. Because of the length of hospitalization and separation of the parents from their infant, the nursing staff would foster the child-parent relationship by:
    ① Encouraging both parents to see the infant during the specified visiting hours
    ② Explaining the process of parent bonding and how the parents should treat the child at home
    ③ Encouraging the parents to touch and hold the newborn as much as possible
    ④ Ignoring the parents' statements indicating their grief at not having a normal baby

243. Sarah tells the nurse that her infant daughter vomits frequently. Knowing this can happen with a child who has a myelomeningocele, the nurse would advise the mother to promote adequate nutrition by:
    ① Holding the infant while supporting the head; offering small frequent feedings
    ② Witholding feedings until the baby stops vomiting, then giving thickened feedings
    ③ Increasing the carbohydrates in each feeding by adding sugar to the formula
    ④ Inserting a nasogastric (NG) tube to give the formula; instructing the mother in the proper care of the NG tube

244. Baby girl Masters is scheduled for insertion of a ventriculoperitoneal shunt to decrease accumulation of cerebrospinal fluid causing hydrocephalus. In planning postoperative care, the nurse knows that the infant would be positioned:
① On the operative side
② In Trendelenburg's position
③ On the nonoperative side
④ In high-Fowler's position

245. Sarah asks the nurse, "Why do you keep measuring my baby's head every day? I thought after the shunt was put in, everything would be all right." The most appropriate response by the nurse would be:
① "The baby's head size should have decreased immediately after surgery. I am checking to see if the shunt helped your baby."
② "By measuring the baby's head, I will know if there is an increase in intracranial pressure."
③ "As cerebrospinal fluid drains from the ventricles of the brain, the head circumference will gradually decrease."
④ "You need not be concerned with what we are doing. Your baby is all right and will be going home soon."

246. Three days following discharge of a newborn with a ventriculoperitoneal shunt, the mother brings her to the emergency room. The infant has a temperature of 104°F (40°C) and has a high-pitched cry. The mother states the infant has had several seizures at home. The infant is admitted with a suspected diagnosis of meningitis. Several diagnostic laboratory tests are ordered, and preparation is made for a lumbar puncture. To prepare the infant for a lumbar puncture, the nurse would:
① Restrain the infant in a side-lying position with the head hyper-extended during the procedure
② Administer 10 mg of Demerol intramuscularly to sedate the infant before the procedure
③ Hold the infant in a sitting position with head flexed during the procedure
④ Place the infant in a mummy restraint and hold neck flexed during procedure

247. The nursery nurse has just admitted a newborn with a congenital disorder in which the abdominal organs have protruded through the abdominal wall and have formed a sac on the abdomen. In developing a plan of care for this infant, it is important for the nurse to know that this is a(n):
① Diaphragmatic hernia
② Umbilical hernia
③ Omphalocele
④ Esophageal atresia

248. Joshua, age 17 months, is admitted to the hospital with a diagnosis of meningitis. In planning care for Joshua, the nurse knows that his symptoms will most likely include:
① Fever, stiff neck, and elevated white blood cells (WBCs) in blood and spinal fluid
② Dyspnea, lethargy, and elevated pulse and blood pressure
③ Vomiting, diarrhea, dehydration, and red raised rash
④ Red raised rash, fever, diarrhea, and elevated WBCs in spinal fluid

249. Jody, age 24 months, has been admitted to the pediatric unit with a diagnosis of meningitis. Of prime importance is nursing observation for seizures. In the event that Jody has a seizure, it is important that the nurse remember to:
① Document and notify the charge nurse immediately
② Restrain the child to prevent injury
③ Insert a padded tongue blade to prevent possible respiratory complications
④ Observe movements and document time and length of seizure

250. After Jody goes home, her mother calls the nurse at the clinic and tells her that Jody is having frequent temper tantrums. Which of the following statements by the nurse best describes the way to handle the situation?
① "Offer her a cookie if she will stop."
② "Ignore Jody until the tantrum is over."
③ "Spank her and send her to her room."
④ "Try to find what the problem is during the tantrum."

251. The physician orders blood cultures to be drawn on an infant with suspected meningitis. Following the puncture for collection of the blood specimens, the nurse would immediately:
① Take the specimens to the laboratory
② Obtain an arterial blood specimen for comparison
③ Apply a warm compress to decrease pain and ecchymosis
④ Apply direct pressure to the area until bleeding has stopped

252. Baby girl Masters, diagnosed with meningitis, is placed in isolation. The baby's mother asks the nurse how long her baby will stay in isolation. The nurse's response is based on the knowledge that:
① Isolation will be maintained until a negative cerebrospinal fluid bacterial growth culture is returned
② Isolation is not necessary 24 hours after antibacterial therapy
③ Preventing the spread of infection is the primary objective in the care of the infant
④ Isolation is maintained until completion of 7 days of IV antibiotics

253. While providing daily care for an infant with meningitis, the nurse would observe for:
    1. Skin integrity, inflammation of IV site, and infiltration of IV
    2. Increase in temperature and urine specific gravity and decrease in urinary output
    3. Change in vital and neurologic signs and increased urinary output
    4. Frequent bowel movements, signs of nuchal rigidity, and hypothermia

254. The physician has ordered 125,000 U of aqueous penicillin q6h intravenously for baby girl Masters, who has been diagnosed as having meningitis. Before each administration of the medication, the nurse would:
    1. Check the IV tube site for signs of phlebitis and infiltration
    2. Flush the IV line with 30 ml of IV fluid to test patency of line
    3. Verify the amount of reconstituted solution to be administered
    4. Ask the mother to leave the room during the procedure

255. With the increasing occurrence of head injuries, it is important for the nurse to know that:
    1. Head injuries are a common cause of mental illness
    2. Concussion is a bruising of cerebral tissue
    3. Negative symptomatology is unrelated to the extent of organic damage
    4. Psychic effects of brain injury are a reaction to the trauma

256. Gerry, age 14, suffered a spinal cord injury following a dive into a shallow pond while on a family outing. Autonomic dysreflexia is common in such patients and is characterized by a sudden elevation in blood pressure, headache, chills, and pallor. In planning care for a patient with a spinal cord injury, the nurse would consider which of the following interventions to lower the blood pressure quickly under such circumstances?
    1. Get the patient to a sitting position
    2. Call the physician immediately
    3. Administer oxygen immediately
    4. Put the patient in Trendelenburg's position

257. In planning to teach patients with spinal cord injuries about the action of certain foods in their bodies, the nurse would make a point to include that the liquid least likely to cause formation of urinary calculi is:
    1. Cranberry juice
    2. Tomato juice
    3. Coffee
    4. Milk

258. Of the following symptoms, which should the nurse watch for in cases of possible spinal cord compression?
    1. Severe headaches
    2. Changes in sensation
    3. Unconsciousness
    4. Convulsions

259. In caring for a patient with head or neck injuries, the nurse is aware that a drug frequently used in the management of such injuries is:
    1. Methylprednisolone (Solu-Medrol)
    2. Dexamethazone (Decadron)
    3. Acetazolamide (Diamox)
    4. Chlorothiazide (Diuril)

260. With some spinal cord injuries, patients often have a great deal of pain. When caring for these patients, the nurse is aware that narcotics are contraindicated for long-term use because of the possibility of:
    1. Respiratory complications
    2. Addiction to narcotic drugs
    3. Abscesses from frequent infections
    4. Circulatory complications

261. In planning care for Jenny, a young asthmatic patient, the nurse would include all of the following nursing care measures *except:*
    1. Monitoring intravenous fluids
    2. Administering aminophylline
    3. Bed rest in supine position
    4. Assisting with intermittent positive-pressure breathing treatments

262. Jenny, age 7, has asthma and was brought to the emergency room while having an acute attack. During the attack the nurse is aware that Jenny's breathing is most likely characterized by:
    1. Noisy inspirations
    2. Wheezing on expiration
    3. Frequent periods of apnea
    4. Labored abdominal breathing

263. Collin, age 3, is admitted to the emergency room in obvious respiratory distress. The admitting physician is talking to the medical student, telling him the child has a respiratory disease that is characterized by spasms of the bronchial tubes caused by hypersensitivity of the airways. In planning care for Collin, the nurse prepares for nursing interventions specific to the diagnosis of:
    1. Pneumonia
    2. Asthma
    3. Cystic fibrosis
    4. Allergic rhinitis

264. The pediatrician orders acetaminophen 40 mg PO. On hand is acetaminophen 160 mg/tsp (5 ml). The nurse would administer:
    1. 0.5 ml
    2. 2 ml
    3. ¼ tsp
    4. ½ tsp

265. Two-year-old Marcus Vasquez was admitted to the pediatric hospital with respiratory difficulty. After Marcus' respiratory problems worsened, the physician performed a tracheostomy. In aspirating Marcus' tracheostomy the nurse should:
    1. Apply suction to the catheter only while withdrawing it
    2. Remove both inner and outer cannula before inserting the catheter
    3. Twirl the catheter rapidly while withdrawing it slowly during removal
    4. Untie the twill neck tapes while cleansing the skin edges of the wound

266. In caring for a child with asthma, the nurse must know that asthma can be caused by extrinsic or intrinsic factors. Intrinsic factors include:
    1. Injury to the nose
    2. Pollen from flowers
    3. Respiratory infections
    4. Allergens in the environment

267. The physician ordered epinephrine (Adrenalin) stat for a child in severe respiratory distress. The epinephrine was ordered to:
    ① Relax the smooth muscles of the bronchi
    ② Produce vasodilation of blood vessels of the skin
    ③ Decrease cardiac output as a result of its vasopressor action
    ④ Stimulate constriction of the smooth muscles of the respiratory tract

268. The physician ordered epinephrine (Adrenalin) to be administered subcutaneously. The injection is administered using a:
    ① 19-gauge, 1-inch needle
    ② 22-gauge, 1-inch needle
    ③ 25-gauge, ⅝-inch needle
    ④ 27-gauge, ½-inch needle

269. Karen, age 5, has been admitted to the pediatric unit with a diagnosis of croup. When planning care for Karen, the nurse would most likely expect the treatment of choice to include:
    ① Warm, humidified air and antibiotics
    ② Humidified oxygen and sedatives
    ③ Humidified oxygen and antiemetics
    ④ Cool, humidified air and syrup of ipecac

270. On the basis of results of a sweat test, chest x-ray examinations, and the decreased amount of duodenal pancreatic enzymes, Sheila is diagnosed as having cystic fibrosis. Which of the following does the nurse correctly recall as the primary factor responsible for the symptoms of cystic fibrosis?
    ① Increased viscosity of mucous gland (exocrine) secretions leads to the mechanical obstruction of the glands
    ② The fetal lungs do not develop properly
    ③ There are multiple untreated episodes of upper respiratory infections
    ④ There are multiple treatments of upper respiratory infections with antibiotics and suppression of the immune system

271. The nurse prepares 4-year-old Sheila, a cystic fibrosis patient, for her bath. The nurse notes several bruises on both of Sheila's lower legs. Sheila's mother states that every time Sheila is bumped or falls down she seems to get another bruise. What is the most likely cause of the bruises on Sheila's legs?
    ① Sheila is developing a neurologic deficit
    ② There is deficient absorption of vitamin K
    ③ Sheila does not have sufficient supervision during play
    ④ At age 4, most children fall and bruise easily

272. What is the primary reason that cystic fibrosis patients do not gain weight even though they may eat voraciously?
    ① They eat the wrong foods for their health problem
    ② They have constant diarrhea because of the use of multiple antibiotics
    ③ They have continual vomiting due to strictures of the upper gastrointestinal tract
    ④ Their intestines are unable to digest fats and proteins

273. A patient is ordered to take a pancreatic enzyme replacement. Which of the following is the best time to take this medication?
    ① With meals or snacks
    ② At bedtime
    ③ Four to six times a day between meals
    ④ In the morning with 8 oz of water or juice

274. In caring for a child with cystic fibrosis, the nurse knows that the foul-smelling, frothy stools often associated with this condition result from large amounts of undigested:
    ① Minerals
    ② Carbohydrates
    ③ Fats
    ④ Vitamins

275. Two-year-old Jenny has otitis media, which is often a common complication of a/an:
    ① Ear injury
    ② External ear infection
    ③ Myringotomy
    ④ Upper respiratory infection

276. Billy, age 2, has been admitted to the pediatric unit with a history of recurring episodes of otitis media. In planning care for Billy, the nurse is aware that repeated episodes of otitis media in infants and toddlers can result in:
    ① Chronic strep throats
    ② Delayed speech development
    ③ Mastitis
    ④ Sleep walking

277. Instructions to the parent of a child with otitis media following a myringotomy should include having the child lie on his or her:
    ① Abdomen
    ② Affected side
    ③ Back
    ④ Unaffected side

278. Mrs. Palmer brought 5-year-old Timmy to the health maintenance organization (HMO) clinic to have his eyes checked. On examination, the nurse finds them to be red and inflamed, with a green crusty discharge. The physician has diagnosed him as having "pinkeye." In planning care for Timmy, it is important for the nurse to know that "Pinkeye" is:
    ① Degeneration of the conjunctiva
    ② Inflammation of the lacrimal sac
    ③ Inflammation of the conjunctiva
    ④ Opacity of the lens

279. In caring for 5-year-old Timmy, who has been diagnosed with pinkeye, the nurse is aware that the medication of choice is usually:
    ① Pilocarpine eye drops
    ② Photocoagulation
    ③ Normal saline eye drops
    ④ Neosporin ophthalmic drops

280. Five-year-old Timmy has been diagnosed with pinkeye. The nurse is teaching Timmy's mother the proper procedure for administering eye drops. Before Timmy's mother puts the medication in Timmy's eyes, the nurse should instruct her to:
    ① Wash the eyes from the inner canthus outward with a cotton ball and warm water
    ② Wash the eyes back and forth several times with a cotton ball and warm water to get all the crusted material off
    ③ Just put in the medication, which will take care of the crusting
    ④ Wash the eyes with hydrogen peroxide to clear away the crusting

281. Five-year-old Timmy has been diagnosed with pinkeye. Mrs. Palmer asks how long she should put the antibiotic into her son's eyes. The nurse's response should be:
    ① "Continue until the medication is finished."
    ② "For 10 days only."
    ③ "Use your own judgment."
    ④ "Continue until 5 days after the eyes appear clear."

282. Mrs. Cleo comes to the well-baby clinic for the first time. She shows a history of a troublesome pregnancy and relates that the baby seemed to move around a lot before she was born and now doesn't seem to be growing. The nurse notes that the baby is small for its age and has altered facial features. In planning care for this mother and baby, the nurse knows these signs and symptoms to be typical of:
    ① Failure to thrive
    ② Hereditary defect
    ③ Cocaine addiction
    ④ Alcohol addiction

283. Baby Scott, age 6 months, is admitted to the emergency room in what appears to be a severe state of dehydration. Nursing assessment of severe dehydration would likely reveal:
    ① An elevated blood pressure; sunken fontanel
    ② A rapid pulse and marked oliguria
    ③ A slow pulse and parched mucous membranes
    ④ Slow respirations and loss of skin elasticity

284. A young mother is concerned with possible adverse effects her child may experience as a result of chicken pox. The nurse knows that chicken pox is associated with:
    ① No serious complications
    ② Loss of hearing
    ③ Loss of visual acuity
    ④ Muscular system involvement

285. When caring for a child with mumps, it is important for the nurse to know that the child must be considered contagious until:
    ① All swelling has disappeared
    ② The rash has completely disappeared
    ③ Temperature subsides
    ④ Two months after onset of symptoms

286. Todd, age 13, is taken to his pediatrician with a suspected case of mumps. Todd's mother appears quite concerned about Todd's condition. To respond appropriately to the mother's concerns, the nurse must know that Todd may be in danger of which of the following complications?
    ① Orchitis
    ② Meningitis
    ③ Myositis
    ④ Pyelonephritis

287. As a nurse in a pediatric clinic, it is important to be knowledgable about child abuse. Which of the following statements is true relative to battered child syndrome?
    ① Child abuse is physical, not emotional abuse
    ② Parents who abuse their children were usually abused children
    ③ Statistics indicate that child abuse is not evident in middle-class families
    ④ Abused children always have congenital defects or other abnormalities

288. In planning care for a child with acquired immune deficiency syndrome (AIDS), the nurse must know that the causative organism of AIDS is:
    ① Cytomegalovirus
    ② Human immunodeficiency virus
    ③ Human papilloma virus
    ④ Herpes virus

289. Jimmy, age 2, has an order for temperature readings q4h. Because of this patient's age, the nurse would take his temperature by which of the following methods?
    ① Axillary/rectal
    ② Oral/rectal
    ③ Rectal only
    ④ Axillary only

290. Of the following data, which would the nurse need to know most in monitoring the respiratory rate of children?
    ① Average respiratory rate for age
    ② The child's developmental level
    ③ Side effects of bronchodilators
    ④ Theophylline level of child

291. To obtain a urine specimen from an infant, the nurse would:
    ① Clean and dry genitalia, perineum, and skin; and apply a self-adhesive plastic bag
    ② Clean and dry perineum and catheterize infant
    ③ Apply disposable diaper and aspirate urine from diaper with needle and syringe
    ④ Place infant on small container to void and pour urine into specimen tube

292. In observing skin conditions, it is important for the nurse to be able to describe the various lesions for documentation. Lesions that are circumscribed elevations of the epidermis, less than 1 cm in diameter, and contain a clear liquid are described as:
    ① Mascules
    ② Vesicles
    ③ Maculopapules
    ④ Papules

293. While assessing a child having a petit mal seizure, the nurse is most likely to observe:
① Body stiffening
② Jerking movements
③ Lip smacking
④ Urinary incontinence

294. The nurse would best protect an infant prone to seizure activity by which of the following nursing interventions?
① Holding the infant's extremities tightly to prevent injury
② Placing clover-hitch restraints on all extremities
③ Placing blankets over the infant to maintain warmth
④ Placing pillows along the sides of the crib

295. A 5-year-old child is taught coughing and deep-breathing exercises before surgery. Which of the following methods used by the nurse would indicate the best teaching approach?
① Placing information in a logical sequence
② Presenting material from simple to complex
③ Building on the child's level of knowledge
④ Using actual equipment for the demonstration

296. When preparing to administer medications, the nurse is aware that the preferred site for administering an intramuscular injection to a toddler is the:
① Deltoid
② Dorsogluteal
③ Vastus lateralis
④ Ventrogluteal

297. The nurse is providing care for 9-month-old Timmy and receives orders to give a preoperative intramuscular injection of a medication. The best site for this injection would be:
① Deltoid
② Ventrogluteal
③ Dorsogluteal
④ Vastus lateralis

298. While administering an intramuscular injection to 9-month-old Timmy, the nurse would most likely need:
① A second individual to secure the child
② Antibiotic ointment for the site
③ A toy to distract the infant during the procedure
④ The patient's hospital number to ensure identification

299. The pediatrician orders aspirin 5 g PO. On hand the nurse has aspirin 300 mg in tablet form. Which of the following would the nurse be correct in giving her young patient?
① ½ tablet
② 1 tablet
③ 1½ tablets
④ 2 tablets

300. Jimmy, age 8, weighs 75 pounds. The nurse is to administer a medication for which the average adult dose is 300 mg. Using Clark's rule, which of the following doses would the nurse be correct in administering to Jimmy?
① 75 mg
② 125 mg
③ 150 mg
④ 200 mg

301. Adam, age 8, is to receive a medication for which the average adult dose is 500 mg. By implementing Young's rule, the nurse would select which one of the following as the correct dose for Adam?
① 200 mg
② 250 mg
③ 325 mg
④ 375 mg

CHAPTER 4

Mental Health Nursing Questions

1. Many psychiatric therapies involve a holistic emphasis. The nurse must understand that the concept of holism is *best* explained by which one of the following statements?
   ① The individual's role in his world determines his health
   ② Illness results from a complex interaction between the mind and body
   ③ The individual is both separate from and part of society
   ④ A community is whole

2. Multifaceted approaches to treatment are used in mental health nursing. In planning patient care, the nurse knows that these approaches comprise which of the following dimensions?
   ① Financial resources, cost effectiveness, efficiency, and efficacy
   ② Bed availability, potential for recovery, potential benefit to society, and therapies available
   ③ Medication, group therapy, millieu therapy, and rehabilitation
   ④ Physical, psychological, cultural, and socioeconomic

3. The determination that an individual's pattern of behavior is evidence of either mental health wellness or illness is made on the basis of which of the following considerations?
   ① Observations of the persons who know the individual best or those who live with him or her
   ② The degree of intelligence and the amount of education the individual has acquired
   ③ The specific behavior, as well as the context in which it takes place
   ④ The degree to which the behavior is pleasing to others

4. Behavior of a psychiatric patient is assessed on the basis of the nurse's understanding that:
   ① Adults must conform to certain societal norms and beliefs
   ② Behaviors of mentally ill individuals are exaggerations of normal human behavior
   ③ Behaviors of mentally ill individuals are sufficiently bizarre that they cannot be understood by a rational person
   ④ Behaviors of mentally ill individuals are the result of failure in his or her moral training

5. Which of the following statements *best* describes mental health?
   ① The absence of worry and pain and the ability to get along with others
   ② A cheerful, positive outlook on life and its problems; the capacity for happiness
   ③ An individual's ability to manage life's problems and to derive satisfaction from living throughout various life stages
   ④ The ability to win power over others; to control the lives of other people

6. Nursing process with the mentally ill patient begins with which of the following?
   ① Establishing firm limits to control the patient's behavior
   ② A thorough assessment, including physical, psychological, and emotional state
   ③ Communicating with the patient so that the patient knows he or she is in good hands
   ④ Finding out the patient's preferences for room assignment

7. To be an effective practitioner in the mental health field, the nurse should possess the ability to:
   ① Point out the patient's moral shortcomings and affect a change in his or her personal value system
   ② Solve one's own personal and family problems without the assistance of others
   ③ Understand oneself, the awareness of how one affects others, and the capacity to treat other people with respect
   ④ Bring others into compliance with society's rules and expectations

8. In caring for patients in a mental health setting, the nurse is aware that communication:
   ① Is talking and listening in an attentive way that is satisfying to parties involved
   ② Is a complex activity resulting in a negotiated understanding between two or more people
   ③ Is an exchange of information
   ④ Consists of verbal and nonverbal messages

9. With a smile on her face, Linda tells the nurse that she has just failed her final exam. This is an example of:
   ① An attempt to be cheerful in the face of adversity
   ② A discrepancy between verbal communication and facial expression
   ③ A lack of seriousness on Linda's part
   ④ An indication that Linda had a desire to fail

10. The nurse finds Amy, a patient on the ward, in her room crying. Which of the following nursing responses should be *most* appropriate?
    ① "Why are you crying?"
    ② "You appear to be feeling sad."
    ③ "What's the matter with you?"
    ④ "Dry up those tears. It's time for group therapy!"
11. Amy, a patient on the ward, tells the nurse she has received a letter from her boyfriend in which he says he wants to break up with her. The *most* appropriate response should be:
    ① "Tell me how you feel about this."
    ② "He must not have loved you enough."
    ③ "You're better off without him."
    ④ "A good-looking girl like you can find a new man in no time!"
12. Dee Ann, a patient on the ward, is very distraught and tells the nurse a rather confusing story of a recent event. The nurse's *best* response is:
    ① "Settle down and tell me this straight."
    ② "You must be very angry."
    ③ "Let me see if I understand what you're telling me."
    ④ "You always overreact."
13. Pat, a patient on the ward, believes that another patient has stolen her watch, and she wants to talk about this with the nurse. The nurse's *best* response is:
    ① "You really can't prove anything."
    ② "Tell me what you believe happened."
    ③ "I'm sure no one here would do a thing like that."
    ④ "No one likes to feel accused."
14. The nurse-patient relationship is marked by which of the following characteristics?
    ① It is a warm, close friendship in which the patient has his or her needs met
    ② It is a reciprocal relationship in which both the nurse and the patient have needs met
    ③ It is a purposeful relationship that has a therapeutic goal for the patient
    ④ It exists solely to permit the patient to depend on the nurse
15. Sam is a patient who is being evaluated for a tumor in the frontal region of his brain. He complains of the odor of cigar smoke in his room. After examining the room and finding no odor, the nurse's *most* important nursing action should be to:
    ① Inform him that you do not smell cigar smoke in the room
    ② Observe, report, and record the clinical symptom
    ③ Ask if he has had an important relationship with a cigar smoker
    ④ Provide a room deodorizer that is more pleasing to Sam
16. Mrs. Paul, age 36, has been on the mental health unit for 3 weeks. In working with Mrs. Paul, the nurse-patient relationship is enhanced when the nurse uses both verbal and nonverbal methods of communication to provide:
    ① Understanding, attention, and recognition
    ② Self-esteem, love, and security
    ③ Persuasive techniques for reducing resistance to therapeutic intervention
    ④ Knowledge of the patient's difficulties
17. A patient asks the nurse to keep a secret and not tell the other staff members what she's about to reveal. The nurse's *most* appropriate response should be:
    ① "Let's move to a more private area."
    ② "Be careful that no one overhears you."
    ③ "I'll have to hear what you have to say before I can promise that."
    ④ "I cannot make that promise. It might be information important for other staff to know."
18. The nurse is meeting with her assigned patient, Mr. Jay. Mrs. Lane, another patient, approaches and interrupts the meeting, stating she must speak with the nurse. The nurse's appropriate response to Mrs. Lane should be:
    ① "Why don't you sit with us until we're finished talking?"
    ② "I'm with Mr. Jay for the next 15 minutes. When our time is up, I'll talk with you."
    ③ "Mrs. Lane, I'm sure you can see that I'm busy right now."
    ④ "You'll have to ask Mr. Jay if it is alright for you to join us."
19. Just as the nurse's contracted time with her patient, Mr. Jay, is up, he says, "I have to tell you something horrible that happened to me yesterday." Which of the following statements is an appropriate response by the nurse?
    ① "You'll have to tell me quickly because our time is up."
    ② "Our time is up; I'm leaving now."
    ③ "I'll give you no more than 5 more minutes to tell me what happened."
    ④ "Our time is up now Mr. Jay. This would be a good place to start at our next session."
20. Mr. Jay is a committed patient. During his contracted time with the nurse, he reveals an elaborate elopement plan. The nurse's *priority* action should be to:
    ① Try to talk Mr. Jay out of eloping
    ② Let Mr. Jay know she understands his feelings
    ③ Tell Mr. Jay that this is serious and the information needs to be reported to other staff
    ④ Tell Mr. Jay that it's important that he discuss his feelings with his psychiatrist at their next session
21. To facilitate a patient's ability to form more healthy relationships, the nurse should:
    ① Encourage the patient to talk with him or her only about the patient's problems
    ② Discourage the patient from forming any close attachments to others to avoid getting hurt
    ③ Let the patient know that the nurse accepts the patient but does not endorse all of his or her behaviors
    ④ Allow the patient to spend time only with other patients with similar problems
22. The role of the nurse in community mental health is *best* described as:
    ① Functioning mostly as a primary therapist
    ② Controlled by physicians and social workers
    ③ Varied according to location and customs
    ④ Stressful and not well-defined by law

23. Which of the following should a community mental health nurse assess that a nurse practicing on an in-patient mental health unit should not?
    ① Sociocultural influences
    ② Client support systems
    ③ Individual psychosocial stressors
    ④ Economic and political factors

24. A patient comes to the local mental health clinic with multiple complaints. The nurse assigned to assess the patient notes the patient's dress, grooming, posture, and facial expressions. These observations help the nurse to assess which of the following?
    ① The patient's emotional state
    ② The patient's thought content
    ③ The patient's general affect
    ④ The patient's level of consciousness

25. During an assessment interview, the patient becomes increasingly confused and seems to have a difficult time paying attention and concentrating. The patient becomes easily distracted when being questioned. The nurse realizes that the patient:
    ① Is probably hallucinating
    ② Is becoming fearful of the nurse
    ③ Does not understand the questions
    ④ Is becoming disoriented

26. A patient being interviewed is becoming agitated but is still able to write her name and draw a circle, square, and triangle on a piece of paper. On the basis of this observation, the nurse can conclude that the patient's:
    ① Mood and affect are stable
    ② Ability to communicate is intact
    ③ Coordination is unaffected
    ④ Agitation is not drug-induced

27. The patient is able to state that she is at the mental health clinic and knows the date and time. She can tell the nurse her own name and recognizes the nurse as a nurse. This patient's ability to do this tells the nurse about her own:
    ① Mental function
    ② Emotional function
    ③ Communication style
    ④ Coping style

28. A patient whose history reflects a reluctance to be hospitalized for a work-up verbalizes anger over a delay in his testing. The nurse's *most* appropriate response should be:
    ① "Believe me, I know just how you feel."
    ② "I'm sorry for the delay, but there are other patients ahead of you."
    ③ "Why don't you read one of these magazines while you're waiting."
    ④ "You seem upset about being here."

29. For the past hour, Mrs. Willis has been observed sitting in the corner of her room, staring out the window. A supportive nursing measure should include:
    ① Asking her if there is something the nurse can do for her
    ② Encouraging her to go to the dayroom and interact with the other patients
    ③ Leaving her alone with her thoughts, but checking on her periodically
    ④ Taking a few minutes to sit with her in case she wishes to talk

30. Mrs. Willis is depressed. She is not eating or sleeping well. As the nurse approaches one morning, Mrs. Willis is sitting on the side of the bed in her night clothes. She states, "I can't go on. I just can't go on." The *best* response by the nurse should be:
    ① "I understand how you feel. We all feel that way from time to time."
    ② "Let me help you shower and dress. It will make you feel better."
    ③ "You'll feel better once you are up and active."
    ④ "You're feeling hopeless and very sad."

31. One morning, as the nurse walks into Mrs. Willis' room, the patient says, "I didn't get any sleep last night. I finally dozed off around 5 AM." The *best* response by the nurse is:
    ① "Don't worry. You'll sleep better at home in your own bed."
    ② "Can you tell me more about what kept you awake?"
    ③ "Why didn't you ask for a sleeping pill?"
    ④ "It's not that bad. You'll be able to take a nap this afternoon"

32. Mrs. Jones is scheduled for gastric intestinal surgery. Which of the following statements by the nurse should encourage Mrs. Jones to verbalize her feelings about her impending surgery?
    ① "Everything will be okay; keep your chin up."
    ② "Things have a way of working out."
    ③ "This must be a difficult time for you."
    ④ "You have a very competent physician."

33. John has an episode of nausea before entering his first group therapy session. He states to the nurse, "I feel worse today than ever before. I wonder why this is happening to me." The nurse's *best* reply should be:
    ① "I'll ask the doctor for some medication."
    ② "I see your symptoms worry you."
    ③ "It will be okay. You'll feel better in a few minutes."
    ④ "Think about something pleasant."

34. Mr. Bell has been pacing up and down the corridor for several hours. The nurse observes him yell at another patient, "Get out of my way, moron." The *most appropriate* nursing response should be to tell him:
    ① That his behavior is unacceptable and won't be tolerated
    ② That, if he doesn't cool it, he'll be put in seclusion
    ③ That if he doesn't stop bothering the other patients, his afternoon privileges will be taken away
    ④ To come to the medication room for his Ativan

35. Mr. McCreary has cancer and a pneumonectomy is performed. Later in the day, a nursing assistant reports that Mrs. McCreary is openly crying. When the nurse approaches, Mrs. McCreary states, "What made my husband so sick? I think God is punishing me for something I did." An appropriate response by the nurse should be:
    ① "Don't worry about what caused this. Pull yourself together and give him support."
    ② "I see no need to blame yourself."
    ③ "You appear to be very distraught."
    ④ "Why do you feel guilty about your husband's illness?"

36. A consistent set of behaviors unique to an individual (i.e., the sum total of the individual's thoughts, feelings, physical characteristics, and sociocultural biases) *best* defines which of the following:
    ① Mental status
    ② Psychological state
    ③ Educational level
    ④ Personality

37. According to Sigmund Freud, the three elements of personality structure are:
    ① Id, ego, and superego
    ② Preconscious, conscious, and unconscious
    ③ Child, adult, and parent
    ④ Oral, anal, and phallic

38. According to Eric Berne, the three elements of personality structure are:
    ① Id, ego, and superego
    ② Preconscious, conscious, and unconscious
    ③ Child, adult, and parent
    ④ Oral, anal, and phallic

39. Personality functions performed by the ID/child should include which of the following?
    ① Societal values; may be judgmental and critical
    ② Objective reality with the needs of the individual; objective and rational
    ③ The perception of the individual's role in his world
    ④ The basic innate psychic energy and drive; the emotional responses of love, anger, and passion

40. Joel has a chemistry test in the morning. His friends want to go to the lake for a party. Joel's decision to study or go to the party is a function of which of the following personality functions?
    ① Id/child
    ② Ego/adult
    ③ Superego/parent
    ④ Unconscious

41. There are negative functions of the superego/parent that include the judgmental, punitive aspects of the personality. The positive aspects are known as:
    ① Maintenance of a positive attitude and a sense of humor
    ② The incorporation of societal values and norms; the inclusion of religious values
    ③ The ability to maintain rational objectivity
    ④ The playful, spirited aspect of the personality

42. Johnny, age 6, is brought to the mental health center because, according to his mother, "He is slow for his age." While observing Johnny during the first interview, the nurse notes that the child is able to tie his own shoelaces. The nurse knows that this is an example of:
    ① Mental illness
    ② Coping behavior
    ③ Cognitive dysfunction
    ④ Autism

43. When caring for a patient who appears to have poor self-esteem, it is important for the nurse to know that poor self-esteem may be described as being the difference between:
    ① Identity and body image
    ② Role and body image
    ③ Ego ideal and perceived self
    ④ Body image and ego ideal

44. Henry Stack Sullivan, a psychoanalytical theorist, is credited with:
    ① Considering birth trauma as a primary factor in personality development
    ② Developing a form of mental exploration and treatment called psychodrama
    ③ Believing that the self-concept or self-image is built to a great extent on the reflected appraisals of significant others
    ④ Developing the belief that critical aspects of personality development are to be found in personal interrelationships

45. The psychoanalytical theorist who founded the client-centered therapeutic school that uses the nondirective interview as a technique is:
    ① Carl Rogers
    ② Harry Stack Sullivan
    ③ Eric Berne
    ④ Erik Erikson

46. Adjustment mechanisms or ego defense mechanisms serve the individual by managing anxiety. These mechanisms become a problem when they:
    ① Cause the individual to draw attention to himself
    ② Interfere with the individual's day-to-day functioning
    ③ Create social embarrassment
    ④ Advance the individual's interest above the interests of others

47. Dee Anne was the victim of abuse in her childhood. After a period of psychiatric care, she is able to recall events of her earlier life so that she can begin to deal with them. Which of the following defense mechanisms was Dee Anne using?
    ① Denial
    ② Rationalization
    ③ Projection
    ④ Repression

48. Dollie had an unpleasant interchange with her mother-in-law. She decides to set the matter aside and go on as if the event had never occurred. The nurse recognizes that Dollie is using which of the following defense mechanisms?
    ① Denial
    ② Suppression
    ③ Repression
    ④ Rationalization

49. Tom and Carol have been married for 10 years. Tom is very attractive and has had a number of affairs with other women. He is very jealous of Carol and frequently accuses her of seeing other men. Which of the following defense mechanisms is Tom using?
    ① Denial
    ② Repression
    ③ Rationalization
    ④ Projection

50. Rob presents himself to his co-workers as morally self-righteous. He is rather judgmental and critical of others and continually portrays himself as superior. Rob's co-workers are surprised when Rob is arrested at work for having robbed a drug store. Rob's ego defense mechanism is:
    ① Denial
    ② Repression
    ③ Reaction formation
    ④ Regression

51. When Kathryn was 3, her family moved to another state. Though she had been fully toilet trained, Kathryn began to have frequent episodes of wetting herself. Kathryn's ego defense mechanism is:
    ① Regression
    ② Denial
    ③ Repression
    ④ Reaction formation

52. Barbara is scheduled for a mastectomy. A well-trained nurse, she studies her anatomy books and knows the procedure in detail. She denies having any feelings about the loss of her breast. Barbara's ego defense mechanism is:
    ① Rationalization
    ② Denial
    ③ Intellectualization
    ④ Fantasy

53. Charles is shaving before going to work. Mike, age 4, comes into the bathroom with his toy razor to join his dad in shaving. Mike is exhibiting which of the following defense mechanisms?
    ① Denial
    ② Identification
    ③ Intellectualization
    ④ Regression

54. Nancy has had a bad day at work but finds it unacceptable to tell her boss how angry she is. She comes home and throws her cat out the door. Nancy's defense mechanism is:
    ① Identification
    ② Displacement
    ③ Introjection
    ④ Reaction formation

55. Celeste went through a painful divorce in which she lost her home and most of her possessions. She spends much of her day imagining herself decorating her lovely home using her unlimited wealth. Which of the following cognitive dimensions is Celeste implementing?
    ① Fantasy
    ② Denial
    ③ Repression
    ④ Reaction formation

56. Five-year-old Tommy is admitted to the hospital. At the end of the day, his parents leave. A short time later, the nurse checks on Tommy and observes that his bed is wet. Which of the following defense mechanisms does Tommy's bed wetting exemplify?
    ① Compensation
    ② Denial
    ③ Projection
    ④ Regression

57. Mrs. Sillers, age 80, has been a resident in Westhaven Nursing Home for the past year, after having lived with her daughter for 5 years. Mrs. Sillers tells the nurse caring for her, "All the people around here mumble when they talk; no one speaks clearly; they ought to take some course in speaking correctly!" The nurse knows that Mrs. Sillers could be using which of the following defense mechanisms?
    ① Projection
    ② Denial
    ③ Withdrawal
    ④ Compensation

58. Mr. McCreary is admitted to the hospital for an open biopsy of the left lung and possible pneumonectomy. During the admission process, the nurse asks Mr. McCreary if he has any questions concerning the surgery. Mr. McCreary says "no" and then starts to talk about his daughter's upcoming wedding. The nurse understands that he is using which of the following defense mechanisms?
    ① Denial
    ② Compensation
    ③ Repression
    ④ Suppression

59. Rose and Sandra have been in a committed relationship for 20 years. They are happy together and have many friends as a couple. Sandra recently experienced a tragedy in which two close members of her family died in a motor vehicle accident. One month after the tragedy, Sandra requests psychiatric care for depression and panic-like symptoms as a result of her grief. In performing a comprehensive nursing assessment, the nurse might view Sandra's homosexual lifestyle in what way?
    ① It is a psychiatric disorder that may require therapy
    ② It is an alternative lifestyle that may be a healthy choice for some individuals
    ③ It is a form of character defect that is an indication of moral inferiority
    ④ It is a lifestyle that undermines the well-being of the traditional family

60. Fred is a newlywed. He is worried because he has been experiencing premature ejaculation. He seeks the nurse's advice in the matter. The nurse knows the *best* response to be:
    ① "This is a result of your being under too much stress. Have you considered attending a stress management class?"
    ② "This is a problem you may find appropriate to discuss with your doctor."
    ③ "Many men experience this. You may find it goes away over time."
    ④ "This is something you will need to discuss with your wife."

61. Feelings of increasing threat, decreasing organization, and rapid verbalization are indicative of which of the following anxiety levels:
    ① Mild
    ② Moderate
    ③ Severe
    ④ Panic

62. It is vital for the nurse to know that fear differs from anxiety in that fear is characterized by which of the following?
① A physical response
② A behavioral response
③ A more specific threat
④ A more emotional response

63. The nurse assesses a patient whose perception appears severely restricted and whose thoughts are distorted and disconnected. The patient's logical processes are impaired. The nurse knows the patient is suffering from which of the following anxiety levels:
① Mild
② Moderate
③ Severe
④ Panic

64. Laura is about to graduate from high school. She is uncertain as to her plans for the future and is struggling with several major decisions at once. She comes to the school nurse's office with complaints of tension, headaches, and sleeplessness. The nurse suspects that Laura is experiencing which of the following?
① Phobia
② Depression
③ Anxiety
④ Fear

65. Edward is experiencing a state of heightened alertness, with mildly increased pulse and blood pressure. He has a project that he must complete in a short time, yet he has to wait for some materials that are necessary to the completion of the project. Which of the following statements is *most* accurate regarding Edward's anxiety?
① It may interfere with the completion of his project
② It is not related to his project; he may have something else on his mind
③ This is a normal level of anxiety that most people would experience in relation to a project
④ It will definitely escalate and interfere with the completion of his project

66. The anxiety level that is optimal for learning is:
① Mild
② Moderate
③ Severe
④ Panic

67. A victim of a recent hurricane that has destroyed his home, Louis is experiencing disturbed perceptions, loss of rational thinking, and an inability to follow the nurse's instructions. This is characteristic of which anxiety level?
① Mild
② Moderate
③ Severe
④ Panic

68. Mrs. Sims has been a patient on the mental health unit for 2 weeks, following admission for extreme anxiety and disruptive behavior. Suddenly, Mrs. Sims yells out, "I'm choking! I'm having a heart attack!" The nurse's response should be:
① "Let me take your blood pressure and pulse and I'll report them to the charge nurse."
② "Does this happen often when you feel anxious?"
③ "Have you had a heart attack in the past?"
④ "Relax, take some deep breaths. Breathe in and breathe out slowly. How do you feel now?"

69. Cathy Mills, the older of two girls in a family, recently went away to college. The younger sister Carol is still at home. Their mother, Mrs. Mills, has grown increasingly anxious and depressed, saying that she can't manage the large house and all its problems. Carol, a typical teenager, is frequently upset over demands made by her mother that she considers unfair. Mr. Mills finally brings his wife and daughter to the clinic because he is fed up with all the wrangling. An appropriate intervention strategy should be to:
① Suggest that Mr. Mills arrange to get some temporary housekeeping help
② Suggest that Carol, as the problem focus, enter long-term therapy
③ Suggest that the physician start Mrs. Mills on tranquilizers
④ Suggest that Mr. Mills enter therapy because he asked for help

70. Mrs. Ahern, age 42, has been on the mental health unit for 3 weeks. She was admitted for anxiety that has prevented her from sleeping at night, functioning at work, and caring for her children. She is disruptive on the unit by overturning tables, throwing magazines, and turning off the TV when others are watching it. Mrs. Ahern's anxiety differs from phobias because it:
① Originates from a specific source
② Originates from an uncertain source and can border on the nonrational
③ Comes from tension that arises from danger
④ Allows avoidance of certain situations

71. A nursing observation that would support evidence of the therapeutic effects of antianxiety drug therapy should be:
① Crying, facial grimaces, and rigid posture
② Anger, aggressive behavior
③ Decrease in blood pressure, pulse, and respirations
④ Verbal statements such as "more worried" or "resting poorly"

72. Mr. Ball is a newly admitted schizophrenic. The nurse observes him pacing up and down the corridor, complaining of a terrible headache. He is unable to concentrate on anything but his unattended apartment. The nurse knows Mr. Ball's level of anxiety is:
① Mild
② Moderate
③ Severe
④ Panic

73. Iorazepam (Ativan) is ordered for Mr. Ball by his physician. A common central nervous system side effect to Ativan is:
    ① Drowsiness
    ② Dry mouth
    ③ Dizziness
    ④ Urine retention

74. Melissa is diagnosed with anorexia nervosa and characteristically performs elaborate rituals with her food. She primarily performs these rituals to:
    ① Reinforce feelings of wellness
    ② Control feelings of anxiety
    ③ Increase calorie expenditure
    ④ Maintain personal boundaries

75. Anxiety related to fear of weight gain is the primary nursing diagnosis for a patient with anorexia nervosa. The best nursing intervention for this diagnosis should be to:
    ① Discuss how she uses weight to control anxiety
    ② Point out how unattractive her extreme thinness is
    ③ Explain that being slightly overweight is more healthy
    ④ Discuss the danger she is in from extreme dieting

76. Sylvia is experiencing a mild level of anxiety before a scheduled job interview. Which of the following behaviors displayed by Sylvia would confirm this for the nurse?
    ① Emotionally overwhelmed
    ② Feelings of tension
    ③ Increased perspiration
    ④ Perceptual awareness

77. Donna is recovering from a major mental illness. Her goal is to live on her own and support herself. Her gathering of her personal resources to accomplish this goal is *most* dependent on which of the following?
    ① Frustration
    ② Anxiety
    ③ Motivation
    ④ Stress

78. Hans Selye identified a response to stress, which he called the:
    ① Alternative lifestyle
    ② General adaptation syndrome
    ③ Frustration
    ④ Anxiety

79. Hallucinations are perceptual experiences and are distressing symptoms that may be present in several types of mental illness. The perceptual experience of hallucinations occurs:
    ① As a result of ingestion of street drugs
    ② In the absence of external stimulus
    ③ As a result of conflict
    ④ As a result of frustration

80. Steve believes that he holds the secret to solving the problem with the hole in the ozone layer. Unfortunately, he says, enemy agents are pursuing him in order to steal his secret. The nurse knows that Steve is experiencing which of the following?
    ① Panic
    ② Stress
    ③ A delusion
    ④ A hallucination

81. Linda is suffering from schizophrenia. She has been hearing voices telling her she is "no good." The nurse notices that Linda is becoming more agitated. She tells the nurse that the voices are louder now and they are telling her to "jump off the bridge over the freeway." The nurse's *priority nursing intervention* should be to:
    ① Involve Linda in group activities so that her mind will be occupied and the hallucinations will be less troublesome for her
    ② Explain to Linda that she is a worthwhile human being and that the staff of the hospital is genuinely concerned about her as a person
    ③ Notify her attending psychiatrist and implement immediate suicide precautions
    ④ Spend time with Linda and teach her techniques for handling the hallucinations

82. The nurse is working the night shift on a general surgery floor. Edna, age 52, had surgery 2 days ago for an acute bowel obstruction. At 3 AM, she calls the nurse to her room to report that she sees green snakes coming from the heater vents. There have been no previous reports of Edna's experiencing visual hallucinations. Your priority nursing intervention should be to:
    ① Turn on the light and reassure her that there are no snakes in the hospital
    ② Notify the charge nurse or her attending physician of her visual hallucinations
    ③ Observe and record the nature and quality of her hallucinations
    ④ Check her chart to see if there is any indication of a history of mental illness

83. Steve tells the nurse that FBI agents are after him and plan to kill him. The *best* nursing action would be to:
    ① Point out the irrationality of his belief and assure him that there are no enemy agents trying to get his secret
    ② Focus on his feelings and encourage ways to verbalize them
    ③ Recognize that there is no verbal response that will make this belief go away, therefore say nothing
    ④ Tell him that his belief is amusing

84. Monique has been admitted of treatment for major depression. She believes that she was never a good mother or wife and that she has let her family down. She believes that she is responsible for any bad luck that has come their way. The nurse understands that Monique is experiencing:
    ① Delusions of grandeur
    ② Delusions of persecution
    ③ Delusions of guilt or sin
    ④ Flight of ideas

85. A patient reports "seeing the face of Satan" on the wall of his room. This is an example of:
    ① Delusion
    ② Illusion
    ③ Hallucination
    ④ Regression

86. John is diagnosed as a paranoid schizophrenic. In planning his care, the nurse should:
    ① Offer him several choices for his morning activity
    ② Discuss his care with the charge nurse while standing outside John's room
    ③ Offer him few choices, as she is aware of ambivalence as a symptom of his disease
    ④ Have a male attendant accompany her when giving care to John

87. John H. arrives in the emergency room seeking help. When asked the date, he says it is April 1886. The nurse can *best* describe John as:
    ① Oriented × 3
    ② Not oriented in time
    ③ Confused
    ④ Dishonest

88. The nurse beings to plan care for a patient who is said to have scattered thought processes. To substantiate this, the nurse should base the observation on:
    ① Frequent changes of topic
    ② Rapidity of speech
    ③ Physical appearance
    ④ Recent history

89. Mr. Swanson was admitted to the mental health unit because his family was concerned that he had been withdrawn, apathetic, and careless of his personal body needs. Since his admission, the nurse notes his behavior as isolated and that he talks aloud to no one in particular. Mr. Swanson's symptoms are characteristic of behavior associated with:
    ① Dissociative reaction
    ② Manic depressive reaction
    ③ Schizophrenia
    ④ Paranoid reaction

90. Which of the following is *most appropriate* when the nurse is aware that a patient is hallucinating?
    ① Tell him that there is no one there
    ② Ask him to describe his feelings at this time
    ③ Use simple statements in communicating with him
    ④ Encourage him to participate in self-care

91. The medication of choice in treating a patient with a diagnosis of schizophrenia comes from the group of antidepressants known as:
    ① Tricyclics
    ② Tetracyclics
    ③ Monoamine oxidases
    ④ Trazdone hydrochlorides

92. Side effects of the antidepressant group monoamine oxidases that the nurse must observe for are:
    ① Lowered blood pressure, increased ocular pressure, and tachycardia
    ② Flushing, diaphoresis, and dry mouth
    ③ Drowsiness
    ④ Confusion

93. In caring for a patient who is receiving monoamine oxidase inhibitors, the nurse is aware that the drug can be dangerous when combined with certain foods. The substance in these foods is called:
    ① Histamine
    ② Phenylalanine
    ③ Lysine
    ④ Tyramine

94. Mr. Edwards has been receiving chlorpromazine (Thorazine) for treatment of auditory hallucinations associated with schizophrenia. Which of the following statements by Mr. Edwards should indicate to the nurse that the chlorpromazine is effective?
    ① "I hear a different voice now."
    ② "I'm not hearing any voices right now."
    ③ "Sometimes I hear voices; sometimes I don't."
    ④ "The voices aren't as loud as they were."

95. Mr. Earl is diagnosed as a paranoid schizophrenic patient. He refuses to eat, telling the nurse the food is poisoned. The *most appropriate* nursing intervention should be to:
    ① Allow food brought from home
    ② Ignore him; he'll eat when he's hungry
    ③ Provide foods in their own containers
    ④ Tell him that feeding tubes are used on patients who don't eat

96. The nurse is sitting with Mr. Earl one day when he turns and says, "Isn't that singing beautiful!" The nurse does not hear anything and concludes that Mr. Earl is probably experiencing a hallucination. The *best response* by the nurse should be:
    ① "I understand you think you hear singing; however, I don't hear anything."
    ② "Tell me the words to the song."
    ③ "What are you talking about? I don't hear any singing."
    ④ "Yes, I'm enjoying the song."

97. Ms. Hamilton is admitted to a psychiatric unit with a 3-month history of depression. Physician's orders include a monoamine oxidase inhibitor and a tyramine-restricted diet. Of the following foods, the nurse knows that Ms. Hamilton is allowed to have:
    ① Chocolate cake
    ② Cottage cheese
    ③ Green beans
    ④ Summer sausage

98. Mrs. Stokes has been hospitalized on a psychiatric unit for 6 years as a committed patient with a diagnosis of schizophrenia. The nurse should expect Mrs. Stokes to be receiving which of the following medications?
    ① Buspirone (Buspar)
    ② Chlorpromazine (Thorazine)
    ③ Lithium carbonate (Lithium)
    ④ Fluoxetine (Prozac)

99. Mr. Moon is a psychiatric patient on chlorpromazine (Thorazine). Which of the following is a central nervous system side effect of chlorpromazine?
    ① Dry mouth
    ② Dyspnea
    ③ Hypotension
    ④ Syncope

100. A patient is diagnosed with schizophrenia. When the nurse is formulating a teaching plan for the patient and his family, what is the *best* thing to tell them about the action of his antipsychotic medication?
    ① The medication works on the nervous system
    ② The medication stabilizes the patient's mood and behavior
    ③ The medication increases the patient's sense of reality
    ④ The medication blocks adrenaline uptake

101. Dave, age 21, is admitted to the mental health unit with a diagnosis of schizophrenia. In the initial interview, Dave's parents indicate he has isolated himself from the family, quit his job, and dropped out of college. The nurse knows which of the following data to be *most characteristic* of schizophrenia?
    ① Unstable mood and delusions of grandeur
    ② Auditory hallucinations and altered thought processes
    ③ Depressive thoughts and low self-esteem
    ④ Lack of judgment and involvement in complicated legal problems

102. Dave, a 21-year-old schizophrenic, is withdrawn, negativistic, and hallucinating. In attempting to activate him, the *most appropriate* nursing intervention should be to:
    ① Invite him to play a simple card game
    ② Insist that he join a group activity
    ③ Explain the benefits of activity
    ④ Mention that his "voices" would want him to participate

103. Dave, a schizophrenic patient, is experiencing racing thoughts, looseness of association, and the belief that he is being controlled by others. He is easily distracted, has trouble with abstract reasoning, and is hearing voices. To help Dave get through his day at his best level of functioning, the nurse plans to:
    ① Provide him with a simple structured schedule to follow
    ② Engage him in talking about the feelings he is experiencing
    ③ Allow him to remain in his room until he feels better
    ④ Offer him the use of mechanical restraints to help him control himself

104. Carolyn is a schizophrenic patient. Following a thorough medical and psychiatric evaluation, Carolyn receives a prescription for haloperidol (Haldol), a major tranquilizer. In planning care with Carolyn, the nurse cautions her to expect which of the following common side effects?
    ① Headache and nausea
    ② Skin rash and itching
    ③ Increased sex drive and breast size
    ④ Dry mouth and blurred vision

105. After the first two doses of haloperidol (Haldol), Carolyn begins to pace and states that she feels "antsy" and can't sit still. Her neck becomes stiff and twists to one side, then her eyes roll upward. These symptoms are consistent with:
    ① A severe allergic reaction
    ② An extrapyramidal reaction
    ③ A worsening of the patient's psychosis
    ④ A rare side effect

106. Carolyn's reaction to haloperidol (Haldol) is most likely to be controlled by which medication?
    ① Acetylsalicylic acid (Aspirin)
    ② Lorazepam (Ativan)
    ③ Benzotropine (Cogentin)
    ④ Lithium carbonate (Lithium)

107. Geoff, age 37, works as an air traffic controller at a local airport. He was recently suspended from his job when he told his supervisor that his co-workers had a plot to steal his wife and kill his dog. Delusions of persecution are associated with which type of schizophrenia?
    ① Catatonic
    ② Disorganized
    ③ Paranoid
    ④ Undifferentiated

108. On admission to the hospital, Geoff is hearing command hallucinations directing him to kill the men whom he believes to be a threat to his family. The *priority* nursing intervention should be to:
    ① Attempt to engage him in therapeutic activities to distract him from these distressing thoughts
    ② Notify all staff immediately so that elopement precautions can be instituted
    ③ Attempt to establish a rapport with the patient, hoping that you will be able to influence him not to kill anyone
    ④ Contact a chaplain who can discuss with the patient the moral consequences of killing

109. Mr. Jones is a paranoid schizophrenic patient discharged from a psychiatric facility 2 months ago with the medication thiothixene (Navane) 30 mg PO hs. He calls the unit and complains that "Every time I turn around, I have to go to the pharmacy to have my prescription filled." He becomes verbally abusive and insists on a 6-month supply of thiothixene so he doesn't have to go to the pharmacy so often. The *best* nursing response to Mr. Jones should be:
    ① "Relax, Mr. Jones. We'll send you a prescription for a 6-month supply."
    ② "You sound upset, Mr. Jones. Why don't you come to the hospital and we'll discuss your problem?"
    ③ "You're on a highly potent medication, Mr. Jones, and the doctors here never prescribe more than a 30-day supply at one time."
    ④ "You're not working, Mr. Jones, so you have plenty of time to go to the pharmacy."

110. Mrs. Kale is a paranoid schizophrenic being treated with chlorpromazine (Thorazine). Which statement by Mrs. Kale would indicate that she has an appropriate understanding of necessary precautions to take while receiving chlorpromazine?
    ① "How can I control this runny nose?"
    ② "I'll be sure to take my medication before each meal."
    ③ "I'll be sure to increase my food intake."
    ④ "Which sunscreen should I buy?"

111. Mr. Sawyer is a schizophrenic patient who experiences delusions of persecution. The nurse recognizes that delusions are a source of protection for the patient and she can expect these delusions to be abandoned under which of the following circumstances?
    ① When the nurse can joke with the patient about his beliefs
    ② When the patient feels safe and secure
    ③ When the patient gains insight into his delusional state
    ④ When the patient is convinced that the nurse likes him

112. Jack, age 20, is having an acute psychotic episode. He is hearing voices that direct him to run from the hospital and jump off a freeway overpass. He is unable to control the impulses that result from the voices he hears. If Jack is placed in seclusion against his will, the nurse is aware that this intervention raises an ethical issue because it is:
    1. Considered to be a crime
    2. A decision based on moral belief
    3. Viewed as control of personal freedom
    4. An obligation of the nurse to protect him from manifestations of illness

113. A patient on the mental health unit is disruptive. He overturns tables and throws anything he can get his hands on at staff, as well as at other patients. Setting limits on the patient's behavior can be done when the nurse:
    1. Considers the morale and safety of other patients
    2. Considers the degree of the staff's responsibility from a legal point of view
    3. Adheres strictly to all rules and regulations
    4. Appreciates the value the patient attaches to each situation

114. A patient is admitted to the mental health unit. During the admission process, the nurse notes that he speaks quite rapidly while frequently changing topics. This patient's speech pattern is described as:
    1. Unintelligible
    2. Disorganized
    3. Variable
    4. Pressured

115. Anna has just been admitted to the psychiatric unit with a diagnosis of bipolar disorder, manic phase. In assessing Anna's emotional status, which of the following should the nurse expect her to say when asked if she is concerned about her family?
    1. "I'm worried about their welfare."
    2. "I'm a failure as a wife."
    3. "Why should I be worried?"
    4. "I just hope they're okay."

116. One of the primary diagnoses for the patient with mania is altered nutrition: less than body requirements related to hyperactivity. The nurse's *best* intervention should be to:
    1. Provide her with small, easily carried foods
    2. Provide large, high-protein meals
    3. Provide a quiet mealtime environment
    4. Provide her with extra vitamin supplements

117. The *best* way for the nurse to see if the manic patient is beginning to attain normal nutritional status is to verify that:
    1. Her appetite is maintained
    2. She eats at scheduled times
    3. Her weight is maintained
    4. Her meals are finished

118. The nurse observes Anna playing cards with another patient, Anna is smiling and conversing quietly. She loses a hand and begins to curse and scream at her partner. This demonstrates which of the following?
    1. Flight of ideas
    2. Ideas of reference
    3. Mood instability
    4. Loose associations

119. The *best* intervention for the nurse when a manic patient is acting out while playing cards with another patient is to:
    1. Ask both of them to leave the game area with you
    2. Ask the other patient to leave the game area
    3. Scold the patient for her inappropriate behavior
    4. Explain the rules of the game to the patient

120. After leaving the unit during a visit, a manic patient's mother calls the nurse from home to report that her son threatened to hit her. Which of the following diagnoses would the nurse add to the patient's care plan?
    1. Ineffective family coping related to hospitalization
    2. Anxiety related to inability to cope with their son's illness
    3. Potential for violence related to unstable mood and affect
    4. Potential for self-injury related to loss of control

121. A patient's mother asks what she should do if her son threatens to hit or hurt her after she takes him home from the hospital. The nurse's *best* response would be:
    1. "Yell for someone's help when he threatens you."
    2. "In a calm voice, direct him to leave the area."
    3. "Ignore his threats. He wouldn't really hit you."
    4. "Call the authorities to have him restrained."

122. When the nurse checks a manic patient's chart for his lithium level, she finds that it is 2 mEq/L. The interpretation/action by the nurse should be:
    1. This level is within therapeutic range; do nothing
    2. This level is below therapeutic range; call the physician
    3. This level is slightly high but does not require action
    4. This level is high; he should be assessed for signs/symptoms of toxicity

123. A patient receiving Lithium complains of blurred vision and frequent urination. The nurse also notices that the patient is having difficulty maintaining his or her balance. Which of the following nursing actions is appropriate?
    1. Administer an antiparkinsonian drug, such as benztropine (Cogentin)
    2. Take the patient's vital signs and administer high-potassium fluids
    3. Hold the patient's next dose of medication and call the physician immediately
    4. Sit with the patient to teach her about the side effects of Lithium

124. The nurse observes that a patient moves very quickly from one idea to another and that there is no connection between them. The nurse knows that the patient is demonstrating:
    1. Confabulation
    2. Primary process
    3. Flight of ideas
    4. Neologisms

125. Jacqueline, age 45, has been admitted for treatment of bipolar disorder, manic phase. She exhibits constant activity and pressured speech. She has been sleeping only 2 hours a night for weeks and is physically exhausted. The *priority* nursing intervention should be to:
    ① Show her to her room and insist that she remain there and take a nap
    ② Show her to her room and remain with her, talking calmly and showing her some relaxation exercises
    ③ Administer the prescribed medication and wait until its effects cause her to become drowsy
    ④ Show her to the dayroom where several patients are engaged in activity

126. The psychiatrist has prescribed haloperidol (Haldol) and lithium carbonate (Lithium) to treat Jacqueline's bipolar disorder. The nurse knows the primary purpose of haloperidol for Jacqueline is to:
    ① Provide sedation
    ② Provide a "chemical restraint"
    ③ Stimulate her appetite
    ④ Alleviate anxiety

127. Lithium, commonly used to treat bipolar disorder, is effective as a mood stabilizer. In planning care for the patient receiving lithium carbonate (Lithium), the nurse should monitor for which of the following side effects?
    ① Food cravings
    ② Fine tremors
    ③ Worsening of psychotic symptoms
    ④ Sensitivity to sunlight

128. Mrs. Hensch is admitted to the psychiatric unit with a diagnosis of bipolar disorder, manic phase. The physician orders lithium carbonate 500 mg PO tid. In planning care for Mrs. Hensch, when should the nurse schedule serum lithium levels to be drawn?
    ① Any time of day
    ② In the evening after the last dose of the day
    ③ In the morning before the first dose of the day
    ④ Only when the previous level exceeds 1.5 mEq/L

129. When monitoring Mrs. Hensch for side effects of lithium carbonate, which of the following manifestations should the nurse observe for?
    ① Dry mouth
    ② Blurred vision
    ③ Dysarthria
    ④ Muscular weakness

130. Mrs. Hensch is receiving lithium carbonate 500 mg PO tid for treatment of bipolar disorder, manic phase. After 3 days of lithium carbonate (Lithium) treatment for Mrs. Hench, Mr. Hench approaches the nurse and says, "I don't see any difference in my wife since she was started on Lithium." The nurse's *best* response should be:
    ① "Let me call the physician to discuss this with you."
    ② "It can take up to several weeks for mood stabilizing effects to occur."
    ③ "We can add a neuroleptic to achieve more rapid treatment."
    ④ "Some bipolar patients require long-term therapy with Lithium."

131. Mrs. Hensch is on salt lithium carbonate 500 mg PO tid. Her last serum lithium level was 0.3 mEq/L 4 weeks ago. On routine rounds, the nurse observes that Mrs. Hensch is lethargic and unresponsive to verbal and tactile stimuli. The nurse's *priority action* should be to:
    ① Call a code
    ② Increase Mrs. Hensch's fluid intake
    ③ Notify the physician
    ④ Take Mrs. Hensch's vital signs

132. Mrs. Hensch is soon to be discharged with the medication lithium carbonate (Lithium) to be taken 500 mg PO tid. Which statement by Mrs. Hensch indicates that she understands the importance of compliance with her medication regime?
    ① "If I miss a dose, I'll have to take an extra dose before I go to bed."
    ② "If I miss a dose, I'll have to go to the lab and have a lithium level drawn."
    ③ "If I miss a dose, I'll have to increase the sodium in my diet."
    ④ "If I miss a dose, what should I do besides notify my physician?"

133. Mrs. Hensch is diagnosed with bipolar disorder, manic phase. Lithium carbonate is prescribed for her, along with a neuroleptic. The nurse understands the action of lithium carbonate (Lithium) to be that of:
    ① Decreasing her depression
    ② Increasing her libido
    ③ Increasing her affect
    ④ Stabilizing her affect

134. Approximately one third of patients with bipolar disorder do not respond to lithium carbonate (Lithium) therapy. Carbamazepine (Tegretol) is sometimes prescribed in such cases. When caring for a patient who is receiving carbamazepine, the nurse should plan to regularly check which of the following diagnostic data?
    ① Blood sugar level
    ② Complete blood count
    ③ Gastric analysis
    ④ Urine for culture and sensitivity

135. Maggie is admitted to the psychiatric unit with a diagnosis of bipolar disorder, manic phase. Maggie is hyperactive, restless, agitated, and hostile. The *priority* nursing diagnosis for Maggie should be:
    ① Altered nutrition: less than body requirements, related to inattention to need for food
    ② Potential for injury: falls, related to hyperactivity
    ③ Potential for violence: self-directed related to hostility
    ④ Sleep pattern disturbance related to hyperactivity

136. During periods of extreme elation and overactivity, the manic patient needs a structured environment. In planning activities, the nurse considers which of the following?
    ① Asking the patient for suggestions in planning unit activities
    ② Keeping her from assuming more responsibility than she can handle
    ③ Putting her in charge of a unit project with a group of patients
    ④ Suggesting activities that require concentration; limiting physical activity

137. Your manic patient has begun to call other patients derogatory names and uses profanity in her conversations. The most appropriate nursing intervention should be to:
    ① Ignore the comments
    ② Tell the patient that her behavior will be reported to the physician
    ③ Set limits to this behavior
    ④ Instruct the other patients to ignore her behavior

138. Jacob has been a severe alcoholic for years. Hospitalized for 3 days, he is in alcohol withdrawal. He complains of bugs and rats crawling on his skin. The nurse knows that Jacob is experiencing which of the following types of hallucinations?
    ① Olfactory
    ② Visual
    ③ Auditory
    ④ Tactile

139. Mr. Jackson was admitted to the mental health unit because he was withdrawn and apathetic. After 3 weeks of taking prescribed medication, he appears to be receptive to further therapy. The *best type* of therapy should include:
    ① Therapeutic group sessions
    ② Transactional analysis group sessions
    ③ Relaxation therapy group sessions
    ④ Reality orientation group sessions

140. Raphel, age 19, is brought to the crisis center after being bailed out of jail for acts of vandalism. His father is requesting a mental health evaluation. The nurse should assess Raphel for what additional characteristics of antisocial personality disorder:
    ① Difficulty maintaining employment
    ② Impulsive, unpredictable behavior
    ③ Dramatic, attention-seeking behavior
    ④ Intentional inefficiency

141. The antisocial personality presents numerous problematic behaviors. The nurse knows that to decrease manipulative behavior, an appropriate nursing intervention should be to:
    ① Immediately set limits on all behavior
    ② Set limits only in those areas necessary to protect the patient
    ③ Let the patient decide the limits to be set
    ④ Allow the community to set limits on the patient's behavior

142. When setting limits on a patient's behavior, the nurse must identify the consequences to the patient should he exceed the established limits. The nurse knows that the *most appropriate* time to establish consequences is:
    ① Just before the anticipated behavior
    ② After the patient has exceeded the set limits
    ③ At the time the limits are set
    ④ When the staff can no longer tolerate the patient's behavior

143. An appropriate goal toward which the patient with personality disorder can work during hospitalization is:
    ① Establishing a stable marital relationship
    ② Planning for productive employment
    ③ Understanding the consequences of substance use
    ④ Finding nondestructive ways to meet needs

144. The primary mechanism by which a patient with a personality disorder will attempt to have needs met by others is:
    ① Manipulation
    ② Projection
    ③ Repression
    ④ Sublimation

145. On the basis of his or her knowledge of the causes of mental illness, the nurse knows that the development of a personality disorder is *most likely* caused by:
    ① A biochemical imbalance
    ② A genetic predisposition
    ③ A parental/family dysfunction
    ④ A birth complication

146. On the basis of her knowledge of personality disorders, the nurse should expect which of the following to be the *primary* problem for these patients during hospitalization?
    ① Participating in activities
    ② Withdrawal from substances
    ③ Observing unit rules
    ④ Relationships with others

147. "Addiction" to a substance means that a person has:
    ① Physiologic dependence
    ② Psychologic dependence
    ③ Both physiologic and psychologic dependence
    ④ Either physiologic or psychologic dependence

148. Of the following systems, which is the most seriously affected by long-term alcohol abuse?
    ① Endocrine
    ② Cardiovascular
    ③ Musculoskeletal
    ④ Reproductive

149. The son of a delirious patient states, "I feel so helpless. I just don't know what to do." Which of the following is the *best way* to help the patient's son deal with his mother's illness?
    ① Reassure him that his mother will be fine in a few days
    ② Suggest that he not visit her until she improves
    ③ Role model how best to interact with his mother
    ④ Refer him to the physician to answer his concerns

150. Sylvia is diagnosed with multiple personality disorder. The nurse understands that the basic explanation of a personality disorder is:
    ① A maladaptation that is most apparent within an interpersonal or social context
    ② The capacity to induce others to feel extreme irritation and annoyance
    ③ A self-centered, inflexible approach to work and interpersonal relationships
    ④ The tendency to be overly concerned with having a good time and entertaining others

151. Art is a 25-year-old outpatient at the local mental health clinic. Although he appears witty and charming, he has had several "scrapes" with the law. He has been unable to hold down a job for any length of time and is a high school dropout. He is an habitual liar and has broken off many relationships with young women. The nurse recognizes these behaviors as consistent with which of the following personality disorders?
   ① Avoidant personality
   ② Schizotypal personality
   ③ Antisocial personality
   ④ Impulsive personality

152. George is identified as having a disruptive lifestyle. The nurse understands that George can be expected to manifest which of the following behaviors?
   ① An illness
   ② A perceptual or affective disorder
   ③ A maladaptive coping style
   ④ A genetically inherited dysfunction

153. Tony is diagnosed as having an antisocial personality disorder. An expected treatment goal for Tony should be:
   ① Success with medication regime
   ② Highly successful group therapy
   ③ Long-term psychotherapy
   ④ Decrease in his anxiety

154. Chip has been a patient on the mental health unit for 1 week and is diagnosed with a paranoid personality disorder. He exhibits mistrust, hypersensitivity, and restricted feelings. The nurse should expect Chip's restricted feelings to be evidenced by which of the following behaviors?
   ① Sentimentality
   ② Lack of a sense of humor
   ③ Self-indulgence
   ④ Attention-seeking behavior

155. An appropriate nursing intervention for a patient with a paranoid personality disorder would be to:
   ① Maintain honest, clear, open communication
   ② Reduce social contact because interactions precipitate further distortions
   ③ Make decisions for him to reduce added stress
   ④ Avoid discussing his treatment plan with him

156. The nurse working in an inner city emergency room is called on to present a community education program on drug abuse. She presents the fact that drugs of the opiate class include medicinal drugs. She discusses heroin, which is also in this class but is not used medicinally in the United States. The nurse will discuss the clinical symptoms of the effect of the opiate class of drugs which include:
   ① Sweating, abdominal pain, and diarrhea
   ② Pinpoint pupils, euphoria, and respiratory depression
   ③ Dilated pupils, drowsiness, and visual hallucinations
   ④ Hypervigilance, hallucinations, and heightened capacity to concentrate

157. Ray is brought to the hospital by two friends. He is a 19-year-old college student who is known to have experimented with drugs. Ray is in a psychotic, violent, and agitated state. His pupils are dilated and he is having vivid visual hallucinations. His skin is flushed and is hot and dry to touch. On the basis of these assessment data, the nurse suspects intoxication with:
   ① Heroin
   ② PCP or Angel Dust
   ③ Barbiturates
   ④ Marijuana or grass

158. Two police officers escort Chuck to the emergency room. Chuck has some minor injuries from an automobile accident that he has caused. After the physician has examined him and his injuries are treated, the physician requests a blood alcohol level. The nurse knows the blood alcohol that legally indicated intoxication is:
   ① 0.25 mg/dl
   ② 0.5 mg/dl
   ③ 0.10 mg/dl
   ④ 0.05 mg/dl

159. Chuck, a newly admitted detox patient, has a hangover. The nurse would expect which of the following signs and symptoms of Chuck's condition?
   ① Prolonged, elevated blood levels of alcohol
   ② Hyperglycemia and decrease in lactic acid in the blood
   ③ Prolonged sense of euphoria
   ④ Headache and irritability

160. Several years ago, Chuck began the use of alcohol. Recently he has been drinking on a daily basis. On the morning following a binge, he has no memory of events of the evening before. Chuck is experiencing which of the following signs of alcoholism?
   ① Social impairment
   ② Wernicke's syndrome
   ③ Blackout
   ④ Selective memory

161. For nervousness, Margaret has been given diazepam (Valium) for several years by her physician. Over the past year, she has begun to use the medication daily. In addition to daily use of Valium, Margaret has begun to drink alcohol daily. The nurse knows diazepam (Valium) to be the second most commonly abused drug classified as:
   ① Amphetamines
   ② Cocaine
   ③ Narcotic
   ④ Sedative/barbiturate

162. Margaret's withdrawal from diazepam (Valium) is complicated by her use of alcohol. The nurse understands that the reason for this is that:
   ① She is becoming an alcoholic and is therefore less motivated
   ② Alcohol and diazepam are cross-tolerant drugs
   ③ She began using the diazepam as a prescription drug and the alcohol is a nonprescription drug
   ④ Once she is no longer receiving diazepam, the alcohol will not be a problem for her

163. Margaret has been in the hospital for 3 days. She is experiencing withdrawal symptoms from alcohol and diazepam (Valium). The nurse should expect to see which of the following symptoms?
① Confusion, disorientation, and stupor
② Irritability, restlessness, and insomnia
③ Gregariousness, euphoria, and irritability
④ Seizures, coma, and death

164. Margaret is withdrawing from alcohol and diazepam (Valium). The *priority* nursing intervention for patients experiencing withdrawal would be:
① Monitoring the vital signs, emotional support, and encouragement
② Insistence on attendance at all group therapy sessions
③ Strict enforcement of mental health unit rules
④ Exploration of feelings about the experience

165. Claire is a dancer in the city ballet. Her profession demands that she keep her weight down. After the birth of her last child, Claire had difficulty losing weight. She acquired some amphetamines from a friend to help her lose weight. After 6 months of steady use, she has become dependent on the drugs. On admission to the hospital, Claire is malnourished and exhausted. On assessment, which additional signs of amphetamine use should the nurse expect to find?
① Mild-mannered and compliant
② Disoriented and disheveled
③ Psychotic and delusional
④ Mildly paranoid and irritable

166. Claire is experiencing amphetamine withdrawal. The nurse knows which of the following to be classic signs of amphetamine withdrawal?
① Chest pain, diaphoresis, and palpitations
② Euphoria, hyperactivity, and alertness
③ Profuse sweating, gooseflesh, and diarrhea
④ Depression, fatigue, and lethargy

167. Yvonne is a successful artist. She began to experiment with cocaine, believing that it improved her ability to be creative in her work. The recent death of a friend from cocaine abuse has convinced her to seek treatment to discontinue using the drug. In addition to cravings from the drug, what should the nurse expect Yvonne to experience during her withdrawal from cocaine?
① Palpitations
② Paranoia
③ Euphoria
④ Depression

168. Warren has been using heroin for several years. He sells drugs and commits other antisocial acts to support his habit. Arrested for robbing a convenience store, he is still intoxicated with heroin when he is involuntarily admitted to the mental health unit. The nurse should expect to see which of the following symptoms of drug intoxication?
① Dilated pupils
② Hostility
③ Pinpoint pupils
④ Profound depression

169. Warren is hospitalized for heroin intoxication. Four hours after admission, what change should the nurse expect to notice in Warren's condition as a result of the beginning of his withdrawal syndrome?
① Dilated pupils
② Hostility
③ Pinpoint pupils
④ Profound depression

170. To relieve some of the serious neurologic symptoms of delirium tremens, the nurse should anticipate the physician ordering which of the following medications while the patient is in withdrawal?
① Disulfiram (Antabuse)
② Calcium
③ Magnesium sulfate
④ Morphine sulfate

171. Mr. Stanley is experiencing delirium tremens. The nurse should implement which of the following *priority actions?*
① Discussing benefits of Alcoholics Anonymous (AA)
② Keeping him awake and oriented
③ Monitoring vital signs
④ Recording hourly outputs

172. Mr. Stanley is recovering nicely from alcohol withdrawal. The nurse attempts a conversation with him. When the nurse begins to speak of alcoholism, Mr. Stanley lapses into a period of silence. To be *most* helpful, the nurse should:
① Sit in silence with him
② Suggest they talk later
③ Change the topic of the conversation
④ Acknowledge his silence and encourage him to speak

173. Beth's father has just been diagnosed with Alzheimer's disease. With which of the following would he experience the most difficulty in stage one of Alzheimer's disease?
① Getting dressed
② Remembering telephone numbers
③ Walking up and down stairs
④ Brushing his teeth

174. Which of the following questions would most effectively allow the nurse to judge the emotional changes that a patient with Alzheimer's disease is experiencing as a result of the illness?
① "Have you noticed any forgetfulness?"
② "Are you still able to care for yourself?"
③ "Is it difficult for you to make decisions?"
④ "Have you been feeling depressed lately?"

175. During his admission assessment, a patient with Alzheimer's disease tells the nurse, "You ask too many questions. Why can't you just leave me alone?" What is the *best* way for the nurse to respond?
① "These are important questions. We have to continue."
② "I know that you don't really feel that way."
③ "You sound upset. Would you like to rest for awhile?"
④ "You know your family wants you to cooperate."

176. While he is waiting to have a computed tomography (CT) scan performed, a patient with Alzheimer's disease becomes anxious and restless and cannot follow the instructions that the staff gives him to prepare for his examination. Which of the following is the *best* nursing intervention at this time?
    1. Allow him to respond to instructions when he feels ready
    2. Give him written rather than verbal instructions
    3. Tell him he will have to leave if he cannot cooperate
    4. Take him to a quiet place to wait for his scan

177. The family of an Alzheimer's disease patient asks the nurse how long it will take him to recover. What is the *best* answer?
    1. "With proper treatment and care, not that long."
    2. "There is no way to tell how long he will be ill."
    3. "He will not be able to regain what was lost."
    4. "He will continue to get progressively worse."

178. Audrey, a 90-year-old widow, is experiencing forgetfulness, confusion, and bouts of disorientation that are worse at night. A medical diagnosis of Alzheimer's disease has been made. The nurse serves the meal and later returns to find the tray untouched. On the basis of the nurse's understanding of this patient's condition, the nurse believes the most likely cause of refusal to eat is that the patient:
    1. Does not care for hospital food
    2. Is too forgetful to remember to feed herself
    3. May believe the food is poisoned
    4. Is too depressed to eat

179. Audrey has Alzheimer's disease. To support her nutritional needs, the nurse's *priority* nursing intervention should be to:
    1. Have a staff member feed Audrey
    2. Have the nutritionist come to talk with Audrey about her food preferences
    3. Have a staff member or a family member remain with Audrey while she is eating
    4. Talk with Audrey about her nutritional needs

180. The nurse observes that, while hospitalized, Audrey naps during the day but tends to become agitated and wander during the night. This behavior, called "sundowning," is common to patients who have organic mental disorders. The *best* nursing intervention for sundowning is to:
    1. Request a sleeping medication from the physician that will enable Audrey to get some rest
    2. Interrupt Audrey's napping in the daytime so that she can rest better at night
    3. Ask Audrey the next morning if anything had bothered her the night before
    4. Have Audrey sleep in a room that is well lit

181. Mr. Touhey has a leg paralysis for which no physiologic cause can be identified. Because of the patient's psychosocial history, the physician suspects a conversion reaction. The nurse understands that a conversion reaction enables an individual to:
    1. Dismiss uncomfortable thoughts or feelings
    2. Find an acceptable excuse for his behavior
    3. Blame someone or something for his action
    4. Express emotions through physical symptoms

182. Jayne, a 34-year-old single parent, is hospitalized for obsessive-compulsive disorder and depression. Jayne's compulsion is washing. She repeatedly scrubs her hands, arrives late for meals, and neglects her nutritional intake. An appropriate nursing intervention to increase Jayne's nutritional intake should be to:
    1. Interrupt the patient's ritual and tell her she must come to the dining room
    2. Tell the patient how silly she's being and that eating is the priority
    3. Instruct her to hurry up; her meal is getting cold
    4. Provide her with nutritious between-meal snacks

183. A short-term goal for an obsessive-compulsive disorder patient should be to decrease the incidence of compulsive behavior. The patient is considered to be responding positively to treatment if he or she:
    1. Outwardly attempts to ignore or suppress impulses
    2. Decreases repetitive performance of ritualistic acts
    3. Verbalizes difficulty in being self-reflective
    4. Expresses a need to control the immediate environment

184. Will was involved in a plane crash 5 years ago. In addition to surviving the crash, he was able to help save the lives of two other people. After the events of the crash, Will returned to his family and his job. On the outside, he had appeared to be doing well. But he has just been admitted to the mental health unit with a diagnosis of post-traumatic stress disorder. The nurse should assess for which of the following symptoms?
    1. Lethargy and disorientation
    2. Paranoia and suspiciousness
    3. Mutism and immobility
    4. Nightmares and anxiety

185. Sally is a buyer for a local department store. She is good at her job, but she annoys her co-workers with her rigid, detail-oriented manner. Sally has definite characteristics of a compulsive personality disorder. Which of the following behaviors should the nurse expect Sally to also demonstrate as a result of this disorder?
    1. Attention seeking
    2. Impulsiveness
    3. Magical thinking
    4. Superior attitude

186. Sally is diagnosed with a compulsive personality disorder. The nurse understands that Sally's interpersonal relationships are most apt to be negatively affected by which of the following behaviors characteristic of compulsive personality disorders?
    1. Perfectionistic
    2. Decisive
    3. Empathetic
    4. Cooperative

187. Which of the following should be the most appropriate nursing intervention for a patient with a compulsive personality disorder?
    1. Teaching relaxation techniques
    2. Avoiding discussion of compulsive behavior
    3. Contracting for amount of time spent doing compulsive behavior
    4. Joining an assertiveness training group

188. The self-concept of the patient with restricting anorexia is based mainly on the idea that thinness will:
    ① Increase their acceptability to others
    ② Increase their mental abilities
    ③ Increase their feelings of power over others
    ④ Increase their feelings of safety

189. Valerie is a 20-year-old college student. Although she is physically attractive, she worries excessively about her weight. Valerie has learned that she can eat anything she wants as long as she can go the the bathroom and make herself vomit after eating. The nurse suspects that Valerie is suffering from:
    ① Anorexia nervosa
    ② Bulimia
    ③ Agoraphobia
    ④ Narcissistic personality disorder

190. Ann plays with her food at mealtime and only occasionally puts a very small amount of food on the tip of the fork to eat. The nurse expects patients with anorexia nervosa to:
    ① Eat large amounts of food periodically
    ② Enjoy eating large amounts of food periodically
    ③ Fear being fat
    ④ Feel hungry constantly

191. Ann, age 16, has been diagnosed with anorexia nervosa. She has lost 24 pounds in 3 months. She weighs 102 pounds and is 5 feet 4 inches tall. Ann tells the nurse that she is still overweight until her hands and feet get smaller. The *priority* nursing diagnosis for Ann is:
    ① Altered nutrition: less than body requirements related to lack of interest in eating
    ② Body image disturbance related to distorted perceptions
    ③ Impaired social interactions related to manipulative behavior
    ④ Potential for violence: self-directed, related to suicidal feelings

192. Ann's parents have agreed to participate in a case conference. Knowing that family dynamics play a role in the illness of the patient with anorexia nervosa, the nurse would expect Ann's parents to display which of the following behaviors?
    ① Immature and eager to please
    ② Overprotective and rigid
    ③ Passive and nonassertive
    ④ Secretive and stubborn

193. An appropriate nursing goal for a patient who is in the terminal stages of an illness should be:
    ① Assisting the patient through each stage of the death and dying process
    ② Reassuring the patient that he or she has nothing to fear in death
    ③ Secluding the patient from others
    ④ Engaging the patient in future planning

194. In evaluating the outcome of care, the nurse reads the following in the care plan: "Patient will understand his medication regimen in 5 days." Although this is a desirable goal, the nurse auditing the care plan knows that:
    ① This goal is not an achievable outcome
    ② This goal is not directly observable
    ③ This goal is unrealistic
    ④ This is a behavioral goal

195. A patient is being prepared for discharge and followup visits at the community mental health center. A goal of community mental health is to:
    ① Quickly return patients to their community
    ② Ensure that the whole community is mentally healthy
    ③ Hospitalize patients away from their communities
    ④ Restructure the community

196. The patient is responding well to drug therapy and is placed in group sessions. Group activities can be expected to be effective if they are:
    ① Democratic in principle, permitting change and providing spontaneity and variety
    ② Scheduled on a fixed agenda
    ③ Practical and presented at the patient's level of function
    ④ Structured to repress aggressive behavior

197. Mr. Smith has an inoperable brain tumor and is in the terminal phase of his illness. While being helped with his morning bath, he begins to talk about dying. The best response by the nurse should be to:
    ① Ask if he would like to see a member of the clergy
    ② Say little and listen to what Mr. Smith has to say
    ③ Act as if she did not hear him and excuse herself from the room
    ④ Encourage Mr. Smith to keep his hope up and think positively

198. Which of the following statements indicates the nurse's understanding of what it means to establish a contract with a psychiatric patient?
    ① It emphasizes what the nurse will do for the patient
    ② It emphasizes what the nurse will not do for the patient
    ③ It states the nurse's level of participation
    ④ It states the patient's responsibilities

199. Mr. Moon is a psychiatric patient with a history of medication noncompliance. The nurse knows the physician will order medications for Mr. Moon in which of the following dosage forms?
    ① Capsule
    ② Liquid
    ③ Tablet
    ④ Parenteral

200. Nancy is depressed over a relationship that ended 2 years ago when she had a miscarriage. She also left her job and is now living with her parents and collecting welfare. She states that she never goes out of the house and feels "terrible all the time." Which of the following should be a top priority outcome for Nancy?
    ① She will return to work within 1 month
    ② She will confront her former fiancé about their broken engagement within 2 weeks
    ③ She will move out of her parents' house and find her own apartment within 5 days
    ④ She will verbalize her feelings about the loss of her baby

201. The nurse is assisting 15-year-old Joanne in her plans for hospital discharge. To reinforce the gains Joanne has made during her hospitalization, the nurse should make which of the following her *highest priority?*
    ① Scheduling regular meetings with Joanne's family
    ② Teaching Joanne about taking medications as prescribed
    ③ Encouraging Joanne's attendance at recreational therapy
    ④ Planning Joanne's return to school after discharge

202. While the nurse is planning for a patient's discharge from alcohol treatment, the patient's mother asks if she will have to make her daughter attend Alcoholics Anonymous (AA) meetings. The nurse should:
    ① Tell the mother that attending AA meetings will help the patient stay sober
    ② Ask the mother how she feels about her daughter attending these meetings
    ③ Emphasize that it is the patient's responsibiity to decide whether to attend AA meetings
    ④ Remind the mother that attending AA meetings is a condition of discharge

203. Sarah is admitted to the hospital with a diagnosis of major depression. She has suffered multiple losses within a 2-year period and states there is nothing left to be taken from her. The *priority* nursing diagnosis for this patient should be:
    ① Altered nutrition: less than body requirements related to loss of appetite secondary to emotional stress
    ② Ineffective individual coping related to internal conflicts
    ③ Sleep pattern disturbance related to emotional stress
    ④ High risk for violence: self-directed related to feelings of loneliness

204. A severely depressed patient is scheduled for electroconvulsive therapy (ECT). While the nurse is preparing the patient for treatment, the patient asks "How long is this procedure going to take?" The *most appropriate* response by the nurse should be:
    ① "Just a few minutes. You'll be finished before you know it."
    ② "It can take anywhere from a few hours to all day, depending on how things go."
    ③ "Actually it only takes a few seconds."
    ④ "The average treatment time is 15 minutes."

205. For a hospitalized patient who has had dysfunctional grieving for 2 years, which of the following times/conditions would be *best* to encourage verbalization of feelings?
    ① At discharge
    ② Monthly, with her social worker
    ③ Daily, with her primary nurse
    ④ Weekly, with her psychiatrist

206. It is important to include the family when teaching a patient about medications, primarily to:
    ① Provide information and support for the patient
    ② Ensure that members of the family will not undermine treatment
    ③ Have the family take responsibility for the patient
    ④ Gain the family's approval for the treatment

207. A patient receiving antipsychotic medication tells the nurse, "I feel so nervous, like I can't sit still." The nurse should suspect that this patient is describing the common side effect of:
    ① Dystonia
    ② Akathisia
    ③ Tardive dyskinesia
    ④ Pseudoparkinsonism

208. A patient's family brings him to the emergency room after he stops taking his antipsychotic medications and starts to hallucinate and become agitated. The emergency room physician orders haloperidol (Haldol) 20 mg intramuscularly. Why does the nurse refuse to give the medication as ordered?
    ① The dose is too low to relieve his symptoms
    ② Haloperidol is only available in oral form
    ③ Haloperidol is an antidepressant and as such is not indicated
    ④ The dose is too high to be given intramuscularly

209. Thirty minutes after a patient receives the antipsychotic drug fluphenazine (Prolixin), his tongue becomes thick, he drools, his jaw becomes rigid, and his speech is slurred. Which of the following prn orders should the nurse give this immediately?
    ① Diazepam (Valium), 15 mg IV
    ② Benztropine (Cogentin), 2mg IM
    ③ Chlorpromazine (Thorazine), 25 mg IM
    ④ Lorazepam (Ativan), 1 mg PO

210. Betty has been hospitalized for 3 days. The nursing team observes that she is not interested in involving herself in the treatment program or in following the unit rules. She clearly prefers some staff members over others. In planning for her nursing care, which consideration is *most important?*
    ① If Betty prefers some staff members over others, those are the ones who should work with her
    ② Patience is required to work with Betty; when she is ready, she will begin to appreciate the value of the treatment program
    ③ The nursing team must confer and decide which rules are important to enforce in Betty's care; all staff enforce the same rules equally and consistently
    ④ Because Betty is an adult, the staff has no responsibility in enforcing any of the rules; Betty will decide for herself when she desires treatment

211. Peggy is a 43-year-old mentally retarded woman who works in a sheltered workshop where she has friends and feels productive. Peggy's mother has just died of cancer. What reaction should the nurse expect to see in Peggy at this time?
    ① No reaction
    ② Tendency to abuse alcohol
    ③ Psychotic depression
    ④ A normal grief reaction

212. Sid has just been told that the illness he is experiencing is inoperable lung cancer. He is advised to get his affairs in order because he has no more than 3 months to live. The nurse should anticipate which of the following reactions from Sid?
    ① Shock and denial
    ② Anger and rage
    ③ Sadness and insomnia
    ④ Acceptance and compliance

213. After Sid's death, Mary, his widow, is experiencing physical symptoms of loss of appetite, nausea, and vomiting. The nurse should assess her stage of grieving as:
① Shock and denial
② Developing awareness
③ Restitution
④ Distorted

214. Neuroleptic malignant syndrome is an unusual reaction to neuroleptic medications (antipsychotic drugs). The nurse should expect a person with this diagnosis to manifest which of the following classic symptoms of neuroleptic malignant syndrome?
① Convulsions, headache, and fever
② Hyperthermia, muscle rigidity, and stupor
③ Severe headache, fever, and neck stiffness
④ Shaking chills, temperature, and hypotension

215. Mr. Harvey is ordered to receive pheneizine (Nardil), a monoamine oxidase inhibitor (MAOI). Which of the following statements by Mr. Harvey should indicate to the nurse that he understands his tyramine-restricted diet?
① "It will take me awhile to develop a taste for hot dogs with sauerkraut only."
② "I like my salads moist. I guess I can use any salad dressing as long as it isn't made with MSG or cheese."
③ "I love pizza, but I guess I can only have it on special occasions now."
④ "My wife and I always have a glass of sherry after dinner. I guess we'll be losing some weight now that we can only have a glass a week."

216. Crisis intervention therapy is short-term. A crisis is usually resolved in which of the following time frameworks?
① 24 to 48 hours
② 2 to 4 days
③ 4 to 6 weeks
④ 6 to 12 months

217. The nurse should expect 7-year-old Sarah's mother to reveal which of the following characteristics of abusive parents?
① Low socioeconomic level
② Realistic expectations of a child's behavior
③ History of abuse as a child
④ Socially interactive

218. Which of the following behaviors in individuals who were abused children should be indications that they suffered *physical* abuse as opposed to other types of child abuse?
① Apprehension when other children cry
② Habit disorder such as rocking
③ Poor peer relationships
④ Developmental lag

219. An appropriate therapy for a sexually abused child that is *least* threatening should be:
① Group therapy
② Hypnosis
③ Art therapy
④ Desensitization therapy

220. Cecelia comes to the clinic after being beaten by her husband. Battered women are most frequently encountered in which of the following settings?
① Emergency rooms
② Obstetric services
③ Mental health clinics
④ Legal aid services

221. Women from lower socioeconomic status (SES) groups are more frequently identified as victims of battering than women from middle or upper SES groups. This is because:
① Women from lower SES groups are more frequently victimized
② Women from middle and upper SES groups conceal their battering
③ Women from middle and upper SES groups obtain better police protection and intervention
④ Men from lower SES groups are naturally more violent

222. Cecelia asks the nurse if her abusive husband can ever change, or should she just "give up hope?" The *best* nursing response is:
① "Leaving is your only real option for survival."
② "You are fooling herself to stay with him."
③ "I understand you are dependent on him."
④ "Batterers can learn more effective ways of relating."

223. Cecelia tells the nurse that her husband gets violent with her after he's been drinking with his friends. Which of the following is the appropriate information for the nurse to give Cecelia regarding the relationship, if any, between abuse and alcohol use?
① If he didn't drink, he wouldn't beat her
② Use of alcohol can increase the likelihood of abuse
③ There is no relationship between these two things
④ Alcohol use is the primary cause of battering

224. The *first priority* for the nurse to address when a battered woman comes for treatment is the woman's need to:
① Feel physically and mentally safe
② Reestablish feelings of control
③ Obtain accurate legal advice
④ Discuss her living situation

225. Mr. Miller is admitted to the unit with a diagnosis of severe depression. His son states that his father always appeared to have poor self-esteem. In planning care for Mr. Miller, the nurse knows that poor self-esteem is described as the difference between:
① Identity and body image
② Role and body image
③ Ego ideal and perceived self
④ Body image and ego ideal

226. Mr. Miles voluntarily admitted himself to a private psychiatric facility for treatment of depression. Three weeks after admission, he decides he wants to leave. Which response by the nurse is *most accurate?*
① "You may sign yourself out against medical advice."
② "You may appeal for discharge through the court."
③ "You're free to leave at any time."
④ "You must give 72 hours' written notice."

227. Mr. King is admitted to a psychiatric facility with a history of depression. He tells the nurse, "I can't eat; I have no appetite." Which of the following responses by the nurse should be *most appropriate?*
   ① "If you have no appetite, how come you're not underweight?"
   ② "You have difficulty eating?"
   ③ "Why do you feel this way?"
   ④ "Why don't you try eating just a little?"

228. Mrs. Gayle is receiving antidepressant therapy. She tells the nurse that the medication she is receiving makes her mouth dry, and she asks the nurse to get her something to drink. The nurse's *best response* should be to:
   ① Tell her there's juice in the refrigerator and she may feel free to help herself
   ② Remind her that she just had a drink a short time ago
   ③ Get her a cup of water from the fountain
   ④ Tell her that it's important that she not concentrate on the side effects of her medication

229. A patient's husband asks what he can do to reduce the likelihood of his wife being hospitalized for depression in the future. Which of the following will the nurse tell him is the *best* preventive measure?
   ① Learn the signs and symptoms of the onset of depression
   ② Keep her busy and distracted from her problems
   ③ Hire household help so she is not stressed
   ④ Give unconditional acceptance of her behavior

230. Una is a 45-year-old mother of four who has been hospitalized for a month for treatment of depression. Her mood has brightened slightly. Just before leaving the hospital on her first weekend pass, she confides to the nurse that she is thinking of killing herself at home. She asks the nurse to hold this information in confidence, asserting that she will no longer trust the nurse if the nurse tells anyone of this plan. Your appropriate nursing response should be to:
   ① Maintain confidentiality in the nurse-patient relationship, refusing to divulge what Una has confided in her
   ② Notify her supervisor immediately so that the weekend pass should be canceled
   ③ Engage Una in discussion of the meaning of suicide in her life to facilitate expression of feelings
   ④ Bring this up in a group therapy session so that the group can assist Una in dealing with her feelings

231. Una's diagnosis is major depression. Her psychiatrist prescribes the tricyclic antidepressant nortriptyline (Pamelor). In addition to administering the medication on time as ordered, the nurse is able to answer Una's questions about the side effects she is experiencing. The nurse's teaching plan for Una should emphasize the need for Una to report the following common side effects:
   ① Rash across her face
   ② Constipation
   ③ Sudden, rapid change in mood
   ④ Jitteriness

232. After 3 weeks of treatment in the hospital for major depression, Una feels much better. She is very appreciative of the nurse's work with her and she wants to call the nurse to have lunch outside the hospital after she is discharged. The nurse's *best response* to Una's request should be:
   ① "It would be a pleasure to have lunch with you. When would you like to go?"
   ② "It would not be appropriate for me to be seen having lunch with a former patient."
   ③ "Our relationship has been a professional one. It would not be appropriate for me to meet you for lunch."
   ④ "Perhaps after you have been out of the hospital for a longer period of time, we could consider having lunch together."

233. Greg, age 6, is hospitalized for treatment of depression. The nurse would expect which of the following treatment modalities to be used for Greg?
   ① Cognitive therapy
   ② Insight-oriented psychotherapy
   ③ Play therapy
   ④ Work therapy

234. After coming on duty, the nurse learns that one of her patients has lapsed into depression after seeming to progress well. The nurse finds the patient sitting in her room with her hands on her lap and her head bowed. The patient does not respond to the nurse's greeting. The *best response* by the nurse should be:
   ① "Chin up, it can't be all that bad."
   ② "I understand that you seem troubled."
   ③ "You must pull yourself together."
   ④ "You were doing so well; what happened to you?"

235. John, a 42-year-old man who recently lost his job, has been drinking more than usual. His father was a suicide victim. Now John reports thinking of suicide. The nurse knows that John is at which level of risk?
   ① Low
   ② Moderate
   ③ High
   ④ Very high

236. When planning care for a suicidal patient, the nurse assists by:
   ① Being aware that most attempts are gestures
   ② Teaching problem-solving strategies to the patient
   ③ Reporting the patient to local authorities
   ④ Asking for the patient's reasons for suicidal thinking

237. Mrs. Mann, age 62, is admitted to the hospital following an unsuccessful suicide attempt. She has been nonresponsive to antidepressant medication and is scheduled for electroconvulsive therapy (ECT). Information in the nurse's pretreatment plan should emphasize which of the following?
   ① ECT cures depression
   ② Memory loss is permanent
   ③ On awakening, the patient will be confused
   ④ Depressive symptoms usually disappear after the first treatment

238. Martha is brought to the hospital after threatening to kill herself. She admits to several years of substance abuse and arrests for shoplifting and prostitution. She has healed scars on her wrists and states that she is angry because "my boyfriend dumped me." The nursing diagnosis with *highest priority* for Martha is:
① Ineffective individual coping related to poor impulse control
② Anxiety related to unstable relationships
③ Knowledge deficit related to effects of substance abuse
④ Potential for violence: self-directed related to impulsiveness

239 Which one of the following is required at all community mental health centers?
① Family therapy programs
② Partial hospitalization
③ Suicide prevention programs
④ Alcohol detoxification

240. All of the statements below indicate that an individual is at some degree of risk for suicide. The nurse knows that the statement that indicates the *highest suicide risk* is:
① "I haven't been able to get the education I've wanted. I can't earn the money I need, and my family doesn't appreciate me. Now and then I feel so frustrated I think of suicide."
② "Since the death of my loved one, life has lost its meaning. I've gotten a large supply of sleeping pills and I will take them tomorrow, which would have been his birthday."
③ "My girlfriend is threatening to leave me because I am so jealous. I told her that if she leaves me, I'll kill myself."
④ "It takes a real man to kill himself. I don't have that kind of courage right now. If things don't get better, I may just have to find it."

241. John has been brought to the hospital following a suicide gesture in which he ingested a quantity of sleeping pills. After gastric lavage is performed and a complete physical examination is accomplished, the nurse makes an assessment of John's suicide gesture. The *most appropriate* question to ask John should be:
① "Don't you realize how you will hurt your family if you kill yourself?"
② "Do you still want to hurt yourself?"
③ "Are you trying to manipulate other people to get your way?"
④ "Why are you being such a big baby?"

242. The head nurse informs the nurse that Mrs. Willis is having suicidal thoughts and instructs the nurse to initiate suicide precautions. The nurse's *first nursing action* should be to:
① Apply ambulatory restraints
② Begin one-to-one observation
③ Place the patient in seclusion
④ Remove dangerous possessions

243. Mrs. Willis has been placed on one-to-one observation for suicidal intentions. Which of the following items should the nurse remove from Mrs. Willis' possession?
① Daily newspaper
② Hairbrush
③ Metal nail file
④ Shoes

244. Glenna, age 18, is brought to the emergency room after having been raped by her date. Her mother asks the nurse for advice in helping her daughter cope with this experience. Which of the following responses by the nurse should be *most appropriate?*
① "It is important to help her move on to new and healthy experiences. She will eventually come to better understand her experience."
② "A period of counseling or therapy might help her and the family recover more fully."
③ "It is sometimes better to let a person work things out by herself."
④ "You might anticipate that Glenna will be reluctant to trust males until she resolves her experience."

245. Marge, age 18, reports being raped at age 11 by a stranger. She speaks of this event with little affect. The characteristic of post-traumatic stress disorder being demonstrated is:
① Anxiety
② Rumination
③ Reliving the event
④ Numbness

246. After initial assessment determines that a rape victim did not suffer any life-threatening injuries, which of the following should be the next intervention for the nurse to perform?
① Prepare her for a vaginal examination
② Give her towels to go and shower
③ Inform her of her rights and options
④ Photograph her cuts and bruises

247. Jason O'Hare is a 60-year-old man who has a history of depression. His physician has ordered electroconvulsive therapy. When planning immediate post-treatment care for Mr. O'Hare, the *priority nursing action* should be to:
① Assist him to become oriented on awakening
② Assure him that memory loss is temporary
③ Implement seizure precautions
④ Monitor intake and output

248. Mrs. Smith's physician is considering electroconvulsive therapy for her. The nurse should expect that Mrs. Smith has which of the following disorders?
① Agonophobia
② Severe anxiety
③ Severe depression
④ Substance dependency

249. Mr. Ball is an alcoholic who arrives at the local emergency room requesting admission for detoxification. He states he has been drinking daily for at least 2 weeks. The nurse should observe Mr. Ball for impending delirium tremens (DTs) and plan to monitor him for which of the following physiologic indications of DTs:

① Constricted pupils, subnormal temperature, and bradycardia

② Hallucinations, fear, and agitation

③ Hypertension, diaphoresis, and elevated temperature

④ Hypotension, tachycardia, and diaphoresis

250. Special legal consideration is given to the relationship between psychiatric nurses and their patients. This is called:

① Privileged communication

② Habeas corpus

③ Malpractice

④ Locus tenens

CHAPTER 5

Comprehensive Examinations

COMPREHENSIVE EXAMINATION ONE: PART 1

1. Mr. Todd, age 54, is admitted to the unit with pain in the calf. Which of the following nursing assessment parameters is *most* significant?
   1. Negative Babinski's sign
   2. Positive Homans' sign
   3. Blood pressure 145/90
   4. Bilateral 1 + edema of ankles

2. Mr. Presley has been hospitalized for over a week for deep vein thrombosis. He is near discharge, and the physician is beginning warfarin (Coumadin) therapy for prophylaxis at home. Which of the following orders would require the nurse to report to the supervising nurse before implementation?
   1. Give all medication ac
   2. Collect daily prothrombin level
   3. Ambulate in the hall bid
   4. Demerol 50 mg IM for pain q4h prn

3. Mr. J. is admitted with pancreatitis. His family tells the nurse he uses alcohol in unknown amounts daily. In addition to safety measures and prescribed care, the nurse should include which of the following in the plan of care?
   1. Report intake and output (I & O) to the supervising nurse q2h
   2. Perform neurologic checks qh
   3. Observe for withdrawal symptoms from alcohol
   4. Provide sedation prn

4. Mrs. Bolling is being discharged after being diagnosed with adult onset diabetes mellitus. She has been stabilized on tolbutamide (Orinase). Which statement shows she has good understanding of this drug's effects and side effects?
   1. "This drug will keep my blood sugar stable all the time."
   2. "I must report the use of this drug to my doctor anytime I am to receive another medication."
   3. "I will need to take this drug after meals."
   4. "I may frequently feel nauseated while I am taking this medication."

5. Mr. Paul is afraid to have the nurse clean around his colostomy stoma during a dressing change. He states that, if the stoma is touched, it will hurt too much. Which of the following statements by the nurse is most appropriate?
   1. "The stoma and the area around it must be cleaned. I'll be as gentle as possible to avoid causing you pain when I touch the stoma."
   2. "This is something that you'll have to get used to for the next several months. I'll be careful."
   3. "I'll be as gentle as possible. You should also know that the stoma has no pain receptors."
   4. "I'm trying very hard to do this correctly. Please tell me if I hurt you."

6. On the fourth day following a colon resection, Mr. Sam's nurse changes the dressing and pouch. The nurse notices that Mr. Sam turns his head and refuses to look at the incision or stoma. What would be the best action by the nurse?
   1. Get a mirror and show Mr. Sam the stoma so he can get used to its appearance
   2. Quickly finish the dressing change so he doesn't have to see the stoma
   3. Ask Mr. Sam if he would like to see or touch the stoma
   4. Start discussing the at-home care of the colostomy

7. On the day Mr. Foster is to be discharged, he confides, "I'm not sure how my wife will like my sleeping in the same bed with her. This colostomy does not sound like a nice thing to have around her." What is the best response by the nurse?
   1. "Some patients find it easier to move to another room or purchase twin beds."
   2. "I'm sure that your wife will get used to it in time."
   3. "I'd be glad to discuss this with her if you would like."
   4. "Moving out of your bed may make your wife feel like you are pushing her away. You should discuss this with her."

8. Before discharge, a patient who has a colostomy asks the nurse to help him review the foods he should eat at home. Which statement by the patient indicates a good understanding of his nutritional needs now that he has a colostomy?
   1. "I should avoid citrus fruits because they contain acetic acid."
   2. "I should avoid foods like cabbage, cucumbers, and radishes because they will make me have more gas."
   3. "I should avoid foods like spinach, oatmeal, and cream of wheat because food high in iron will make me constipated."
   4. "I should avoid juices like apple and cranberry because they may cause diarrhea."

9. The afternoon following an incomplete abortion and a dilatation and curettage (D&C), Mrs. Jones confides to the nurse, "This baby meant so much to my husband and me. We were so excited about having a baby and had already started thinking about decorating a nursery and everything. I feel so disappointed and hurt." What is the *best* response by the nurse to Mrs. Jones?
   1. "I know you feel bad now, but as time goes by you will feel better."
   2. "Somehow nature takes care of problems. There had to be something wrong with how the baby was growing."
   3. "I can see that you feel bad about this. Let's talk about it."
   4. "If you give your body about 6 months to recuperate, you should be able to get pregnant again."

10. Mrs. Jenkins' fifth child has Down's syndrome, and she is having difficulty accepting the baby. During the early neonatal period, which nursing action would be the *most helpful* to Mrs. Jenkins and the baby?
    1. Keeping the baby in the nursery for care
    2. Assisting Mrs. Jenkins to hold and cuddle the baby
    3. Leaving Mrs. Jenkins and the baby alone so she can begin grieving
    4. Completing the infant care in an Isolette for Mrs. Jenkins

11. Following an 18-hour induced labor, Mary Simmons, age 38, delivers her fourth child. Soon after birth, the pediatrician informs Mrs. Jenkins that the baby is suspected of having Down's syndrome. Which of the following factors most likely contributed to the development of Down syndrome?
    1. Pitocin induction
    2. Prolonged labor
    3. Maternal age
    4. Multiparity

12. Jim, age 22, is brought into the emergency room by his wife. She reports that Jim had been with friends who were using LSD. She says that Jim is having "a bad trip." Which of the following symptoms should the nurse expect to find in this patient?
    1. Slurred speech, blurred vision, light-headedness, ringing in the ears, loss of coordination, and excessive nasal secretions
    2. Drying of the mouth, increased appetite, reddening of eyes, and short-term memory impairment
    3. Tremendous confusion, unpleasant sensory images, and extreme panic
    4. Stomach pains, chills, hallucinations, headache, and delirium tremens

13. All states in this country require that 1% silver nitrate or penicillin drops be instilled into every newborn's eyes. The *primary* reason is to prevent:
    1. Gonorrheal infection of the eyes
    2. Syphilitic infection of the eyes
    3. Development of retrolental fibroplasia
    4. Development of cataracts

14. A nursing mother often does not menstruate for several months after delivery or until she discontinues breast-feeding. Of the following information, which would be appropriate for the nurse to offer in planning care for this nursing mother?
    1. Although she is breast-feeding, ovulation is not suppressed, and pregnancy is possible
    2. Ovulation is suppressed, and pregnancy is not possible while breast-feeding
    3. Breast-feeding should be stopped if she does not menstruate in 3 months
    4. The uterus will not return to normal size while breast-feeding

15. Marti, age 22, is brought into the emergency room by friends. Marti is hallucinating and is frightened of everyone. The nurse discovers that Marti has taken LSD 3 hours ago. What terminology is also used for hallucinogens or psychedelics?
    1. Bennies, speed, hash
    2. Buttons, PCP, acid
    3. H, smack, junk
    4. Rainbows, downers, M

16. When assessing the patient's lochia, the nurse notes a foul smell. Which of the following actions would be most appropriate for the nurse to take?
    1. Do nothing because this is normal
    2. Administer vaginal douches
    3. Report this immediately because the patient could have an infection
    4. Count the perineal pads used

17. Niki Neal, age 68, was admitted with pitting edema of both ankles and dyspnea. Her orders include bed rest, oxygen at 4 L, morphine sulfate 5 mg SC q4h, Lasix 40 mg PO stat, and a chest x-ray examination stat. The diagnosis was pulmonary edema. Mrs. Neal is restless and thrashes in bed. On the basis of written physician's orders, the nurse should:
    1. Administer morphine sulfate 5 mg subcutaneously
    2. Increase the amount of oxygen from 4 to 8 L
    3. Talk with her to decrease her level of anxiety
    4. Elevate both legs

18. Paula, age 19, is brought into the emergency room by friends. She is hallucinating and acts frightened of everyone. The nurse discovers that she has taken LSD several hours ago. If Paula continues to use LSD for an extended period of time, she should be warned that she may:
    1. Become physically addicted
    2. Suffer symptoms of withdrawal such as agitation, insomnia, and seizures
    3. Have children with birth defects
    4. Suffer from acute organic brain syndrome

19. While the nurse is working in the emergency room, Scott, age 26, is brought in by friends. He is hallucinating, and the nurse discovers that he has been using LSD. What statement made by the nurse would be *most* beneficial to help Scott recover and regain control?
    1. "You're all right; don't worry."
    2. "You're having a bad trip, and the main reaction is about over."
    3. "You were using acid and shouldn't have."
    4. "You've taken a psychedelic and are suffering a mild psychosis that will only last a short time."

20. Christine, age 18, is brought into a local clinic by friends. The nurse discovers she has taken LSD. On recovery, Christine says that she enjoys taking LSD because it helps in numerous ways. Which statement by Christine would be most doubtful as to why she enjoys taking the drug?
    1. It seems to increase creativity
    2. It seems to make time pass more slowly
    3. It seems to make sounds be portrayed in color
    4. It seems to create visual hallucinations

21. An antibiotic, ordered for a pediatric patient, comes in liquid form. The label reads 125 mg/5 ml. The physician orders 150 mg q6h. How many ml would the nurse give for each dose?
    1. 0.5 ml
    2. 5 ml
    3. 6 ml
    4. 10 ml

22. Teaching the mother of a child being discharged on antibiotic therapy should include giving the antibiotic:
    1. Until the child feels better
    2. Only while the child is awake
    3. Every 6 hours until all the medication has been taken
    4. Every 6 hours until the fever remains below 99° F (37.2° C) for 2 days

23. Mrs. Sims calls about her child's appointment to receive her 15-month measles, mumps, and rubella immunization (MMR). The child is coughing, running a fever of 102° F (38.8° C), and vomiting. The nurse should instruct Mrs. Sims to:
    1. Keep the appointment and let the physician decide about administering the injection
    2. Give the child two baby aspirins and report for the injection at the appropriate time
    3. Skip the injection; because of the illness, she will not be able to receive the vaccine at 15 months
    4. Skip the injection at this time and call after the fever has decreased to reschedule the appointment

24. The nurse would caution a concerned parent not to be alarmed about which of these side effects of her child's recent immunization?
    1. Convulsions, fine tremors, and malaise
    2. Malaise, soreness, and a raised red area at the injection site
    3. Urticaria, arthritic-type pain, and severe vomiting
    4. Temperature of 104° F (40° C), whelps over the entire body, and malaise

25. Linda Johnson, age 22, is admitted to the hospital for acute appendicitis. Admission testing reveals that she also has active pulmonary tuberculosis. To plan the nursing care for Miss Johnson, the nurse must be aware of the route of tuberculosis transmission. Which of the following statements is *most accurate?*
    1. A single contact with an infected person will usually cause the disease
    2. Feces and stool can also contain the organism for pulmonary tuberculosis
    3. A tine tuberculin test or tuberculin skin test (Mantoux test) can cause a person to develop active tuberculosis
    4. Tuberculosis is spread via aerosolization such as coughing, sneezing, or singing

26. Miss Johnson reports that she was tested for tuberculosis several years ago because her grandmother had it. She further stated that she thought the test was negative. What would indicate a positive response to the tuberculin skin test (Mantoux test)?
    1. An area of induration appearing at the site of the intradermal injection 48 to 72 hours after administration
    2. A maculopapular rash appearing on the inner aspect of the forearms 36 to 72 hours after the test
    3. A reddened, raised area on the deltoid muscle where the injection was given
    4. An increased cough and sputum production 24 to 72 hours after the test is administered

27. While Miss Johnson is in surgery for an appendectomy, the nurse plans for her postoperative recovery and gets her room ready. Because Miss Johnson's tuberculosis is active and she will need to do deep breathing and coughing exercises following surgery, what type of precautions should the nurse be prepared to take?
    1. Isolation; the nurse need only wear a mask, carefully washing her hands after providing care
    2. Isolation; the nurse must wear a mask, gown, and gloves while providing care
    3. Isolation is not necessary; the patient must wear a mask while in the hospital
    4. No specific precautions are needed, only good hygiene by both the patient and nurse

28. The nurse is aware that her patient, age 23, with a diagnosis of active tuberculosis will need specific instruction about good nutrition, including the four food groups. Why is this instruction particularly important for the patient?
    ① The patient will be unable to cook at home for the next few weeks and will need to rely on others to bring meals
    ② Patients with tuberculosis usually have anorexia, nausea, and weight loss; they need proper nutrition to heal
    ③ Because of age, the patient often relies only on "fast foods" for nutrition
    ④ The medication needed to treat the patient's tuberculosis often causes patients to experience a rapid weight gain

29. Just before discharge, Miss Johnson tells the nurse that she is anxious to return to work because she needs the income to pay her hospital bills and living expenses. What can the nurse tell Miss Johnson about returning to work while being treated for tuberculosis?
    ① She should be able to return to work about 3 to 4 weeks after beginning therapy and will need follow-up treatment for 1 year
    ② She will be able to return to work after completing a year of therapy at home
    ③ She will be able to work after a year's therapy in a special tuberculosis hospital/sanitorium
    ④ She will be able to return to work as soon as she is started on therapy and feels well enough to work

30. Mrs. Adele Henson, age 26, is admitted to the gynecologic unit for a dilatation and curettage (D&C) following an incomplete abortion of a desired pregnancy. Following the D&C, Mrs. Henson's hematocrit is 29%, and her hemoglobin level is 8.5 g/dl. How should the nurse interpret these laboratory findings?
    ① Higher than normal
    ② Average
    ③ Lower than normal
    ④ Life-threatening

31. Considering a patient's hematocrit of 29% and hemoglobin of 8.5 g/dl, what postoperative nursing measures should most concern the nurse?
    ① Intake of oral fluids
    ② Adequate pain control
    ③ Ambulation
    ④ Assessment of voiding

32. A patient is ordered to take ferrous sulfate following surgery. Which of the following statements made by the patient indicates an understanding of the nurse's instructions about this medication?
    ① "I can only take the pill between meals to promote absorption."
    ② "I must take the pill with a laxative to prevent constipation."
    ③ "I must take the pill only with meals or a snack."
    ④ "I can only take the pill with liquids."

33. Discharge nutritional counseling for a patient with low postoperative hemoglobin and hematocrit levels should include an emphasis on which of the following types of foods?
    ① Citrus fruits
    ② Milk and other dairy products
    ③ Breads and pasta
    ④ Leafy green vegetables

34. Florence Cox, age 63, has a medical history of peptic ulcer disease. During a recent upper GI series, it was discovered that Miss Cox has cancer of the stomach. She is admitted to the hospital for gastrectomy surgery. On the second postoperative day, Miss Cox's Levine tube has drained only a small amount of clear greenish-tinged fluid. The *most appropriate* nursing action should be to:
    ① Do nothing; this amount of drainage is expected with this type of surgery
    ② Call the physician immediately to report an impending complication
    ③ Irrigate the tube with 100 ml of normal saline solution to ensure patency
    ④ Connect the tube to high suction on the Gonco machine for 15 minutes

35. Following a partial gastrectomy, a patient has physician's orders to receive vitamin B_{12} injections. The primary reason for this is to:
    ① Provide relief from gastric irritation and distention
    ② Assist in the repair and healing of the gastric mucosa
    ③ Stimulate appetite and decrease anorexia
    ④ Provide the body with the factor necessary to promote red blood cell production

36. In planning care for a patient diagnosed with ulcerative colitis, it is important that the nurse knows that the term ulcerative colitis is defined as:
    ① An inflammatory process in the sigmoid colon
    ② An ulcerative disorder of the terminal ileum
    ③ Inflammation and ulceration of the colon and rectum
    ④ A condition with alternating bouts of diarrhea and constipation

37. When obtaining patient data related to bowel history, it is important for the nurse to know that the earliest warning sign of cancer of the large intestine is:
    ① Change in bowel patterns
    ② Weight loss
    ③ Clay-colored stools
    ④ Flatulence when eating certain foods

38. The nurse is assisting the physician with a procedure requiring a sterile field and sterile tray. The nurse notices that the sterile drape has been soiled with povidone iodine (Betadine) as it was poured into the cup on the sterile tray. The *most appropriate* nursing action should be to:
    ① Prepare another sterile field with a new sterile tray
    ② Say nothing and watch to be sure that the physician does not use the contaminated part of the field
    ③ Inform the physician that he contaminated the field and will have to start over; provide the new sterile tray
    ④ Remove the soiled drape; place a new one onto the field as the tray is held with gloved hands

39. To prevent the spread of organisms and protect other patients, the nurse should always do which of the following?
    ① Use sterile gloves
    ② Use isolation gowns
    ③ Practice proper handwashing
    ④ Provide nonsterile gloves to the family

40. Mr. Hodge has diarrhea of unknown origin and fever. He is on body surface isolation. To perform his dressing change, the nurse should don:
    ① Mask and gloves
    ② Gown and gloves
    ③ Mask and gown
    ④ Gloves, gown, and shoe covers

41. A 23-year-old man is brought into the emergency department dead on arrival from drowning. The bereaved family arrives within minutes after the ambulance and requests to see the body immediately. The nurse's response should be to:
    ① Allow the family to see the body as requested
    ② Tell the family that viewing the body will make the grieving more painful
    ③ Suggest waiting until the mortician has cared for the body
    ④ Suggest that the family call other close relatives or friends to be with them when they see the body

42. Mr. Johnson, age 82, comes into the clinic with a piece of steel embedded in his right foot. He has a history of diabetes and hypertension. In setting up the supplies for the physician to anesthetize the foot, the nurse should offer which of the following?
    ① Benzalkonium (Zephiran)
    ② Benzoin spray
    ③ Lidocaine with epinephrine
    ④ Lidocaine without epinephrine

43. The nurse knows that mental illness may be evidenced by:
    ① A pattern of behavior disturbing to the individual or the community in which one lives
    ② The development of mature patterns of problem solving
    ③ The ability to cope with crisis
    ④ Having satisfying work and work relationships

44. Betty, a personal friend, says during coffee that she is very stressed with her job. The nurse knows that stress can be best defined as:
    ① Another way of coping with anxiety; used to block conscious awareness
    ② A specific response of the body to any demand made on it
    ③ A universal emotion; a general state of apprehension
    ④ Anything that interferes with goal achievement

45. Judy, a co-worker, says her job is very stressful. The nurse is aware that:
    ① Health factors do not directly affect a person's response to stress
    ② The nurse should be a resource in helping Judy develop maladaptive patterns of behavior
    ③ Most changes in situations or events are not directly related to stress
    ④ The meaning an individual gives to stress determines whether the person feels distress

46. The process of constructing plausible reasons to explain and justify one's behavior is a commonly used defense mechanism of:
    ① Reaction formation
    ② Compensation
    ③ Conversion
    ④ Rationalization

47. The Lamaze instructor teaches mothers about the various positions the fetus may assume while in utero. To fully explain a "breech position," she states that the presenting part is the:
    ① Back
    ② Shoulder
    ③ Buttocks
    ④ Head

48. A patient is admitted in active labor with a known breech presentation. She was formerly scheduled for a cesarean section (C-section). In planning care for this patient, the nurse knows that if her membranes rupture, she would be at risk for which of the following?
    ① A prolapsed cord
    ② Hemorrhage
    ③ A precipitus delivery
    ④ A nuchal cord

49. The external fetal-maternal monitor is applied to a patient's abdomen. The phonotransducer indicates a fetal heart rate (FHR) of 140 beats/min. The labor room nurse knows the normal range for the FHR is:
    ① 70 to 90 beats/min
    ② 80 to 120 beats/min
    ③ 120 to 160 beats/min
    ④ 170 to 190 beats/min

50. A patient is in the early stage of labor and is 2 cm dilated and 50% effaced. As the nurse times contractions, the patient asks him or her what effacement really means. The nurse explains that effacement is the:
    ① Position of fetus
    ② Size of the fetus
    ③ Irregular contractions of the uterus
    ④ Thinning and shortening of the cervix

51. The nurse verifies rupture of the membranes (ROM) by testing the:
    ① Fluid in the vagina with Nitrazine paper and obtaining an alkaline reaction
    ② Fluid in the vagina with Nitrazine paper and obtaining an acid reaction
    ③ Condition of the vagina
    ④ Urine for protein

52. Linda, age 16, reports to the office for a routine visit and lab work and has been taking anticonvulsants for her seizures. Linda reports that because she has not had a seizure in a year and does not feel that she needs to take the medication every day, she skips a dose now and then. The nurse's reply should be:
    ① "You should be more careful in your drug treatment regimen."
    ② "I know that you are glad that the seizures are under control now."
    ③ "It is important that you follow your treatment plan on a strict basis and avoid skipping any doses."
    ④ "It may help you to buy a pill organizer that allows you to place the medicine necessary for each day of the week."

53. Connie, age 3, is seen at a clinic and is diagnosed with an upper respiratory infection. Symptoms of an upper respiratory infection include which of the following?
    ① Dehydration, vomiting, and irritability
    ② Fever, sore throat, and sneezing
    ③ Restlessness, fever, and pulling at the ears
    ④ Vomiting, pale color, and sharp abdominal pains

54. Mr. McCrain, an elderly patient confined to bed, is suffering from emphysema and receiving oxygen therapy. On entering his room, the nurse notices flames coming from a garbage can. The nurse's initial response should be to:
    ① Push the fire alarm in the hall
    ② Alert the house supervisor immediately
    ③ Remove the patient and turn off the oxygen
    ④ Use the water pitcher to pour water in the garbage can

55. The nurse notices after report that one of the other nurses on the unit is talking excessively. She complains of not sleeping well last night, appears restless, and has slight hand tremors when pouring her medication. The nurse knows that this co-worker has been going through some difficult times in her personal life lately. The nurse might suspect her co-worker of misuse of which of these agents?
    ① Alcohol
    ② Diphenhydramine (Benadryl)
    ③ Amphetamines
    ④ Sympathomimetic drugs

56. A new patient, Mr. Nell, arrives on the floor and the nurse helps the charge nurse admit him. After the health history is taken, Mr. Nell states that he cannot remember if he is allergic to any medications but thinks he might be. On the basis of this information, the nurse would want to have on hand which classification of drug in case of an allergic reaction?
    ① Ganglionic agents
    ② Sympathomimetic drugs
    ③ Parasympathetic blocking agents
    ④ Neuromuscular blocking agents

57. In assessing Mrs. Snow on early morning rounds, the nurse notices that bowel sounds are hypoactive and hypoperistalsis is evident. When the patient's medications are reviewed, the nurse notices that she is receiving an anticholinergic antidiarrheal. The best nursing action should be to:
    ① Hold the dose and call the physician
    ② Give one fourth of the ordered dose and encourage PO fluids
    ③ Give one half of the ordered dose and encourage PO fluids
    ④ Give the ordered dose and assess bowel sounds in 1 hour

58. The nurse's neighbor calls the nurse about a headache and asks if she should take a pain reliever. She mentions that she is breast-feeding her baby. The nurse's advice should be to:
    ① Take the drug and watch the baby closely for side effects
    ② Take half the drug instead of the whole dose and watch for side effects
    ③ Check with the physician because some drugs are excreted in breast milk
    ④ Take the medication as needed; it shouldn't harm the child

59. For a toothache, Mrs. Hill, age 23, is given the antibiotic erythromycin to be taken tid for 10 days. Which set of instructions offered by the nurse would be correct to give her while taking this antibiotic?
    ① Take the antibiotic until the tooth stops hurting
    ② Take the antibiotic on an empty stomach, perhaps 1 hour before meals
    ③ Regardless of allergies, erythromycin is a relatively safe drug
    ④ Concurrent use of this drug with oral contraceptives may render the contraceptives ineffective

60. Which of the following nursing diagnoses would be top priority for a patient receiving neuromuscular blocking agents?
    ① Alteration in thought processes
    ② Alteration in respiratory function
    ③ Alteration in tissue perfusion
    ④ Altered level of consciousness

61. Mr. Jack calls the nurse from home and states that he has gained 10 lb since his discharge 4 days ago from the hospital. He is taking his diuretic faithfully, but is concerned about what to do. The nurse's *first* action should be to:
    ① Tell him to report to the hospital immediately
    ② Assess for consistency in his routine to monitor his weight
    ③ Encourage him to make an appointment with his doctor as soon as he can
    ④ Tell him to decrease his fluids and weigh himself again in the morning

62. Paul Watson, age 74, is diagnosed with bilateral senile cataracts and is scheduled for surgery. He is admitted to the surgical unit because he also has congestive heart failure and is receiving multiple cardiac medications. Mr. Watson is able to see only shadows. He delayed having this surgery because, he says, "I was afraid. Since I have this heart problem, I just figured I was going to die." Which of the following represents an *appropriate* response by the nurse?
    ① "This must be frightening for you."
    ② "People do not die from cataract surgery."
    ③ "I can understand how you feel. I'd be afraid of dying too."
    ④ "How did you live at home when you couldn't see?"

63. Mr. Watson, a patient with congestive heart failure, has been taking digoxin 0.125 mg orally when at home. The nurse realizes that to administer this medication in the hospital she must complete which of the following actions?
    1. Place the patient on a cardiac monitor
    2. Obtain the radial pulse and notify the physician of the results
    3. Obtain the apical pulse for 60 seconds and withhold the medication if the pulse is below 60
    4. Check Mr. Watson's mouth after administration to be sure he has swallowed the medication

64. Margaret, age 92, has recently moved into a nursing home. A nurse caring for Margaret learns that the patient is very "down" and feels worthless and unloved by her family. Margaret's family reports that she has made a previous suicidal gesture. Which is an *appropriate* nursing intervention at this time?
    1. The nurse should directly ask Margaret if she has thoughts or plans about committing suicide
    2. To prevent giving her ideas of self-harm, the nurse should avoid bringing up the subject of suicide
    3. The nurse should indicate that she knows others who have felt as Margaret does
    4. The nurse should outline some alternative measures to suicide during periods of depression

65. Mrs. Furlow was admitted to the unit following an attempted suicide with sleeping pills. Her husband had arrived home early from a business trip and discovered her deeply sedated. In evaluating this patient's level of risk for future suicide attempts, the nurse is aware that this attempt:
    1. Was not planned out thoroughly
    2. Was intended to bring about emergency care and intervention
    3. Was most serious, because a lethal method was used and there appeared little chance for discovery
    4. Was less serious, because she used pills rather than a gun or more lethal method

66. Mrs. Furlow is profoundly depressed and has not responded to conventional therapy. The physician elects to begin electroconvulsive therapy (ECT). Following the procedure, the patient is somnolent and does not remember the occupational therapist's name the next day. The nurse is aware that:
    1. These are expected behaviors following ECT
    2. ECT can cause minimal damage to the frontal lobe
    3. This is an adverse response and should be reported
    4. ECT will cause a permanent loss in some parts of the patient's recent memory

67. A patient states, "I have heart trouble because I don't eat right, but I don't have time to worry about eating well." The nurse identifies his response as:
    1. Suppression
    2. Rationalization
    3. Displacement
    4. Conversion

68. A nurse preparing to take a patient's fetal heart rate palpates the abdomen to determine fetal position. This procedure is called:
    1. Homans' sign
    2. Leopold's maneuver
    3. Chadwick's sign
    4. Ritgen's maneuver

69. Sara is a 25-year-old gravida 3 para 1 who is admitted to labor and delivery with ruptured membranes. She is having contractions 6 to 7 minutes apart, lasting 30 seconds. The nurse obtains Sara's temperature, pulse, blood pressure, respirations, and fetal heart rate on admission because:
    1. This information is part of the admission record
    2. Obtaining this information is a hospital policy
    3. A baseline is necessary for further assessment
    4. The nursing care plan depends on this information

70. In her eighth month of pregnancy, Mrs. White is admitted through the emergency room with a diagnosis of eclampsia with convulsions. The nurse might expect the physician to order:
    1. A magnesium preparation
    2. A potassium preparation
    3. A sodium preparation
    4. A calcium preparation

71. Sheila Sims, age 4, has had multiple episodes of upper respiratory infections (URIs) since birth. She is thin and in the 30th percentile on the pediatric growth charts for height and weight. Sheila is in the pediatrician's office for a checkup. Which comment made by Sheila's mother indicates the need for immediate follow-up?
    1. "When I kiss Sheila, she tastes salty."
    2. "Sheila drinks plenty of fluids."
    3. "Sheila occasionally wets the bed at night."
    4. "Sheila really seems to dislike vegetables."

72. Besides the appearance of a high sodium and chloride content in sweat, what additional information should the nurse be sure to obtain when cystic fibrosis is suspected?
    1. The type of diapers or underpants the child wears at night
    2. The time the child goes to bed and wakes up in the morning
    3. The kind of bowel movements the child has
    4. The kinds of food the child enjoys eating

73. Pulmonary therapy is ordered for Tara, a patient with cystic fibrosis. Her mother was taught the techniques of postural drainage and breathing exercises. Which of the following responses by the mother indicates an understanding of these techniques?
    1. "Therapy should be done immediately before meals to open air passages and make eating easier."
    2. "Therapy should only be done if Tara has difficulty breathing."
    3. "Therapy should not be done immediately before or after meals."
    4. "Therapy should only be done if Tara feels like she wants it."

74. Mrs. Underwood brings her daughter Melissa, age 18 months, to the emergency room because she believes Melissa has broken her arm while trying to get out of her crib. While Melissa is sobbing, the nurse notices several bruises on both of her upper arms in addition to what appears to be a broken forearm. The nurse begins to collect information. Why does the nurse realize that it is important to obtain a well-documented history from the mother?
    ① Infants and toddlers do not normally sustain fractures while climbing into or out of a crib
    ② Melissa is crying and cannot talk to the nurse
    ③ The nurse needs to know what kind of first aid was given to Melissa
    ④ The nurse needs to determine Melissa's state of health and need for a tetanus immunization

75. Melissa Underwood is a patient in the pediatric unit. On the basis of the admitting diagnosis, the psychosocial and physical assessment data, and the presence of an old, healing fracture found on x-ray examination, the physician and nurse suspect child abuse. In addition to the medical treatment of this child, which of the following nursing actions should also be initiated?
    ① An appointment should be made with the family pediatrician
    ② Child protection services should be notified
    ③ Family counseling services should be recommended to Mrs. Underwood
    ④ The mother should be counseled in the emergency department before Melissa's discharge

76. Ms. Brown is being admitted to the unit with cholecystitis and a bipolar manic disorder. She is scheduled for a gallbladder series in the morning. She arrives in a wheelchair, claiming she is a great actress like Betty Davis and will remember all of the little people in her future. She asks the nurse to draw her bath and have the kitchen send up pheasant for her supper. The nurse's *best* response is:
    ① "Mrs. Brown, I'll check your diet orders."
    ② "Mrs. Brown, I'll get you some more lithium."
    ③ "I'll be glad to draw your bath, but you must get into bed as soon as you are through. We have to prepare for your exam in the morning."
    ④ "Mrs. Brown, you are in the hospital. I need to get some information from you and discuss your scheduled procedures, then I will help you bathe."

77. Sarah, age 35, is an outpatient in a mental health clinic. She exhibits a range of behaviors and presents characteristics of poor impulse control. She exhibits a total disregard for rules and regulations. Sarah is expressing the characteristics of which mental disorder?
    ① Personality disorder
    ② Panic disorder
    ③ Thought process disorder
    ④ Bipolar affective disorder

78. Kay, age 20, is brought to the emergency room. Her parents report that she is a heroin addict. When Kay leaves the hospital, she needs to learn new social and living skills. This is primarily because she previously has been living in a state of:
    ① Fear of authorities
    ② Minimal contact with friends and family
    ③ Preoccupation with obtaining and taking drugs
    ④ False sense of security

79. Mr. Link puts on his call light and complains of his arm burning severely at the IV site that contains potassium. He says he cannot tolerate the pain anymore. The nurse should *first:*
    ① Assess the site, discontinue the IV, and notify the team leader
    ② Assess the site, slow the IV until it is infused, and notify the team leader
    ③ Slow the IV, assess the site, and notify the team leader
    ④ Tell him the physician ordered the medication, assess the site, and keep the IV rate the same

80. After a patient receives a calcium channel blocker, her blood pressure drops to 78/50. She says she feels all right but was dizzy when she stood. The nurse should take which nursing action while notifying the physician?
    ① Place her in a low-Fowler's position and increase her IV fluids
    ② Place her in a high-Fowler's position and increase her IV fluids
    ③ Place her in Trendelenburg's position and increase her IV fluids
    ④ Place her in reverse Trendelenburg's position and decrease her IV fluids

81. A nurse's aide on the unit mentions that Mrs. Johnson has a pulse rate of 42 beats/min. She checked the radial pulse for 15 seconds. She asks the nurse to check the pulse rate again to confirm her findings. The nurse should assess:
    ① The radial pulse for 1 minute
    ② The apical pulse for 15 seconds
    ③ The apical pulse for 1 minute
    ④ The radial pulse in each arm for 15 seconds

82. Which of the following conditions is an example of a patient response that a nurse can treat independent of physician or nursing orders/supervision?
    ① Sepsis
    ② Hypertension
    ③ Fatigue
    ④ Pneumonia

83. Mrs. Davis has angina pectoris and is now diagnosed with a myocardial infarction. Administering oxygen to Mrs. Davis is related to which of the following patient problems?
    ① Chest pain
    ② Alteration in myocardial perfusion
    ③ Anxiety
    ④ Alteration in heart rate

84. The nursing staff has reviewed Ms. C's progress to date and has written several short-term goals. Of the following outcome (goal) statements, which one is *most appropriately written?*
    ① The nurse will walk the patient whenever necessary
    ② The patient will take 15 steps, unassisted, by 5/19
    ③ The patient will be given a complete bath every day
    ④ The patient will want to be discharged by 5/16

85. A patient says he is scared about his upcoming hernia repair. He is having second thoughts about going ahead with the surgery. He states he is fearful about telling the physician that he has changed his mind. Which of the following *best* describes the nurse acting as a patient advocate?
    ① The nurse informs the surgeon that the patient does not want to go ahead with the surgery
    ② The nurse discusses the reasons for the surgery with the patient
    ③ The nurse agrees to accompany the patient to the surgical suite
    ④ The nurse tells the patient that most people are anxious about surgical procedures

86. Recent modern developments in the treatment of mental illness include:
    ① Gradual re-entry of patients back into their homes, enabling certain change in society's attitudes, discovery of tranquilizing drugs, and development of support systems
    ② Ostracization, mistreatment, and banishment from the community as a result of the individual being possessed by supernatural spirits and forces
    ③ Deinstitutionalization, concept of humors, ostracization from society, mistreatment, and major change in attitude of society
    ④ Returning patients to their homes as quickly as possible, development of support systems, and discovery of tranquilizing drugs

87. Bill has a history of difficulty with personal relationships; he does not grow or learn from experience or punishment; he has no real loyalties to any person, group, or code; and he has a tendency to rationalize behavior. Bill demonstrates which type of personality disorder?
    ① Abusive personality
    ② Paranoid personality
    ③ Borderline personality
    ④ Antisocial personality

88. Mr. Anderson, age 80, has recently moved into a nursing home. While visiting with him, a nurse notes that he is depressed. The geriatric nursing assistants have expressed frustration working with him because of his depression. The nurse may need to explain to the assistants that it may be difficult to maintain an effective relationship with this patient when he is depressed primarily because:
    ① People who are depressed are very lazy
    ② His poor personal grooming results in disgust from others
    ③ Independence and pride prevent him from asking for any kind of assistance
    ④ His pessimism arouses frustration and anger in others

89. Mr. Norris, age 62, has recently moved into a nursing home. While visiting with Mr. Norris, a nurse learns he is very depressed and feels worthless and unloved by his family. Mr. Norris is receiving medication amitriptyline (Elavil) prescribed by his physician. When would this drug be most likely to achieve the goal of lifting Mr. Norris' depression?
    ① After a 6- to 7-week period
    ② In 2 to 4 weeks
    ③ Within a few days
    ④ Almost immediately

90. Mrs. P. has a cataract extraction with an intraocular lens implant. Immediate postoperative care includes having the patient:
    ① Turn, deep breathe, and cough
    ② Lie in high-Fowler's position with knees flexed
    ③ Lie on the unoperated side and in low-Fowler's position
    ④ Lie on the operated side and in high-Fowler's position

91. In caring for a patient who has had cataract surgery, the nurse should observe for what complication that might occur?
    ① Refractive errors
    ② Conjunctivitis
    ③ Retinal detachment
    ④ Optic atrophy

92. Randy, age 19, was injured in a motor vehicle accident. X-ray examination reveals a comminuted fracture of the left arm. Randy's arm is in a long arm cast. The *most* effective way to control swelling in the left arm is through:
    ① Cast application
    ② Medication therapy
    ③ Elevation of the extremity
    ④ Heated massage q4h

93. Nursing interventions following the application of a cast include:
    ① Helping the drying process by using a heat lamp positioned 24 inches away
    ② Handling cast with the fingertips rather than the flat part of the hand
    ③ Making a "window" to ensure the relief of pressure
    ④ Keeping the cast exposed to air

94. A patient with a fractured left arm is placed in a long arm cast. Which of the following findings is indicative of neurovascular dysfunction?
    ① Foul odor coming from the cast
    ② Pain, pallor, or paresthesia
    ③ Drainage or new stains on the cast
    ④ Elevated temperature and pulse rate

95. Appropriate nursing interventions for the patient in skeletal traction include:
    ① Restricting movement and turning until the pin is removed
    ② Releasing traction weights q8h
    ③ Manipulating slipped pins back into place
    ④ Ensuring that the weights hang freely

96. Which of the following actions should the nurse initiate if she suspects that a child's condition may be the result of an abusive situation?
    ① Ask the mother to go to the waiting room
    ② Undress the child and help her into a hospital gown
    ③ Send for any of the child's old medical records and x-ray studies
    ④ Call the hospital business office for a bill estimate to give to the mother

97. All of the following observations in a newborn infant are important. Which one should take *highest* priority in terms of planning his care?
    ① Skin eruptions
    ② Frequent crying
    ③ Cyanotic hands and feet
    ④ Respiratory difficulties

98. A patient asks the nursery nurse what the "white spots" on her baby's nose are. The nurse tells her that plugged sebaceous glands on the nose and cheeks of the newborn are called:
    ① Vernix caseosa
    ② Milia
    ③ Lanugo
    ④ Mongolian spots

99. A 22-year-old undergoes a variety of tests for evaluation of a persistent dry cough, night sweats, and weight loss. Testing reveals that he is HIV positive. The positive HIV result indicates:
    ① An infection of unknown etiology
    ② The presence of AIDS-related complex
    ③ That he has a definitive diagnosis of AIDS
    ④ Exposure to the virus known to cause AIDS and antibody development

100. An HIV-positive patient shows the nurse two reddish-purple bumps on the top of his mouth. This finding is most probably which opportunistic infection associated with immunosuppression?
    ① Tuberculosis
    ② Herpes simplex
    ③ Kaposi's sarcoma
    ④ *Pneumocystis carinii*

101. Which of the following precautions reflects an understanding of the methods of transmission of the AIDS virus?
    ① Precautions are limited to individuals with respiratory problems
    ② Necessary precautions should be taken with any patient known to be HIV positive
    ③ Precautions should be used with all patients, assuming that they could be HIV positive
    ④ Only needle and blood precautions are necessary

102. Tammy is brought to the emergency room by her mother, who thinks that the child has a fractured arm. The nurse also notes several bruises that do not appear to be related to a broken arm. Considering Tammy's injury, which of the following questions would be most helpful during the nurse's data collection?
    ① "Where are Tammy's toys located?"
    ② "At what age did Tammy begin to climb and walk?"
    ③ "What time does Tammy usually get up in the morning and go to bed?"
    ④ "What usual methods of discipline do you use for Tammy?"

103. Jimmy Johnson, age 16, has just been diagnosed as having insulin-dependent diabetes mellitus. If Jimmy receives NPH insulin at 7AM, when would he be most likely to have a hypoglycemic reaction?
    ① 8 AM to 11 AM
    ② 12 noon to 3 PM
    ③ 5 PM to 11 PM
    ④ 12 midnight to 4 AM

104. A call is placed to a clinic by a mother who says her 16-year-old daughter has a boyfriend who has mononucleosis. When asked the symptoms of this condition, the nurse should indicate which of the following?
    ① Chronic infections, urinary tract infections, pneumonia, weight loss, and hepatosplenomegaly
    ② Fatigue, enlarged lymph nodes, fever and sore throat, and stiff neck
    ③ Polyphagia, polyuria, fatigability, and polydipsia
    ④ Changes in behavior patterns, poor academic performance, and wearing long-sleeved blouses

105. Five-month-old Chad is admitted to the hospital because of severe diarrhea. The nurse would describe Chad as having diarrhea on the basis of:
    ① Color and consistency of stools
    ② Consistency and frequency of stools
    ③ Amount and color of stools
    ④ Frequency and amount of stools

106. Mrs. Peterson has just had her second child and has a 2-year-old daughter at home. She is afraid her 2-year-old will be jealous of the baby. Of the following suggestions, which one is *most appropriate* for the nurse to include in her conversation with Mrs. Peterson?
    ① "Divide your time equally between the two children."
    ② "Ignore any signs of jealousy to diminish the behavior."
    ③ "Give your daughter undivided attention, for a short period, several times a day."
    ④ "Keep the children apart to prevent your daughter from harming the baby."

107. Mrs. C is being discharged with her first child. She tells the nurse she is afraid she might not know how often to feed the baby. The nurse responds that it is generally agreed that an infant should be fed:
    ① On a demand schedule when he becomes hungry
    ② Every 4 hours even if he has to be forced to eat
    ③ At least every 2 hours for the first 2 months of life
    ④ At the convenience of the mother

108. Mrs. Bowen asks the nurse when her baby's umbilical cord will drop off. The nurse answers that the cord will normally drop off when the infant's age is between:
    ① 3 and 4 days
    ② 7 and 10 days
    ③ 12 and 14 days
    ④ 15 and 20 days

109. Four-month-old Brent is admitted to the hospital because of severe diarrhea. When providing treatment, the nurse should initially plan to:
① Offer Pedilyte (electrolyte solution) and clear liquids progressing up to half-strength formula
② Observe closely, keep baby NPO, and follow isolation procedures
③ Note time, type, and character of vomitus; weigh daily; and check patency of IV
④ Provide large amounts of fluids, remove all blankets, and monitor temperature hourly

110. Jenny, age 7 months, has severe diarrhea and is brought to the local neighborhood clinic. The nurse should expect that in addition to dehydration, Jenny also has:
① An electrolyte imbalance
② Retention of urine
③ Hyperactive reflexes
④ Pulmonary congestion

111. Three-month-old Betty Lou is admitted to the hospital with a diagnosis of diarrhea. Betty Lou is very irritable and is kept NPO. Which nursing intervention would be most beneficial for her irritability?
① Putting a mobile above the crib
② Talking quietly to the infant
③ Giving a pacifier
④ Placing Betty Lou with other infants

112. Nursing interventions for a child with upper respiratory tract infection may include:
① Antibiotics, ear drops, encouraging fluids, and eliminating environmental allergies
② Providing emotional support for the parents, decreasing fluids, positioning on the side, and decreasing stimuli
③ Antipyretics, bed rest, oral decongestants, cool air humidifier, proper nutrition, and encouraging fluids
④ Breathing exercises, liquid diet, steroid medications, bronchodilator medications, and intermittent positive-pressure breathing treatments

113. A 60-year-old black male is admitted to the hospital. He has a long history of hypertension. His BUN and creatinine levels are markedly elevated. A diagnosis of chronic renal failure is made. The chronic renal failure is *most probably* related to:
① Aging
② Diuretic use
③ Hypertension
④ Prostate problems

114. As the nurse is finishing her shift assessment, a patient who is HIV positive begins crying. He states he has lost most of his close friends and that his family doesn't want to see or talk to him anymore. What should be the nurse's *best* action?
① Tell him not to worry; there are many community agencies that can help
② Guide the conversation toward the acceptance phase of his illness
③ Encourage him to establish a relationship with another patient
④ Sit down and listen to his concerns and frustration

115. A 30-year-old is HIV positive. Significant others include his mother, father, two sisters, his lover, and a cat. He is now ready for discharge. He asks questions about living in a household with other individuals. Which of the following statements by the patient indicates his understanding of teachings relative to home care?
① "I'll have someone clean the cat's litter pan."
② "I'll use gloves when preparing meals."
③ "My clothes and bed linens should be washed and dried separately."
④ "I'll avoid contact with others so the risk of AIDS transmission will be decreased."

116. After checking for placement of an enteral feeding tube, the nurse prepares for the next enteral feeding of Ensure 480 ml. The residual feeding is assessed, and 500 ml is aspirated from the stomach. The nurse should proceed as follows:
① Hold the feeding and notify the physician
② Give the 480 ml of feeding as scheduled
③ Hold this feeding and give extra the next feeding
④ Give half of the feeding and the other half in an hour

117. A nurse developed low back pain after lifting some equipment at work. A diagnosis of herniated intervertebral disk is made. Bed rest and methocarbamol (Robaxin) are ordered. The desired effects of the medication are achieved if which of the following occurs?
① Her anxiety is lessened
② She sleeps more restfully at night
③ A decrease in muscle spasms occurs
④ Pain radiation to upper back is reduced

118. A patient with complaints of low back pain is admitted for evaluation. Which question by the nurse would obtain the *best* assessment data?
① "Do you feel like you need to urinate?"
② "Does the pain interfere with your daily activities?"
③ "Describe your pain and any associated feelings of discomfort."
④ "Is there any increase in pain when you have a bowel movement?"

119. A myelogram is ordered for a patient with low back pain that has not responded to bed rest. Which of the following *best* describes the procedure?
① A contrast medium is injected via a lumbar puncture
② Small needles are inserted into the back muscles being evaluated
③ An amplified recording of the electrical activity of the brain is obtained
④ A noninvasive, painless procedure provides cross-sectional views of the spine

120. During the postoperative period following a lumbar laminectomy at the L4-L5 level, nursing care should include:
① Instructing the patient to turn as a unit
② Maintaining the patient's legs in an adducted position
③ Limiting range-of-motion exercises to the lower extremities
④ Turning the patient from side to side using the log-rolling technique

COMPREHENSIVE EXAMINATION ONE: PART TWO

121. Bob is admitted to the hospital for treatment of cirrhosis of the liver. The nurse who admits Bob says to the nursing assistant that Bob must be an alcoholic. This is an example of:
    ① A mental set
    ② An ideology
    ③ A halo effect
    ④ A stereotype

122. Lori, age 67, has a history of Parkinson's disease. During assessment, which of the following signs can the nurse anticipate Lori to exhibit?
    ① Impaired physical mobility and verbal communication with muscle rigidity, tremors and akinesia
    ② Exaggerated sense of euphoria, salivation, and decline in cognitive memory and perceptual abilities
    ③ Headache, dizziness, seizures, aphasia, and personality changes including fear and anxiety
    ④ Nausea and vomiting, lethargy, disorientation; may appear dazed or unconscious

123. Fred Townsend, age 87, has recently moved into a nursing home and is feeling depressed. His physician has prescribed amitriptyline hydrochloride (Elavil). An adverse effect of this antidepressant may be:
    ① Diarrhea
    ② Insomnia
    ③ Hypertension
    ④ Urinary retention

124. The older adult may perform certain cognitive tasks more slowly because of:
    ① Increased motor response to sensory stimulation
    ② Increase of visual and auditory acuity
    ③ Loss of the family unit
    ④ Recent memory loss

125. Avoiding injury in the older adult involves:
    ① Eating low-energy food; daily outdoor exercise; keeping at least one room warm
    ② Using higher light intensity; avoiding objects on floor; avoiding use of blues and greens
    ③ Using direct lights, exposed light bulbs; using white surfaces
    ④ Keeping room temperature somewhat lower than usual; preparing signs with light backgrounds and dark lettering; daily contact with another person

126. Fern, age 49, is admitted to the hospital for treatment of cirrhosis of the liver. After several days in the hospital, Fern complains of "bugs all over my bed." When completing her charting, how should the nurse best express Fern's behavior?
    ① Seeing "bugs" on her bed
    ② Out of contact with reality
    ③ Restless and disoriented; hallucinating
    ④ Agitated; auditory hallucination

127. Mrs. Roberts has been admitted to the hospital for treatment of cirrhosis of the liver. Her husband does not believe her intake of a six-pack of beer daily has any connection to her liver disorder. The defense mechanism that Mr. Roberts is exhibiting is:
    ① Reaction formation
    ② Displacement
    ③ Denial
    ④ Rationalization

128. Mr. Pauling, a long-time alcoholic, is going home on a weekend pass. His physician has ordered disulfiram (Antabuse A). Which statement made by the patient shows understanding regarding his medication?
    ① "I can drink, but if my blood alcohol level gets above 0.1, then I will be ill."
    ② "The Antabuse will keep me from wanting a drink and I can more effectively participate in AA and other therapy."
    ③ "I should not take any over-the-counter cough syrups."
    ④ "The Antabuse will alter my metabolism so the alcohol will have no effect on my system."

129. Mrs. Furlow has a depressive disorder and has been ordered to receive amitriptyline (Elavil). After 4 days she says, "I don't believe this helps; I don't feel any different." The nurse's *best* statement should be:
    ① "I will check the dosage to see if it is therapeutic."
    ② "I know you feel frustrated, but we are doing all we can."
    ③ "Tricyclic antidepressants may require 3 to 4 weeks before any significant effect can be noticed."
    ④ "You may have some benefits you haven't noticed."

130. A patient in a psychiatric unit is a substance abuser and has been avoiding talking about his abuse of chemicals. He says, "I am just bored," or "I can get along fine," or he makes similar statements when asked about his use of chemicals. The nurse recognizes that:
    ① He is attempting to manipulate her into not confronting him
    ② Denial is a common defense mechanism for substance abusers
    ③ Strict limits on activities may be needed so he will communicate more effectively
    ④ Alteration of this patient's reward system may be needed to verbalize his feelings

131. Thirteen-month-old Kerri is admitted to the hospital with a fracture of the right femur. She is accompanied by both parents, each of whom provides a different story. Child abuse is suspected. The nurse should be alert to which of the following that may indicate abuse?
    ① Thumb-sucking
    ② Underdevelopment for her age
    ③ Interacting well with others
    ④ Eating well without urging

132. An 18-year-old male patient has 85% burns on the entire posterior aspects of his body to the mid-axilla on each side. He is complaining of severe pain and requests medication. The physician has ordered meperidine (Demerol) and hydroxyzine (Vistaril) intramuscularly for his complaints of pain. The nurse should use which site for the injection?
   ① Deltoid
   ② Dorsogluteal
   ③ Ventrogluteal
   ④ Vastus lateralis

133. A nurse wonders what the repercussions of reporting child abuse are, especially if abuse was not the cause of injury. An emergency room nurse correctly informs her that:
   ① Nurses will be held accountable in court if the injury was not caused by abuse
   ② Nurses reporting suspected child abuse cases are protected from civil action
   ③ The parents may obtain legal services and file suit in civil court against the nurse
   ④ The nurse can be discharged as a hospital employee if abuse is not the cause of the injury

134. Cindy, a secretarial stenographer, is admitted to the emergency department with a history of increased seizure activity during the last 48 hours. Nursing diagnosis for Cindy, or a patient with seizures, may include, but *need not be* limited to:
   ① Ineffective airway clearance, anxiety, and potential for injury
   ② Altered nutrition, potential for powerlessness, and loss of body control
   ③ Constipation related to intestinal mobility, and potential for aspiration
   ④ Anxiety as a result of cognitive impairment, functional incontinence, and potential for injury related to cognitive problems

135. Barbara is a 42-year-old rehabilitation counselor who is seen at a local clinic for a routine follow-up visit. She reports that because she had not been having effective control of seizures, her physician prescribed another medication, carbamazepine (Tegretol). Barbara indicates that this new medication was enabling good control. Carbamazepine is prescribed for what type of seizures?
   ① Petit mal, akinetic
   ② Grand mal, focal
   ③ Grand mal, petit mal
   ④ Grand mal, psychomotor

136. A patient has been diagnosed by his physician as having congestive heart failure. He can best avoid weight from fluid retention by:
   ① Taking his prescribed diuretic before bedtime
   ② Limiting his salt intake
   ③ Reducing all food intake
   ④ Following a high-calorie diet and forcing fluids

137. Mrs. P has an obsessive compulsive disorder. The nurse knows that Mrs. P has begun to identify her feelings when she states:
   ① "I don't use compulsive activities as often in the hospital"
   ② "I try to involve myself in other activities when obsessive thoughts enter my consciousness."
   ③ "I will never have compulsive behavior again."
   ④ "Anxiety is so unpredictable that I stay prepared all the time."

138. Mary, age 32, has a history of multiple sclerosis. Signs and symptoms of multiple sclerosis are:
   ① Impaired chewing and eating, excessive sweating, and tremors
   ② Aphasia, syncope, and seizures
   ③ Blurred vision, dysphasia, and ataxia
   ④ Splenomegaly, hepatomegaly, and elevated white blood count

139. Mr. Warren, age 72, has been admitted to the hospital. His symptoms include rapid, shallow, dyspneic respirations. He has been diagnosed by his physician as having congestive heart failure. What cardiac drug would the nurse expect to be ordered in Mr. Warren's case?
   ① Inderol
   ② Aspirin
   ③ Lanoxin
   ④ Atropine

140. Mr. Gray, age 32, has delusions of persecution involving the CIA and the KGB. Following occupational therapy one day, Mr. Gray asks if he can work on his wood-burning activities on the unit. The nurse's *primary* consideration in response is:
   ① Encouraging participation in activities to accomplish goals
   ② Concern for patient safety
   ③ Unit rules on activities
   ④ Other patients' response to Mr. Gray's privileges

141. Brenda Kayn, a 26-year-old schizophrenic, is discussing her relations with her estranged husband. She discusses making a complete break and then discusses their future while she laughs and cries throughout the conversation. The nurse recognizes this as:
   ① Apathy
   ② Ambivalence
   ③ Paranoia
   ④ A simple defense mechanism

142. Mrs. Harris, a 54-year-old disorganized schizophrenic, is walking around complaining of hornets stinging her all over her body. The nurse should note which of the following actions on the plan of care?
   ① Keep the patient away from areas where insects may be present
   ② Discuss with the patient the sensation of stinging hornets
   ③ Place medication on sting areas
   ④ Frequently assess the skin for integrity

143. A skin infection that is characterized by red vesicular lesions often seen in newborn nurseries and is caused by *Streptococcus* or *Staphyloccus* bacteria is known as:
   ① Infantile eczema
   ② Pediculosis
   ③ Urticaria
   ④ Impetigo

144. The nurse knows that physiologic jaundice, which is often seen on or about the infant's third day of life, indicates:
    ① An incompatibility of mother and infant blood
    ② Damage to infant's liver
    ③ Destruction of the excessive number of red blood cells present at birth
    ④ Improper care of infant at birth

145. The newborn's movements are jerky and uncoordinated. The nurse understands that this is a result of:
    ① A warm, comfortable environment
    ② An immature nervous system
    ③ No muscle tone
    ④ Injuries received during birth

146. The newborn's skin is bright red as a result of:
    ① Irritation during delivery
    ② Large amounts of pigment characteristic of all newborns
    ③ Anemia, which is common in newborns
    ④ The large number of red blood cells present in the infant's blood

147. Mr. Hix tells the nurse that he will be the most popular patient in the unit once everyone gets to know him. The nurse responds, "Mr. Hix, it sounds like you are concerned with how others feel about you." The technique the nurse used is:
    ① Seeking clarification
    ② Encouraging comparisons
    ③ Summarizing
    ④ Focusing

148. Mrs. Patrick is a patient with a depressive disorder. She is sitting in the dayroom knitting when the nurse approaches her to ask if she would like to talk. When she doesn't respond, the nurse replies, "I'll just sit down with you for a while in case you feel like talking." The nurse is using which of the following techniques when dealing with the patient?
    ① Open-ended questions
    ② Empathetic understanding
    ③ Therapeutic use of self
    ④ Reflection

149. Susan, a recent nursing graduate, would like to work with physically challenged patients. Rehabilitation nursing is defined as:
    ① The medical-surgical specialty concerned with the physiologic and pathologic changes in later maturity
    ② The blend of nursing and public health, promoting prevention, education, and maintenance
    ③ The nursing process of maximizing the use of an individual's capabilities or resources to foster optimal growth and functioning
    ④ The practice in which a nurse assists the individual in the performance of those activities contributing to health or its recovery, or peaceful death

150. Jason, age 20, enters an outpatient clinic in an agitated state. He reports that his best friend has been diagnosed as HIV positive. The nurse knows that AIDS is best described as:
    ① A disease of the immune system
    ② A chronic and incurable disease that is multicausal in origin
    ③ A neoplastic immunodeficiency disease
    ④ An inflammatory skin response to certain allergenic offenders

151. Derrick, age 51, is admitted to the hospital for treatment of cirrhosis of the liver. Noncaffeinated beverages are substituted for his usual colas and coffee. This is done because:
    ① Regular colas and coffee have a diuretic effect that interferes with hydration
    ② A transfer of the patient's oral dependency needs to take place
    ③ Regular caffeinated coffee and colas aggravate tremors and interfere with sleep
    ④ Patients tend to transfer their addiction to coffee instead of to alcohol

152. Diane is admitted to the hospital for treatment of cirrhosis of the liver. She is prescribed large doses of niacin. Diane should be observed for side effects of niacin that include:
    ① Retention of body fluids
    ② Eyelid irritation
    ③ Swelling of the tongue
    ④ Flushing of the skin

153. Mrs. F is admitted to the unit following an attempt at suicide. In planning suicide precautions for Mrs. F, the nurse should include:
    ① Providing occupational therapy to keep her active and to keep her thoughts away from suicide
    ② Sedation when the patient shows agitation and anxiety
    ③ Limiting her activities to her room or to strictly supervised activities
    ④ Walks and outdoor activities to promote physical fitness

154. Joanne was brought to the emergency room by her roommate after she stayed up all night telephoning the police to report that she was being spied on by aliens who had taken over their town. The idea that aliens are spying on her is an example of:
    ① Loose association
    ② Autistic thinking
    ③ Persecutory delusion
    ④ Conversion reaction

155. A patient says that she is frightened of aliens. The *best* response by the nurse should be:
    ① "I don't see anything like that."
    ② "Where do you see them, exactly?"
    ③ "I understand that you are feeling afraid."
    ④ "Don't worry, you'll feel better soon."

156. Marina Sims, age 13, comes to the school health office to see the nurse. Marina tells the nurse that she has some questions about "being a woman" and that she cannot talk about this with her mother because her mother doesn't understand her. Which of the following statements about early adolescent development helps the nurse understand Marina's statement?
    ① Marina is developing a disrespectful attitude toward her mother
    ② Young adolescents sometimes normally reject parental efforts at guidance
    ③ Seeking independence from the family is normally a task of late adolescence
    ④ Professional therapy is often needed at this age to control the adolescent child

157. Fourteen-year-old Teri is wearing clothes in the newest fashion with her hair stylishly combed. She states that looking attractive at school is very important to her. What understanding of adolescent development should the nurse have before responding to Teri?
- ① Teri is unduly influenced by peer pressure at this age
- ② Teri is behaving in a narcissistic manner
- ③ Peer responses are normally important to early adolescents
- ④ Promiscuous tendencies are evident in Teri's attitude

158. A 13-year-old tells the school nurse that her menses began 6 months ago but that her periods are irregular. What advice can the nurse *appropriately* give the adolescent?
- ① For the first year or so after menses begins, periods are commonly irregular
- ② Something may be wrong; it is best to schedule an appointment with a physician
- ③ She should not worry so much about menses; nature and time takes care of minor problems
- ④ She should ask her mother for advice

159. Sue, age 13, asks the nurse if soaking in a tub bath is "okay" during menses because she heard that water could be harmful at that time. What would be the *best* response by the nurse?
- ① "It is always better to take a shower during menses rather than a tub bath."
- ② "Tub bathing, as well as showering, is a good hygiene practice during menses."
- ③ "Immersion in water is not safe during menses."
- ④ "It's best to take a sponge bath during menses to avoid contamination of the perineal area."

160. In prenatal clinics, the nurse is responsible for teaching patients the danger signals of pregnancy. Which of the following symptoms is *not* considered a danger signal of pregnancy?
- ① Excessive swelling of the feet
- ② Persistent vomiting
- ③ Increased vaginal discharge
- ④ Persistent headaches

161. A patient has been diagnosed with placenta previa. Considering the diagnosis, the nurse expects to find the patient complaining of which of the following?
- ① Abdominal pain
- ② Painless vaginal bleeding
- ③ Uterine tenderness
- ④ Tetanic contractions

162. While caring for a patient diagnosed with placenta previa, the nurse must be especially observant for increased vaginal bleeding. Placenta previa is a complication of pregnancy indicating:
- ① The placenta separates prematurely from the uterine wall
- ② The placenta has one umbilical vein and two arteries
- ③ The placenta adheres high on the wall of the uterus
- ④ The placenta lies low in the uterus or completely covers the cervical os

163. The nurse is giving Baby Boy Zellers his *first* oral feeding of sterile water. The infant quickly starts to cough and choke. He sounds as if he has moist respirations. His color is pink, and he has appropriate reflex responses. The *first* thing the nurse should do is:
- ① Stop the feeding and try again in ½ hour
- ② Stop the feeding, burp the baby, and resume feeding
- ③ Stop the feeding, and notify the physician or the nurse in charge
- ④ Understand that this is normal, as all babies need to learn how to suck and swallow

164. If the nurse observes an infant gagging on mucus and becoming cyanotic, she should *first:*
- ① Call the charge nurse
- ② Aspirate the pharynx with a bulb syringe
- ③ Raise the baby's head and pat the infant on the back
- ④ Give oxygen by positive pressure

165. Which of the following techniques is *most* important in preventing infections in the newborn nursery?
- ① Sterilize all baby linen
- ② Use scrub attire for all nursing personnel
- ③ Wash hands before and after each infant contact
- ④ Have individualized newborn equipment

166. John is a 32-year-old truck driver who is admitted to the hospital with a fractured hip. Appropriate nursing diagnoses would include:
- ① Anxiety, knowledge deficit, and potential for injury
- ② Sleep pattern disturbance, activity intolerance, and altered thought processes
- ③ Pain, impaired physical mobility, and altered peripheral tissue perfusion
- ④ Knowledge deficit, alteration in self-concept, and impaired physical mobility

167. Mrs. Bee, age 71, uses timolol (Timoptic) for glaucoma at home. While visiting her on a home visit, the nurse observes that the patient's apical pulse rate is 50 beats/min. What action should be taken?
- ① Contact Mrs. Bee's physician and discuss her heart rate and parameters for continuation of the medicine
- ② Instruct Mrs. Bee to continue the drug as prescribed and continue to monitor the heart rate
- ③ Tell Mrs. Bee to stop taking the drug and to discuss it with her physician during her next weekly appointment
- ④ Tell Mrs. Bee to stop taking the drug, then reassess her pulse rate the next day

168. The physician orders nitroglycerin ointment for his patient to prevent any further chest pain. Soon after applying the ointment to the patient, the nurse begins to have heart palpitations and feel faint. After noticing the ointment on her hands, the nurse realizes that she is probably experiencing:
- ① A local effect
- ② A systemic effect
- ③ An additive effect
- ④ A teratogenic effect

169. An 85-year-old stroke patient has an order for turning q2h. When the nurse goes into the room to turn her, the family refuses and states that she has "had enough" and that she needs to rest. The nurse should:
① Call for assistance and turn the patient; instruct the family that physician orders must be followed
② Wait an hour or so and hope the family members will change their mind; if not, insist that the patient be turned
③ Explain that it is the physician's order and must be continued; family members will need to speak to the physician on his next rounds
④ Explain the importance of turning to the family and arrange for the patient to rest uninterrupted for the next 2 hours

170. Triazolam (halcion) 0.25 mg is ordered qh for rest. It comes in 0.125 mg tablets. How many scored tablets should be given?
① ½ tablet
② 2 tablets
③ 2½ tablets
④ 4 tablets

171. A patient, Mrs. B, is being discharged. During preparations for the discharge, Mrs. B's daughter voices concern over use of the wrist restraints and posey vest. The nurse should instruct the daughter to:
① Use the restraints only at night
② Loosen the posey vest and turn the patient every 6 to 8 hours
③ Release the restraints every few hours, checking for circulation to the hands
④ Release the restraints q2h or more often and check for circulation to the hands

172. A patient has a physician's order to force fluids to 4340 ml q24h. How many 8-oz glasses of liquid can she have over a period of 24 hours?
① 10
② 18
③ 22
④ 26

173. Sally is completely incoherent. Her roommate asks the nurse whether she should contact Sally's parents to come to the hospital. The nurse's best response would be:
① "It's better for them not to see her when she is so confused."
② "Please call them; perhaps they can give us some helpful information."
③ "No; she is an adult and responsible for her own care."
④ "No; that would violate her confidentiality."

174. The nursing diagnosis that should receive priority for a thought-disordered patient in the emergency room is:
① Ineffective individual coping related to disordered thought processes
② Anxiety related to perceived environmental threat
③ Violence, potential for, related to confusion
④ Knowledge deficit related to new onset of illness

175. The drug that the nurse would most likely administer in the emergency room to a patient with a thought disorder is a/an:
① MAO inhibitor
② Tricyclic antidepressant
③ Hypnotic
④ Antipsychotic

176. The psychiatrist in the emergency room decides that Joanne needs to be admitted to the hospital. She refuses to sign herself in, saying "it is a plot by the aliens." Her parents ask what the possible options are in this situation. Which is the *best* answer for the nurse to give?
① Joanne can be sent home with her roommate because she does not want to stay in the hospital
② Her parents can sign her out of the hospital if they are willing to take responsibility for her safety
③ Joanne will be kept in the emergency room under nursing supervision until she feels better
④ Joanne can be involuntarily committed to the hospital if the physician judges that she is a danger to herself

177. Mrs. Gray brings her 1-month-old son, Lee, to a well-baby clinic. Which of the following developmental achievements is normal for Lee?
① Smiling and laughing out loud
② Rolling from back to his side
③ Holding a rattle for a short period of time
④ Turning his head from side to side

178. Mrs. Nelson brings her 4-month-old infant, Pat, into a well-baby clinic. Pat appears healthy. What would you *not* expect Pat to be demonstrating at 4 months of age?
① Responding to pleasure with smiles
② Grasping a rattle
③ Sitting up without support
④ Turning himself from his side to his back

179. Mrs. Oltman brings her 5-month-old infant, Benjamin, into a well-baby clinic. Ben appears healthy, and Mrs. Oltman asks when she should wean Ben from breast feeding. The nurse should inform her that Ben will show readiness to be weaned when he is:
① Sleeping through the night
② Taking solid foods well
③ Eating on a regular schedule
④ Around 6 months of age

180. Nancy, age 4, has been exposed to chicken pox while in daycare today. The nurse knows that clinical signs and symptoms should include:
① Severe cold with high temperature, nasal congestion, cough, and conjunctivitis
② Headache, stiff neck, malaise, sore throat, and coryza
③ Slight fever, anorexia, and malaise
④ Low-grade fever, malaise, edema, and pain in salivary glands

181. To appropriately teach prenatal patients good health behaviors, it is important for the nurse to know that the fetus is most susceptible to malformation from teratogens during the:
① First trimester
② Second trimester
③ Third trimester
④ Last half of pregnancy

182. In preparing to teach a class on nutrition in a prenatal clinic, the nurse knows it is suggested that the pregnant mother increase her caloric intake by:
    ① 300 calories per day
    ② 500 calories per day
    ③ 800 calories per day
    ④ 1200 calories per day

183. In early labor, Mrs. Peters is very anxious about the outcome of this pregnancy. She asks the nurse, "Do you think that the baby will be okay?" The nurse should respond appropriately by saying:
    ① "Oh, I wouldn't be too concerned. Your other children are fine."
    ② "I really don't know. I hope so."
    ③ "Yes, I'm sure you're worried. Would you like to talk about what concerns you have?"
    ④ "Why would you be concerned? You have a very good physician."

184. During one of her prenatal visits, Mrs. Bayer complains of "heartburn." She claims that it happens every day and she really does not want to eat because of it. The nurse's *best* response should be to advise Mrs. Bayer to:
    ① Eat one large meal in mid-day
    ② Eat frequent, small amounts of foods that are not greasy or fried
    ③ Take ½ tsp of sodium bicarbonate in water to relieve the heartburn
    ④ Buy an antacid in the drugstore and follow the directions on the label

185. Mrs. Johnson is 5 months' pregnant and has some problems with constipation. The nurse would teach her that she could decrease constipation by:
    ① Eating an adequate diet that includes fluids, fresh fruits and vegetables, and fiber
    ② Administering a Fleets enema when necessary
    ③ Maintaining good posture while standing and working
    ④ Using a glycerine suppository as necessary

186. Knowing that the average adult dose of a medication as listed in drug literature is based on an adult who weighs 150 lbs and is between the ages of 18 and 65, the nurse should be *most* concerned about delivering the average adult dose to which of the following?
    ① A 16-year-old who plays football and weighs 200 lbs
    ② An adult of normal weight and height who has a liver disease
    ③ An elderly lady, age 85, who is dehydrated and has an emaciated appearance
    ④ A 69-year-old gentleman who is in relatively good health except for degenerative arthritis

187. Mr. Joseph had a barium enema yesterday. On rounds today, the nurse should be most concerned in assessing for which of the following?
    ① Whether a bowel movement has occurred since the test
    ② Bowel sounds and any complaints of pain or discomfort
    ③ Color, amount, and consistency of the last bowel movement
    ④ Whether the patient is passing flatus, how much, and how often

188. While making rounds, the nurse notices that the Salem Sump is not draining into the suction apparatus properly for a new postoperative patient. The nurse should perform which of the following measures?
    ① Irrigate the blue pigtail with air
    ② Irrigate the blue pigtail with water
    ③ Disconnect the suction and irrigate with air through the tube
    ④ Disconnect the suction and irrigate with water through the tube

189. Hal was receiving an antibiotic supplied in 50-mg capsules. How many capsules should be given per dose if 0.2 g PO is ordered daily in four divided doses?
    ① ½
    ② 1
    ③ 2½
    ④ 4

190. Mr. C.D. is a 55-year-old factory line worker, a heavy smoker, and obese. He is admitted with the diagnosis of Buerger's disease. When assessing Mr. C.D. for symptoms typical of Buerger's disease, the nurse should observe for:
    ① Leg pain at rest (not associated with activity)
    ② Redness and pain along a vein pathway
    ③ Dilated veins and ankle edema
    ④ A positive Homans' sign

191. In preparing a patient for testing related to Buerger's disease, the nurse explains that the three diagnostic tests are Doppler ultrasonography, arteriography, and:
    ① Echocardiography
    ② Stress test
    ③ Electrocardiogram
    ④ Oscillometry

192. When documenting the type of pain in a patient with Buerger's disease, the term that most accurately describes such pain is:
    ① Claudication
    ② Intermittent claudication
    ③ Homans' sign
    ④ Hyperemia

193. In providing nursing care for a patient with Buerger's disease, the nurse should stress:
    ① Restricting salt and eggs in the diet
    ② Substituting margarine for butter
    ③ Wearing cotton socks and gloves
    ④ Avoiding smoking and cold temperatures

194. After a patient is admitted to the inpatient psychiatric unit, she asks if she can keep her personal belongings. What is the *best* response for the nurse to make?
    ① "Of course you can. This is not a prison."
    ② "Of course not this is a psychiatric unit."
    ③ "You will be allowed to keep anything that is not harmful to you or anyone else."
    ④ "Everything will be sent home with your family to keep until your thinking is clearer."

195. To provide effective intervention for the most serious side effects of antipsychotic medications, the nurse should:
    ① Recommend high-calorie snacks between activities
    ② Administer antiparkinsonian drugs as ordered
    ③ Restrict potassium intake at meals and snacks
    ④ Provide extra exercise periods as requested by patient

196. Jimmy, age 5, has been exposed to chicken pox while in school today. His mother inquires how long from exposure to onset of symptoms. The correct response would be:
    ① 2 to 5 days, sometimes longer
    ② 2 to 3 weeks
    ③ 4 to 15 days
    ④ 12 to 26 days

197. Four-month-old Sara is seen at a local clinic because of severe diarrhea. Because of Sarah's diarrhea, she presents signs and symptoms of dehydration that include:
    ① Slow, labored breathing, bulging anterior fontanel, glassy eyes, and low-grade fever
    ② Rapid shallow breathing, depressed anterior fontanel, hollow eyes, and high fever
    ③ Failure to gain weight, delayed motor activities, and inadequate growth weight
    ④ Anemia, listlessness, and an appearance of malnourishment

198. Eight-month-old Brad is brought into a physician's office because he has had diarrhea for the past 24 hours. Potential causes for Brad's *acute* diarrhea could include:
    ① Cystic fibrosis, celiac disease, or carcinoid tumors
    ② Parasites, protein-calorie malnutrition, or chronic pancreatitis
    ③ Irritable colon syndrome, hyperthyroidism, or immune deficiencies
    ④ Changes in formula, milk protein allergy, or URI (upper respiratory tract infection—otitis media)

199. Jamie, age 2, is brought into the clinic for a well-baby check-up. Jamie's physical growth would be expected to show:
    ① A decrease in rate of growth, but an increase in rate of development
    ② A gain of less than 5 lb and less than an inch in height each year
    ③ An increase in rate of growth and a decrease in rate of development
    ④ A rapid language development, and talking to himself and other people

200. Jim Smith, age 50, was involved in a motor vehicle accident. During the accident, the buckle on the seatbelt caused a blunt injury to his bladder. Following an anterior repair of his bladder, Mr. Smith is admitted to the surgical unit. During the transfer of Mr. Smith from the operating room to his bed, he complains of nausea and begins vomiting. Which of the following should be the *first* nursing action?
    ① Obtain the antiemetic medication as ordered
    ② Turn his head to the side
    ③ Quickly place him on the bed
    ④ Notify the team leader or physician

201. Mr. B, recovering from bladder surgery, is ordered promethazine (Phenergan) 50 mg intramuscularly for nausea. What is the best method for administering this medication?
    ① The ventrogluteal site should be chosen for the injection
    ② Hold the syringe at a 45-degree angle
    ③ Mark the site for the injection with an index finger
    ④ Use a ⅝ inch needle for greater patient comfort

202. Mr. P returns from bladder surgery with a Foley catheter. What is the *best* procedure in caring for his catheter?
    ① Extra tubing should be coiled to prevent urinary stasis
    ② For sanitary reasons, disconnect the drainage bag and drain the urine in the bathroom
    ③ The drainage bag should be attached to the bed at a level lower than the bladder
    ④ Tape the catheter to the patient's thigh for comfort

203. Mr. White has a large abdominal dressing and a closed suction drain following an anterior repair of the bladder. During the first evening after surgery, the nurse notes a 2 cm spot of blood on the abdominal dressing. What should her next action be?
    ① Notify the team leader or physician immediately
    ② Remove the dressing and inspect the wound
    ③ Reinforce the dressing with a sterile ABD pad
    ④ Mark the spot and assess the dressing for further bleeding

204. A patient weighs 260 lbs and is 6 ft tall. On the third postoperative day, which of the following signs would indicate a postoperative complication?
    ① The catheter is draining very light yellow urine
    ② The patient requests a medication for incisional pain
    ③ The dressing becomes damp with serosanguinous drainage
    ④ The patient complains about his full-liquid diet

205. Mr. Samuels two days postoperatively begins to cough and tells the nurse, "I just felt something 'give away' under this bandage." What *appropriate* action should the nurse take next?
    ① Ask the patient why he coughed so hard
    ② Check the incision
    ③ Reassure the patient that he is 'okay'
    ④ Obtain the ordered pain medication for the patient

206. Kassie is an active 2-year-old. Three characteristic behaviors Kassie may exhibit are:
① Display of negativism, ritualism, and temper tantrums
② Display of stranger anxiety, cries easily, laughs easily
③ Reaction to adult anger, has definite social attachments, and presents imitative and repetitive speech
④ Development of imagination, acute awareness of sexuality, and learning through play

207. In caring for a 2-year-old the nurse should be aware that the most common accidents for a child this age involve:
① Falls, drownings, and suffocations
② Suffocations, burns, and falls
③ Foreign body aspiration, injury from toys, and burns
④ Falls, lacerations, and abrasions

208. Julie, age 2, has been exposed to chicken pox while in daycare today. If Julie develops varicella, which of the following patient teachings should the nurse offer Julie's mother?
① Keep Julie in bed; photophobia is common, so keep window shades down and lights dim
② Keep Julie isolated; relieve her discomfort with Tylenol; avoid giving her spicy or sour foods
③ Keep Julie hospitalized and isolated; avoid sudden noises
④ Keep Julie in strict isolation at home until crusts form

209. Before bathing Brian, age 5, the nurse suggests to his mother that she step out to have coffee and stretch during the boy's morning care. On seeing his mother leave the room, Brian begins to cry and ask for her repeatedly. The nurse should offer assurance to him, knowing that he is likely experiencing:
① Temper tantrum
② Loss of self-image
③ Separation anxiety
④ Dependent coping mode

210. The nurse has an order for acetaminophin (Tylenol) chewable tablets, two PO q4h. for T > 101° F (38.3° C) for a pediatric patient. The nurse assistant reports a rectal temperature of 39.2° C. The nurse would proceed with which of the following?
① Give two Tylenol tablets
② Give one Tylenol tablet
③ Do not give any Tylenol tablets
④ Check the temperature orally first

211. Mrs. John tells the nurse that she is really disappointed now that she can't breast feed her daughter because of a cesarean delivery. The nurse's *best* response should be:
① "Mrs. John, you can still breast-feed your baby. We will help you do this."
② "Yes, Mrs. John, it is more difficult to breast-feed if you have had a cesarean section."
③ "Mrs. John, some mothers do and some don't. It depends on how you feel about it."
④ "Mrs. John, you are going to need time to recover. It might be best if you thought of yourself first."

212. Several hours after delivery, Mrs. Sutter's uterus is firm and lies to the right side of her abdomen. The most likely reason for this uterine position is that the patient's:
① Stomach is overdistended
② Uterus is returning to a normal position
③ Urinary bladder is distended
④ Uterus is filling with blood

213. Mrs. Smith, a 2-day postpartum patient, has been crying most of the evening. The nurse notes a decrease in her verbalizations and less eye contact than before. The *most appropriate* nursing action should be to:
① Avoid any discussion of what is bothering her
② Question her concerning mental illness history
③ Tell her to discuss this with her physician, enabling him to order tranquilizers
④ Offer support and try to discover her concern through therapeutic communication

214. Mrs. Booth, a postpartum patient, complains to the nurse, "My stitches really hurt." Which action would be most appropriate for the nurse to take *first?*
① Apply wet dressings
② Examine the perineum
③ Apply a heat lamp
④ Notify the nurse in charge

215. Mrs. Bowen, a postpartum patient, asks the nurse when she may resume sexual intercourse. The nurse responds that it is a common practice to recommend that sexual intercourse be avoided after delivery for a period of approximately:
① 2 weeks
② 4 weeks
③ 6 weeks
④ 12 weeks

216. Mrs. Gloria Turner, age 44, is admitted to the gynecology unit for an exploratory laparotomy and possible abdominal hysterectomy. Mrs. Turner brings her laboratory workup with her. The nurse notes that her potassium level is 3.0 mEq/L. What action should the nurse take?
① Notify the team leader or physician
② Tape the laboratory results on the patient chart
③ There is no needed action
④ Give Mrs. Turner a drink of orange juice

217. The physician orders Mrs. Turner to have an IV of 5% dextrose in lactated Ringers solution. The IV is to run at 125 ml/hr. The IV tubing has a ratio of 15 gtt/ml. An infusion pump is not currently available; so the IV will run by gravity. The IV should be running at how many gtt per minute?
① 15 gtt/min
② 25 gtt/min
③ 31 gtt/min
④ 46 gtt/min

218. The nurse observes Mrs. Turner's IV for signs of possible infiltration. Which of the following descriptions most likely indicates that the IV is infiltrated?
    ① Blood backflows into the tubing when the IV bag is lowered
    ② The IV appears to be dripping too slow
    ③ The skin around the infusion site is cool to touch and slightly swollen
    ④ The connection between the IV catheter and the tubing is leaking

219. Mrs. Watts is ordered to have a retention catheter inserted before surgery. Which catheter should the nurse select for this procedure?
    ① Straight catheter, 16 to 18 gauge
    ② Foley catheter, 14 to 16 gauge, with a 5 ml balloon
    ③ Foley catheter, 8 to 12 gauge, with a 10 ml balloon
    ④ Coude catheter, 14 to 18 gauge, with a 10 ml balloon

220. On the morning of Ms. Vep's scheduled surgery, the nurse is to administer preoperative medication. Which of the following nursing actions is appropriately completed after the medication is given?
    ① Change the patient's gown
    ② Give the last preoperative instructions
    ③ Have the patient sign the consent form for surgery
    ④ Pull up the bed side rails

221. As the nurse is preparing to give the preoperative medication, her patient states, "I'm afraid of the anesthesia, going to sleep and maybe having trouble waking up, or getting sick." What is the *best* response by the nurse?
    ① "Tell me more about this worry."
    ② "There is nothing to be afraid of, this is done every day."
    ③ "You have an excellent anesthesiologist. He'll take good care of you."
    ④ "I'll call your physician."

222. Sherry Jones, age 18, comes to the health clinic complaining of "blisters" on her perineal area and difficulty voiding. The physician diagnoses active genital herpes and *Trichomonas vaginalis*. Ms. Jones is ordered to take acyclovir (Zovirax) 200 mg five times per day. What instructions should the nurse give Ms. Jones about this medication?
    ① This medication is the only cure for genital herpes
    ② Ms. Jones should decrease her fluid intake because voiding will irritate her lesions
    ③ The lesions should resolve in 2 to 6 weeks
    ④ No showers or tub baths should be taken while the lesions are present

223. The nurse decides to instruct Ms. Jones, diagnosed with active genital herpes, on safe sex practices. Which of the following instructions indicate that the patient understands the nurse's teaching?
    ① "Condoms need only be worn when the lesions are present."
    ② "I should not have sex at all if the lesions are present."
    ③ "The use of a diaphragm will help prevent the transmission of herpes."
    ④ "There is no relationship between genital herpes and an increased risk of cervical cancer."

224. Ms. Teppen is ordered to take metronidazole (Flagyl) 250 mg tid for 7 days. Which of the following statements made by Mrs. Teppen indicates her understanding about this medication?
    ① "I can discontinue the medication if the symptoms disappear."
    ② "I should not take alcohol while I'm using this medication."
    ③ "It is probably not necessary to treat my sexual partner with this medication."
    ④ "I should avoid dairy products, which could cause nausea while using this medication."

225. Before administering acyclovir (Zovirax) and metronidazole (Flagyl), the nurse should confirm that:
    ① The patient's hemoglobin level is above 15 gm/dl
    ② The patient is not pregnant
    ③ The patient is not allergic to eggs
    ④ The patient is able to tolerate a normal diet

226. Mrs. Joan Thomas, age 33, is admitted to the hospital with a diagnosis of thrombophlebitis. While assessing Mrs. Thomas, the nurse is aware that the problem of thrombophlebitis most commonly occurs:
    ① In superficial peripheral veins
    ② In deep leg veins
    ③ As a result of exercising while pregnant
    ④ Only in large arteries

227. A patient with thrombophlebitis is ordered to receive heparin 10,000 U q8h subcutaneously. Which of the following techniques should be used in the administration of this medication?
    ① A 22-gauge needle should be used for the injection
    ② The deltoid muscle is the best injection site
    ③ The syringe should not be aspirated after the needle is inserted
    ④ The site should be carefully massaged after the injection

228. Mrs. Jones complains of a headache and asks the nurse for an aspirin. The nurse, aware that the patient is receiving heparin, would take which of the following actions?
    ① Notify the physician for an aspirin order
    ② Tell Mrs. Jones that ibuprofen works better for headaches than does aspirin
    ③ Inform Mrs. Jones that aspirin will interfere with her therapy and notify the physician for another order
    ④ Tell Mrs. Jones that the headache is an expected side effect of her heparin therapy

229. In planning care for a patient with a diagnosis of thrombophlebitis, the nurse should include which of the following measures?
    ① Notify physical therapy that the patient will need exercises several times a day
    ② Observe for the symptoms of pulmonary embolism
    ③ Reduce fluid intake in order to reduce the circulatory volume
    ④ Keep the affected leg completely flat in bed

230. Mrs. Louise Hartly, age 28, reports to the urology clinic with a history of repeated urinary tract infections (UTIs). She states that she has had these many times before and has taken "lots of antibiotics." She believes she currently has another infection. While obtaining the nursing assessment from Mrs. Hartly, which of the following symptoms would the nurse expect her to most likely report?
    1. Feeling faint or dizzy while in the bathroom
    2. Inability to void when away from home
    3. A "burning" sensation when voiding
    4. Unusual thirst

231. Which of the following statements would indicate a patient's understanding of instructions that would aid in preventing the recurrence of urinary tract infections or cystitis?
    1. "I must remember to void after sexual intercourse."
    2. "I can wear only nylon underpants with a cotton crotch."
    3. "I must always wipe in a back-to-front manner after voiding."
    4. "I must use deodorant perineal pads during menses to reduce the amount of bacteria on the skin."

232. The physician orders a urine culture for his patient. What is the best method to use to obtain a specimen for this test?
    1. Ask the patient to void in the bedpan to obtain the entire amount of urine
    2. Obtain a clean-catch urine specimen
    3. For the cleanest urine specimen catheterize the patient
    4. Obtain a 24-hour urine specimen

233. Mrs. Hartly's urine culture reveals the presence of *Escherichia coli (E. coli)* and *Candida* in her urine. What is the most likely cause of the presence of the *Candida* organism?
    1. Increased intake of yogurt with an active culture
    2. Multiple uses of antibiotics
    3. Use of deodorant soaps
    4. Use of scented toilet paper

234. Because of Mrs. Smith's history of recurrent urinary tract infections, a cystoscopy is scheduled. This procedure is to be done in the clinic using a local anesthetic. What instructions should the nurse give Mrs. Smith following the procedure?
    1. The patient should wear a perineal pad after the procedure to absorb the bloody drainage
    2. Mrs. Smith should drink plenty of fluids after the procedure
    3. To recuperate fully, Mrs. Smith will not be able to return to work for several weeks after the procedure
    4. If Mrs. Smith has difficulty voiding after the procedure, she should soak in a warm bubble bath

235. Methenamine (Urised) 1 g qid is prescribed for a patient with a urinary tract infection. Which of the following statements by the patient indicates an understanding of the instructions given by the nurse about this medication?
    1. "I will expect my urine to be a red-orange color from the medication."
    2. "I should reduce the amount of fluids I take so that the medication will remain in the bladder longer."
    3. "My urine may appear pink or slightly bloody as a result of the cleansing action of this medication."
    4. "My urine will appear to have a blue or blue-green coloration."

236. Approximately 1 year ago, Mrs. Joyce Lowrey, age 50, was diagnosed as having ovarian cancer with distant metastases (stage iv). Since her initial diagnosis, she has undergone chemotherapy and radiation therapy. She is now admitted to the hospital with respiratory distress. What should the *priority* nursing action be on Mrs. Lowrey's admission to the hospital?
    1. Resumption of her physician-ordered chemotherapy
    2. Pain relief
    3. Assistance with breathing
    4. Orienting her to the unit and her room

237. A patient has a diagnosis of ovarian cancer and has undergone chemotherapy and radiation therapy. Two days after her admission with respiratory distress, Mrs. Lowrey is able to breathe without a great deal of difficulty. While assisting her with morning care, the nurse notes that Mrs. Lowrey is very quiet, difficult to engage in any conversation, and seems "lost in her thoughts." The nurse recognizes this as part of the grief process. Mrs. Lowrey seems to be in which stage of the grief process?
    1. Denial
    2. Anger
    3. Bargaining
    4. Depression

238. During the evening visiting hours, the family remains out in the hall across from a patient's room. The nurse hears the family arguing, "This is your fault, you didn't take care of her well enough," "No, this is your fault, you are only concerned with yourself." The family continues bickering for 10 minutes before entering the patient's room. What would be an appropriate nursing diagnosis for this family?
    1. Anxiety related to the patient's medical diagnosis
    2. Hopelessness related to patient illness
    3. Altered family processes related to inadequate coping behaviors
    4. Social isolation as a result of many hospital visits and length of the patient's illness

239. During the evening shift, Mrs. Peters asks the nurse for assistance with writing a living will. The nurse recognizes which of the following as the primary purpose of a living will?
    ① It provides that the family may make all decisions regarding the patient's health care when the patient is no longer able to decide for himself or herself
    ② It provides for the distribution of all the patient's material possessions
    ③ It states exactly what measures are to be taken to save the patient's life
    ④ It provides that extraordinary measures not be taken to save a patient's life if he or she becomes terminally ill

240. Several evenings before Ms. Dancer's death, she confides to the nurse, "I just keep on hoping that someone will find a cure for this so I can continue to raise my family." What should be an appropriate response by the nurse?
    ① "I'll keep praying for you. There must be a cure somewhere."
    ② "I'll try to do everything I can to help you and keep you comfortable."
    ③ "I just read an article in a nursing journal about all the work being done at another hospital. I'll see what I can find out."
    ④ "Try to have more peace of mind with what you have accomplished."

COMPREHENSIVE EXAMINATION TWO: PART I

1. The nurse is caring for Mr. F during a blood transfusion. He has been receiving blood for an hour. As the nurse assesses Mr. F's vital signs, he complains of the following. Which complaint demands priority intervention by the nurse?
    ① A "cool" sensation at the site
    ② The need to void
    ③ The need to sit up to "get breath"
    ④ A slow-dripping IV

2. Mrs. Trent is admitted to the hospital with chest pain and has physician's orders to receive topical Nitro-Bid q8h. She is scheduled for several tests to determine the cause of her chest pain. What nursing intervention does the nurse take when administering Nitro-Bid to an ambulatory patient?
    ① Weigh the patient, because the dose is based on weight
    ② Check the most recent laboratory tests for nitrate levels
    ③ Obtain the blood pressure and pulse rate after the patient lies down
    ④ Monitor the ECG tracing

3. A patient is admitted with pain in the lower right quadrant and rebound tenderness. As symptoms indicate appendicitis, the nurse should also note an elevated:
    ① Red blood cell (RBC) count
    ② Hemoglobin level
    ③ Serum lipase level
    ④ White blood cell (WBC) count

4. Caffeine-containing beverages are avoided by patients with peptic ulcer disease because caffeine:
    ① Depresses the central nervous system
    ② Dehydrates the body
    ③ Delays production of gastric secretions
    ④ Stimulates gastric secretions

5. If Mr. Hill's duodenal ulcer perforates, which one of the following symptoms is he *most likely* to exhibit?
    ① Clay-colored stools
    ② Coffee-ground emesis
    ③ Boardlike abdomen
    ④ Distention after eating

6. The family of a patient admitted with depression asks if she "will ever get sick like this again." The *most* appropriate answer for the nurse to give them is:
    ① "No, she will not be sick like this again."
    ② "Her chances of having another episode are increased."
    ③ "No; if it happens again it will be worse."
    ④ "Not if she takes medications and has electroconvulsive therapy."

7. The physician decides to give electroconvulsive therapy (ECT) to a patient who has not responded to medication. Which of the following is the *most appropriate* nursing action to take with a patient immediately following an ECT treatment?
    ① Give extra fluids because the patient has been NPO
    ② Encourage rapid ambulation
    ③ Reorient the patient to time, place, and person
    ④ Give the patient a small high-protein meal

8. Diane's physician has prescribed a monoamine oxidase inhibitor for her depression. Which of the following should the nurse tell Diane regarding her medication?
    ① She will need to have frequent blood tests done
    ② She will experience some gastrointestinal distress
    ③ She will need to avoid chocolate and red wine
    ④ She will experience visual changes

9. Mark Gordon, age 5, is admitted to the emergency department. He is lethargic and is coughing and wheezing with nasal flaring, moist breath sounds and an increase in respiratory and heart rates. The nurse's *first* intervention should be to:
    ① Elevate the head of the bed
    ② Administer oxygen as needed
    ③ Administer aerosol treatment
    ④ Monitor respiratory rate q2h

10. The nurse discusses motor skill development with a mother, explaining that at about 7 months of age her child will *most likely* be able to:
    ① Walk with assistance
    ② Feed herself with a spoon
    ③ Stand holding onto furniture
    ④ Sit alone using hands for support

11. The nurse would instruct the mother to instill ear drops in her 5-month-old child's ear by grasping the:
    ① Auricle and gently pulling down and back
    ② Auricle and gently pulling upward
    ③ Pinna and gently pulling backward and up
    ④ Pinna and gently pulling downward

12. The nurse should instruct a mother of a child who has otitis media to examine the ear for:
① Warmth
② Cilia
③ Color
④ Drainage

13. Jeanette Carter, a 5-month-old, 12-lb infant, was brought to the pediatric clinic and diagnosed as having acute otitis media, which is most commonly secondary to:
① Mastoiditis
② Scarlet fever
③ Measles (rubeola)
④ Respiratory infections

14. A congenital disorder that occurs as a result of a chromosomal abnormality affecting chromosomes in the number 21 position is:
① Down's syndrome
② Patau syndrome
③ Turner syndrome
④ Klinefelter syndrome

15. Sally is 17 weeks' pregnant, and her physician ordered an alpha-fetoprotein (AFP) level. Her results show that AFP levels are elevated, and the physician has just explained the need for further diagnostic evaluation. She asks, "Is my baby sick? Will he be okay?" The nurse's best response is:
① "Your baby will be fine; let's talk about the next step."
② "There is nothing we know right now. Try to calm down until we find out."
③ "You sound very concerned; let's talk about what you are feeling."
④ "You sound upset about your baby. Lets talk about dealing with a child who has congenital problems."

16. Mrs. J is in the OB-GYN office for her first visit. She says she may be pregnant. Which of the following assessment areas are presumptive signs of pregnancy?
① Breast changes
② Goodell's sign
③ Positive urine pregnancy test
④ Darkened, vascular vaginal area

17. The nurse is helping Mrs. J figure her expected date of confinement (EDC). The first day of her last menstrual period (LMP) was October 4. Using Nägele's rule, the nurse would conclude Mrs. J's due date is:
① March 7
② July 11
③ August 7
④ January 8

18. When Mrs. J's fundal height is at the umbilicus, the nurse would know that this patient is most likely at which week of pregnancy?
① Tenth
② Twelfth
③ Twentieth
④ Thirtieth

19. Mrs. F complains of the following symptoms at 22 weeks of pregnancy. Which of the following is cause for *immediate* concern?
① Absence of fetal movement
② Swelling in the feet and ankles
③ Weight gain of 3 lb over the last month
④ Clear watery discharge from the vaginal area

20. Mrs. Myers returns from surgery, having had a cholecystectomy. Her postoperative orders include keeping her NPO and connecting her nasogastric tube to low intermittent suction. Ten hours after surgery, Mrs. Myers' abdomen is distended. The *priority* nursing action should be to:
① Advance the position of the nasogastric tube 2 inches
② Irrigate the tube with 30 ml of normal saline solution
③ Check the suction equipment
④ Call the physician

21. Mrs. Rosendale has diverticulitis. Which one of the following menus would be *most* consistent with her diet instructions?
① Turkey on whole wheat bread and an apple
② Ham omelet and ice cream
③ Cream of shrimp soup and canned pears
④ Strawberry yogurt and chocolate chip cookies

22. Jason Daley, age 27, is admitted to short-stay surgery for an inguinal hernia repair. Which of the following factors *does not* predispose a patient to hernia formation?
① Congenital defects
② Obesity
③ Appendicitis
④ Defect in the muscular wall

23. In planning nursing care for a patient in sickle cell crisis, the nurse knows that the treatment plan will include:
① Chemotherapy
② Supportive therapy for presenting symptoms
③ Fluid restriction
④ Active range-of-motion exercises

24. While taking the medical history during the admission of Mr. Adam, the nurse discovers that he is an alcoholic taking disulfiram (Antabuse) prescribed by the treatment center he has been attending. In providing patient teaching to a patient taking the drug disulfiram, the nurse would explain that it is important to avoid any medications in which of the forms listed below?
① Tinctures
② Oral solutions
③ Enteric coated tablets
④ Sustained release action tablets

25. The charge nurse starts an aminophylline drip (1 g in 500 ml) as ordered at 30 gtt/min. The nurse wants to chart the milligrams of aminophylline the patient is receiving per minute. In calculating the milligram per minute, if the drop factor is 60 gtt/ml, which of the following is correct?
① 0.05 mg/min
② 1 mg/min
③ 2 mg/min
④ 3 mg/min

26. For the nursing diagnosis "ineffective airway clearance related to increased secretions," a nursing intervention is to "assess respirations and sputum." This nursing intervention statement is:
    ① Incomplete without a physician's order
    ② Appropriate for the nursing diagnosis
    ③ Inappropriate for the nursing diagnosis
    ④ Too general to be effective in giving care

27. Ann, age 25, has been transferred from the intensive care unit, where she has been receiving thrombolytic therapy for 2 weeks for an extensive blood clot in her leg. On entering Ann's room, the nurse finds her upset and crying. An appropriate nursing intervention for Ann should be to:
    ① Call her physician and suggest an antidepressant prn
    ② Allow her time to cry and express her feeling, while providing her with support
    ③ Call her family to bring her make-up, gowns from home, and a depilatory to remove the hair from her legs
    ④ Ask her family to talk to her and find out why she is crying

28. Mrs. Gates was admitted with weakness and pain in the left leg and placed on bed rest. The nurse should inform the nursing assistants to avoid which of the following?
    ① Bathing the patient's legs
    ② Assisting the patient to shower
    ③ Turning the patient on the right side
    ④ Massaging the right leg during the bath

29. The physician has ordered fluid restriction for a patient. The order reads "Limit fluid to 1400 ml/24 hrs." The nurse would inform the patient and place a sign in the room indicating which of the following distributions?
    ① Day shift, 700 ml; evening shift, 300 ml; night shift, 400 ml
    ② Day shift, 700 ml; evening shift, 700 ml; night shift, 0.0 ml
    ③ Day shift, 1000 ml; evening shift, 200 ml; night shift, 100 ml
    ④ Day shift, 700 ml; evening shift, 500 ml; night shift, 200 ml

30. Immediately after returning to his room from the recovery room, a patient complains of severe pain at his incision site. He has a narcotic analgesic ordered for pain q4h prn. The nurse should withhold the medication if:
    ① Vital signs were equal to or within the range before surgery
    ② Oxygen were still being administered and respirations were 18
    ③ Pain medication was administered in the recovery room an hour before returning to the room
    ④ Proper positioning and preparation of a quiet environment did not provide relief

31. Codeine is available in vials containing 30 mg/ml. If gr ¾ is ordered q4h prn, how many milliliters should be administered per dose? (Use 1 gr = 60 mg)
    ① 1.5 ml
    ② 2 ml
    ③ 2.5 ml
    ④ 3 ml

32. Mr. Jay's assessment after receiving a narcotic for his incisional pain reveals a blood pressure of 100/60, a pulse of 68, and shallow respirations at 8/min. The physician is notified and orders a narcotic antagonist naloxone [Narcan]. After administering naloxone, the nurse should expect the return of the pain and should assess for:
    ① A further drop in blood pressure
    ② A drop in the pulse rate
    ③ An increase in respirations in about 15 to 20 minutes
    ④ A decrease in respirations in about 15 to 20 minutes

33. After being admitted to the unit, a patient refuses to get out of bed to shower, have breakfast, or join in unit activities. The *best action* for the nurse to take is:
    ① Ignore her lack of participation
    ② Set small goals and stay with her while she does them
    ③ Encourage her to be active but do not force her
    ④ Restrict her phone calls until she follows the rules

34. Which of the following nursing diagnoses addresses the *highest priority* for a patient hospitalized with the symptoms of depression?
    ① Anxiety related to unfamiliar environment
    ② Fluid volume deficit related to limited intake
    ③ Nutritional deficit related to limited intake
    ④ Ineffective family coping related to hospitalization

35. Diane's family asks when her symptoms of depression are going to get better. What is the nurse's *best response*?
    ① "As soon as she makes up her mind to get better."
    ② "There is no way to tell how long she will be depressed."
    ③ "We need more information to determine how long she might be ill."
    ④ "We will know better in another week."

36. During Diane's admission assessment, she tells the nurse that she has not been eating, has been unable to sleep through the night for the past 3 months, and cannot seem to concentrate on any task long enough to finish it. The symptoms that Diane is describing are *most likely* a result of:
    ① An affective disorder
    ② A personality disorder
    ③ A substance abuse disorder
    ④ A thought disorder

37. In planning nursing care for a child with whooping cough, the nurse needs to consider that the child with whooping cough:
    ① Is severely ill
    ② Usually has to be hospitalized in the intensive care unit
    ③ May become physically exhausted from coughing
    ④ Does not require medical treatment

38. The nurse is explaining to her patient that the communicable disease that affects the parotid glands near the ear and jaw is called:
    ① Measles
    ② Mumps
    ③ Scarlet fever
    ④ Chicken pox

39. The nurse explains to a patient that German measles are also known as:
    ① Red measles
    ② Roseola
    ③ Scarlet fever
    ④ Rubella

40. Which of the following immunizations should the nurse recommend to the mother of a child before he starts kindergarten?
    ① Diphtheria-pertussis-tetanus (DPT) injections only if he did not receive them during infancy
    ② DPT injections, even if he had them during infancy
    ③ Chicken pox vaccination
    ④ Immunization against cholera

41. Kara, age 11, is admitted to the hospital with the symptoms of severe abdominal pain, vomiting, and a temperature of 101° F (38.3° C). The physician diagnosed her as being in a sickle cell crisis. The nurse knows that sickle cell anemia results from:
    ① An infection in the blood
    ② Failure to follow a correct diet
    ③ Malformed cells clumped together
    ④ White blood cells attacking red blood cells

42. When administering nose drops to an infant pediatric patient, the nurse should:
    ① Hold the infant in a sitting position during and after the procedure
    ② Place the infant on his abdomen after instilling the drops
    ③ Hold the infant with his head down lower than his body maintaining this position for several minutes
    ④ Place the infant on his side during and after the procedure

43. Mrs. K has been admitted with a threatened abortion. Her symptoms include cramping with moderate bleeding. In addition to bed rest and vital sign assessment, the nurse's *major* goal for the patient should be to:
    ① Prepare for immediate surgery
    ② Replace electrolytes promptly
    ③ Provide supportive emotional care
    ④ Prepare for oxytocin administration

44. Mrs. K has been scheduled for a stat cesarean delivery because of abruptio placentae. As the nurse assists in transporting her to the delivery room, she should expect to observe in this patient:
    ① Profuse vaginal bleeding
    ② A tense painful abdomen
    ③ Strong, spasmodic contractions
    ④ Painless, bright red vaginal drainage

45. Ms. Jones is 2 days postpartum and is not breast-feeding. As the nurse checks on this patient during routine rounds, the patient states she has noticed more bleeding on her pads. The nurse's *first action* should be to:
    ① Assess vital signs including blood pressure
    ② Turn her on her side
    ③ Encourage fluids PO
    ④ Palpate her fundus and massage until firm

46. Which of the following characteristics should the nursery nurse observe for when an infant is suspected of having Down syndrome?
    ① Blue hands and feet; irregular respirations at birth
    ② The presence of inner epicanthal folds; small ears
    ③ Head circumference larger than chest circumference
    ④ Infant arms and legs flexed on the chest and abdomen

47. When Down's syndrome is suspected, the nursery nurse should carefully assess which of the following?
    ① Heart sounds
    ② Cognitive deficits
    ③ Visual impairments
    ④ Hearing impairments

48. Mrs. Jenkins, whose newborn has been diagnosed with Down syndrome, asks the nurse, "How retarded will my baby be? What will he be able to do?" Which of the following statements is the *best response* by the nurse?
    ① "Only genetic counseling can determine the extent of the disability."
    ② "Most children with Down syndrome eventually become self-sufficient."
    ③ "Children with Down syndrome are generally severely retarded."
    ④ "It is not possible to determine the extent of the disabilities at this time."

49. Which of the following responses by a mother indicates her understanding of discharge instructions for her baby, born with Down syndrome?
    ① "The baby should be fed a little more often in order to gain weight."
    ② "The baby should be dressed very warmly to prevent colds."
    ③ "The baby should not have visitors for several weeks."
    ④ "The baby has a higher risk of upper respiratory infections than do other babies."

50. The nurse administered a theophylline preparation PO to a 3-year-old with asthma. Vital signs are temperature 100.1° F (37.8° C) axillary, apical pulse 90, respirations 28. One hour after the administration of theophylline (Theo-Dur), the nurse notes the patient has a pulse of 110. The nurse identifies this as:
    ① An expected outcome
    ② A side effect
    ③ The desired effect
    ④ A toxic effect

51. To determine if a mother understands the instructions concerning her infant's immunizations and feeding, the nurse should:
    ① Instruct the mother to call with any questions
    ② Link sensory perceptions
    ③ Interpret all medical terms for the mother
    ④ Check for communication barriers between herself and the mother

52. Thirteen-month-old Sally is admitted to the hospital with a fracture of the right femur. She is accompanied by both parents, each of whom provides a different story. Child abuse is suspected. The nurse knows that legal aspects of child abuse require that she:
    ① Report her findings to a physician
    ② Report this as a known or suspected case of child abuse
    ③ Exercise caution; reporting does not grant immunity from civil suits
    ④ Exercise caution; this is considered privileged communication

53. Eighteen-month-old Mary is brought into the emergency room by both parents. She is diagnosed as having a fracture of the right humerus. Her parents tell differing accounts of the accident; child abuse is suspected. When interviewing the parents, the nurse is aware that which of the following is *most typical* of parents who abuse their children?
    ① There are step-parents involved
    ② The parents have numerous children spaced closely
    ③ The parents were older when having their first child
    ④ One or both parents were abused as children

54. A disorder characterized by abdominal organs protruding through an abnormal opening in the abdominal wall and forming a sac lying on the abdomen is:
    ① Esophageal atresia
    ② Omphalocele
    ③ Hirschsprung's disease
    ④ Pyloric stenosis

55. Which of the following is the most important aspect of the relationship of the nurse to the patient in crisis?
    ① The nurse provides primary emotional support for the patient
    ② The nurse identifies the most appropriate resources for the patient
    ③ The nurse assists the patient to regain equilibrium
    ④ The nurse supports the patient's significant others

56. The *most appropriate* short-term goal for the patient to work on in a situational crisis is:
    ① To improve her relationship with her own family
    ② To return her to her precrisis level of function
    ③ To decrease her incidence of physical symptoms
    ④ To explore her feelings about her losses

57. A patient has admitted that he does not take the prescribed fluphenazine (Prolixin) every day. What is the *best way* for the nurse to increase the likelihood that he will be more compliant about taking his medication following discharge?
    ① Ask his family to administer his medication
    ② Ask him to come to the clinic to get his medication
    ③ Ask him when the best time is for him to take his medication
    ④ Inform him that his physician can prescribe an injectable form

58. Which of the following is an appropriate goal for a psychiatric patient to increase his socialization?
    ① Join a singles dating service
    ② Join a social skills outpatient group
    ③ Volunteer in his local community
    ④ Become more involved in his church

59. A patient asks the nurse if he can "have a date" after his discharge from the hospital. The *best response* by the nurse would be:
    ① Nothing; ignore the question
    ② Nothing; she shouldn't speak to him again until discharge
    ③ To go over the goals of their relationship
    ④ To tell him she is upset by his request

60. The nurse finds her patient huddled in his room with a frightened look on his face. He says, "The voices are back, telling me to do bad things." The nurse's *best response* is:
    ① "Listen to my voice, not to what they are telling you."
    ② "We'll put you into seclusion until the voices stop."
    ③ "I don't hear anything like that."
    ④ "Let's go find something for you to do."

61. Mrs. Chae, age 39, is scheduled for a tubal ligation tomorrow. The health history reveals that she smokes two packs of cigarettes a day, is overweight by 50 lb and is a borderline hypertensive. Following surgery, *the priority* nursing *diagnosis* for Mrs. Chae is:
    ① Ineffective individual coping related to lack of support system
    ② Impaired physical mobility: ambulation related to abdominal discomfort
    ③ Potential ineffective airway clearance related to smoking
    ④ Alteration in nutrition: greater than body requirements, related to excessive caloric intake

62. Mr. Johnson, age 83, has a history of congestive heart failure and beginning renal failure. The nurse should be *most* concerned about which principle of drug action?
    ① Absorption
    ② Distribution
    ③ Metabolism
    ④ Excretion

63. Before administering the bronchodilator metoproterenol sulfate (Alupent), the nurse should obtain a relevant nursing history, note the character of the sputum, and obtain which of the following?
    ① Baseline temperature
    ② Baseline heart rate
    ③ Sputum specimen for culture
    ④ Blood specimens ordered

64. Phenobarbital is ordered gr $\overline{ss}$ per feeding tube bid. An elixir of 30 mg/7.4 ml is supplied. Using the conversion 1 tsp = 5 ml and 1 gr = 60 mg, how many tsp should the nurse give?
    ① 1 tsp
    ② 1.5 tsp
    ③ 2 tsp
    ④ 2.5 tsp

65. The nurse administers the same medication to Mr. Jones that he has been taking at home. He states that the medicine still works, but lately it seems to take more of the drug to be effective. The nurse should consult the physician after suspecting which of the following?
    1. Tolerance
    2. Additive effect
    3. Idiosyncratic reaction
    4. Psychological dependence

66. Which of the following agents is/are used to promote fertility?
    1. Rho-gam
    2. Ergot alkaloids
    3. Androgens
    4. Human chorionic gonadotropin

67. On the third day of hospitalization, Mr. S voices several complaints. The complaint that should alert the nurse to possible digitalis toxicity would be:
    1. "My back hurts today."
    2. "I'm so nauseated and I have no appetite."
    3. "I feel like I've put on 5 pounds."
    4. "I'm too tired to sleep well at night."

68. After administering one nitroglycerin tablet sublingually to a patient, a nurse evaluates his condition and finds that he is still complaining of pain and has a blood pressure of 80/50. The nurse would *first*:
    1. Wait another 3 minutes and take the blood pressure again before giving another dose of nitroglycerin
    2. Call the physician immediately and withhold the second dose of nitroglycerin
    3. Elevate his feet (unless contraindicated) and give another dose of nitroglycerin
    4. Elevate his feet (unless contraindicated), withhold the medication, and notify the physician

69. Mr. Tom complains of severe chest pain, and the nurse prepares to administer his *first* dose of nitrate. The nurse should follow which of these procedures?
    1. Take his pulse and blood pressure, then administer a transdermal patch
    2. Take his pulse and blood pressure, then administer sublingual nitrate
    3. Administer sublingual nitrate immediately, then take his pulse and blood pressure
    4. Before administering the nitrate, obtain a detailed medical history to be sure the pain is related to angina

70. Laboratory reports reveal that a patient has leukopenia. Specific nursing interventions will include:
    1. Avoiding injections or rectal temperatures
    2. Provisions for adequate periods of rest
    3. Protecting from infections
    4. The liberal use of antiemetics

71. A patient receiving external radiation therapy is concerned about being "radioactive." The nurse tells the patient that:
    1. The external radiation effects are generalized to all body systems
    2. He is radioactive only while he is receiving the therapy
    3. Only his urine and bodily secretions are radioactive
    4. He is not radioactive

72. In reviewing breast self-examination (BSE) information, the nurse instructs the patient to:
    1. Conduct the examination before her menstrual period
    2. Check the breast while positioning herself in both a supine and erect position
    3. Perform the examination on a weekly schedule
    4. Use the palm of the hand for the examination

73. The test that is used to determine if a breast lump is benign or malignant is the:
    1. Biopsy
    2. Ultrasonography
    3. Xeroradiography
    4. Computed tomography (CT)

74. A right modified radical mastectomy is scheduled. The patient tells the nurse that she is anxious and afraid of the surgery. She is fearful that she might even die during the procedure. What would be the nurse's *best* response?
    1. "Why are you afraid of the surgery?"
    2. "Try to get as much rest as possible before surgery."
    3. "Those must be frightening feelings. Tell me more about them."
    4. "Don't worry, you won't die. That type of procedure is quite perfected and often done."

75. Postoperative care following a right modified radical mastectomy will include:
    1. Limiting movement of the right arm
    2. Keeping the right arm below heart level
    3. Instructions to use her left arm for such activities as hair brushing
    4. Posting signs warning against taking blood pressure or drawing blood from the right arm

76. Combination intravenous chemotherapy is planned for a patient with cancer. The patient asks why there are numerous side effects associated with the administration of the medications. The nurse's response is based on the knowledge that:
    1. Side effects are limited to single-agent chemotherapy
    2. Rapidly dividing normal and abnormal cells are destroyed
    3. Chemotherapeutic drugs administered intravenously have less side effects
    4. Side effects will be minimal if the medications are given as a one-time dose

77. A patient has hypothyroidism. When collecting admission information, the nurse should expect the patient to complain about:
    1. Exophthalmos
    2. Fine tremors
    3. Heat intolerance
    4. Facial puffiness

78. A nursing intervention in the plan of care for a patient with hypothyroidism should include:
    1. Providing a calm, nonstimulating environment
    2. Providing high-calorie dietary supplements
    3. Providing a warm environment
    4. Urine testing for glucose

79. Kevin, age 2, is brought into the well-baby clinic for a checkup. The average vital signs for a 2-year-old should be:
    ① Heart rate 110; respirations 25, blood pressure 96/68
    ② Heart rate 120, respirations 35, blood pressure 70/50
    ③ Heart rate 88, respirations 19, blood pressure 110/70
    ④ Heart rate 100, respirations 21, blood pressure 105/70

80. A child is seen in the pediatric clinic for iron deficiency. The physician prescribes an iron supplement. Home care instructions for the patient include teaching the mother to:
    ① Mix the iron product with the child's milk to disguise the flavor
    ② Use a dropper to drop the medication directly into the child's mouth
    ③ Place the medication on a cookie and have the child eat the cookie
    ④ Mix the iron product with juice to disguise the flavor and have the child use a straw

81. Cindy Johnson, age 5, was admitted to the hospital for diagnostic studies and heart surgery for repair of tetralogy of Fallot. The nurse should expect a child with tetralogy of Fallot to exhibit which of the following clinical manifestations?
    ① Skin with bluish tint; favoring of squatting position
    ② Skin with natural pink color; clubbing of fingers and toes
    ③ Retarded growth, but usually normal in intelligence
    ④ Hypertension in upper extremities and hypotension in lower extremities

82. Steven was diagnosed with chronic schizophrenia 10 years ago. He was admitted to the hospital today after he began hearing voices at work telling him to "end it all." Which of the following is the *most likely reason* for Steven's relapse?
    ① Changes in his living environment
    ② A change to a high-protein diet
    ③ Noncompliance in taking antipsychotic medications
    ④ An argument with his girlfriend

83. Which of the following is the *most* important factor for the nurse to remember when planning how best to work with adolescent patients?
    ① Their general dislike of adults
    ② Their need to experiment with substances
    ③ Their level of cognitive ability to consider consequences
    ④ Their natural mistrust of health-care providers

84. A 16-year-old is brought to an outpatient clinic for alcohol counseling. She admits to drinking but denies she has a problem, stating that she hates her parents. According to Erickson, the developmental issue facing this patient is:
    ① Autonomy vs. shame and doubt
    ② Industry vs. inferiority
    ③ Intimacy vs. isolation
    ④ Identity vs. identity diffusion

85. Which of the following possible nursing interventions for a victim of rape should be implemented *first?*
    ① Discuss evaluation for sexually transmitted diseases
    ② Discuss the possible need for postcoital contraception
    ③ Discuss community resources and possible referrals
    ④ Discuss and identify her immediate needs and concerns

86. When the emergency room nurse goes to interview a rape victim, she finds the patient to be calm, able to answer questions without hesitation, and in apparent control, with no evidence of anger, fear, or tearfulness. What is the *most likely explanation* for her behavior?
    ① She has calmed down since being raped
    ② She is in a state of emotional shock
    ③ She agreed to have sex with her assailant
    ④ She is using intellectualization to cope

87. According to experts who have studied its incidence and occurrence, rape is *best* defined as:
    ① An act of sexual frustration
    ② An act of sexual aggression
    ③ An act of sexual dominance
    ④ An act of sexual ambivalence

88. Mary Jane comes to the emergency room for treatment after coming home from her class to find a man in her apartment who raped her. The nurse knows that rapists and their victims come primarily from which population group?
    ① Poor and lower-class whites
    ② Young blacks between 25 and 35 years of age
    ③ All ethnic and socioeconomic groups
    ④ Single urban Latinos

89. A patient in active labor requests medication for pain, and the physician orders meperidine (Demerol) 50 mg IM. The nurse should know that:
    ① This is not a correct dose
    ② The newborn infant will require Narcan
    ③ Meperidine is given only orally
    ④ Meperidine is a narcotic analgesic

90. Mrs. Smith is pregnant with her first child and asks the nurse about where conception takes place. The nurse notes this as an opportune teaching moment and responds that conception takes place in the:
    ① Uterus
    ② Corpus luteum
    ③ Vagina
    ④ Fallopian tubes

91. A woman is admitted to the hospital with a diagnosis of threatened abortion. She is on complete bed rest. Which of the following nursing actions would be a *priority* in caring for this patient?
    ① Save any tissue passed vaginally
    ② Place the patient in semi-Fowler's position
    ③ Provide a nonstimulating environment
    ④ Force fluids

92. In caring for a patient in the early period after vaginal delivery, which of these measures by the nurse is *most essential?*
    ① Keep environmental stimulation at a minimum
    ② Offer her frequent sips of water
    ③ Be certain that the uterus remains contracted
    ④ Take her temperature q4h

93. A 19-year-old male is hospitalized for an appendectomy. Nursing history reveals that he has a seizure disorder and that he has seizures when he is sick. The patient has a generalized seizure when the nurse is in the room. Which of the following nursing actions is appropriate during the seizure?
    ① Insert a padded tongue blade
    ② Notify the physician immediately
    ③ Remain in the room with the patient
    ④ Restrain his extremities if possible

94. A patient has a generalized seizure. After the seizure activity ceases, the nurse should implement which nursing action *first*?
    ① Insert an airway
    ② Position him on his side
    ③ Take a set of vital signs
    ④ Begin oxygen administration

95. When the patient returns from the postanesthesia unit following a craniotomy for a frontal lobe tumor, his wife asks about the swelling around his eyes. Which of the following is the *most* appropriate action by the nurse?
    ① Notify the physician immediately
    ② Keep the bed in a flat position at all times
    ③ Ask the patient's wife to bring dark eye glasses for her husband
    ④ Reassure the wife that the edema is normal and will subside in a few days

96. The nurse monitors the postoperative intracranial surgery patient for signs of increased intracranial pressure. An early indication is:
    ① Drowsiness
    ② Elevated temperature
    ③ Decreasing pulse rate
    ④ Irregular respirations

97. Following surgery, the nurse is caring for a patient who has had intracranial surgery. A possible pituitary problem is suspected when the nurse notes which of the following?
    ① An increased temperature
    ② Sluggish pupil reaction to light
    ③ Clear drainage on the head dressing
    ④ Increased output of low-specific gravity urine

98. When checking the head dressing following intracranial surgery, the nurse notes the presence of clear drainage from the ear. The patient is also complaining of a postnasal drip. Which nursing action is *most* appropriate?
    ① Notify the physician
    ② Circle the drainage, noting date and time
    ③ Recognize that this is normal mucus drainage
    ④ Reinforce the dressing until the physician arrives

99. A 55-year-old patient is admitted for observation. History reveals changes in level of consciousness and a possible cerebrovascular accident (CVA). The plan of care includes assessment of the patient's level of consciousness using the Glasgow Coma Scale. With this tool, the nurse assesses the patient's:
    ① Emotional reactions
    ② Intellectual functioning
    ③ Best motor and verbal responses
    ④ Lower extremity strength and gait

100. Assessment of the patient admitted with a history of a stroke reveals a right hemiplegia. To avoid aspiration, the patient would be instructed to *avoid:*
    ① Sitting up for meals
    ② Lying down immediately after meals
    ③ Swallowing with his head slightly flexed
    ④ Placing liquids in the left side of the mouth

101. Bladder retraining is to be started because the patient developed incontinence as a result of a stroke. Which of the following actions is usually included in a training program?
    ① Limit fluid intake during the day
    ② Offer the urinal q2h
    ③ Check for residual urine after each voiding
    ④ Use disposable adult diapers to protect the skin

102. The nurse should teach Mrs. Brown that the *best* way to ensure the infant has an adequate breast milk supply is for her to:
    ① Follow a daily exercise program
    ② Drink generous amounts of milk each day
    ③ Eat a high-protein diet
    ④ Allow the infant to empty each breast at each feeding

103. Mrs. Bowen is breast feeding her baby. The nurse should teach Mrs. Bowen that at the end of a feeding session, she should release baby Bowen from the nipple by putting gentle downward pressure on the infant's:
    ① Lips
    ② Nose
    ③ Chin
    ④ Forehead

104. As a pregnancy progresses, normal changes in hemoglobin and hematocrit occur. The nurse expects:
    ① Hemoglobin to increase and hematocrit to decrease
    ② Hemoglobin to decrease and hematocrit to increase
    ③ Both hemoglobin and hematocrit to become slightly lower as a result of increased blood volume
    ④ Both hemoglobin and hematocrit to become slightly higher as a result of decreased blood volume

105. The nurse has been evaluating a patient's understanding of the physician's health teaching during the prenatal period. Which statement made by the patient indicates a need for further teaching?
    ① "I can get calcium from milk, cheese, and yogurt."
    ② "I can continue to have sexual intercourse throughout the pregnancy."
    ③ "I will eliminate my alcohol intake."
    ④ "I will decrease my smoking to a pack a day."

106. Ms. H has a discharge order that includes a buccal tablet. The nurse knows the patient understands the correct method of administration when she says:
    ① "I will let the tablet completely dissolve in my mouth."
    ② "I will follow the tablet with 8 oz of water."
    ③ "I will allow the tablet to dissolve between my cheek and gum."
    ④ "I will place the tablet under my tongue."

107. After teaching a patient about diabetes mellitus, the nurse knows he understands his condition when he states that diabetes mellitus is the result of:
    1. Eating too much sugar and carbohydrates
    2. Eating less sugar and carbohydrates
    3. Decrease or no production of insulin
    4. Increase or more production of insulin

108. Timolol maleate (Timoptic) is an agent used for long-term control of glaucoma. The nurse should know the action of this drug causes:
    1. Miosis
    2. Mydriasis
    3. Diaphoresis
    4. Diuresis

109. The nurse should be prepared to assist the patient with gout to accept a dietary modification that will restrict foods high in:
    1. Purines
    2. Fats
    3. Carbohydrates
    4. Calcium

110. In caring for a patient with pernicious anemia, the nurse evaluates the patient's response to therapy, which includes the patient's response to:
    1. Transfusions of whole blood
    2. Transfusions of packed cells
    3. Injections of iron dextran (Imferon)
    4. Injections of vitamin B$_{12}$

111. While observing a patient receiving a blood transfusion, the nurse must be prepared for a possible reaction. Which of the following differentiates a hemolytic reaction from an allergic or pyogenic reaction?
    1. Urticaria and pruritus
    2. Fever and chills
    3. Hypertension and low back pain
    4. Oliguria and hematuria

112. The nurse is assigned to a patient who is to receive a unit of whole blood. The nurse observes the patient carefully for any signs of incompatibility during transfusion, which is indicative of an antibody and antigen reaction more commonly known as:
    1. Achromia
    2. Agnosia
    3. Agglutination
    4. Anticoagulation

113. Rehabilitation of a patient with a myocardial infarction is flexible to meet the patient needs. The nurse should anticipate the effect of activity and reevaluate the rehabilitation program if the patient:
    1. Complains of dyspnea on exertion
    2. Expresses denial of condition
    3. Refuses to accept dietary restrictions
    4. Expresses lack of knowledge of prescribed medication

114. When checking patient response to initial nitrate therapy, which of the following adverse reactions would the nurse commonly note?
    1. Hypertension
    2. Headache
    3. Bradycardia
    4. Drowsiness

115. A patient, Mrs. Miller, has ankle edema. The physician orders the nurse to weigh her every day. Mrs. Miller asks why she is being weighed every day. The *best explanation* is that:
    1. The physician wants to know her weight every day so he can change medication dosages if necessary
    2. It is necessary to determine if her low-calorie diet is effective
    3. The physician wants to know if she has congestive heart failure
    4. Comparison of daily weights is a good indication of whether she is losing excess fluids

116. Mrs. Shelby has experienced severe diarrhea for several weeks since being prescribed her drug regimen. The nurse should be *most* concerned about which of the following?
    1. Drug absorption
    2. Drug elimination
    3. Drug metabolism
    4. Drug distribution

117. While working as a staff nurse on the same unit for 5 days, the nurse notices that several of the patients on the unit have developed urinary tract infections after being catheterized by the same nurse. The nurse should do which of the following to convey her concerns?
    1. Report the incident to the physician on the next rounds
    2. Confront the nurse and suggest that she has used an inappropriate technique
    3. Follow the proper chain of command and report the incident so that Quality Assurance can follow up
    4. Try to enter the room the next time this nurse performs a catheterization in order to observe her technique

118. Which of the following statements is considered correct, factual recording of patient data in the nurse's notes?
    1. "Mr. Dell is aggressive and obnoxious today."
    2. "Patient stated something about wanting to die."
    3. "Patient is hard to please and refusing any efforts to make him comfortable."
    4. "Patient refused lunch and did not engage in conversation. Observed staring blankly at wall."

119. Mr. Helps, age 23, was seen in the emergency room after falling into a hay bailer and suffering multiple lacerations. He was given a tetanus toxoid and discharged. He asked when he would need another tetanus shot. The nurse should tell him the injection he received is good for:
    1. 3 years
    2. 10 years
    3. Lifetime
    4. Until the next accident

120. Which of the following patients is at greatest risk of developing an infection?
    ① A terminally ill child receiving care at home
    ② A nursing student rotating clinical areas within the agency
    ③ A pediatric patient receiving treatment for a simple laceration in the emergency department
    ④ An acutely ill elderly patient admitted to a medical floor until a bed is available in the intensive care unit

COMPREHENSIVE EXAMINATION TWO: PART 2

121. In the nursing care plan for Mrs. Ball, who is suffering from an infected decubitus ulcer, the nurse would list which of these interventions as an independent nursing action?
    ① Arrange for a whirlpool bath qd by physical therapy
    ② Turn q2h (8 AM, 10 AM, 12 noon, etc), rotating right, left, and back
    ③ Administer penicillin PO q6h at 6 AM, 12 noon, 6 PM, 12 AM
    ④ Cleanse with hydrogen peroxide and apply Betadine q4h and with each dressing change

122. Mr. Snell, a 43-year-old executive with four children, has been brought into the hospital because of a severe motor vehicle accident. He suffered extensive trauma to the chest. He states he is comfortable, with only slight shortness of breath, but is very anxious. He knows that he almost died and talks about it constantly. *From highest to lowest priority,* how should Mr. Snell's problems be ranked?
    ① Fear, anxiety, gas exchange
    ② Anxiety, gas exchange, fear
    ③ Gas exchange, fear, anxiety
    ④ Fear, gas exchange, anxiety

123. The physician orders a loading dose of aminophylline. The order reads "aminophylline 250 mg in 100 ml D₅W to infuse at 33 gtt/min, followed by an aminophylline drip." The drop factor is 10. The charge nurse hangs the loading dose. How long will this intravenous piggyback take to infuse?
    ① 20 min
    ② 30 min
    ③ 45 min
    ④ 60 min

124. Mr. Sam is scheduled for a chest x-ray examination tomorrow morning. He is in respiratory isolation due to his constant coughing and suspected tuberculosis. The nurse would initiate which of these plans?
    ① Place a mask and gown on the patient as he travels to the radiology department
    ② Notify the charge nurse about scheduling a portable chest x-ray examination
    ③ Contact the infection control nurse about the scheduled test
    ④ Contact the radiologists and suggest that the technicians wear a mask during the procedure

125. Missy has a laceration to the lower part of her leg and an ulcer at her ankle that needs irrigating every day. The nurse should prepare her for the treatment by placing her in which position?
    ① Lying down flat on the stretcher
    ② Dangling her leg over the side of the stretcher
    ③ Lying down with the foot of the stretcher elevated
    ④ Sitting in a chair with the leg elevated on the stretcher

126. Kay, age 17, is having contractions at 36 weeks' gestation. She asks if this is premature labor or false labor. The nurse tells her false labor:
    ① Often begins in the back
    ② Has a regular pattern
    ③ Often eases with ambulation
    ④ Is easily controlled with breathing techniques

127. Mrs. Davis, a 35-year-old multipara, is at term. She is traveling through town and comes to a rural emergency department. She is having contractions every 4 minutes for 50-second durations. She states that the physician told her she has a marginal placenta previa. Which of the following is *most important* for the nurse to note on her plan of care?
    ① Schedule for ultrasound immediately
    ② No vaginal examinations
    ③ Pad count
    ④ Type, cross and give 2 units of packed red blood cells

128. Which of the following nursing assessments is a *priority* following spontaneous rupture of membranes?
    ① Station
    ② Contractions
    ③ Fetal heart tones
    ④ Maternal vital signs

129. You are caring for Mrs. J, a patient in the third stage of labor. Signs of placental separation include:
    ① Increase in vaginal bleeding
    ② Shortening of the umbilical cord
    ③ Softening of the uterus
    ④ Increase in pulsations of the umbilical cord

130. Mrs. J is in active labor. She is in a supine position, on a uterine and fetal monitor. Vital signs show a pulse of 88, blood pressure of 130/82, and respirations of 24. Her labor progresses and 2 hours later the nurse notes a pulse of 98; and blood pressure of 102/70. The nurse's next action should be:
    ① Place the patient in modified Trendelenburg's position
    ② Turn patient to left side
    ③ Administer oxygen and notify the physician
    ④ Check for fetal heart rate changes

131. A rape victim asks the nurse what her options are if she is pregnant as a result of her assault. Which of the following is the *most appropriate* answer?
    ① The physician can prescribe hormone therapy
    ② Pregnancy as a result of rape is unlikely
    ③ An early abortion is her only option
    ④ She will be given a spermicidal douche

132. During a physical examination, an 8-year-old girl describes several incidents of sexual abuse by one of her teachers. Which of the following is the *first priority* of the nurse in this situation?
    ① Explain the psychological effects of sexual abuse to her parents
    ② Prepare her for a pelvic examination by a physician
    ③ Inform local child protection authorities
    ④ Suggest that her parents confront the teacher

133. The *most important* nursing intervention care in a situation of suspected child abuse in a school is:
    ① Discourage the keeping of secrets in the family
    ② Assure the safety of the patient and other students
    ③ Help the child express her feelings about the abuse
    ④ Have the teacher removed from his or her position

134. When assessing a child's emotional response to alleged abuse, the nurse would be most likely to find that the child:
    ① Expects her parents to support and not blame her
    ② Uses familiar rituals to decrease her anxiety
    ③ Uses rationalization to cope with the abuse
    ④ Feels responsible for not stopping the abuse

135. An abused child's mother cries and tells the nurse that she "feels upset and responsible" for what has happened. What is the *best response* for the nurse to make to this statement?
    ① "Don't blame yourself. It could happen to anyone."
    ② "She's young, so it won't affect her that much."
    ③ "If you don't act upset, she won't be upset."
    ④ "It sounds like you feel you weren't there for her."

136. Liz, age 5, is admitted to the hospital for removal of her tonsils and adenoids. Before surgery, the nurse should keep an accurate record of the child's temperature and vital signs. This is done primarily because:
    ① The child needs intravenous fluids before surgery
    ② Hemorrhage is quite common in tonsillitis before surgery
    ③ An elevated temperature or changes in vital signs may mean an infection and a need to postpone surgery
    ④ Any change in vital signs or temperature may indicate need for immediate surgery

137. A patient returns from surgery following a tonsillectomy and adenoidectomy. In planning nursing care, the nurse knows the *best position* for this patient immediately after surgery is the:
    ① Prone position
    ② Side-lying position
    ③ Lithotomy position
    ④ Fowler's position

138. While caring for a fresh postoperative tonsillectomy and adenoidectomy patient, the nurse knows that the most common postoperative complication of a tonsillectomy is:
    ① Hemorrhage
    ② Abdominal pain
    ③ Loss of hearing
    ④ Loss of speech

139. Which of the following signs would alert the nurse that a postoperative tonsillectomy and adenoidectomy patient is bleeding excessively?
    ① Flushed face; bright red bleeding; loss of consciousness
    ② Tarry stools; restlessness; loss of consciousness
    ③ Frequent swallowing; restlessness; bright red bleeding
    ④ Elevated temperature; decreased respirations; decreased pulse

140. When Liz, a postoperative tonsillectomy and adenoidectomy patient, is allowed liquids, it would be best to give her:
    ① Fresh orange juice
    ② A popsicle or Gatorade
    ③ Hot tea or coffee
    ④ Ice cream

141. Mrs. Matlock has been diagnosed with a deep vein thrombosis and is being placed on strict bed rest with close observation. As the nurse prepares the thrombolytic agent, Mrs. Matlock asks what the medicine does and how it will help her leg. The nurse explains by stating:
    ① "The medicine thins the blood so that it will not clot anymore."
    ② "The agent inhibits the aggregation of platelets in the bloodstream."
    ③ "The medicine will prevent the formation of fibrin, which forms clots."
    ④ "The agent helps to dissolve the clot and will provide relief of the discomfort in your leg."

142. The nurse is to give heparin 8000 U SQ. The label reads 5000 U/2 ml. How many ml should the nurse administer?
    ① 0.06 ml
    ② 0.6 ml
    ③ 0.625 ml
    ④ 1.6 ml

143. Nursing implications for a patient on heparin include:
    ① Rotating sites in the abdomen if ordered subcutaneous
    ② Rubbing the site after a subcutaneous injection
    ③ Administering the medicine intramuscularly in the arm
    ④ Administering a continuous infusion by gravity

144. The nurse would explain to a surgery patient about to be discharged when to report to the physician concerning changes in the incision. The nurse's explanation should include reporting:
    ① Any coolness or swelling at the incision site
    ② Soreness and bruising at the incision site
    ③ Signs of inflammation or infection
    ④ Redness, warmth, or severe pain at the incision site

145. While assisting a diabetic patient with morning care, the nurse notices her toenails are long and unkempt. After talking to her about her nails, the nurse realizes she does not understand correct foot care for a diabetic patient. The nurse should instruct the patient to:
    ① Assess her feet occasionally for cuts
    ② Wear clean socks and carefully trim her nails
    ③ Wear socks if preferred and trim her nails when desired
    ④ Assess her feet occasionally and wear clean white socks

146. Mrs. Brown is a 2-day postoperative patient who received a shunt in her right arm for dialysis due to renal failure. She is scheduled to begin dialysis when the incision heals. Which of the following should be reported *immediately?*
   1. Abnormal blood pressure in the right arm
   2. Absence of a thrill over the shunt
   3. Complaint of soreness in the right arm
   4. Fear of catching AIDS from the dialysis procedure

147. Mrs. Blakely is being discharged on a monoamine oxidase inhibitor. During the patient teaching session, the nurse should instruct the patient to:
   1. Avoid bananas and yogurt; take the medicine prn
   2. Avoid seasonings and milk; be compliant in taking the medication
   3. Avoid aged cheese, red wines, and beer; be consistent in taking the medication
   4. Avoid colas and fruit; be consistent in taking the medication

148. Mr. Adam has been receiving a CNS depressant every 8 hours for several days. Upon entering the room to give him the 9 AM dose, the nurse notices that his pulse and respirations are slow, he is drowsy and difficult to awaken. Upon further examination, the nurse notices that his pupils react sluggishly to light. The nurse should:
   1. Withhold the medication, raise the side rails, and call the physician
   2. Withhold the medication and observe him carefully over the next few hours
   3. Administer the medication and observe him carefully over the next few hours
   4. Administer the medication, raise the side rails, and instruct him not to get out of bed

149. Mr. McGehee is to receive intermittent feedings q4h through the Levine tube. The physician orders a total of 2800 calories and no more than 3000 ml in 24 hours. The feeding comes in 240-ml cans with 1 ml = 1 calorie. How many cans should be given q4h?
   1. 1.5 cans
   2. 2 cans
   3. 2.5 cans
   4. 6 cans

150. Mrs. Boss reports that her father has not had a formed bowel movement in several days and that he passes small amounts of water only. The nurse should proceed with which of the following?
   1. An order for a laxative
   2. An order for an antidiarrheal
   3. Assessment for a fecal impaction
   4. Assessment of the daughter's concern

151. The physician orders a 1-day postoperative patient to sit in a dangling position for breakfast and sit in a chair for lunch. The patient asks if he can shower after breakfast. The *most appropriate* nursing response should be:
   1. "A shower will be alright, but I would like to assist you in dressing."
   2. "As long as you feel up to it, you may shower. Warm water may make you feel better."
   3. "Surgery often makes patients feel dizzy the first few times they get up; let's wait until you've been up longer."
   4. "You cannot take a shower until your dressing and stitches are removed completely by the doctor, probably before you go home."

152. The respiratory therapist enters and explains the use of a triflow to a surgery patient who is a smoker. When the therapist leaves, the patient states the triflow is not needed and is a waste of money. The nurse should explain that the triflow:
   1. Is a standard procedure for patients his age
   2. Provides better aeration to the lungs after surgery
   3. Is needed to expand the alveoli after surgery because of the anesthetics given and his smoking history
   4. Loosens the secretions that could exist as a result of the anesthetics given in surgery and his smoking history

153. The physician orders carbamazepine (Tegretol) 1.2 g/day in three divided doses. The medication is supplied in 100-mg tablets. How many tablets should be given per dose?
   1. 2 tablets
   2. 3 tablets
   3. 4 tablets
   4. 6 tablets

154. Patient teaching for a patient receiving an anticonvulsant should include which of the following?
   1. Refraining from driving if drowsiness and dizziness occur
   2. Taking the medicine between meals and with milk
   3. Stopping the medication if drowsiness occurs, and calling the physician
   4. Use of sunscreen for photosensitivity only if the sun is extremely hot

155. After performing range of motion on a 19-year-old paraplegic, the nurse notices that his right foot is in a plantar flexion most of the time. The nurse should initiate which of the following interventions?
   1. Position the patient in proper alignment while he is asleep; increase his exercise while he is awake
   2. Inform the charge nurse of the need for intervention; increase exercise
   3. Offer the range of motion more frequently; change the type of exercise
   4. Place a foot board at the end of the bed; position the feet in a dorsal flexion position

156. A 24-hour-urine collection for creatinine clearance is ordered. The test is scheduled to end at 9 AM. The nurse would:
    ① Discard the 9 AM voiding and send the entire specimen to the laboratory
    ② Collect a final voiding at 9 AM and send with all the other collected urine to the laboratory
    ③ Instruct the patient to collect a specimen at 8:30 AM before sending it to the laboratory at 9 AM
    ④ Instruct the patient to obtain a clean-catch, midstream urine for the final urine specimen

157. Which of the following problems commonly results from chronic renal failure?
    ① Anemia
    ② Hypotension
    ③ Hypokalemia
    ④ Weight loss

158. The patient is started on hemodialysis three times a week. An arteriovenous fistula is created in the right arm. Specific nursing interventions include:
    ① Palpating the access for a thrill
    ② Keeping the right arm in a dependent position
    ③ Taking the blood pressure in the affected arm
    ④ Teaching the patient to keep the arm protected and covered

159. Which of the following statements is *most* descriptive of hemodialysis?
    ① Blood is circulated through a filter by the patient's own arterial system
    ② Removal of chemical substances from the blood through a vascular access
    ③ Removal of toxic substances from the body through the peritoneal cavity
    ④ The process is continuous through a permanent peritoneal catheter

160. Dietary management for the patient with chronic renal failure usually includes:
    ① Providing high-carbohydrate liquid supplements
    ② Restricting protein, sodium, and potassium
    ③ Increasing protein and sodium intake
    ④ Decreasing fat intake

161. Tony, a newborn, has tested positive for phenylketonuria (PKU). The nurse knows that a sample of Tony's blood will contain abnormal amounts of:
    ① Tyrosine
    ② Phenylalanine
    ③ Phenylpyruvic acid
    ④ Phenylalanine hydroxylase

162. Phenylketonuria (PKU) is caused by an inherited error of metabolism which, if untreated, will result in:
    ① Hepatic coma
    ② Renal shutdown
    ③ Mental retardation
    ④ Epileptic seizures

163. In planning a diet for a patient with phenylketonuria, the nurse knows that the diet therapy will be based on the knowledge that the nutrients to be controlled are:
    ① Fats
    ② Minerals
    ③ Proteins
    ④ Carbohydrates

164. Melissa is admitted to the hospital after losing 25% of her normal body weight in a 2-month period. The diagnosis is restricting anorexia. What is the nurse's *first priority* for this patient?
    ① Exploring her feelings about her body
    ② Assessing her physiological status
    ③ Discussing her relationship with her family
    ④ Planning a meal and exercise schedule

165. Which of the following is the *most appropriate* short-term goal for a person with restricting anorexia?
    ① To encourage expression of feelings
    ② To alter the patient's body image
    ③ To promote peer relationships
    ④ To restore safe nutritional status

166. Shirley's son brings her to the emergency department for evaluation after she becomes suddenly ill. The examining physician makes a diagnosis of delirium. Which of the following statements made by the patient's son best supports this diagnosis?
    ① "Mom has become so forgetful over the past 6 months."
    ② "She was perfectly fine until late this afternoon."
    ③ "Maybe we should expect this; she's 75."
    ④ "My uncle's death has made her very depressed."

167. Which of the following assessment findings would *most likely* be associated with a diagnosis of delirium?
    ① Patient has been taking antibiotics for a sinus infection
    ② Patient has been taking furosemide (Lasix) for congestive heart failure
    ③ Patient had a hip replacement 12 months ago
    ④ Patient has lost 10 pounds over the past year

168. Shirley is admitted with a diagnosis of delirium, secondary to dehydration. Which of the following nursing interventions would be the *most appropriate* for her in her present condition?
    ① Acquaint her with the unit and her room
    ② Have her son leave a list of family numbers
    ③ Explain the use of the call light and side rails
    ④ Reorient her frequently to person and place

169. Which of the following nursing diagnoses should receive priority for a patient who is delirious?
    ① Self care deficit related to confusion
    ② Activity intolerance related to weakness
    ③ Alteration in comfort related to dry mucous membranes
    ④ Potential for injury related to impaired judgment

170. Which of the following questions asked by the nurse is *most appropriate* to reassess the level of orientation of a patient hospitalized for delirium?
    ① "Can you tell me what time of day it is?"
    ② "Can you tell me how you are feeling right now?"
    ③ "What did you have for breakfast yesterday?"
    ④ "What would you do if there was a fire?"

171. Mrs. Roberts asks if she can use a bottle prop when she is too busy to feed the baby. The nurse should base her response on the knowledge that bottle propping is:
    ① All right if the mother stays with the baby
    ② Considered dangerous because the baby might aspirate some of the formula while sucking
    ③ A safe and time-saving practice for busy mothers
    ④ Better than holding the baby during feeding

172. Mrs. Eve is a young mother, who is very apprehensive with her first child. She tells the nurse that her 3-week-old baby girl sleeps most of the day. As a nurse and neighbor, the nurse should inform her that newborns:
    1. Should have only brief naps
    2. Sleep all day and stay awake most of the night
    3. Need at least 12 hours of sleep in a 24-hour period
    4. Usually sleep about 18 to 20 hours during the first month

173. The condition of a pediatric patient with croup has improved with treatment, and he is ready for discharge from the hospital. To promote rest, which of these instructions should the nurse give the mother?
    1. Sedate him every 4 hours
    2. Place him in a dark room
    3. Allow him to stay with her at all times
    4. Provide a quiet environment as much as possible

174. In caring for a child with croup, it is necessary for the nurse to know that croup is characterized by:
    1. An infection of the pharynx
    2. Spasms of the larynx with partial obstruction of the respiratory tract
    3. Contractions of the trachea
    4. Inflammation of the lung tissue

175. An infant patient is scheduled to receive ampicillin 250 mg orally. The label on the bottle reads "125 mg/5 ml." How much does the nurse administer?
    1. 1.5 ml
    2. 4 ml
    3. 2.5 ml
    4. 10 ml

176. A 35-year-old insulin-dependent diabetic is admitted to the hospital because her blood sugar has been difficult to regulate. The nurse knows that significant hyperglycemia is often manifested by:
    1. Dehydration, nausea/vomiting; elevated serum glucose levels
    2. Pale, cool, clammy skin; restlessness and irritability
    3. Lowered serum glucose levels; negative urine glucose
    4. Drowsiness, moist skin, perspiration, and tremors

177. In which situation would the nurse anticipate using NPH insulin?
    1. For "sliding scale" coverage
    2. For managing acute hypoglycemia
    3. For daily injection to control disease
    4. In the emergency of diabetic ketoacidosis

178. The nurse is reviewing foot care with a patient with diabetes. Instruction should be given to:
    1. Keep the toenails short and rounded at the edges
    2. Apply alcohol after washing her feet every day
    3. Keep her feet warm at night by using a heating pad set on low
    4. Select absorbent socks/stockings that allow for toe motion

179. The nurse and a diabetic patient are reviewing exchange lists for meal planning. The patient shows an understanding of instructions by which of the following statements?
    1. "I should cut out desserts other than fresh fruit."
    2. "I should decrease my food intake during periods of heavy exercise."
    3. "I should use only designated dietetic foods."
    4. "I should schedule regular meals."

180. Bradley Smith, newly admitted to the newborn nursery, had an initial Apgar score of 4. The nurse interprets the Apgar score to indicate:
    1. A vigorous newborn
    2. A depressed newborn
    3. Respiration had to be initiated
    4. A respiratory rate of 20

181. The nurse may obtain a Moro's reflex by implementation of which of the following nursing actions?
    1. Grasping the newborn's hand
    2. Stimulating the newborn's feet
    3. Creating a banging noise
    4. Turning the newborn's head to the right side

182. The nurse is working for Dr. Paul and is preparing an obstetrical patient for a physical examination. The patient, Mrs. G, states that she has been having nausea and vomiting for the past 2 months. The term the nurse would note on the patient's medical record to indicate this would be:
    1. Pernicious vomiting
    2. Vomitus marinus
    3. Morning sickness
    4. Hyperemesis gravidarium

183. The physician orders a pregnancy test to be done to determine the presence of a hormone that is excreted in the urine only during early pregnancy. In filling out the requisition form for the laboratory, the nurse should mark which hormone?
    1. ACTH
    2. FSH
    3. HCG
    4. TSH

184. A pregnancy test is done, and the results are positive. The physician tells the nurse to position the patient for a vaginal exam. The nurse should place her in what *preferred* position?
    1. Horizontal recumbent
    2. Supine position
    3. Dorsal recumbent
    4. Lithotomy

185. Mrs. G returns for a follow-up obstetrical visit about 4 months into her pregnancy. The nurse checks her weight and blood pressure. She notes that the patient has gained 10 lb since her last visit and that her blood pressure is 200/90. Mrs. G states that her fingers and feet have become swollen. The nurse knows that these symptoms may be an indication of:
    1. Pre-eclampsia
    2. Eclampsia
    3. Hypertension
    4. Hypersthenia

186. While teaching Mrs. G, a patient with symptoms of preeclampsia, about high blood pressure, water retention, and weight gain during the last trimester of pregnancy, the nurse should instruct the patient about:
    ① Bed rest and decreasing her caloric intake
    ② Moderate exercise and decreasing her caloric intake
    ③ Bed rest and decreasing her salt intake
    ④ Moderate exercise and decreasing her salt intake

187. Regina's mother asks if her daughter will ever be "cured" of her alcohol addiction. The nurse's *most appropriate* answer *should* be:
    ① "Yes, after she is sober for a long period of time."
    ② "No, because alcohol addiction is a chronic illness."
    ③ "Alcohol addiction is not a disease."
    ④ "Yes, if she does not already have permanent damage."

188. Which of the following is of *primary importance* during the detoxification phase of the substance-addicted patient's hospitalization?
    ① Increase interpersonal skills
    ② Encourage group participation
    ③ Increase patient's sense of responsibility
    ④ Prevent or treat symptoms of acute withdrawal

189. Bernice comes to her physician's office complaining of recurring headaches and abdominal pains. She states that her youngest son just left for college, that her mother-in-law has just moved into her home, and that she and her husband are fighting constantly. She says, "I just can't take it anymore!" The problem that Bernice presents is an example of a(n):
    ① Depressive episode
    ② Anxiety disorder
    ③ Situational crisis
    ④ Schizophrenic relapse

190. The way in which patients in a situational crisis handle their current problem is *most determined* by:
    ① The level of support from their family
    ② The way that they have coped in the past
    ③ Their ability to change their life-style
    ④ The amount of therapy they receive

191. The immediate short-term goal for a patient in situational crisis should be to:
    ① Explore family relationships
    ② Decrease any somatic symptoms
    ③ Get him or her started with insight-oriented therapy
    ④ Encourage him or her to verbalize concerns

192. A patient in a situational crisis asks why the physician can't give her something like Valium to make her feel better. The nurse knows that the most important reason antianxiety drugs such as this are not prescribed to patients in crisis is:
    ① They have a high potential for abuse
    ② They do not address the underlying problem
    ③ They cause personality changes
    ④ They do not effectively treat the symptoms

193. Mrs. Grissom, a postpartum patient with an episiotomy, has a heat lamp ordered to the perineal area. To provide this treatment the nurse should:
    ① Warm up the heat lamp thoroughly before applying heat
    ② Use a 60-watt bulb
    ③ Place the light 18 to 24 inches from the site
    ④ Allow the patient to use the light for 30 min

194. Ms. F is 3 days postpartum. She had a normal labor, delivered an 8-lb 4-oz boy and had an episiotomy. She has not had a stool since delivery. In an effort to assist her with her elimination needs, the nurse should provide:
    ① Adequate analgesia to allow comfortable bowel elimination while the episiotomy heals
    ② Adequate fluids and exercise to promote peristalsis and soft stools
    ③ Rest and calories to promote healing
    ④ Laxatives and sitz baths to promote elimination

195. Mrs. Hill had an emergency cesarean section under general anesthesia for cephalopelvic disproportion (CPD) at 3 AM this morning. She was delivered of an 8-lb 12-oz live female infant with an Apgar score of 6. When the nurse first enters Mrs. Hill's room, she asks, "Is my baby all right?" The nurse's *best response* should be:
    ① "I really don't know. When you see the nurse from the nursery, why don't you ask her?"
    ② "I'm sure the pediatrician will be in soon to give you a progress report."
    ③ "The nursery report this morning said she was progressing well. I will ask the nurse from the nursery to come and speak with you soon."
    ④ "Oh, I would not be too concerned. We give such good care that all our babies do real well."

196. Mrs. Brickman, a cesarean patient, asks why she cannot have something to drink, stating, "I have not had any water since 6 hours before I had my C-section." She begs you for some ice water. The nurse's *best response* should be:
    ① "Mrs. Brickman, I know you are very thirsty. I will give you mouth care and I'm sure you'll feel better."
    ② "Mrs. Brickman, I know you are very thirsty and I would like to give you some water. But it is important that you not have anything by mouth until we know that you can digest it properly."
    ③ "The physician's order said you cannot have any water until at least tomorrow, and then we will only start with ice chips first."
    ④ "The IV handles all of your fluid needs, so why don't you rinse your mouth with mouthwash?"

197. Ms. Aaron, a 1-day postoperative cesarean patient, is reluctant to cough and deep-breathe because her "stomach hurts." Which of the following should the nurse do to help Ms. Aaron cooperate with this nursing measure?
    ① Maintain Mrs. Aaron in a dangling position before the procedure
    ② Check her last pain medication time to see if she could have something to relieve the pain
    ③ Explain the reasons why coughing and deep-breathing are necessary; stay with her and encourage her while she is trying to deep-breathe
    ④ Tell Mrs. Aaron she will come back later when Mrs. Aaron is feeling better

198. For a patient who abuses substances, inflicts frequent self harm, has multiple abusive/unstable relationships, and frequently threatens suicide, the nurse should suspect which of the following disorders?
    1. Character disorder
    2. Anxiety disorder
    3. Borderline personality disorder
    4. Substance abuse disorder

199. Which of the following statements is the *best indication* that a patient with bipolar disorder has improved enough to be safely discharged to outpatient treatment?
    1. "I'm going to take lithium until I feel better."
    2. "I'm going to keep my therapy appointments every week."
    3. "I'm going to pursue my dream of taking over IBM."
    4. "I'm going to begin a new diet and redecorate my house."

200. A 32-year-old female is a homemaker and the mother of two boys. She complains of fatigue, nervousness, and irritability. A tentative diagnosis of hyperthyroidism is made. A finding that the nursing assessment is *most* likely to reveal is:
    1. Anorexia
    2. Weight gain
    3. Constipation
    4. Heat intolerance

201. Early signs of exophthalmos are observed in the patient with hyperthyroidism. Which symptom is typical of this condition?
    1. Blurring of vision
    2. Protrusion of the eyeballs
    3. Watery discharge from the eyes
    4. Inability to distinguish colors

202. The plan of care for the patient with hyperthyroidism should include:
    1. Limiting caloric intake
    2. Providing for a restful environment
    3. Application of emollients for dry skin
    4. Maintaining the room temperature at above normal levels

203. A patient with hyperthyroidism begins taking propylthiouracil (PTU). The nurse should instruct the patient to report a(n):
    1. Pulse rate above 100
    2. Increased body weight
    3. Metallic taste in her mouth
    4. Sore throat, rash, or fever

204. A patient's hyperthyroidism is not controlled with medications, and a subtotal thyroidectomy is performed. Postoperatively, the nurse assesses the patient's wound for bleeding. Which technique is *most* appropriate?
    1. Inspect dressing for any dried blood
    2. Monitor the hemoglobin and hematocrit levels for changes
    3. Loosen dressing on both ends and check the wound directly
    4. Slip hand behind patient's neck and check for blood on back of neck and bed linens

205. A patient who had a subtotal thyroidectomy is brought back to the nursing unit from the postanesthesia care unit. The nurse asks the patient to state her name and repeats this request frequently. The *primary* reason the nurse includes this intervention in the postoperative plan of care is to monitor for signs of:
    1. Hemorrhage
    2. Laryngeal nerve damage
    3. Lower airway obstruction
    4. Level of consciousness change

206. A 70-year-old patient is being treated for chronic glaucoma. Data from the history would *most* likely reveal that the patient had:
    1. Acute attacks of eye pain
    2. A loss of her peripheral vision
    3. Tearing and redness after reading
    4. A decreased ability to focus on near objects

207. The nurse is teaching the patient how to instill eye drops. The nurse should tell the patient to:
    1. Apply light pressure to the eye after instilling the drops
    2. Cover the eye for at least 10 minutes after the drops are instilled
    3. Place the eye drops in the conjunctival sac that is made by gently pulling the lower eyelid outward
    4. First remove any excess fluid by wiping the eye from the outer to inner canthus

208. A 20-year-old male college student is brought to the hospital following an accident. He states that he is unable to move or feel his legs. His neck has been immobilized. Initial diagnostic studies indicate a C5-C6 fracture. Crutchfield tongs are inserted, and 10 lb of traction applied. The parents ask the nurse about the seriousness of the injury. The nurse's *best* response is to:
    1. Inform them that their son will be confined to a wheelchair and will require mechanical ventilation
    2. Reassure the family that he will be back to his preinjury status but it will take a couple of months
    3. Inform the parents that it is too early to know the full extent of the injury
    4. Reassure the parents that their son will be back in college soon

209. The incorporation of Crutchfield tongs and traction into the plan of care following an acute cervical injury/fracture is to:
    1. Allow the patient to maintain normal head and neck movement
    2. Align the injured vertebrae and reduce muscle spasm
    3. Provide support for the lower extremities
    4. Prevent the development of spinal shock

210. Neurological assessment of the lower extremities of a patient with an acute spinal fracture at the cervical level would reveal:
    1. Absent deep-tendon reflexes
    2. Hyperactive deep-tendon reflexes
    3. Increasingly higher levels of sensory paralysis
    4. Absent temperature sensation bilaterally above the injury

211. A finding characteristic of spinal shock is:
    ① Hypertension
    ② Bradycardia
    ③ Spasticity
    ④ Seizures

212. A spinal cord—injured patient is now ready for the application of a Halo brace. Which of the following *best relates* to the use of the Halo fixation device?
    ① Infection is less of a problem because skull pins are not required
    ② The patient will have normal head and neck range-of-motion capability
    ③ The patient must remain in bed so that the weights can hang freely
    ④ Stabilization of the spine is provided without the use of a frame or special bed

213. In preparation for a patient's home care following a cervical spinal injury, the nurse is teaching the patient and his family how to recognize signs and symptoms of complications that can develop because of his spinal injuries. He is encouraged to increase his intake of fluids *mainly* because:
    ① The replacement is needed for fluids lost during perspiration
    ② Fluids decrease the incidence of pulmonary infection
    ③ Fluids decrease the formation of urinary calculi
    ④ Fluids reduce the possibility of spinal shock

214. Otitis media is a common complication of an upper respiratory infection in infants. It occurs primarily because:
    ① The sinuses of an infant are not fully developed
    ② The digestive system is not fully developed
    ③ The infant's eustachian tube is shorter, wider, and straighter than that of an adult
    ④ The infant's eustachian tube is longer and more narrow than that of an adult

215. Jimmy, age 16 months, was admitted to the hospital. He is experiencing dyspnea, he looks slightly cyanotic, and he has a temperature of 103° F. The physician has diagnosed him as having a severe upper respiratory infection and orders a Croupette with oxygen. A Croupette is *best described* as:
    ① An aerosol therapy that deposits medication into the airway
    ② A plastic tent designed to provide cool, moist air and oxygen for the patient to breathe
    ③ Prepared by placing a blanket over the sides of the crib and placing a steam pot nearby
    ④ A plastic tent designed to keep air warm and moist inside the tent

216. To promote comfort and optional functioning to a child who is placed in a Croupette, which of these actions would be *most appropriate* for the nurse to take?
    ① Change the bed linens and the patient's gown as often as necessary to keep him dry and comfortable
    ② Establish continuous drainage from the ice chamber as the ice melts
    ③ Restrain the child to prohibit changing position in bed
    ④ Maintain child in a prone position

217. Upper respiratory infections are potentially more serious in infants than in adults primarily because:
    ① Infants cannot be given a well-balanced diet
    ② Infants have no ability to build up an immunity to disease
    ③ Most infants cannot be given antibiotics
    ④ The air passages of an infant are very small and easily obstruct with mucus

218. Susie, age 15, visits the clinic for a physical examination required to play sports. The physician orders a clean-catch specimen for a urinalysis. The nurse should instruct Susie to:
    ① Void a small amount in the toilet, then a small amount in the cup; cleanse her hands with the wipe
    ② Cleanse with the wipes; void a small amount in the toilet and a small amount in the cup; urinate the remainder in the toilet
    ③ Urinate a small amount in the toilet, stopping in midstream; cleanse from front to back with each wipe, then urinate the remainder in the cup provided
    ④ Use each individual wipe only once, cleansing from front to back; urinate a small amount in the toilet, stopping in midstream; urinate the remainder in the cup provided

219. Mr. Harold Beare, age 52, comes to the physician's office for a routine health screening. He weighs 210 lb and is 5 ft 10 in tall. He works a 45-hour week as a warehouse foreman. His primary source of exercise is his employment. He smokes one pack of cigarettes per day and usually eats at home. The nurse assists in Mr. Beare's assessment by taking his blood pressure. Where should the nurse listen with the stethoscope to best hear the blood pressure sounds?
    ① Over the radial artery
    ② Over the brachial artery
    ③ Over the outer aspect of the antecubital fossa
    ④ One half inch below the edge of the cuff

220. A friend's daughter comes home with a note that she has head lice. The mother doesn't know what to do other than buy some lindane (Kwell) to shampoo her daughter's hair. The nurse should also advise the mother to:
    ① Shampoo the hair for 15 minutes before rinsing
    ② Shampoo the hair again the next day and repeat the same process
    ③ Use a comb dipped in vinegar to comb out the nits after the shampoo
    ④ Wash linen and clothing only if desired; the head lice was confined to the child's hair

221. Mrs. Bee calls in a panic-stricken voice stating that her 2-year-old daughter has just ingested "some" Clorox. The mother states that she has syrup of ipecac at home. The nurse should instruct her to:
    ① Administer 10 ml of syrup of ipecac with milk
    ② Administer 10 ml of syrup of ipecac with water
    ③ Not give syrup of ipecac; bring her daughter to the emergency room
    ④ Not give syrup of ipecac; observe her daughter at home for the next hour

222. A child is to receive D₅RL at 50 ml/hr. A 500-ml bag of solution is available for the charge nurse to start the IV. How many hours will it take to infuse the 500 ml?
① 4 hours
② 6 hours
③ 10 hours
④ 15 hours

223. On entering the patient's room, the nurse finds 9-month-old Sam being rocked by his mother. The mother is crying softly. After the nurse checks the vital signs, she asks the mother, "How is the baby doing today?" The mother replies, "I thought he was going to die when his respirations were so fast this afternoon." What is the *best response* by the nurse?
① "Yes, we too thought he would die."
② "It must have been very frightening for you."
③ "Don't be silly, we don't let 9-month-old kids die."
④ The nurse should say nothing and just finish the assessment

224. Mrs. Jancy's son, who has been hospitalized for a week with bronchitis and pneumonia, is being discharged today. The physician orders an antibiotic q6h, an expectorant q4h, and an antitussive prn. The nurse should instruct her to give the child the:
① Expectorant and the antitussive together when needed
② Antibiotic as prescribed, but the other two only when needed for coughing
③ Expectorant during the night and the antitussive during the day if the child is coughing
④ Expectorant during the day and the antitussive during the night if the child is coughing

225. The *most* accurate method of evaluating fluid status in the patient with chronic renal failure is:
① Intake and output
② Daily BUN levels
③ Daily weight
④ Skin turgor

226. A 60-year-old being treated through the outpatient clinic is receiving external radiation therapy to the chest area. The skin over the treatment area is dry and red. The nurse instructs him in skin care. Which of the following statements indicates that he understands the teaching?
① "I will apply lotion to the dry areas daily."
② "I will make an effort to wear loose-fitting clothing."
③ "An astringent will be used after washing the site thoroughly."
④ "To help strengthen the skin, I will use rubbing alcohol on the area."

227. An insulin-dependent diabetic tells the nurse she is thinking about beginning an exercise program and asks about the role of exercise in relation to her diet and medication. The nurse's response is based on the knowledge that:
① Exercise prevents hypoglycemia attacks
② Fruit or juice should be limited before exercising
③ The blood sugar should be monitored before and after exercise
④ Physical exercise is discouraged for insulin-dependent individuals

228. A patient is started on thyroid replacement therapy. Which of the following would indicate an undesirable effect from taking levothyroxine (Synthroid)?
① Chest pain
② Constipation
③ Decreased activity
④ Sore throat and fever

229. The nurse suspects that tetany may be occurring if following a thyroidectomy the patient complains of:
① Joint pains and backache
② Excessive perspiration
③ Her fingers tingling
④ Voice weakness

230. The physician has prescribed pilocarpine eye drops for the patient with glaucoma. This medication is given to:
① Dilate the pupil
② Decrease inflammation
③ Promote drainage of aqueous humor
④ Increase the production of aqueous humor

231. A patient with a history of seizures takes phenytoin (Dilantin). Which statement made by the patient indicates that he understands self-care related to his anticonvulsant medication?
① "I will take an additional dose when I feel stressed."
② "I will only consume a moderate amount of alcohol."
③ "I will keep my medication with me at all times."
④ "I will need an ongoing plan of oral hygiene."

232. A patient who has had a stroke is attempting to feed himself. He becomes easily frustrated as he tries to explain what he wants to eat. He cries and throws down his fork. This behavior supports a nursing diagnosis of:
① Anxiety, severe
② Diversional activity deficit
③ Sensory-perceptual alteration
④ Coping, individual ineffective

233. A patient is to receive a blood transfusion. The nurse will be monitoring his vital signs. Thirty minutes after the transfusion started, the patient complains of respiratory distress and dyspnea. His pulse rate increased from 80 to 110. These symptoms *most* likely indicate what type of problem?
① Febrile reaction
② Allergic reaction
③ Hemolytic reaction
④ Circulatory overload

234. A patient is started on iron therapy. A liquid preparation is prescribed. Which patient statement indicates the need for additional teaching?
① "I will take the medication with meals."
② "A straw is necessary to prevent teeth staining."
③ "I'll report diarrhea and light-colored stools."
④ "Taking orange juice will help with absorption of the medication."

235. The nurse is reviewing the results of the CK-MB enzymes 6 hours after the admission of a patient with an acute myocardial infarction (MI). The nurse notes that the enzymes are elevated. These findings are indicative of the:
   ① Presence of infection
   ② Location of the myocardial infarct
   ③ Evolution of the myocardial infarct
   ④ Effects of heart disease on the kidneys

236. The nurse evaluates the success of the postoperative interventions to maintain oxygenation. She knows that which of the following is indicative of decreased oxygen level?
   ① Bradycardia
   ② Ruddy complexion
   ③ Decreased breath sounds
   ④ Mental confusion, drowsiness

237. The nurse begins teaching the patient with angina about the use of nitroglycerin (NTG) sublingual. Which statement indicates that the patient understands how to use the medication?
   ① "I'll take it after doing any exercising."
   ② "I'll take it at bedtime to prevent nighttime attacks."
   ③ "I'll take it every 6 to 8 hours to prevent any chest pain."
   ④ "I'll take it as soon as I notice any sign of chest pain."

238. A patient with a pneumothorax has had a chest tube in place for 32 hours. Which finding would indicate that his lung has re-expanded?
   ① Fluctuation in the water-seal chamber
   ② Drainage changes in color from red to yellow
   ③ Absence of bubbling in the water-seal chamber
   ④ Continuous bubbling in the water-seal chamber

239. Discharge teaching has been completed for the patient who has had a total laryngectomy. Which statement indicates a need for additional teaching about home care?
   ① "When coughing, I will cover my stoma instead of my mouth."
   ② "I will check my stoma for signs of redness or swelling."
   ③ "I will clean the stoma area daily with a deodorant-type soap."
   ④ "A protective cover will be needed when I shave or have my hair cut."

240. Considering Mr. Wilson's age of 52, which of the following blood pressure values should the nurse recognize as abnormal and report?
   ① 128/84
   ② 136/74
   ③ 118/64
   ④ 132/94

CHAPTER 6

Answers and Rationales for Review Questions

All questions have been classified by cognitive level, nursing process, patient need, and level of difficulty. These classifications are provided following the question number.

The first word signifies the cognitive level of the questions: knowledge, comprehension, or application. The second word indicates the phase of the nursing process: assessment, planning, implementation, or evaluation. The third word indicates the type of patient need and is abbreviated as follows: environment = safe, effective care environment; physiological = physiological integrity; psychosocial = psychosocial integrity; health = health promotion/maintenance.

The letters in parentheses indicate the difficulty of the question. The letter *a* signifies that more than 75% of students should answer the question correctly; *b* signifies that between 50% and 75% should answer correctly; and *c* signifies that between 25% and 50% should answer correctly.

Rationales for all four answer choices for each question are provided. The rationale for the correct answer is listed first, followed by rationales for the incorrect answer choices.

Medical-Surgical Nursing

1. Comprehension, assessment, physiological (b)
   3 Pain and stiffness that is more severe in the morning and less at the end of the day are classic symptoms of rheumatoid arthritis.
   1 This is classic of osteoarthritis, not rheumatoid arthritis.
   2 She may experience a low-grade fever throughout the day, not only at night.
   4 This is classic of osteoporosis, not rheumatoid arthritis.
2. Application, implementation, health (c)
   3 Giving aspirin will reduce inflammation and decrease pain and stiffness in the morning.
   1 A warm bath would relax muscles and decrease pain and stiffness. A cool bath is contraindicated.
   2, 4 This type of exercise is too strenuous for rheumatoid arthritis.
3. Application, implementation, environment (a)
   2 When the patient is in the prone position, he/she cannot flex the hips or knees; therefore, flexion deformities would be prevented.
   1 High-Fowler's position could actually cause flexion deformities of the hip.
   3 Sims' position could cause knee and hip deformities.
   4 Trendelenburg's position is not used in rheumatoid arthritis because it is not a comfortable position, and it will not prevent flexion deformities.

4. Application, implementation, health (c)
   4 Aspirin is an antiinflammatory; acetaminophen (Tylenol) is an analgesic. Aspirin is the drug of choice for rheumatoid arthritis.
   1 Because of No. 4, these drugs are not interchangeable.
   2 Rheumatoid arthritis patients need both antiinflammatory and analgesic properties in drugs.
   3 Statement is not true; irrelevant.
5. Knowledge, assessment, physiological (a)
   1 Arthritis refers to inflammatory changes in the synovial joints as a result of failure in the immune system.
   2 There may be acute phases to arthritis, but the disease is mainly chronic.
   3 Arthritis is inflammatory rather than infectious.
   4 This disease does not affect immovable joints.
6. Comprehension, assessment, physiological (a)
   2 Chronic inflammatory reaction in the synovial membrane affects freely movable joints.
   1 This is characteristic of osteoarthritis.
   3 This is characteristic of osteoporosis.
   4 This is characteristic of osteomyelitis.
7. Comprehension, implementation, environment (b)
   4 Active/passive exercising allows continued movement of the joints to prevent complications and assists in reducing pain.
   1 Bed rest limits activity and contributes to complications even with range-of-motion exercises.
   2 Balanced, rather than limited, activity with rest is needed to prevent complications even if it does tire her.
   3 Immobility leads to joint damage and deformity.
8. Application, implementation, environment (a)
   2 Medication is given with meals so that food in the stomach can help prevent gastric irritation.
   1 Gastric irritation occurs when no food or milk products coat the stomach lining.
   3 There is an increased risk of irritation of the gastric lining at bedtime, when no food or milk coats the stomach lining.
   4 This is an inappropriate response; medication is needed on a regularly scheduled basis.
9. Comprehension, planning, health (a)
   4 Restores and maintains function of the affected parts while preventing further debilitating complications.
   1 Bed rest increases the opportunity for further debilitating complications.
   2 Feeding meals encourages patient dependency rather than maximal functioning.
   3 Total care not only promotes dependency but decreases the needed stimulation of doing things for herself and feeling a useful purpose in life.

10. Application, implementation, psychosocial (b)
    3 Encourage the patient to talk about the cure, to express her feelings about her diagnosis, and to keep her physician informed.
    1 There is danger in following programs that promise false cures.
    2 This response does not allow her to express her feeling.
    4 This response does not allow her to share the information she has found and logically discuss the implications of the "cure."

11. Knowledge, assessment, physiological (a)
    2 Gout is the metabolic disorder of purines, which break down into uric acids.
    1 This is osteoporosis.
    3 This is systemic lupus erythematosus.
    4 This is osteoarthritis.

12. Comprehension, planning, physiological (a)
    1 Gout is the accumulation of uric acid as a result of the body's inability to metabolize purines.
    2, 3, 4 These nutrients are not related to gout.

13. Knowledge, assessment, physiological (a)
    3 Acute pain results from the accumulation of uric acid salts deposited in a joint, most frequently in the great toe.
    1 This is an objective symptom; gout does not necessarily affect all joints at the same time.
    2 These are subjective symptoms of scleroderma.
    4 This is a subjective symptom associated with osteoarthritis.

14. Application, implementation, health (b)
    4 Organ meats are high in purines, which break down into uric acid.
    1, 2, 3 These foods would not be restricted.

15. Knowledge, planning, physiological (a)
    1 Allopurinol inhibits the formation of uric acid.
    2 Corticosteroids are antiinflammatory agents and would be used in treatment of lupus erythematosus.
    3 Acetaminophen (Tylenol) is an analgesic.
    4 Estrogen replacement is recommended for osteoporosis.

16. Comprehension, assessment, physiological (b)
    1 A herniated intervertebral disk can occur suddenly (from lifting, twisting, or trauma) or gradually (from degenerative changes).
    2 These are signs and symptoms of a fracture.
    3 These signs and symptoms may indicate osteogenic sarcoma.
    4 These signs and symptoms may indicate multiple myeloma.

17. Comprehension, assessment, environment (c)
    2 Magnetic resonance imaging (MRI) uses magnetic forces to image the body structures. Computed axial tomography (CT or CAT scan) provides a three-dimensional picture of the structures being studied. A complete history and physical examination are essential.
    1 These are tests indicated for seizure disorders.
    3 These are tests indicated for various tumors of the bone.
    4 These are tests indicated for degenerative joint disease (osteoarthritis).

18. Comprehension, planning, physiological (b)
    4 This is the expected nursing care for this diagnosis. Other nursing interventions include documenting effectiveness of analgesics, and providing the patient and family with information about procedures to help reduce anxiety.
    1 This is nursing care for spinal cord injury.
    2 This is nursing care for rheumatoid arthritis.
    3 This is nursing care for gouty arthritis.

19. Application, implementation, health (c)
    3 Laminectomy involves excision of the ruptured portion of the nucleus pulposus.
    1 This is the surgical procedure for diskectomy.
    2 This is the surgical procedure for spinal fusion.
    4 This drug dissolves the nucleus pulposus; the procedure *cannot* be performed on patients with nerve involvement. Mr. Smith would *not* be a candidate.

20. Comprehension, implementation, physiological (c)
    4 Assessment should be completed for erythematous purulent exudate from the wound. Because ventilation is vital, the nurse should assist the patient to turn, cough, and deep-breathe q2h. In transferring the patient out of bed, the nurse should limit the sitting position to a period of time; the straight-back chair allows for **greater** comfort in and out of the sitting position. The patient may be permitted to walk as much as possible.
    1 This is nursing care for cardiovascular accident (CVA).
    2 This is nursing care for spinal cord injury.
    3 This is nursing care for fractures and fractured hip.

21. Comprehension, implementation, health (a)
    1 The nurse should review with the patient the physician's orders. After discharge information has been discussed, the nurse should evaluate the patient's comprehension by asking questions. Patient teaching, patient's condition and method of discharge should be charted.
    2 These are dismissal instructions for patients with dislocations.
    3 This is nursing care for patients with total knee replacement.
    4 This is nursing care for a patient with Parkinson's disease.

22. Knowledge, planning, physiological (a)
    1 Articulates with the femur above and talus below, supporting the entire body.
    2 The tibia is located at the lower aspect (medial side) of the leg.
    3 The tibia is surrounded by a lot of muscular tissue.
    4 It's the distal end of the fibula that is connected to the tibia.

23. Knowledge, assessment, physiological (a)
    4 This describes a complete type fracture in which the break is clean through the bone.
    1 The torsion fracture coils around the bone.
    2 This describes a comminuted-type fracture.
    3 The telescoped fracture is an impacted-type fracture.

24. Comprehension, planning, environment (a)
    3 Decreased circulation is a major complication needing close attention.
    1 This is a factor but not a major one.
    2 This is important, but it is not a major consideration.
    4 This is not an important factor.

25. Application, implementation, psychosocial (b)
    3 The nurse should be factual and supportive, getting him to talk about his concerns.
    1 This response gives false assurance.
    2 This response gives inaccurate information.
    4 This comment stops the patient from asking questions and leaves him unsupported.

26. Comprehension, implementation, physiological (b)
    2 This provides good alignment and support for calcification and healing to the fracture.
    1 This is not a major goal.
    3 This is not an appropriate response.
    4 This is not applicable to this situation.

27. Application, implementation, environment (a)
    1 This decreases pressure on the skin when elevating the body.
    2 The nurse should not put anything between the cast and the skin that may increase pressure on the skin.
    3 This adds pressure in the groin area by the cast edge.
    4 This causes potential for disproportionate pressure by the cast.

28. Application, implementation, health (c)
    4 The nurse should use a new sterile 4×4 pad for each area and move from the center of the wound outward to prevent contamination of the wound from organisms on the skin surface.
    1 The nurse is moving from a dirty area and will contaminate the wound; see No. 4 rationale.
    2 The nurse should use different pads/wipes to prevent cross-contamination; see No. 4 rationale.
    3 The nurse will not be moving the debris from the wound with this technique; and will only cross-contaminate with use of a circular motion; see No. 4 rationale.

29. Application, planning, health (c)
    4 Patients are often immunosuppressed and have decreased resistance; strict asepsis is needed to minimize exposure to microorganisms.
    1 Preparing supplies is important, but most important is to prevent contamination of supplies.
    2 Drainage tubes will be checked as part of the assessment, but reducing the spread of microorganisms takes priority.
    3 Giving assistance to patient's needs will be done, but most important in planning wound care is to avoid a wound infection.

30. Application, implementation, environment (c)
    4 The nurse should begin at the lowest point (distal part) and bandage in a direction toward the heart to prevent venous congestion and swelling in unbandaged area.
    1, 3 Not bandaging toward the heart will result in venous congestion.
    2 The distal part (hand) will swell as a result of uneven compression on tissue and blood vessels.

31. Application, assessment, environment (c)
    2 A patient with a new cast should be assessed at least every hour for 24 hours.
    1 Less frequent assessment of a cast may be safe in some situations but not necessary q15min.
    3, 4 The cast is assessed q4h for another 2 or 3 days after the first 24 hours.

32. Application, implementation, environment (c)
    4 Petals are trimmed strips of tape inserted over the edges of a cast that smooth and repair cast edges temporarily to protect the integrity of the skin.
    1 Petaling will not keep the cast from becoming wet.
    2 Petaling will not keep the cast from becoming too tight; it only stops irritation that results when the cast is too tight.
    3 Petaling will not keep debris from getting under the cast.

33. Comprehension, planning, physiological (a)
    1 The abducted position keeps the prosthesis in the appropriate alignment.
    2 The adducted position would dislodge the prosthesis from alignment.
    3 The flexed position is contraindicated; the hip should not be flexed.
    4 The prone position is inappropriate because just the leg alone could not be positioned in this manner.

34. Application, implementation, environment (a)
    2 The patient should be placed on the unaffected side with appropriate supports to maintain proper alignment of the prosthesis.
    1 It is contraindicated to place a patient on the affected side because this may cause the prosthesis to become dislodged.
    3, 4 These are inappropriate because it could cause flexion of the hip, could result in possible flexion of the hip.

35. Comprehension, planning, physiological (a)
    4 This is the usual time allowance for a hip prosthesis.
    1 This applies to a hip pinning.
    2 The patient is not allowed full weight bearing until 4 weeks.
    3 Partial weight bearing is in 10 to 14 days; it may not be necessary to use crutches in 3 to 6 months.

36. Application, implementation, psychosocial (b)
    1 This statement allows the patient to express his feelings more.
    2, 3 This statement provides false assurance.
    4 This statement avoids the patient's feelings and does not allow him to express himself.

37. Comprehension, assessment, physiological (b)
    1 Assessment of pain characteristics, including location, is most important to assess before considering the administration of any pain medication.
    2, 3, 4 These are not the first step.

38. Comprehension, evaluation, physiological (c)
    3 The main support of the compression bandage is to reduce edema and promote venous return.
    1, 2, 4 These do not primarily affect wound healing.

39. Comprehension, evaluation, environment (b)
    1 Alcohol is drying and will promote skin breakdown on the residual limb.
    2 This is a good exercise to toughen the residual limb.
    3 Good hygiene with mild soap and water is appropriate skin care.
    4 Range of motion to the joints above and below the residual limb is important to prevent contractures.

40. Application, implementation, environment (c)
    4 The tripod position, with the crutches 6 inches apart and 6 inches from the feet, is the beginning position for all gaits.
    1 The crutch and the unaffected leg must ascend first to afford greatest support.
    2 The major part of the weight is maintained with the hands. Weight on the axilla can lead to brachial injury or paralysis.
    3 If the patient constantly looks down, he will lose his balance and fall.

41. Comprehension, planning, environment (b)
    2 Frequent turning decreases the incidence of complications, provides good circulation, and maintains good skin integrity.
    1 Referring to an adjustment period produces anxiety and fear.
    3 The patient may experience phantom pain.
    4 This increases the incidence of complications, poor circulation, and poor skin integrity.

42. Comprehension, assessment, physiological (b)
    4 This action assesses the arterial blood flow to both legs; doppler pressure measurements can also be implemented.
    1 There is a need to increase the collateral circulation to the leg; elevation is not recommended.
    2 Blood work will not directly provide this information.
    3 Movement is needed to increase the collateral circulation to the leg.

43. Comprehension, implementation, environment (b)
    3 If bleeding does occur, it will drain down under the residual limb.
    1 This will cause discomfort. Elevating the foot of the bed slightly should assist circulation and decrease bleeding.
    2 This causes flexion of the hip, which can further cause contractures.
    4 There is no therapeutic advantage to this procedure.
44. Comprehension, assessment, physiological (c)
    1 Because of the level of amputation, the flexor muscles get stretched when the hip is flexed.
    2 Because of the location of the incision, strong sutures and a pressure dressing are usually in place to decrease chances of hemorrhage.
    3 Because of the type of surgery, antibiotics are usually given both before and after surgery, decreasing the incidence of infection.
    4 Good preventive postoperative care decreases the incidence of this.
45. Application, implementation, health (c)
    2 Elastic wraps shape the residual limb into a cone to facilitate proper fitting of the prosthesis.
    1 Because of the location of the incision, strong sutures, not the use of elastic wrap, decrease the chance of hemorrhage.
    3 This is not a primary consideration.
    4 This is an inappropriate response; there is no direct relationship between elastic wraps and decreasing the chance of infection.
46. Comprehension, evaluation, health (c)
    4 Normal muscle facilitates power and increases tolerance for the use of the prosthesis.
    1 It is necessary to equalize the weight to both legs and to avoid overburdening the normal leg.
    2 This is an inappropriate response; there will be limited muscle in the amputated side.
    3 This is an inappropriate response; emphasis is on strengthening the residual limb.
47. Application, implementation, environment (a)
    3 Epistaxis is the term used for nose bleed. The first emergency action the nurse can perform is to try to control the bleeding by applying pressure to the bridge of the nose.
    1 This is not an immediate action of the nurse because information can be obtained from a family member by another health-care worker.
    2 Fear and anxiety are not life-threatening; however, these should be alleviated as quickly as possible.
    4 Assessing vital signs and level of consciousness is usually done q15min; however, control of bleeding takes priority until the nurse can be relieved by another person.
48. Application, implementation, environment (a)
    3 Fowler's position with the head leaning forward prevents the patient from swallowing the blood draining from the nose that could cause nausea and vomiting.
    1, 2, 4 These are contraindicated because they would not allow the patient to expectorate the blood; they could cause blockage of the airway.
49. Knowledge, assessment, environment (a)
    2 Hoarseness and voice changes are early signs of laryngeal cancer.
    1 Pain is a late symptom of laryngeal cancer.
    3 Weight loss is a late symptom of laryngeal cancer.
    4 Difficulty swallowing (dysphagia) is a late symptom of laryngeal cancer.

50. Comprehension, implementation, physiological (a)
    4 After total laryngectomy, the patient breathes through a permanent tracheostomy stoma.
    1 Because of removal of the entire larynx, the patient's breathing pattern is altered, and breathing is through a permanent tracheostomy stoma.
    2 The patient's breathing pattern is altered as a result of extensive surgery.
    3 The tracheostomy is permanent following a total laryngectomy.
51. Application, implementation, environment (b)
    1 The suction is turned off as the catheter is inserted to avoid irritation of the trachea and additional loss of oxygen.
    2 Suctioning does not relate to blocking of the catheter.
    3 Having the suction on or off does not relate to an infectious process.
    4 Having the suction on or off does not relate to "kinking" of the catheter.
52. Comprehension, assessment, physiological (b)
    3 Increasing respirations and use of accessory muscles to facilitate breathing indicate the need for suctioning due to blockage of tube by mucus.
    1 Pulse and respiratory rate would increase rather than decrease.
    2 Increased swallowing and moisture on neck dressing may indicate bleeding.
    4 Pain and dry hacking cough are more indicative of lower airway infection.
53. Application, implementation, physiological (b)
    2 Prolonged suctioning may cause mucosal damage.
    1 Continuous suctioning may cause mucosal damage.
    3 If suction is applied, the catheter may "grab" mucosa and cause damage.
    4 The patient should be placed in semi-Fowler's position.
54. Comprehension, implementation, physiological (b)
    2 This position best minimizes the risk of aspiration in the immediate postoperative period.
    1 The supine position does not promote maintenance of a patent airway in the immediate postoperative period.
    3 Positioning the patient with the head down does not promote maintenance of a patent airway in the immediate postoperative period.
    4 In the immediate postoperative period, the patient is partially anesthetized, and in this position the patient would be at increased risk for aspiration.
55. Application, planning, health (b)
    1 Because water could easily enter the stoma during showering, the patient will need to wear some type of protection.
    2, 3, 4 No specific modifications are indicated.
56. Knowledge, planning, physiological (a)
    4 This results in ventilation and stasis of fluid in the lungs.
    1, 2, 3 These are contributory factors, not primary.
57. Application, implementation, environment (a)
    2 Lying on the affected side helps to splint the chest and assist in coughing.
    1 Because it is painful to breathe, the patient will avoid deep-breathing.
    3 Coughing increases the pain if there is no chest support.
    4 In this position the patient will be unable to give support to the affected side. This will not help the amount of pain the patient is experiencing.
58. Knowledge, planning, environment (a)
    2 Body fluid that is lost normally is not replaced by intake of food and fluids.
    1 Edema, not dehydration, occurs.
    3 Uremia, not dehydration, occurs.
    4 Incontinence, not necessarily dehydration, occurs.

59. Comprehension, planning, physiological (b)
    1 Increased fluids increase output and filtration of body wastes through the kidneys.
    2 Fluids alone will not contribute to proper nutrition.
    3 Waste products are not diluted but are excreted from the body.
    4 An indirect contributory factor; not the main purpose for forcing fluids.
60. Knowledge, planning, environment (a)
    3 These tests are a microscopic examinations to determine organisms present.
    1 This confirms existence of disease; it does not determine causative organisms.
    2, 4 These are inappropriate tests for diagnosis.
61. Comprehension, evaluation, physiological (a)
    3 Acetaminophen (Tylenol) is an antipyretic medication that relieves fever by central action in the hypothalamic heating regulating center.
    1 Acetaminophen has no direct effect on kidney function.
    2 Acetaminophen has no direct effect on sputum reduction.
    4 Acetaminophen has no effect on fluid retention.
62. Knowledge, assessment, environment (a)
    4 Oxygenated blood is circulating faster to get to the top of the lungs, thus causing an increased pulse rate.
    1, 2, 3 These are not the predominant factor.
63. Comprehension, assessment, physiological (a)
    1 On the affected side, there will be little or no movement of the chest wall; on the unaffected side, breathing will appear normal.
    1, 2 These are not usual symptoms of pneumothorax.
    3 Pain is a symptom, but position is not an aggravating factor.
64. Comprehension, evaluation, environment (b)
    3 To prevent the backflow of drainage from the collection system, the system should be kept below the chest level.
    1 The drainage chamber is never emptied; the chest tube should be removed before this chamber is filled.
    2 This is not necessary. A patient must lie on the affected side only if he has a lobectomy.
    4 This is not necessary. As long as the drainage system is below chest level, the patient may be out of bed as the physician allows.
65. Application, implementation, environment (b)
    1 The most important initial action is to prevent air from entering the chest cavity and disturbing negative pressure balance.
    2 No. 1 must be done before notification of the team leader.
    3 This is not necessary at this point.
    4 This is never done; not within a nurse's scope of practice.
66. Comprehension, planning, physiological (a)
    4 Patients must be considered as individuals; their care must be flexible to meet their individual needs and problems.
    1, 2, 3 These are incorrect statements.
67. Knowledge, planning, physiological (a)
    1 Pneumothorax occurs when air or gas accumulates within the pleural cavity. This leads to partial or complete collapse of the lung.
    2 Pneumonia is inflammation of lung tissue.
    3 Epistaxis is the term for a nose bleed.
    4 Hemothorax is the term for blood in the pleural space.

68. Comprehension, assessment, physiological (a)
    2 Bright-red frothy sputum is indicative of a punctured lung because air is entering the chest and lung tissues.
    1 This is usually indicative of congestive heart failure.
    3 This is usually indicative of an infectious process within the pulmonary system. This could also indicate other disease processes. The word purulent indicates infection.
    4 This is not an appropriate symptom regarding lung injury.
69. Comprehension, planning, physiological (a)
    3 This is the space between the visceral lining and the pleural lining. The tubes allow drainage of secretions, blood, and air.
    1, 2, 4 These are inappropriate to allow for lung expansion.
70. Comprehension, planning, physiological (c)
    1 Chest tubes are inserted between the ribs into the pleural space to allow drainage of secretions, blood, and air.
    2 The negative pressure within the thoracic cavity is restored when the lung is expanded.
    3 Atmospheric pressure rushing into the thoracic cavity causes the lung to collapse.
    4 The thoracic cavity pressure is normally negative as opposed to the atmospheric pressure. The pressure is not equal.
71. Comprehension, implementation, physiological (b)
    2 This bottle is used to allow the flow of secretions and air by gravitation.
    1 Suction is possible by a second or third bottle and sometimes may be connected to a suction machine.
    3, 4 These are inappropriate for this situation.
72. Comprehension, implementation, environment (b)
    2 This allows for drainage of secretions, blood, and air via gravity.
    1 This is contraindicated because the drainage would flow back into the thoracic cavity, causing further complications.
    3 This is contraindicated because drainage would re-enter the pleural space. Rationale is the same as for No. 1.
    4 The level is of primary importance to prevent complications and respiratory distress.
73. Knowledge, implementation, physiological (a)
    4 Close observations of both the patient for respiratory distress and the underwater-seal drainage for proper functioning is the primary responsibility of the nurse.
    1 This is contraindicated; bottles are kept lower than the patient to facilitate proper drainage.
    2 This does not apply.
    3 The bottles should not be emptied without special precautions because of the danger of breaking the closed underwater-seal drainage system.
74. Application, implementation, environment (b)
    4 Unless contraindicated, this should be done to prevent spontaneous pneumothorax and further complications.
    1, 2, 3 These should not be the immediate actions.
75. Knowledge, assessment, environment (b)
    1 Dyspnea, chest pain, and decreased movement of the involved chest wall are usual clinical manifestations.
    2 Pain is not relieved with leaning forward. Insertion of a chest tube is usually required.
    3 Breath sounds are usually decreased on the affected side.
    4 Breath sounds may be absent on the affected side.

76. Knowledge, planning, physiological (a)
    4 A pneumothorax is a collection of air between the chest wall and the lung. The chest tube will release air from the pleural cavity.
    1 In this situation, the chest tube is inserted to remove air, not to instill medication.
    2 Following chest surgeries, a chest tube is often used to drain secretions.
    3 With a hemothorax, a chest tube would drain blood.

77. Comprehension, implementation, physiological (b)
    2 Marking the level of drainage and noting the time should be done according to prescribed protocol. Changes in the amount or characteristics of drainage can be noted/reported.
    1 The practice of "stripping" chest tubes is controversial and needs a specific order. It is not usually necessary when chest tubes are used to drain air.
    3 Lifting the bottle(s) would allow air/fluid to be pulled back into the pleural cavity.
    4 The bottle(s) should be placed below the level of the patient's chest so air/fluid is not pulled back into the pleural cavity. Drainage is also facilitated.

78. Application, assessment, physiological (c)
    3 Fluctuations in rising with inspiration and falling with expiration should be observed in patients who are breathing spontaneously.
    1 When the system is working effectively, intermittent bubbling is seen in the water seal.
    2 Continuous and constant bubbling usually indicates an air leak. The source should be determined; retaping all connections may be necessary.
    4 Fluctuation of the fluid in the water seal chamber should remain constant.

79. Application, implementation, environment (c)
    3 Forced expiratory efforts against a closed airway help to create positive pleural pressure and decreases the likelihood that air will enter the pleural space.
    1 This does not facilitate creation of positive pleural pressure. Air could enter pleural space on tube removal.
    2 Air could enter pleural space as the tube is removed.
    4 Pursed-lip breathing involves slow exhalation. Chronic obstructive pulmonary disease patients are frequently helped with this type of breathing.

80. Knowledge, planning, health (a)
    3 The test consists of the tubercle bacillus extract being injected intradermally in the inner aspect of the upper arm; 48 hours is the amount of time needed for the extract to permeate the system.
    1, 2 This is too short a period of time; see response to No. 3.
    4 This is too long a period of time for the extract to take effect.

81. Comprehension, assessment, physiological (b)
    1 A productive cough with rusty-colored sputum (indicating slight bleeding in the respiratory tract) are common symptoms.
    2 Fever is usually normal during the day, but it elevates in the late afternoon and evening.
    3, 4 These are not symptoms of tuberculosis.

82. Comprehension, assessment, physiological (b)
    3 Coughing from the diaphragm will generate sputum as deeply as possible from the respiratory tract.
    1 Abdominal breathing is too shallow to encourage the expectoration of sputum.
    2 This will destroy bacteria that are an important part of the specimen.
    4 A high-Fowler's position is preferable to encourage the expectoration of sputum.

83. Comprehension, planning, physiological (c)
    4 This is the most realistic goal because it takes about 2 weeks for therapeutic blood levels of medication to develop.
    1, 2, 3 These would be unrealistic because the therapeutic blood levels of medication are not reached.

84. Application, implementation, health (c)
    3 This is an expected reaction. The drug should not be discontinued because of this.
    1 The dose should not be increased without the physician's order.
    2 This is unnecessary in relationship to the drug.
    4 The physician must be notified before this is done.

85. Comprehension, assessment, physiological (b)
    1 The *Mycobacterium Tuberculosis* in the system may be in either an active or arrested state.
    2 The Mantoux test does not necessarily mean an active case of TB, because exposure can cause a positive test reaction.
    3 Incorrect response.
    4 Being exposed to TB does not necessarily mean active disease is present.

86. Comprehension, planning, environment (b)
    4 With less movement, secretions are not coughed up and are not contaminated with food and fluids.
    1, 3 These are inappropriate responses.
    2 This is not necessarily the case.

87. Comprehension, planning, health (a)
    2 These procedures decrease the spread of the infection.
    1 Contact with people is important for the patient.
    3, 4 These are not primary concerns.

88. Application, implementation, health (b)
    1 These medications inhibit the enzyme needed for the growth of the bacilli.
    2, 4 The treatment regimen is usually 9 months or longer.
    3 These drugs nearly, but never completely, eliminate viable bacilli.

89. Comprehension, evaluation, health (b)
    3 The lesion will heal by fibrosis and calcification but remains in an arrested or inactive state.
    1 The disease becomes arrested or inactive.
    2 This is not necessarily so, because disease in an arrested or inactive state can reactivate.
    4 Reinfection can occur, giving rise to a progressive form of the disease.

90. Knowledge, assessment, environment (a)
    3 Elevated temperature and night sweats are symptoms characteristic of tuberculosis.
    1 This is characteristic of asthma.
    2 This is characteristic of cerebral anoxia.
    4 This is a term meaning blood in the pleural space.

91. Knowledge, assessment, physiological (b)
    3 Koch's bacillus is the causative organism of tuberculosis. AFB stands for acid-fast bacillus.
    1 Shigella is a bacterium that causes bacillary dysentery.
    2 The gas bacillus is a spore-forming type of organism that is responsible for gas gangrene.
    4 The Epstein-Barr virus is responsible for infectious mononucleosis.

92. Knowledge, implementation, physiological (a)
    3 The intradermal method injects the medication into the dermis, making a small bleb resembling a mosquito bite.
    1 The intramuscular method injects medication into muscle tissue.
    2 The subcutaneous method injects medication into subcutaneous tissue.
    4 The Z-track method is used to inject medication deep into muscle tissue; it prevents leakage of medication into the surrounding tissues.

93. Application, implementation, physiological (a)
    1 A 15-degree angle of the needle allows insertion just under the skin.
    2 This is not an appropriate angle for an injection.
    3 This is an appropriate angle for a subcutaneous injection.
    4 This is an appropriate angle for an intramuscular injection.
94. Comprehension, implementation, physiological (a)
    3 The site of injection should not be rubbed; it should be marked to be read in 48 hours.
    1, 2, 4 These are contraindicated for a skin test injection.
95. Comprehension, implementation, health (a)
    2 A positive tuberculosis (TB) skin test indicates exposure to the TB organism and is not diagnostic in itself.
    1 A positive TB skin test does not indicate infection or necessitate admission to the hospital.
    3 This is not correct because a positive TB skin test does not ensure immunity. To say not to worry gives false assurance.
    4 A positive TB skin test is not the same as an allergic reaction; however, it should not be repeated. It should be followed by an x-ray examination.
96. Knowledge, planning, physiological (a)
    3 Asthma involves recurring episodes of increased tracheal/bronchial responsiveness to various stimuli.
    1 This is the definition of emphysema.
    2 This is the definition of bronchiectasis.
    4 This is the definition of pulmonary tuberculosis.
97. Knowledge, assessment, health (a)
    2 Cigarette smoking is the highest risk factor for the development of emphysema.
    1 Although pneumonia can precipitate severe hypoxia in a patient with emphysema, it is not a risk factor.
    3 Air pollution can be a risk factor for the development of emphysema, but smoking is a greater risk factor.
    4 This is not a risk factor for emphysema.
98. Comprehension, implementation, environment (a)
    1 Theophylline (Theodur) relaxes smooth muscle in the bronchi so that ventilation becomes easier.
    2, 3, 4 These are not actions of this medication.
99. Knowledge, assessment, environment (a)
    2 Aminophylline, because it relaxes smooth muscle, may cause hypotension as a side effect.
    1 Tachycardia is a side effect.
    3 Restlessness is a side effect.
    4 Nausea and anorexia are side effects; weight gain is not.
100. Comprehension, assessment, physiological (b)
    4 Because of chronic hypoxia and labored breathing, the chest develops a barrel-like configuration and the fingertips become blunted and clubbed.
    1 Pigeon chest is a congenital deformity; it is not usually the result of a chronic respiratory disease.
    2 The hair would become dry and sparse as a result of conditions other than emphysema.
    3 Moist shiny skin is not a manifestation of emphysema.
101. Application, implementation, environment (a)
    3 When suctioning a patient, it is important to give oxygen before and after because suctioning removes oxygen as well as secretions. The length of time to suction would be 10 to 15 seconds. At least 5 minutes should elapse between each suctioning.
    1 Thirty seconds is too long; this would remove oxygen from the system.
    2 Coughing and deep breathing should not be performed as part of the suctioning procedure. Oxygenation is the last step.
    4 Twenty-five seconds is too long and would remove oxygen from the system. The last step is to oxygenate.

102. Comprehension, planning, environment (b)
    3 After the procedure, the patient is not allowed oral fluids until the gag reflex has returned. A topical anesthetic is used before the bronchoscope is introduced.
    1 Sputum collection is not part of the standard postoperative bronchoscopy orders.
    2 The procedure allows for a direct visualization of the larynx, trachea, and bronchi. A flexible fiberoptic bronchoscope is usually used. No surgical incisions are necessary.
    4 Voice restriction is associated with laryngoscopy.
103. Knowledge, planning, physiological (a)
    4 The entire lung is removed in a pneumonectomy.
    1 In a wedge resection, a specific diseased portion is removed.
    2 When one or more lung segments are surgically removed, the procedure is called a segmental resection.
    3 Removal of one lobe of the lung is termed a lobectomy.
104. Comprehension, implementation, physiological (b)
    2 The remaining lung can expand better in the semi-Fowler's position.
    1 Chest drainage tubes are not usually used. These permit serous fluid to accumulate in the space.
    3 Anticoagulant medications are not usually indicated following lung surgery.
    4 Lungs can expand better in the semi-Fowler's position than in the supine position.
105. Comprehension, assessment, physiological (c)
    4 There is an accumulation of serous fluid in interstitial lung tissue.
    1 This is characteristic of arterial respiratory distress.
    2 This is characteristic of chronic obstructive pulmonary disease.
    3 This is characteristic of pulmonary emboli.
106. Comprehension, assessment, physiological (b)
    3 Bronchial structures become engorged with fluid as a result of interstitial edema.
    1 Pulmonary means lungs; therefore, there is accumulation of fluid in the lungs.
    2 Edema means swelling; therefore, there is an increase, not a decrease, of fluid.
    4 Edema means swelling, and pulmonary refers to lungs.
107. Application, implementation, environment (b)
    2 Body weight indicates the effectiveness of a diuretic used to reduce alveolar and systemic edema by increasing urinary output.
    1 Monitoring intake and output alone does not indicate reduction of alveolar and systemic edema.
    3 These procedures will not rid the fluid in body tissue.
    4 These procedures alone will not accurately indicate fluid reduction in body tissue.
108. Application, implementation, psychosocial (c)
    1 To assist the patient in good oxygen/carbon dioxide exchange, the nurse should implement nursing measures to decrease the patient's anxiety and inform the charge nurse.
    2 Medication can assist respirations to a point; anxiety reduction treats the major cause of distress.
    3 Such a direct response may increase her anxiety even more.
    4 This does not provide the immediate assistance needed.
109. Comprehension, planning, health (a)
    4 The nasal cannula allows her more freedom to move around, eat, and talk while getting the oxygen needed.
    1 The face mask fits too snugly, is too confining, and adds to her feeling of suffocation.
    2 The oxygen tent is too constricting and anxiety-producing.
    3 The nasal catheter traumatizes nasal mucosa.

110. Application, evaluation, environment (c)
    4 These symptoms indicate a decrease in potassium, a side effect of too much fluid loss.
    1 Hematuria is not a side effect of this medication.
    2 These are side effects that bear watching, but they are not significant.
    3 Diarrhea by itself is not indicative of a problem.
111. Knowledge (b)
    1 Anatomically, the tricuspid valve is located between the right atrium and right ventricle.
    2 Anatomically, the bicuspid valve is located between the left atrium and left ventricle.
    3 The aortic valve guards the opening between the left ventricle and the aorta.
    4 The mitral valve is also known as the bicuspid valve.
112. Knowledge (a)
    2 The sinoatrial node is located in the wall of the right atrium.
    1 The left atrium does not contain a primary conduction node, but it does contain conduction fiber.
    3 The left ventricle does not contain a primary conduction node, but it does contain conduction fibers.
    4 The right ventricle does not contain a primary conduction node, but it does contain conduction fibers.
113. Comprehension, assessment, physiological (a)
    1 Intermittent claudication results from inadequate circulation to the muscles as a result of decreased blood supply to the extremities.
    2, 3, 4 These have no direct relationship to intermittent claudication.
114. Comprehension, planning, environment (b)
    3 Heat increases vasodilation, thus improving circulation.
    1 This has no relationship to the disease process.
    2 This increases the chance for emboli because of decreased blood flow.
    4 Bathing with warm water increases circulation and decreases chances of emboli.
115. Comprehension, planning, health (b)
    2 Smoking causes vasoconstriction, which decreases the blood supply to the extremities.
    1 Alcohol has no direct relationship to dilation or constriction of blood vessels.
    3 Caffeine is a stimulant that doesn't directly affect dilation or constriction of blood vessels.
    4 Tannic acid and the amount of caffeine present don't directly affect dilation or constriction of blood vessels.
116. Application, implementation, psychosocial (b)
    4 This response gives the patient the opportunity to talk more about what is bothering him.
    1 Putting him off doesn't help his concerns or the stress they may be causing.
    2 Making such a decision for him is inappropriate.
    3 This is an inappropriate, judgmental response.
117. Comprehension, assessment, physiological (a)
    4 Angina pectoris is the result of insufficient oxygen to the myocardium and is usually related to stress, exercise, or heavy meals.
    1 This is the definition of arteriosclerosis.
    2 This is the causative factor in a myocardial infarction.
    3 This is related to congestive heart failure.
118. Comprehension, assessment, physiological (b)
    2 Angina pectoris usually occurs during exertion and usually subsides with rest and vasodilators.
    1 This is typical of pain with a myocardial infarction.
    3 Although this may be present with angina, it is typical of pain with a myocardial infarction. The key is to distinguish between the two conditions.
    4 Radiating pain is typical for both angina and myocardial infarction; however, this kind of pain seems more common with angina.

119. Comprehension, assessment, physiological (b)
    2 Sharp, burning substernal pain radiating to the jaw, shoulder or left arm are most common descriptions of anginal pain.
    1, 4 These are not descriptive of anginal pain; wrong location.
    3 This is more descriptive of a myocardial infarction.
120. Comprehension, evaluation, health (c)
    2 All packaged and processed foods could contain sodium. It is important to read the ingredients of these foods on the label. If sodium is listed near or at the beginning of the ingredients, the food is high in sodium and must be avoided. Also, processed foods are likely to contain hidden sources of sodium such as monosodium L-glutamate (MSG)—a flavor enhancer.
    1 Vegetables are usually canned with salt and are higher in sodium than are fresh vegetables.
    3 Beef that has not been processed is low in sodium; cheese is very high in sodium.
    4 Fruit is canned with sugar, not salt; therefore, it is low in sodium.
121. Comprehension, evaluation, health (c)
    3 A burning sensation under the tongue is an expected reaction and means that the medication is effective. These pills should not be destroyed.
    1 Nitroglycerin may be taken prophylactically to prevent the onset of angina before physical activity.
    2 This is proper storage of nitroglycerin.
    4 Nitroglycerin must be taken in this manner, 5 minutes apart.
122. Comprehension, assessment, physiological (b)
    4 Angina means pain, and pectoris refers to the chest.
    1 This symptom most likely occurs in a heart attack.
    2 Cyanosis is not necessarily a symptom of angina.
    3 Exercise usually precedes an angina attack.
123. Application, evaluation, health (b)
    2 Nitroglycerin dilates the coronary arteries, bringing blood and oxygen to the heart muscle.
    1 Nitroglycerin dilates; it does not constrict.
    3 This is not related to the situation.
    4 Nitroglycerin has no specific effect on chest muscles.
124. Application, planning, physiological (a)
    1 Although the patient takes the nitroglycerin as needed, the amount taken must be documented on the record.
    2 It is not necessary to take the blood pressure q6h.
    3 This is not necessarily a dependency drug.
    4 It is the nurse's responsibility to monitor nitroglycerin use.
125. Comprehension, planning, psychosocial (a)
    3 Relieving the patient's anxiety helps to reduce the stress that may bring on further anginal episodes.
    1 Although this is important, relieving anxiety may reduce the need for vasodilators. Assuring the patient that the medication will be given promptly is a means of relieving anxiety.
    2 This should not be a primary goal, but it is included as follow-up instructions.
    4 Monitoring the weight is not necessary unless edema is present. This might indicate further problems.
126. Application, implementation, physiological (b)
    3 This would most accurately and completely document an anginal episode. It is especially important to document activity in relation to the anginal episode.
    1, 2, 4 These do not completely document all areas.

127. Knowledge, planning, physiological (b)
    2 Nitroglycerin is a vasodilator; doses may be taken 5 minutes apart, three times if necessary.
    1 This drug is an antihypertensive.
    3 This drug is a cardiotonic.
    4 This drug is a vasoconstrictor.
128. Application, implementation, environment (a)
    1 This includes all aspects that would be considered for patients with angina pectoris.
    2 It would be impossible to *avoid* emotions; it is more accurate to learn to deal with emotions of anxiety. Avoiding exercise would not be appropriate for most conditions.
    3 This does not include all aspects to be considered for angina pectoris; patients are also cautioned to avoid eating heavy meals and extreme changes in temperature.
    4 This does not include all areas necessary for follow-up.
129. Knowledge, assessment, physiological (c)
    3 Angina pectoris is characterized by the inability of the coronary arteries to meet the oxygen demand of the myocardial muscle, a condition leading to pain (angina).
    1 Necrosis would be indicative of myocardial infarction, not angina.
    2 Although the friction of an enlarged epicardium rubbing against the pericardial sac may cause pain, it is not typical of anginal discomfort.
    4 Vasospasm of a coronary artery is transient and reversible; it is not generally relieved by decreasing activity, as it is in the case of angina.
130. Knowledge, assessment, physiological (a)
    1 Protein is an abnormal finding in urine. It may indicate renal pathology.
    2 Urine is naturally acidic.
    3 Urine ranges in color from pale straw color to amber, depending upon its concentration.
    4 Normal urinary output on a daily basis ranges from 1200 to 2500 ml.
131. Application, implementation, physiological (b)
    3 The main action of nitroglycerin is the promotion of coronary-vasodilation.
    1 Nitroglycerin does not cause venous pooling in the body, but rather helps in eliminating such because of its vasodilation effects.
    2 Nitroglycerin does not vasoconstrict; it dilates.
    4 The administration of nitroglycerin may lower the blood pressure, but this is not considered to be the *main* function of this drug.
132. Comprehension, assessment, physiological (b)
    3 Although the exact cause of hypertension is not known, heredity plays an important role because of familial tendencies.
    1 This has no effect on hypertension.
    2 Overweight is a predisposing factor to hypertension.
    4 Parents with hypertension would more directly predispose a patient to this disease, because they were a much closer relation to the patient.

133. Application, implementation, psychosocial (a)
    2 The nurse lets the patient express all her feelings and gives her reassurance.
    1 This is not the best time to teach the patient.
    3 The patient is concerned about her condition and needs to be reassured.
    4 By avoiding the subject, the patient might think that the nurse does not care.
134. Application, implementation, physiological (b)
    3 Using the method, desired over available, the nurse would calculate the following: 1 g = 1000 mg; 1000 mg divided by 250 mg = 4 tablets.
    1 This dose is only 250 mg.
    2 This dose is only 750 mg.
    4 This amount exceeds the required dose.
135. Comprehension, assessment, physiological (b)
    4 There are few symptoms associated with the disease, so the patient does not feel ill. Patients find side effects of the medication to be too bothersome.
    1 This is becoming true, but No. 4 is more accurate.
    2 With hypertension, there are not very many symptoms present.
    3 Because the patient was taking the medication, he/she most likely received instructions from the prescribing physician or his/her nurse.
136. Application, implementation, environment (c)
    1 Constriction of the arterioles occurs in these patients. The heart exerts more pressure to circulate, thus an elevation of systolic/diastolic pressure occurs.
    2 Caffeine does not contribute to increased cholesterol.
    3 Caffeine does not harden the vessels.
    4 Caffeine constricts; it does not dilate.
137. Comprehension, implementation, health (a)
    2 Mr. Clover has a borderline blood pressure reading for hypertension. Smoking increases his risk of coronary artery disease by causing arterial vasospasm.
    1 The normal adult will require 8 hours of sleep to maintain health.
    3 This is not an appropriate suggestion; it is not physiologically necessary.
    4 An exercise program would be helpful to Mr. Clover.
138. Comprehension, assessment, physiological (a)
    2 A typical sign of primary hypertension is a chronically elevated diastolic pressure. Usually a diastolic pressure of 90 mm/Hg is the cutoff.
    1, 4 These are not applicable.
    3 Diastolic pressure is primarily involved.
139. Knowledge, implementation, physiological (a)
    3 Hypertension is a lifelong problem that can be controlled with diet, medications, and other therapies.
    1 Hypertension cannot be cured, just controlled.
    2 Needs to be treated (see No. 3).
    4 If diet, medication, and general treatment plan are followed, hypertension should not be fatal, unless there are other problems.
140. Application, planning, physiological (a)
    2 Pretzels are high in sodium content.
    1, 3, 4 These are low in salt.
141. Comprehension, planning, physiological (a)
    1 The purpose in treating hypertension is to minimize the has damage occurred the blood vessels.
    2 This is not applicable at this time.
    3 It is not advisable to lower blood pressure below normal level.
    4 Because there are no early symptoms, some damage has already occurred and cannot be repaired.

142. Comprehension, planning, physiological (a)
    2 A low to moderate sodium diet is recommended because of tendency to retain fluids.
    1 A bland diet is more often associated with gastric problems.
    3, 4 These are contraindicated in hypertension.

143. Comprehension, implementation, health (b)
    2 A gradual weight loss program, with a loss of no more than 2½ lb per week, is the most effective.
    1 A very rapid weight loss is not recommended.
    3 A vegetarian diet is not necessary.
    4 1000 calories per day is not sufficient for an adult male.

144. Knowledge, assessment, physiological (b)
    2 The symptoms accompanied by cyanosis are suggestive of a myocardial infarction.
    1, 3, 4 With these conditions, the patient usually does not have cyanosis, a condition which indicates lack of oxygen to the tissues.

145. Knowledge, assessment, physiological (a)
    1 These are subjective data because the patient must express these to the nurse. They cannot be observed by the nurse.
    2, 3, 4 These are objective data that can be observed by the nurse.

146. Comprehension, planning, physiological (b)
    4 The primary goal is to provide complete bed rest to promote healing of the damaged myocardium.
    1 This is important, but immediate attention should be to provide rest for the damaged myocardium.
    2 A gradual increase of activities may begin the second day, but initially bed rest is most important.
    3 To provide diversional activity is not a primary goal; this is, however, included as part of the nursing care.

147. Comprehension, implementation, physiological (b)
    4 The description of the type of chest pain is significant to assist in diagnosing a myocardial infarction, angina pectoris, or congestive heart failure.
    1, 2, 3 These relate to symptoms of congestive heart failure.

148. Application, planning, health (b)
    2 Assessment of the patient's knowledge is always the first step in health teaching.
    1 The patient should be assessed for knowledge of nutritional needs before patient teaching.
    3 The patient's knowledge level should be assessed first.
    4 The patient may not know what to ask concerning his illness.

149. Application, assessment, physiological (b)
    3 Mr. Garcia should be on a low-fat diet to help lower his cholesterol level.
    1 Some foods may not contain cholesterol (found in animal foods) but may have a high level of fat content such as vegetable oil. A low-fat diet best reduces cholesterol levels.
    2 A soft, high-protein diet is not needed.
    4 This diet is not necessary.

150. Knowledge, planning, environment (b)
    1 Nitroglycerin tablets are only effective when administered sublingually.
    2 Liquids should not be taken with nitroglycerin.
    3 Nitroglycerin is not taken with food. It is inactivated in the stomach.
    4 It is not necessary to take nitroglycerin at bedtime, unless the patient is experiencing angina.

151. Comprehension, assessment, environment (c)
    2 The pain associated with an acute myocardial infarction is usually not relieved with rest, nitroglycerin, or changes in position.
    1 The pain of a myocardial infarction is typically not relieved with rest.
    3 Pain is often described as severe, squeezing, or crushing.
    4 The pain of a myocardial infarction is usually not relieved with the administration of nitroglycerin.

152. Comprehension, assessment, physiological (c)
    1 Symptoms of acute pulmonary edema include rapid onset of severe dyspnea, coughing, and orthopnea. This is often followed by the production of frothy, pink-tinged sputum. Heart failure is a potential complication following a myocardial infarction.
    2 Findings of cardiogenic shock include falling blood pressure; tachycardia; weak pulse; cool, clammy skin; and decreasing urinary output.
    3 With pulmonary embolism, signs and symptoms usually include onset of shortness of breath with or without pleuritic chest pain.
    4 Right-sided failure is characterized by pitting edema, distended neck veins, fatigue, and increase in the size of the abdomen.

153. Comprehension, implementation, physiological (b)
    1 In an upright position, full expansion of the lungs is facilitated. Decreasing venous return reduces the cardiac workload.
    2 Rest is important in reducing oxygen requirements, but relieving the dyspnea would not be helped by placing the patient in the supine position.
    3 Measures to decrease, not increase, venous return should be implemented.
    4 With the patient's head down, additional respiratory distress would occur.

154. Comprehension, assessment, environment (b)
    4 Echocardiography is a noninvasive test that is used to evaluate changes in the heart's structure and function.
    1 The chest x-ray examination provides information about respiratory disorders.
    2 The electrocardiogram (ECG) provides specific information about the electrical forces of the heart.
    3 Serial blood cultures provide information about infections.

155. Application, planning, physiological (c)
    4 The goal for these nursing interventions is that the patient will adjust to changing energy levels and will learn to conserve energy.
    1 These are the nursing interventions for a patient with depression.
    2 These are the nursing interventions for hypertensive crisis (a sudden, severe elevation of blood pressure with systolic greater than 200 mm Hg and diastolic greater than 120 mm Hg).
    3 These are the nursing interventions for secondary polycythemia. This is a compensatory response to hypoxemia, which may result from chronic obstructive pulmonary disease (COPD) or congenital heart disease.

156. Comprehension, assessment, physiological (b)
    4 Decreased cardiac output causes blood to dam up in left side of the heart; blood can't be pumped effectively, resulting in lung congestion.
    1 This may be a contributing factor, but it is not the primary cause.
    2 This is not a primary cause. Etiological factors associated with congestive heart conditions are coronary occlusion, myocardial infarction, vascular heart disease, and pericardial inflammatory condition. The underlying mechanism in congestive heart failure involves failure of the heart's pumping mechanism to respond to the body's metabolic changes. Congestive heart failure is also attributed to hypertension, stress, hyperthyroidism, hemorrhage, anemia, or fluid-replacement therapy.
    3 This may be a result; however, it is not a primary cause.
157. Knowledge, assessment, physiological (a)
    2 Paroxysmal nocturnal dyspnea (waking up at night with shortness of breath) is a common sign of early congestive heart failure as a result of decreased cardiac output.
    1 These are signs of pulmonary edema, a life-threatening complication of CHF.
    3 These are symptoms of emphysema.
    4 These are symptoms of pulmonary tuberculosis.
158. Knowledge, planning, physiological (b)
    3 This results from the inability of the heart to function as a pump.
    1 This is a symptom of myocardial infarction.
    2 This is a symptom of endocarditis.
    4 This is a symptom of an aneurysm; an aneurysm can result from trauma, congenital weakness, arteriosclerosis, or infection.
159. Application, assessment, physiological (c)
    2 This is most characteristic when lungs are congested.
    1 These sounds are associated with pneumothorax.
    3 These are sounds of chronic obstructive pulmonary disease.
    4 This is not expected when auscultating.
160. Comprehension, assessment, health (a)
    1 Inflammation is the body's reaction to injury or irritation, not to an invasion of pathogenic microorganisms.
    2 Allergy is an antigen-antibody reaction of the body to a substance, causing the body to be hypersensitive to that substance.
    3 Infection occurs when the body is invaded by microorganisms and illness develops.
    4 Immunity is the body's ability to have a resistance to a specific disease. Resistance can be the result of either active or passive immunity.
161. Application, implementation, health (a)
    3 Exercise and support hose help reduce the complication and possibility of clots in the lower extremities.
    1 Exercise usually increases rather than decreases circulation.
    2 Exercise does not prevent abdominal edema.
    4 Exercise does not necessarily reduce edema of the extremities.
162. Knowledge, assessment, physiological (a)
    2 Citrus fruits in their natural state are least likely to contain large amounts of sodium.
    1 Baking soda has a high sodium content.
    3 These choices contain sodium.
    4 Canned meats are high in sodium.
163. Knowledge, planning, physiological (a)
    4 Digitalis strengthens and tones the heart muscle.
    1 Antianxiety drugs are used to lessen the tension or anxiety when required.
    2, 3 These do not strengthen or tone heart muscle.

164. Comprehension, assessment, physiological (b)
    4 These symptoms are the results of pulmonary congestion in the interstitial spaces and alveoli.
    1 Dyspnea is experienced, but not necessarily on exertion.
    2 Orthopnea, not necessarily angina, is experienced.
    3 Sputum is frothy, not tenacious.
165. Comprehension, planning, physiological (a)
    2 The gain or loss of body weight usually indicates a gain or loss of body fluid.
    1 This is not an indication for daily weights.
    3 This is not applicable.
    4 Loss of appetite does not necessarily mean a loss of weight.
166. Comprehension, assessment, physiological (c)
    1 This causes a backup of blood into the lungs.
    2 This does not affect the backup of blood into the lungs.
    3, 4 There is no backup of blood flow into the lungs.
167. Comprehension, assessment, physiological (c)
    4 Increased pulmonary pressure occurs with fluid buildup in the lungs (pulmonary edema).
    1 Fatigue does occur, but it is not a significant indication of complications.
    2 Restlessness may occur without indicating a major problem.
    3 This is not indicative of the diagnosis.
168. Comprehension, planning, environment (b)
    3 Maintaining skin integrity, rest, and position for easier breathing are important considerations.
    1 This is not commonly considered.
    2 Stabilization of the condition is needed first, before ambulation.
    4 The nurse must avoid increasing the strain on the heart; increasing fluid intake will also increase fluid buildup in the lungs.
169. Application, evaluation, environment (c)
    1 This provides for systemic monitoring of fluid intake and output.
    2 This is indicative, but daily weights are needed for closer monitoring.
    3, 4 Activity is not a factor in fluid balance.
170. Application, planning, health (c)
    3 Patients with valvular disease need prophylactic antibiotic therapy before dental or surgical procedures to reduce their risk of developing endocarditis.
    1 Although activity may be restricted for a short time, the patient does not usually need to continue with a sedentary life-style.
    2 Dehydration is not an associated problem.
    4 The patient must watch for signs and symptoms of infection, but wearing a mask in crowds is not practical or appropriate.
171. Knowledge, planning, physiological (a)
    4 Rheumatic fever is seen in children between 5 and 14 years of age.
    1 It is more prevalent in children.
    2 It is no more prevalent in males than it is in females.
    3 It is no more prevalent in females than it is in males.
172. Application, implementation, environment (b)
    2 The patient will be awake during the procedure and can view the monitor.
    1 There may be discomfort as a result of the procedure, but there should be no pain.
    3 The NPO order is for 6 to 8 hours before the procedure.
    4 Blood samples from the various chambers of the heart are obtained.

173. Comprehension, evaluation, physiological (c)
    1 The P wave is caused by the atria thereby recording the impulse from the sinoatrial node.
    2 The Q, R, S, and T waves are related to the contraction of the ventricles.
    3 It is not the P wave that diagnoses myocardial infarction.
    4 P wave records impulses, not lesions.

174. Application, implementation, physiological (a)
    3 This represents the pressure within the artery between beats.
    1 Refractory period refers to skeletal muscle fiber.
    2 Systole represents the ventricles contracting.
    4 Atrial systole refers to the contraction of the atria.

175. Comprehension, evaluation, physiological (c)
    1 Scar tissue forms, affecting the functioning of these valves.
    2 The tricuspid valve is not affected.
    3 The pulmonary valves are not affected.
    4 These valves are not affected.

176. Comprehension, assessment, physiological (b)
    1 Plaque formation occludes major coronary arteries, obstructing the blood supply to the myocardium.
    2, 3 ASHD does not affect the lungs.
    4 Endocarditis is a bacterial infection with no direct relationship to sclerotic vessels.

177. Application, implementation, environment (a)
    4 This artery provides the best pulsating sound and is easily accessible.
    1 The radial artery's pulsating sound is not clear and strong.
    2 This artery can be used but not usually unless the brachial site is unavailable.
    3 The location of the femoral artery is not convenient for this procedure.

178. Application, implementation, environment (a)
    2 Bed rest assists in maximizing cardiac function; penicillin and aspirin are given to minimize the inflammatory process.
    1 Dietary implications are not a factor.
    3 Steroid therapy is used with complications such as arthritis or congestive heart failure.
    4 This is treatment for anginal pain; not applicable.

179. Knowledge, planning, physiological (a)
    4 There is an obstruction or cutting off of the blood supply to the coronary artery or its branches.
    1, 2 These are not related to the situation.
    3 The coronary arteries can become occluded by a thrombus or emboli.

180. Comprehension, planning, physiological (a)
    2 This grafts healthy vessels around the area of the occlusion.
    1 Inappropriate response.
    3 No stimulation of the heart muscle is needed.
    4 This procedure is known as an endarterectomy.

181. Knowledge, assessment, physiological (b)
    2 A cardiac catheterization is an invasive test using radiopaque dye to visualize the patency of the coronary vessels.
    1 The test will not determine the actual amount of blood entering the right atrium.
    3 Left ventricle pressure may be measured during the procedure, but is not the primary purpose of the test.
    4 Ventricle contractility may be measured in terms of an ejection fraction, but the most common purpose of catheterization is to determine blockage.

182. Knowledge, assessment, physiological (c)
    4 Contrast media contains iodine, which is also found in seafood.
    1 There is no correlation between the contrast medium and the intake of foods high in fat.
    2 Antihistamines do not affect the contrast medium.
    3 Weight gain or loss is not relevant to the use of a contrast medium.

183. Comprehension, implementation, environment (b)
    1 A potential complication is the formation of an arterial thrombus that is so large it occludes or partially occludes the artery. The pulse distal to the catheter entry site should be assessed frequently the first few hours following the procedure.
    2 The extremity used for the catheter insertion is immobilized and kept in a straight position.
    3 Hyperextension and flexion of the extremity are to be avoided.
    4 Fluids are usually encouraged to aid in removing the contrast medium from the body, especially from the kidneys.

184. Application, assessment, psychosocial (b)
    4 Nicotine acts as a vasoconstrictor that results in poor circulation to the extremities.
    1 There is some connection that needs further explanation.
    2 This is not applicable.
    3 Arteriosclerosis does not directly affect the lungs.

185. Knowledge, assessment, physiological (b)
    1 Because of lack of blood supply to lower extremities, the patient with arterial insufficiency may experience loss of hair on the extremity.
    2 This would be a sign of varicose veins, not arterial insufficiency.
    3 This is normal.
    4 This is more like the symptoms of venous disease.

186. Knowledge, assessment, environment (c)
    4 Lack of pedal pulse means that there is a gross lack of blood supply to the extremity. This must be reported immediately.
    1 This is an indicator of arterial insufficiency, but it is not as severe as No. 4.
    2, 3 These are normal.

187. Comprehension, evaluation, physiological (b)
    2 The temperature of the patient's leg gives an indication of blood supply to the leg.
    1 Vital signs should be taken more often initially to monitor for bleeding or hypovolemia.
    3 Not relative to circulation assessment.
    4 Not necessary immediately following surgery.

188. Comprehension, assessment, physiological (b)
    3 Homans' sign is elicited by dorsiflexing the foot and is considered positive when pain is present.
    1 Platelets (thrombocytes) are necessary blood constituents of the clotting process, but they are not specifically elevated in thrombophlebitis.
    2 Chvostek's sign is a contraction of facial muscles in response to a light tap over the facial nerve in front of the ear.
    4 Anemia is a reduction in the number of erythrocytes and levels of hemoglobin and hematocrit; it is not a manifestation of thrombophlebitis.

189. Knowledge, planning, physiological (c)
    2 The cardinal symptoms of a blood clot in a vein are pain, heat, redness and swelling.
    1 Fever, nausea and vomiting may be associated with an infectious process, but they are not specific for thrombophlebitis.
    3 These gastrointestinal symptoms are not related to venous obstruction.
    4 Anorexia may occur as a result of the pain involved in vascular obstruction. This answer, however, is not inclusive of the primary symptoms of thrombophlebitis.
190. Knowledge, assessment, psychosocial (b)
    3 The inflammation and clot formation are associated with venous stasis.
    1 There is no ulcer present.
    2 There is inflammation, but the condition involves a clot.
    4 Phlebitis is an inflammation of the vein.
191. Application, evaluation, physiological (b)
    1 Chest pain is exhibited if the embolism is lodged in the lungs. Severe pain can lead to shock and depletion of proper circulation.
    2 Areas involved would be cyanotic and cold; patient would complain of a tingling sensation or numbness.
    3 The patient's pulse would be elevated.
    4 The patient would show apprehension and sudden onset of dyspnea.
192. Knowledge, implementation, physiological (a)
    4 This is a blood clot that circulates in the blood and more commonly lodges in the lungs.
    1 An embolism travels.
    2 Most emboli arise from deep-vein thrombi.
    3 Emboli can lodge in different vital organs.
193. Knowledge, assessment, health (a)
    2 Early ambulation and exercise promote circulation.
    1 This is not given in this situation.
    3 Massage helps to relax, providing some circulation; however, it is not the best choice.
    4 Encourage movement in bed to prevent venous stasis.
194. Application, implementation, environment (a)
    1 Massaging the legs could dislodge the thrombus that becomes an embolus, which can circulate in the blood to the vital organs.
    2 This could help circulation and relaxation.
    3 The patient has no limitation of activity in bed.
    4 Elevating the head does not affect this condition.
195. Application, implementation, environment (a)
    1 Because circulation is poor, there is a good chance of burns to the extremities.
    2 Snug shoes will further impair circulation.
    3 Legs should be elevated periodically to improve circulation.
    4 Avoid extreme cold weather to prevent further constriction and impairment of circulation.
196. Comprehension, assessment, physiological (b)
    1 Assessment of the patient's description of the pain would be the first step in the nursing process. Subjective data from the interview should be obtained first.
    2, 3, 4 These would be done after No. 1. They are based on objective data.
197. Comprehension, assessment, physiological (b)
    4 Thrombophlebitis, as do other venous disorders, causes edema and redness of the lower extremity because of venous pooling.
    1, 3 A sign of arterial, not venous, disease.
    2 Redness, not ecchymosis, would be present.

198. Application, implementation, environment (b)
    4 Elastic stockings support the leg and encourage venous blood return. They should be worn at all times.
    1 This is not necessary, because no wound is present.
    2 The affected extremity should not have change of motion. Inflamed parts must be at rest.
    3 Warm compresses are preferred to encourage venous circulation.
199. Comprehension, evaluation, health (a)
    3 Green leafy vegetables are a source of vitamin K, which enhances the clotting process and should be avoided.
    1, 2, 4 These are not good sources of vitamin K.
200. Comprehension, assessment, physiological (c)
    2 When the valves are no longer able to function, the venous return of blood becomes sluggish and blood accumulates in the veins.
    1 There is no infection involved.
    3 This condition is not considered congenital.
    4 There is no deposit of materials in the veins.
201. Knowledge, assessment, physiological (b)
    1 Varicose veins are dilated and tortuous veins that are a result of a backflow of blood because of inadequate closure of valves.
    2 The increased amount of blood causes further dilation of the veins.
    3 Because of elasticity, the veins become longer as well as larger.
    4 There is no bacteria involved.
202. Application, implementation, physiological (a)
    3 Thrombolytic drugs are used to promote the digestion of fibrin to dissolve the clot(s).
    1 There is no correlation with antibiotics in this case.
    2 There is no indication for use of vitamins.
    4 These are used for chemotherapy.
203. Application, assessment, environment (c)
    4 Iron is a component of hemoglobin. A deficiency of iron affects the ability of the red blood cells to carry oxygen to the tissues. The red blood cells contain decreased levels of hemoglobin.
    1 Impaired production of blood-forming elements is associated with aplastic anemias.
    2 White blood cells protect the body against disease.
    3 Platelet destruction and bleeding are related to coagulation disorders.
204. Application, planning, physiological (b)
    4 Fatigue is a common symptom associated with iron-deficiency anemia. Because of chronic tissue hypoxia the patient has an activity intolerance.
    1 Pain is not associated with iron-deficiency anemia.
    2, 3 These are not specific for iron-deficiency anemia.
205. Application, planning, physiological (b)
    4 Nursing interventions focus on balancing activity and rest periods.
    1 Absolute bed rest is not needed.
    2 This is not a specific intervention for iron-deficiency anemia.
    3 The patient needs more rest periods than increased periods of exercise.
206. Comprehension, evaluation, health (b)
    4 Green leafy vegetables are a good source of iron.
    1 These are not a problem for iron deficiency anemia.
    2 Although eggs do contain some iron, green vegetables are a higher source.
    3 Milk does not contain iron. A quart of milk is unnecessary for adults.

207. Knowledge, assessment, physiological (c)
    4 Sickle cell anemia is a hereditary trait that occurs mostly in the black population.
    1 Sickle cell anemia is not a viral disease.
    2 It is not a bacterial disease.
    3 The disease is not caused by blood transfusions.
208. Comprehension, assessment, environment (b)
    1 In acute leukemia, there is an abnormal overproduction of a specific white blood cell, usually at an immature stage.
    2 Decreased T-lymphocytes are associated with immune disorders.
    3 A marked increase in hematocrit is associated with the blood disorder polycythemia vera.
    4 A low level of hemoglobin is associated with iron-deficiency anemia.
209. Comprehension, planning, environment (c)
    2 Because of the thrombocytopenia (lower-than-normal number of platelets), the patient is at risk for bleeding. Patient should be taught about bleeding precautions.
    1, 3, 4 These choices address precautions to be taken when the patient is at risk for infection because of neutropenia or leukopenia.
210. Application, implementation, physiological (c)
    2 Patients with leukopenia are at increased risk for infection. When the WBC count is low or there are large numbers of immature white cells, the usual signs of infection (redness, heat, swelling) are not manifested. The presence of fever is very significant, and efforts must be made to find the source of the infection.
    1 Rectal temperatures are not necessary. Patients receiving chemotherapy are also at risk for thrombocytopenia and rectal temperatures are not recommended.
    3 Bleeding is associated with thrombocytopenia.
    4 Although fluids are important, on the basis of the situation this is not the action that is most warranted.
211. Application, implementation, environment (b)
    3 A vial of medication, even if new, should be cleansed with an antiseptic before inserting the needle for withdrawal.
    1 To prevent further contamination to broken skin, sterile gloves would be best during dressing change.
    2 An IV where the site is is red and warm should be discontinued, not slowed down.
    4 A new isolation gown should be worn every time a nurse enters the patient's room.
212. Comprehension, planning, physiological (b)
    3 The human immune deficiency virus (HIV) attacks the immune and nervous systems.
    1 Mononucleosis causes increased fatigue.
    2 Herpes simplex produces blister-like lesions.
    4 Hepatitis B virus affects the liver.
213. Comprehension, planning, environment (b)
    1 The major source of HIV transmission is in blood and body fluid.
    2 This is not medically necessary, nor is the social isolation good for the patient psychologically.
    3 This is not medically indicated.
    4 This is not medically necessary because transmission is from blood and body fluids.
214. Application, implementation, health (b)
    2 Health maintenance is needed.
    1, 3 These produce psychosocial isolation.
    4 Health maintenance is the primary focus.

215. Comprehension, evaluation, psychosocial (b)
    1 Sharing feelings demonstrates that the patient trusts the nurse.
    2 This avoids personalizing the issue.
    3 This avoids personalizing the issue and establishing trust between patient and nurse.
    4 This is not significant in relation to establishing closeness or trust.
216. Knowledge, assessment, health (b)
    4 These are the major routes of AIDS transmission.
    1, 2, 3 Although HIV has been isolated in these routes of transmission, the primary routes remain sexual, blood, and transplacental.
217. Comprehension, assessment, health (c)
    2 The enzyme-linked immunosorbent assay (ELISA) is an AIDS virus antibody test that detects the organism causing the disease. For most persons, this test could detect marker antibodies at or about 10 to 12 weeks after exposure. Some persons may not experience marker antibodies for as long as 6 months after exposure.
    1, 3, 4 Although these diseases are often *associated* with AIDS, the ELISA is not specifically for them.
218. Knowledge, planning, health (a)
    3 This establishes rapport and provides accurate information and potential support groups.
    1 They may have been using the same needles while experimenting with drugs.
    2 The HIV virus is not transmitted by visiting with others.
    4 These tests may be appropriate at a later date, following discussion with Melissa and obtaining a proper history.
219. Comprehension, assessment, physiological (c)
    4 Karposi sarcoma, which manifests itself as purplish skin lesions, is a common symptom in homosexual men with AIDS.
    1 Patients with AIDS usually have chronic diarrhea, not constipation.
    2 This is not a usual symptom of AIDS.
    3 The temperature of AIDS patients is usually elevated, not subnormal.
220. Comprehension, assessment, physiological (b)
    3 Oral candidiasis causes painful lesions in the mouth and throat.
    1, 2, 4 These are not signs of candidiasis.
221. Application, implementation, environment (a)
    4 Chlorine bleach is the best disinfective against the AIDS virus, which could be found in body fluids.
    1, 2 This is not necessary. Blood and body fluids are the infective material. Gloves, gown, mask, or goggles should be used only when there is danger from contact with body fluids.
    3 AIDS patients may be in semiprivate rooms and share bathrooms because blood and body fluids are the only mode of transmission.
222. Knowledge (a)
    1 The liver aids in the process of digestion but is *not* considered a primary organ in the gastrointestinal (GI) system.
    2 The ileum is the distal portion of the small intestine and is considered a primary organ in the GI system.
    3 The stomach is regarded as a primary organ and acts as a reservoir for food, allowing for continuation of digestive processes.
    4 The sigmoid colon is part of the large intestine that terminates in the rectum and is considered a major organ of the GI system.

223. Knowledge (a)
    3 A strangulated hernia is an emergency situation in which the blood supply of the protrusion is eliminated, resulting in potential gangrene.
    1 An incarcerated hernia is edema of the protruding structures, which eliminates the possibility of returning the structures to the involved cavity.
    2 An incisional hernia occurs through the scar of a surgical incision when healing has been impaired.
    4 An umbilical hernia usually occurs because the umbilical orifices fail to close after birth. Obesity and prolonged abdominal distention can also result in an umbilical hernia.
224. Knowledge, implementation, environment (a)
    2 An upper gastrointestinal (GI) series assists in identification of pathology of the esophagus and stomach as the patient swallows barium liquid.
    1, 3, 4, These do not relate to the purpose of a GI series.
225. Comprehension, implementation, environment (b)
    4 The appropriate preparation for both upper GI series and barium enema is to keep the patient NPO and to give enemas usually until clear, to visualize the lower colon.
    1 The patient is to be NPO after midnight.
    2 This is the preparation of a patient for an oral cholecystography.
    3 This is part of the procedure for a liver biopsy.
226. Application, planning, environment (a)
    3 An endoscopy is considered an invasive procedure; preparation is similar to preparing a patient for surgery.
    1 This refers to an oral cholecystography.
    2 This refers to a T-tube cholangiography.
    4 This applies to noninvasive procedures such as ultrasounds and computed axial tomography (CAT) scans.
227. Comprehension, implementation, physiological (a)
    2 The patient's gag reflex is temporarily anesthetized; therefore, the patient is to be NPO until the gag reflex returns.
    1, 4 This is contraindicated until the gag reflex returns.
    3 There is no time limit as to when the patient can have food or liquids. The only criteria is to wait for the gag reflex to return.
228. Comprehension, assessment, physiological (b)
    1 Gastric ulcer pain is more frequent when the stomach is empty and hydrochloric acid is secreted. Food relieves this.
    2 Pain in gastric ulcer disease is relieved by vomiting because hydrochloric acid is expelled.
    3 Food relieves the pain of gastric ulcers.
    4 Pain may occur during the night but also when the stomach is empty during the day.
229. Comprehension, evaluation, physiological (c)
    4 Sudden onset of intense abdominal pain is a sign that the ulcer has perforated and peritonitis is developing.
    1 Body temperature may rise.
    2 This is not a sign of perforation.
    3 Vomitus would be grossly bloody, not blood tinged.
230. Application, implementation, environment (c)
    3 Nasogastric tubes must always be connected to low intermittent suction. High suction would disturb acid/base balance.
    1 This is not an independent nursing action. Fluids are not given with a nasogastric tube.
    2 Normal saline only must be used as an irrigant to preserve acid/base balance.
    4 Cantor tubes, not nasogastric tubes, are advanced hourly.

231. Comprehension, evaluation, health (c)
    4 Carbohydrates, particularly refined carbohydrates, are contraindicated in dumping syndrome because they are absorbed quickly, causing an increase in dumping syndrome symptoms. Fats delay absorption.
    1, 2, 3 These will prevent premature emptying of the stomach.
232. Application, implementation, environment (b)
    3 The warm moist urine could foster growth of microorganisms, resulting in an inappropriate diagnosis and treatment for the patient.
    1 A urine specimen does not need to be warm when it arrives in the laboratory.
    2 The specimen could be spilled, but this would not be the most important concern.
    4 The microorganisms will continue to grow instead of die.
233. Comprehension, planning, environment (b)
    1 The endoscope will be passed into the stomach; no food or fluid should be present to obstruct the view.
    2, 3, 4 These are not needed; it is the stomach that will be viewed.
234. Application, implementation, physiological (b)
    2 Drug therapy will decrease or neutralize the normal gastric acidity.
    1 After medication therapy, a high-fat, high-carbohydrate diet is needed.
    3 A high-fat, high-carbohydrate diet is needed for gastric juices to digest over a longer period of time and thus decrease gastric acidity.
    4 The diet should be low in protein and milk products to decrease the need for high levels of gastric juices.
235. Comprehension, planning, physiological (c)
    3 This decreases acid production by the parietal cells of the stomach.
    1 This procedure, known as an antrectomy, is not necessary.
    2 This procedure, known as a gastric resection, is not necessary.
    4 This procedure, known as a gastrectomy, is not necessary.
236. Comprehension, planning, physiological (c)
    4 Rapid gastric emptying is the result of a bolus of hypertonic food that increases motility and peristalsis and thus changes blood glucose levels.
    1 This is only a partial causative factor.
    2, 3 These are inappropriate responses.
237. Application, implementation, physiological (c)
    1 This decreases or slows the emptying time of the stomach.
    2 Reclining before meals is not helpful to the condition.
    3 The nurse should teach the patient to avoid fluids during meals to decrease motility and peristalsis after eating.
    4 A decreased amount of carbohydrates will slow the emptying time of the stomach.
238. Comprehension, assessment, physiological (b)
    4 It is not uncommon for the ulcerative colitis patient to experience 10 to 12 bloody stools per day.
    1 Constipation is not a symptom.
    2 Bright dark-red bleeding is more common than tarry stools.
    3 Pain is located in the lower abdomen.
239. Comprehension, evaluation, health (b)
    1 Oatmeal and orange slices are high in fiber. Most ulcerative colitis patients have a lactose intolerance; milk should not be included.
    2, 3, 4 These are low-residue foods.

240. Comprehension, assessment, physiological (a)
    1 Because the feces is coming from the ileum, the consistency is semiliquid with mucous shreds from the lining.
    2 Blood should not be present. Semiformed feces would come from an ascending colectomy.
    3 This would be characteristic of a sigmoid colectomy.
    4 Blood should not be present in the stool after an ileostomy.
241. Knowledge, assessment, physiological (a)
    3 Edema and redness means that there is an adequate blood supply to the stoma. The stoma will shrink slowly as time goes by.
    1 Light pink indicates lack of blood supply.
    2 This could mean blockage or other problems.
    4 This could mean constriction of the blood supply.
242. Comprehension, assessment, physiological (b)
    3 The contents of the stomach are aspirated to determine the amount of hydrochloric acid present.
    1 Gastric refers to the stomach and does not involve analysis of stools.
    2 Ulcerative colitis does not involve pus in the stomach.
    4 The test does not involve the lower gastrointestinal tract.
243. Knowledge, planning, physiological (a)
    1 Histamine is normally present in the body but when given stimulates the production of gastric secretions.
    2 Belladonna inhibits gastric secretions, which is contrary to the purpose of a gastric analysis.
    3 Atropine blocks vagal effect rather than stimulates it as diagnostic test requires.
    4 Paregoric diminishes digestive secretions, which is contraindicated in this test.
244. Comprehension, planning, environment (a)
    3 The causative factor of stress is considered with rest and privacy for toileting.
    1 Rest is needed, but privacy for toileting is an important factor.
    2 Restrictions may be needed to decrease stress and provide rest that is needed.
    4 This does not allow for rest and privacy in toileting.
245. Comprehension, evaluation, health (a)
    1 This would indicate less irritation or active disease process within the colon.
    2 Hardening is not a factor in the disease process.
    3 Normal stools are not present in the disease process.
    4 A decrease is indicative, but a decrease in pus, blood and mucus is also a factor.
246. Comprehension, implementation, physiological (a)
    4 Psychosomatic factors may cause or aggravate the mucosa or submucosa of the colon.
    1 This is not a contributory factor.
    2 Increased motility of the intestine is not characteristic of the disease.
    3 In most cases it is a viral, not a bacterial, infection.
247. Comprehension, assessment, physiological (a)
    1 In the colon tiny abscesses form, producing purulent drainage; capillaries become irritated and bleed with sloughing of the mucosa, producing mucus.
    2 Disease of the colon does not allow the formation of a hard stool.
    3 Normal-type stools are nonexistent with an active disease process.
    4 This is possible, but stools would include mucous, pus, and blood.

248. Application, assessment, physiological (b)
    2 A liquid light-brown stool is expected from a transverse colostomy in the immediate postoperative period.
    1 Bloody stool with clots is not a normal expectation of a colostomy, even in the postoperative period.
    3 A semisolid stool is expected after the patient has a normal food intake.
    4 A solid stool is not normally produced by a transverse colostomy. Blood is also not a normal expectation.
249. Application, assessment, physiological (c)
    4 A purple discoloration may indicate inadequate circulation to the stoma; therefore the physician should be notified
    1 The nurse's notes may not be immediately read by the physician; this may leave the patient's problem untreated for some time.
    2 A purple discoloration on the stoma does not necessarily indicate simple bruising; it may indicate inadequate circulation to the stoma.
    3 A petroleum dressing will do nothing to treat the problem.
250. Comprehension, implementation, physiological (a)
    2 Placement is of prime importance to avoid aspiration of liquids into the lungs.
    1 Patency is important but should be determined after placement is checked.
    3 This is an important nursing measure, but it is not the primary intervention.
    4 Nasogastric tubes are *not* clamped prior to instillation of liquids; however, they should be clamped after instillation of medications to facilitate absorption.
251. Comprehension, assessment, physiological (c)
    4 Stool is passed through the narrowed colon to form a thin stool before exiting through the rectum.
    1, 2, 3 These are not the appropriate locations for such a stool.
252. Comprehension, planning, environment (a)
    2 This will clean out the lower bowel for visualization of the lower colon.
    1 This will not clean out the lower bowel
    3 This is not appropriate for this procedure.
    4 Both methods are not needed.
253. Comprehension, assessment, psychosocial (b)
    2 Use of an open-ended question gets her to tell the nurse more about what she is thinking.
    1 This is an inappropriate response; it prevents establishing an effective relationship with the patient.
    3 This does not allow her to express her concerns.
    4 This response prevents establishing therapeutic communication.
254. Comprehension, assessment, physiological (c)
    1 The sigmoid colostomy removes the specific area involved.
    2 This is not appropriate; it involves the small intestine.
    3 The colectomy is removal of the area that is not involved.
    4 This is not the area where the involvement is located.
255. Knowledge, evaluation, physiological (a)
    4 Cramping does occur when fluid is first introduced.
    1 The level of the container does not affect cramping.
    2 Cramping normally occurs so there is no need to discontinue the procedure.
    3 This will not allow irrigation and will not change the cramping effect.

256. Comprehension, planning, environment (b)
 3 This is the immediate postoperative need of the patient; other needs include wound care, pain management, and prevention of infection.
 1 It is too early to include this now.
 2 This is not appropriate to discuss at this point.
 4 It is too early to identify these.
257. Comprehension, implementation, environment (a)
 2 This is adequate placement for the solution to reach the stool.
 1 This is not in far enough; solution will drain out.
 3, 4 This is too far in for the solution to irrigate colon.
258. Knowledge, evaluation, psychosocial (a)
 2 This indicates denial of both the colostomy and the need for self-care.
 1 It is not unusual to have not gained full appetite back yet.
 3, 4 This is appropriate after having such a procedure.
259. Application, planning, health (c)
 2 This allows the patient input into decisions about his or her care.
 1 This doesn't allow for the patient's individual needs.
 3 This is not an important factor at this time.
 4 The patient is the primary focus at this point.
260. Knowledge, assessment, physiological (a)
 1 Chole (gall) lithiasis (stone) is the correct term.
 2 Cholecystitis is the term for inflammation of the gallbladder.
 3 Nephrolithiasis is the term for renal calculi.
 4 Glomerulonephritis is the term for inflammation of the nephrons of the kidneys.
261. Knowledge, assessment, physiological (a)
 4 Bile is essential for the breakdown of fats; therefore the inability to digest fats properly is noted, along with the accumulation of bile, causing jaundice.
 1 This is indicative of heptatits.
 2 This is indicative of peritonitis.
 3 This is indicative of cirrhosis.
262. Comprehension, planning, physiological (a)
 2 Chole (gall) cyst (bladder) ectomy (removal of) is the correct term.
 1 This is the term for removal of the colon.
 3 This is the term for removal of the stomach.
 4 This is the term for removal of a kidney.
263. Comprehension, planning, physiological (a)
 2 This is a specially designed tube resembling a T that is placed in the common bile duct to facilitate drainage of bile.
 1 This is appropriate for a thoracotomy.
 3 This is appropriate for wound drainage.
 4 This is appropriate to provide an artificial airway.
264. Knowledge, planning, health (a)
 4 These choices offer the least fat content.
 1, 2, 3 These choices offer more fat content than choice No. 4.
265. Application, assessment, environment (b)
 2 Nausea, bloating, and vomiting may occur due to impaired fat digestion and impaired bile flow.
 1 Bile pigments may be present in urine, giving it a very dark color.
 3 Stools may become grayish or "clay-colored" because of the absence of bile pigments.
 4 Abdominal pain may occur after eating fatty foods, not carbohydrates.

266. Application, planning, environment (b)
 3 The patient should be NPO for 10 to 12 hours beforehand or food may stimulate the gallbladder to contract and expel the contrast media.
 1 If an oral contrast media is used, an IV is not usually needed.
 2 The area does not need to be prepped or shaved for an x-ray examination.
 4 The patient should be NPO for 10 to 12 hours before the test.
267. Application, implementation, physiological (b)
 4 To prevent damage to the gastric mucosa, low intermittent suction should be used.
 1 Irrigation is not necessary unless the nasogastric tube is clogged.
 2 Wrapping the tube will serve no purpose in preventing postoperative nausea and vomiting.
 3 The patient will be NPO following surgery.
268. Application, implementation, physiological (b)
 1 The dressing will need to be changed because even small amounts of bile leakage around the T-tube will irritate the skin.
 2 Reinforcing the dressing can still leave bile drainage on the skin.
 3 This is inappropriate general postoperative care.
 4 The patient will need appropriate analgesia, not usually sedation.
269. Application, planning, health (b)
 3 This position will prevent the backflow of bile into the common bile duct.
 1 Tight clothing or a binder can cause pressure and irritation of the wound site.
 2 Showers are preferred because running water will prevent the possibility of bacteria entering the wound.
 4 Without clarification of this statement, the patient may consider all signs of redness and tenderness normal, even those associated with a developing infection; and so may not report the symptoms to the physician.
270. Comprehension, assessment, physiological (b)
 3 This indicates the inability of liver cells to remove bile pigment from circulating blood.
 1 This is not directly related to the pancreas.
 2 This is not directly related to the intestines.
 4 Inappropriate response; the cause is known.
271. Comprehension, planning, environment (b)
 1 This is a disease transmittable through direct contact with body fluids and secretions.
 2 IV antibiotics are not generally ordered unless severe infection is present.
 3 Universal precautions are a higher priority.
 4 Contrary to treatment because altered nutrition usually occurs and increased fluid intake will be needed.
272. Comprehension, planning, physiological (c)
 2 This indicates the inability of the liver to metabolize bile, which causes the elevation of bilirubin, SGOT, and serum glutamic pyruvic acid (SGPT).
 1 There is no direct relationship to these.
 3 An elevation of serum glutamic oxaloacetic transaminase (SGOT) is noted, but there is a decrease in serum albumin.
 4 A decrease is noted in the serum albumin, but there is no direct relationship to hemoglobin noted in the test results.
273. Comprehension, planning, physiological (b)
 2 Bed rest is necessary to decrease physical debilitation.
 1 Diet of choice is low in fat.
 3 Inappropriate response; diet is an integral part of the treatment plan.
 4 This would increase physical debilitation.

274. Knowledge, assessment, environment (a)
    3 Stool is clay-colored as a result of poor metabolism of the affected liver.
    1 This is usually the color of a normal stool.
    2 Black stool could be indicative of bleeding, but is also noted in patients who are taking iron preparations.
    4 This could be indicative of a disease process, but not in this case.

275. Comprehension, assessment, psychosocial (b)
    2 Codependency is defined as a set of maladaptive and/or immature responses, behaviors, and feelings experienced by someone closely associated with an actively chemically dependent person. Commonly reported symptoms include a self-esteem that relies heavily on feeling needed by others, the need to control others, and the tendency to develop complicated relationships with chemically dependent people.
    1 Sam may feel he is doing this as a caring husband; however, he may in fact be contributing to the problem itself.
    3, 4 Incorrect answers; these are not examples of this type of behavior.

276. Knowledge, assessment, physiological (c)
    3 A sign of acute pancreatitis is an elevated serum amylase level. Serum amylase levels increase within 24 to 48 hours of the onset of the condition and can range from 300 to 800 Somogyi units, although there is no apparent relationship between the severity of the disease and elevation of enzyme levels.
    1 The abdomen becomes hard and rigid.
    2 Bloody urine is not a usual sign.
    4 Elevated serum creatinine is indicative of poor kidney function, not poor pancreatic function.

277. Comprehension, evaluation, health (b)
    3 Steamed vegetables and skimmed milk are fat-free foods.
    1 Tuna salad is made with mayonnaise, which is a fat.
    2 Hamburger is usually a high-fat meat.
    4 Cheese is a high-fat food. Usually butter or margarine is added in the grilling process.

278. Comprehension, planning, physiological (b)
    3 Leukocytosis indicates an abnormal increase in the number of circulating white blood cells, a condition that often accompanies bacterial, but not usually viral, infections.
    1 Agranulocytosis is an abnormal condition of the blood characterized by a severe reduction in the number of granulocytes.
    2 Leukopenia is an abnormal decrease in the number of white blood cells to fewer than 5000 cells/m³.
    4 Aplastic anemia is a deficiency of all of the formed elements of the blood, representing a failure of the cell-generating capacity of the bone marrow.

279. Comprehension, evaluation, physiological (a)
    1 Peritonitis is an inflammation of the parietal and visceral surfaces of the abdominal cavity caused by bacterial infection.
    2 Ileitus is an inflammation of the ileum.
    3 Colitis is an inflammatory condition of the large intestine.
    4 Diverticulitis is an inflammation of one or more diverticula; penetration of fecal matter through the thin-walled diverticula causes inflammation and abscess formation in the tissues surrounding the colon.

280. Comprehension, planning, environment (b)
    4 An ice bag to the abdomen is ordered to safely relieve the pain.
    1 Narcotics mask the symptoms, especially of a ruptured appendix.

2 Heat on the abdomen increases circulation to the area and can contribute to a ruptured appendix.
    3 A cleansing enema contributes to rupture of the appendix.

281. Knowledge, planning, physiological (a)
    1 There is undefinitive speculation that acute appendicitis is from a hardened mass of stool or foreign body.
    2, 3, 4 These bear no relationship to appendicitis.

282. Knowledge, implementation, environment (a)
    3 This provides the patient with information about what he should expect after surgery, thereby decreasing his anxiety level and soliciting his assistance.
    1, 4 These are not immediate concerns.
    2 The pain caused by the appendicitis should be gone.

283. Comprehension, assessment, physiological (c)
    1 Although all the answers are signs of increased intracranial pressure, changes in levels of consciousness are the earliest sign.
    2, 3, 4 See No. 1.

284. Comprehension, assessment, physiological (a)
    3 Vital sign changes in intracranial pressure (ICP) include elevated blood pressure, bradycardia, slow irregular respirations, and elevated temperature.
    1, 2, 4 These are not indicative of vital sign changes in ICP.

285. Application, implementation, environment (a)
    4 The supine position with the head elevated 30 degrees allows for proper drainage of cerebral edema and will help reduce intracranial pressure (ICP).
    1, 2 These will not help reduce ICP.
    3 This will increase ICP.

286. Knowledge, assessment, physiological (c)
    2 The Glasgow Coma Scale has been designed to quantitatively relate consciousness to motor, verbal and eye-opening responses. Higher scores indicate increased degrees of arousal. A score of 14 to 15 indicates a patient is not neurologically impaired.
    1 Depending on the system used, scores of 9 or more do not qualify as coma; however, it is the examiner who determines the best response the patient can make to a set of standardized stimuli.
    3 Depending on the system used, a score less than 7 is accepted to indicate a coma.
    4 Determining a patient's orientation via a "best" verbal response is only one of the three responses tested using the Glasgow Coma Scale.

287. Comprehension, assessment, physiological (a)
    1 These are subjective in that the patient would have to tell the nurse these symptoms.
    2, 3, 4 These are objective in that they are seen and measurable.

288. Application, assessment, physiological (b)
    2 Rechecking assures equipment is functioning, and reporting to the immediate supervisor (charge nurse) brings prompt attention to the changes because these changes indicate increased intracranial pressure.
    1, 3 Delay of reporting could have serious consequences, and therefore it is not correct procedure.
    4 These changes are significant and need to be reported.

289. Comprehension, planning, environment (a)
    4 Trendelenburg's (shock position) is contraindicated because it would increase the flow of blood to the cranium.
    1, 2, 3 These positions may be permitted.

290. Comprehension, planning, physiological (b)
    4 Although all of the answers could cause anxiety before the surgery, the patient's fear of the unknown would be the priority concern and could be relieved by the nurse explaining all procedures.
    1, 2, 3 These are not priority concerns.

291. Comprehension, assessment, environment (c)
 1 Dilated fixed pupils are the most ominous sign of neurological damage and increased intracranial pressure (ICP).
 2 Widening pulse pressure is a sign of ICP.
 3 This is not the most critical sign.
 4 These are normal vital signs.

292. Comprehension, assessment, physiological (c)
 2 This could mean injury to the spinal cord and leakage of cerebral spinal fluid.
 1, 4 These are not common complications.
 3 This would be a normal sign.

293. Application, implementation, environment (b)
 4 Priority interventions during a seizure would be to remove harmful objects and protect the patient from injury.
 1 It is not necessary to monitor vital signs during a seizure.
 2 The nurse would be unable to open the patient's jaws; airways only are used in the mouth.
 3 Although a side-lying position is important, safety is priority.

294. Comprehension, evaluation, health (c)
 2 Gingival hyperplasia is a side effect of phenytoin (Dilantin) and should be reported to the physician for treatment.
 1 Weight loss is a side effect of phenytoin.
 3 Pink urine is a common harmless side effect of Dilantin. It does not mean that the drug should be stopped.
 4 The patient must be stabilized on the drug for 2 years before driving a car or participating in hazardous activities.

295. Application, assessment, environment (c)
 1 This seizure activity is associated with complex distortion of thinking and feeling, as well as partially coordinated motor activity.
 2 This seizure activity is characterized by peculiar generalized tonelessness.
 3 This seizure activity may or may not be progressive.
 4 This seizure activity is characterized by mild or rapid forceful movements.

296. Application, assessment, environment (b)
 3 A complete health history is necessary to document any history of seizures.
 1 A skull series of x-ray examinations is a diagnostic study and not a nursing assessment; it will not provide necessary data because most seizures are not the result of musculoskeletal injury.
 2 The neurological examination is not a nursing assessment; it is rather a diagnostic study. A complete neurological examination will not demonstrate necessary information to diagnose seizure activity.
 4 This is a laboratory study, not a nursing diagnosis. It will not provide pertinent information for accurate diagnosis.

297. Comprehension, assessment, physiological (b)
 4 Status epilepticus is a medical emergency and requires medical and nursing intervention to prevent death from brain damage that is a result of prolonged hypoxia and exhaustion.
 1 Grand mal seizure activity is characterized by loss of consciousness for several minutes.
 2 Psychomotor seizures are characterized by a sudden change in awareness associated with a complex distortion of feelings and thinking and partially coordinated motor activity.
 3 Petit mal seizures are characterized by sudden impairment in or loss of consciousness, with little or no tonic-clonic movement.

298. Knowledge, planning, physiological (a)
 3 The oil-retention enema softens and lubricates to help in an easier defecation for a patient of this age and condition.
 1 A Fleet enema would be safe, but it is not the best answer for this patient. Straining may still occur if the stool is hard and difficult to pass.
 2 Saline is not recommended in cardiac patients because of the possibility of electrolyte and fluid changes.
 4 This amount is too much for a patient her age and may place too much strain on an already weakened heart.

299. Application, implementation, physiological (b)
 4 This is the result of prolonged hypoxia and exhaustion.
 1 Status epilepticus does not cause toxic disturbances.
 2 Status epilepticus does not cause metabolic problems.
 3 Status epilepticus does not cause hypertension.

300. Comprehension, implementation, health (b)
 3 Most states now require medical proof that seizures are under control.
 1 Driving during daylight hours does not decrease seizure activity.
 2 Driving laws vary concerning specific regulations. This is not the most common requirement.
 4 It is recommended that the patient carry an identification card; however, this is not legally required.

301. Application, planning, health (b)
 4 The warning feelings some people experience are odd sensations such as unpleasant odors, spots before their eyes, flashing lights, vertigo, tingling, or numbness.
 1 This occurs during the recovery stage, in the postictal period. During this time there are common complaints of headaches and muscle aches.
 2 This is sometimes reported postictally.
 3 Hallucinations are not reported in most seizure activities.

302. Knowledge, assessment, physiological (a)
 2 Complaints of headache are common.
 1, 4 These are not typically associated with seizures.
 3 This is not typical postictally.

303. Comprehension, implementation, environment (c)
 4 Most seizure disorders can be controlled partially or completely by anticonvulsants. These drugs also act to raise the seizure threshold. The choice of medication depends on the type of seizures.
 1 Digitalis preparations and atropine are examples. They are used to slow and strengthen the heartbeat and increase the heart rate.
 2 Anticonvulsants are central nervous system (CNS) depressants.
 3 Antispasmodics are used to treat muscle spasms and are *not* anticonvulsants.

304. Comprehension, assessment, environment (b)
 3 Hypertension is a major risk factor associated with a cerebrovascular accident (CVA) or stroke. Other risk factors are emboli, intracranial hemorrhage, diabetes mellitus, increased blood viscosity, and cardiac disease.
 1, 2, 4 These individuals do not have known risks.

305. Comprehension, planning, health (b)
 3 Multiple sclerosis is a progressive degenerative disease in which the myelin sheath of the brain and the spinal cord are destroyed.
 1 This is characteristic of a type of seizure in epilepsy.
 2 This is characteristic of Parkinson's disease.
 4 This is characteristic of Meniere's syndrome.

306. Comprehension, assessment, physiological (b)
    2 Loss of muscular activities is a result of interference of nerve impulses.
    1 This is characteristic of a grand mal seizure.
    3 This is characteristic of a head injury.
    4 This is characteristic of Parkinson's disease.
307. Application, planning, health (a)
    1 The patient should remain active as long as possible and continue daily activities without becoming fatigued.
    2 This is recommended in Parkinson's disease.
    3 The patient is not to assume complete bed rest until complete loss of muscular function necessitates it. The drug therapy of choice is corticosteroids, which are antiinflammatory agents, not antibiotics.
    4 The diet recommended is high calorie, high vitamin, and high protein.
308. Knowledge, implementation, physiological (a)
    3 Proper supports and body alignment are important to prevent decubitus ulcers and contractures that are a result of loss of muscle tone.
    1 The patient should be encouraged to maintain social activities as long as possible. Occupational activities may have to be changed if necessary. Appropriately trained persons would best meet these needs of the patient.
    2 The patient should be encouraged to avoid treatments that promise a cure, because there is no cure.
    4 The patient should avoid complete bed rest unless absolutely necessary. Encourage patient to be independent as long as possible.
309. Application, implementation, health (b)
    1 At the present time there are no drugs that can stop the degenerative process of multiple sclerosis.
    2, 3, 4 These are included in the education for patients with multiple sclerosis.
310. Comprehension, planning, environment (b)
    4 This provides necessary exercise that is recommended for patients with Parkinson's.
    1 This does not provide exercise.
    2 In this activity, dexterity may be a problem; also, it does not provide needed exercise.
    3 This does not provide needed exercise.
311. Comprehension, planning, environment (a)
    3 The nurse should encourage daily exercise as tolerated to prevent pneumonia and to maintain joint mobility. Encourage participation in previous work, as well as social and diversional activities to avoid social withdrawal.
    1 Many patients with Parkinson's disease live for years.
    2 At this time there is no known way to stop progression of this disease.
    4 There is no known cure at this time.
312. Comprehension, planning, environment (c)
    1 This is the nursing diagnosis for low back pain. Pain in the lower back may be caused by a variety of diseases.
    2 There is a potential for powerlessness imposed by progressive physical deterioration, loss of body control, and/or threat to physical integrity. The goal is for the patient to demonstrate an optimal level of mobility.
    3 The goal with this nursing diagnosis is to meet the patient's self-care needs by such measures as encouraging self-care as tolerated; promoting adequate pulmonary function by encouraging coughing and deep-breathing exercises; maintaining a well-balanced soft diet; and providing small feedings as indicated.
    4 This is an appropriate nursing diagnosis for Parkinson's disease. The goal is for the patient or significant other to demonstrate understanding of home care and follow-up instructions through interactive discussions and actual return demonstration.

313. Knowledge, assessment, physiological (a)
    4 This is the disorder in adults that results from excessive secretion of the growth hormone.
    1 This is the disorder of hypopituitarism.
    2 This is the disorder of hyperthyroidism.
    3 This is the disorder of excessive production of the growth hormone in children.
314. Comprehension, assessment, health (b)
    1 These features are typical in an adult as a result of closure of the epiphyses of the long bones.
    2 These are subjective symptoms, not observations.
    3, 4 These are objective symptoms of gigantism.
315. Comprehension, implementation, psychosocial (b)
    4 Coarse facial features and broad hands, fingers, and feet may make one avoid social contacts.
    1 These are observations after a thyroidectomy if parathyroids have been accidentally removed.
    2 These are dietary changes with hypoparathyroidism patients.
    3 These are observed with adrenalectomy patients.
316. Comprehension, assessment, physiological (b)
    1 Hyperactivity and excitability are some of the classic signs of hyperthyroidism.
    2, 3 These are signs of hypothyroidism.
    4 This is not a sign of thyroid dysfunction.
317. Application, implementation, environment (b)
    3 This position will prevent stress on the suture line and will prevent postoperative bleeding.
    1 This position would cause too much stress on the suture line.
    2 The head must be kept straight after surgery to prevent bleeding. A side-lying position is contraindicated.
    4 The prone position would cause stress on the suture line.
318. Comprehension, implementation, environment (b)
    4 This is to be prepared in case of excessive swelling of the throat that may occur resulting in an emergency situation.
    1 This is not needed because in most cases the patient would be too warm (not of an emergent nature). Anyway, the blanket would cool off rapidly at the bedside.
    2 These are not used; seizures are unlikely.
    3 This is not commonly needed for a thyroidectomy patient postoperatively (not of an emergent nature).
319. Application, implementation, health (b)
    3 Keeping the head straight after surgery prevents stress on the suture line and prevents bleeding.
    1 The patient should be able to swallow right after surgery.
    2 This is not a priority in the early postoperative period.
    4 Coughing is contraindicated right after surgery because it could cause bleeding.
320. Comprehension, implementation, environment (b)
    2 Patient is instructed not to cough because it could cause bleeding.
    1 Fluid intake is necessary and can be given in spite of sore throat.
    3 This fails to facilitate breathing for the patient and does not allow for easier observation of respiratory complications.
    4 Caution must be exercised with morphine because it depresses respirations.
321. Comprehension, assessment, physiological (b)
    4 Tetany manifested by involuntary tremors may be a sign of decreasing calcium levels.
    1, 2, 3 These are signs of hypocalcemia.

322. Comprehension, evaluation, physiological (b)
 1 The medication actually blocks the production of thyroid hormones, thus decreasing the activity of the gland.
 2, 3 The medication decreases, rather than increases, the activity of the gland.
 4 Activity has no effect on the pancreas.
323. Knowledge, planning, health (a)
 4 Graves' disease is a disorder characterized by pronounced hyperthyroidism; usually associated with an enlarged thyroid gland and exophthalmus.
 1 Myxedema is the most severe form of hypothyroidism. It is characterized by swelling of the hands, face, feet and periorbital tissues and may lead to coma and death.
 2 Cretinism is a condition characterized by severe congenital hypothyroidism; often associated with other endocrine abnormalities.
 3 Colloid goiter involves a greatly enlarged, soft thyroid gland in which the follicles are distended with colloid.
324. Knowledge, implementation, environment (a)
 3 One of the functions of the thyroid gland is to regulate metabolism.
 1 This is not an endocrine gland but one of the largest pair of salivary glands that lie at the side of the face just below and in front of the external ear.
 2 The parathyroid gland is an endocrine gland which helps to maintain the level of blood calcium and ensures normal neuromuscular irritability, blood clotting, and cell membrane permeability.
 4 The pituitary gland is an endocrine gland supplying numerous hormones that govern vital processes such as growth and development, milk secretion, and contraction of smooth muscle.
325. Knowledge, planning, physiological (a)
 2 Overproduction of the thyroid hormone thyroxin increases the activity of the thyroid gland.
 1 Basal metabolic rate would be high, not low.
 3 Thyroxin levels would be high, not low.
 4 Thyroxin levels would be high; see rationale to correct answer, No. 2.
326. Application, assessment, environment (b)
 2 Tetany can be caused by the parathyroid gland having been removed inadvertently or by excessive edema that can occlude parathyroid functioning.
 1 There is no direct relationship to the urinary system that would cause problems.
 3 This is to be expected as a result of edema in the throat.
 4 This could be a result of poor fluid intake because of edema of the throat; if observed, this should not become a major complication.
327. Application, planning, environment (a)
 1 Iodine can be irritating to the lining of the stomach and is difficult to absorb; additional fluids are necessary.
 2 Empty stomachs have a high potential for irritation.
 3 The medication is being given for a purpose; giving it on a prn basis does not meet that purpose.
 4 Iodine preparations should not be given on an empty stomach because of irritability and poor absorption.
328. Application, evaluation, environment (b)
 1 Increased pulse rate is a result of a release of large amounts of thyroid hormone into the bloodstream.
 2 The pulse rate would increase.
 3 The large amount of thyroid hormone released should increase respirations.
 4 The increased amount of thyroid hormone released should elevate the temperature.

329. Application, implementation, environment (b)
 3 Regular insulin starts to work in ½ to 1 hour. When a mix of NPH and regular insulin is given in the morning, breakfast must be given within a ½ hour of administration of the insulin.
 1 Regular insulin peaks in 2 to 3 hours. Not eating before this time could cause hypoglycemia.
 2 So that there is food for it to work on, regular insulin is always given before meals.
 4 Regular insulin peaks in 2 to 3 hours.
330. Comprehension, assessment, physiological (b)
 2 Lethargy leading to coma develops because of metabolic acidosis (ketoacidosis).
 1, 4 These are not symptoms of ketoacidosis.
 3 This may be a symptom of hypoglycemia, not ketoacidosis.
331. Application, implementation, health (c)
 4 Capillary blood glucose should always be tested before strenuous activity. Because exercise burns glucose and lowers blood glucose levels, it is important to assess the blood glucose level before exercising so that food and insulin could be adjusted to prevent hypoglycemia.
 1 Although testing the blood glucose level after exercise could be done, it is not the most important time to do this.
 2 Two hours after meals, blood glucose levels would be at their highest; this is not the best time.
 3 Although the level could be taken before lunch, this is not the best time.
332. Application, implementation, health (a)
 4 As blood glucose levels fall, the first symptom that the patient develops is hunger.
 1 Flushed face may be a sign of hyperglycemia.
 2 Diplopia is not a symptom of hypoglycemia.
 3 Slurred speech is not an early symptom of hypoglycemia; it may be a sign of hyperglycemia.
333. Comprehension, evaluation, health (b)
 2 Hamburger and peanut butter are both in the meat group. They may be exchanged.
 1 Fruit salad is in the fruit group.
 3 Tomato soup is in the vegetable group.
 4 Corn muffin is in the bread group.
334. Comprehension, evaluation, physiological (c)
 1 Exercise burns glucose; therefore, insulin needs may decrease.
 2, 3 Less insulin is required (see No. 1).
 4 Untrue statement. Food alone cannot control diabetes or affect insulin requirements. The combination of food, exercise, and insulin is needed.
335. Application, planning, environment (c)
 2 NPH insulin peaks in approximately 4 to 12 hours after administration. Insulin reactions may occur at this time if there is not enough carbohydrate to maintain blood glucose levels within normal range. A split dose of NPH insulin before breakfast and at bedtime could lead to an insulin reaction at 4 to 5 PM and/or during the night.
 1 This is too soon for the morning NPH insulin to peak.
 3 One hour after breakfast is too soon for morning NPH insulin to peak; 1 hour after dinner is too soon for the afternoon NPH insulin to peak.
 4 One hour after lunch is too soon for morning NPH insulin to peak. Because the patient is still metabolizing carbohydrates from lunch, an insulin reaction at this time is unlikely.

336. Comprehension, assessment, environment (b)
    1 Obesity and genetics are the primary risk factors in the development of type II diabetes.
    2 Eating many sweets does not cause diabetes.
    3, 4 These are symptoms of type II diabetes; they are not risk factors.
337. Application, implementation, physiological (b)
    4 Drinking alcohol when taking Micronase can make the drug more potent, increasing the risk of hypoglycemia.
    1 Insulin may be adjusted according to capillary blood glucose levels. Micronase is given in a standard dose.
    2 Exercise should be performed after meals, not after taking Micronase.
    3 Micronase should be taken before breakfast.
338. Comprehension, evaluation, physiological (a)
    4 The action of Micronase is to stimulate the pancreas to produce more insulin and to increase the sensitivity of insulin receptors on the cell.
    1 Oral hypoglycemics are not insulin and cannot replace it.
    2 Oral hypoglycemics have no digestive action.
    3 Oral hypoglycemics have no effect on weight.
339. Comprehension, planning, environment (b)
    2 Maintaining ideal body weight is essential in the control of type II diabetes.
    1 Insulin is not necessary. Achieving ideal body weight through diet and exercise would be the primary method of control.
    3 The ideal diabetic diet is 60% complex carbohydrate.
    4 This is unnecessary for a type II diabetic unless the conditions are out of control. Not a priority at this time.
340. Comprehension, planning, physiological (b)
    3 There is a decreased production of insulin needed to metabolize carbohydrates.
    1 This condition does not interfere with the body's ability to absorb minerals.
    2 This condition does not interfere with the body's ability to absorb vitamins.
    4 Diabetes mellitus involves the pancreas and the lack of insulin secretion by the beta cells.
341. Comprehension, assessment, physiological (c)
    4 This is the normal amount of glucose that is found in the bloodstream as an end product of digestion.
    1, 2, 3 Incorrect amount.
342. Knowledge, planning, environment (a)
    3 Orinase stimulates the beta cells in the pancreatic islets to produce insulin so that glucose metabolism occurs.
    1 There is no medication classified as an "oral" insulin.
    2 The medication must be taken on a regular basis in order to be effective.
    4 There are different types of oral hypoglycemics; not all diabetics require the same type of medication or need them at all.
343. Comprehension, assessment, environment (a)
    4 An increase of acetone in the body accounts for fruity smelling breath and hot dry skin.
    1, 2 These are indicative of hypoglycemic reaction.
    3 The systolic blood pressure drops and circulatory collapse may occur.

344. Application, planning, environment (c)
    1 Oral hypoglycemic agents stimulate the pancreas to produce insulin; exercise and dietary control of metabolism are also needed.
    2 Adult-onset diabetes in overweight men needs exercise and dietary control, but the disease usually can be controlled without insulin.
    3 Insulin replacement is needed when diet and oral hypoglycemic agents can't control the disease.
    4 Weight loss is indicated, but stimulating insulin production is most needed at this point.
345. Comprehension, evaluation, health (c)
    2 Too little insulin causes ketoacidosis from high glucose level; coma may occur if the condition is untreated.
    1 Incorrect response. Too much insulin decreases the glucose level in the body and causes a hypoglycemic reaction.
    3 Incorrect response; there is a presence of ketone bodies.
    4 Absence of appetite usually occurs.
346. Knowledge, assessment, physiological (a)
    2 An abnormally high glucose level in the blood and glucose in the urine are characteristic symptoms of diabetes mellitus.
    1 Hypoglycemia is an abnormally low glucose level in the blood, making this statement incorrect.
    3 Hypoglycemia is an abnormally low glucose level in the blood, and hypokalemia is an abnormally low potassium level in the blood.
    4 Hyperglycemia is correct, but glycogen is the product of the breakdown of carbohydrates and is stored in the liver and muscles.
347. Comprehension, assessment, physiological (b)
    3 The skin becomes dry and flushed and the patient usually complains of extreme thirst with diabetic acidosis (coma).
    1 The skin is not moist, but dry; not pale, but flushed. A gradual loss of appetite, not extreme hunger, occurs with diabetic acidosis.
    2 The skin is dry, but not pale. Extreme hunger makes this response wrong. The patient usually has a gradual loss of appetite.
    4 The skin is flushed and anorexia may be present. The skin is dry, not moist with diabetic acidosis.
348. Comprehension, assessment, physiological (a)
    1 Increased levels of glucose in the blood are a result of insufficient insulin to help the body use glucose.
    2 This would be the result of excess insulin in the blood.
    3 This would result in hypoglycemia.
    4 Pancreatic juices play a role in digestion of foods, not in the body's use of glucose.
349. Knowledge, assessment, physiological (b)
    2 These symptoms along with Kussmaul's respirations and an increased pulse rate are later symptoms of diabetic acidosis.
    1, 3, 4 These are symptoms of insulin shock.
350. Knowledge, assessment, physiological (c)
    4 Ketoacidosis is the accumulation of glucose and waste products from the increased metabolism of fats and proteins.
    1 Insulin reaction occurs when the body has increased insulin in the blood.
    2 Hypoglycemia is an abnormally low level of glucose in the blood.
    3 Diabetic retinopathy is a severe complication of diabetes in which there are pathological changes involving the optic nerve that can lead to blindness.

351. Comprehension, assessment, physiological (b)
    2 Fragile skin that is prone to breakdown is a classic symptom of Cushing's syndrome.
    1 Cushing's syndrome usually causes weight gain from retention of sodium and water.
    3 Cushing's syndrome causes hypertension because of retention of sodium and water.
    4 Cushing's syndrome causes hyperglycemia and can induce diabetes.

352. Comprehension, planning, environment (c)
    3 Depression is a sign of Cushing's syndrome. Increased mental stability would be an appropriate goal.
    1 Patient's with Cushing's syndrome need to be on a low sodium diet.
    2 Because they retain fluids, patients need fluid restriction.
    4 Weight loss is a more appropriate goal.

353. Comprehension, planning, health (b)
    1 Because sodium and water are retained as a result of the increase in cortico steroid levels, a low-sodium diet is an important intervention in Cushing's syndrome.
    2 High protein is not necessary; calcium should not be decreased because of bone softening from the disease.
    3 This would irritate skin that is prone to breakdown.
    4 Blood glucose levels are important, but urine glucose levels are unnecessary and inaccurate.

354. Comprehension, planning, physiological (b)
    1 Overstimulation by the pituitary hormone ACTH produces an overabundance of the hormone in the cortex of the gland.
    2 Incorrect response; hypoplasia is a decreased amount of the hormone produced.
    3, 4 Inappropriate; the question does not state "secretions from which part of the gland."

355. Comprehension, assessment, physiological (b)
    3 Muscle weakness is a result of muscle wasting away; osteoporosis is a result of abnormal calcium absorption.
    1 Hypertension is more the case with peripheral edema and weight gain.
    2 Increased appetite and weight gain are more usual. Muscle weakness does occur.
    4 Moon face does occur from overabundance of the hormone, but hypertension is indicated because of weight gain and edema.

356. Comprehension, planning, physiological (b)
    1 This procedure is necessary to maintain fluid balance.
    2, 4 These are not a primary concern.
    3 Sugar is not excreted in urine.

357. Comprehension, planning, environment (b)
    3 Adrenocorticotropic hormone (ACTH) is released by the anterior portion of the pituitary gland, which regulates functional activity of the adrenal cortex.
    1 The adrenal cortex secretes cortisol and androgens; the adrenal medulla secretes the catecholamines epinephrine and norepinephrine.
    2 Growth is a factor related to the thyroid hormone.
    4 ACTH stimulates growth of the adrenal gland cortex and the secretion of corticosteroids.

358. Application, implementation, environment (c)
    4 Accurate records of intake and output provide information about fluctuation and instability of the adrenocortical hormones, thus preventing complications.
    1 Included in all for postoperative management but not the most significant in this case.
    2, 3 These are not the highest priority in this case.

359. Comprehension, evaluation, physiological (c)
    1 Addison's disease is adrenocortical insufficiency when adrenal glands do not secrete adequate amounts of ACTH.
    2, 3 These do not directly involve the parathyroid.
    4 This does not involve the thyroid gland.

360. Application, implementation, health (c)
    2 Stress is the major precipitating factor in adrenal crisis.
    1 Salt intake should be restricted.
    3 Moderate activity with some rest periods is required.
    4 There is no interference with insulin production from the pancreas.

361. Comprehension, implementation, environment (b)
    4 Cystoscopic examination allows visualization of the inside of the bladder.
    1 The size, shape and location of the kidneys are usually determined by an intravenous pyelogram.
    2 The prostate gland is usually not visualized with contrast media and cannot be seen on cystoscopic examination.
    3 Visualization of the ureters requires the use of a contrast media. A cystoscopic examination does not require the use of a contrast media.

362. Knowledge, planning, environment (a)
    1 The examination of the kidneys, ureters and bladder (KUB) provides proper visualization of the structures to confirm the suspected diagnosis.
    2 The cystourethrogram is a radiograph of the urinary bladder and urethra; it is insufficient to confirm diagnosis.
    3 Cystometry is a study of bladder function.
    4 Proctoscopy is an examination of the rectum with an endoscope.

363. Knowledge, planning, environment (a)
    3 The purpose of the urine culture is to identify the organism in the genitourinary (GU) tract and to determine which antibiotics they are sensitive to.
    1 This would be a routine urinalysis.
    2 This would be a urine cytology test.
    4 This is not a purpose of the urine culture and sensitivity.

364. Application, implementation, environment (a)
    4 To properly collect a 24-hour urine specimen, the patient discards the first void. Timing begins when the patient collects the total amount of voiding for 24 hours.
    1 This is not a 24-hour specimen; separate containers not necessary.
    2 This is not a 24-hour specimen; all urine is to be collected after the patient discards the first void.
    3 This is not a 24-hour specimen; this is the procedure for maintaining strict intake and output.

365. Knowledge, assessment, environment (b)
    3 Intravenous urogram (pyelogram) is the test that allows for visualization of the size, shape and structure of the kidney, ureters, and bladder. It also determines if the bladder empties sufficiently in a post-void film.
    1 Cholecystography is an x-ray examination using a contrast substance to evaluate the functioning of the gallbladder and to detect disease or gallstones.
    2 Cystography is an examination of the urinary bladder using a contrast medium introduced through a urethral catheter.
    4 Retrograde pyelography is a more sophisticated test of the urinary system whereby a contrast medium is injected directly into the ureters through catheters introduced through a cystoscopy; this test is generally used to confirm findings suspected on the intravenous urogram.

366. Knowledge, assessment, physiological (a)
    2 Severe flank pain and hematuria are cardinal symptoms of renal calculi.
    1 These may be symptoms of incontinence and/or infection.
    3 Frequency and dysuria are indicative of cystitis.
    4 Urgency and polyuria may be associated with an endocrine disorder.

367. Comprehension, assessment, physiological (b)
    1 Severe, colicky flank pain, radiating to the testes, is a common symptom of renal calculi in male patients.
    2 This is not a symptom of renal calculi.
    3 These are more common symptoms of urinary tract infection.
    4 This may be a symptom of bladder cancer.

368. Knowledge, planning, physiological (a)
    4 Renal colic is a spasm in the tubular structure of the ureter that causes pain.
    1 The kidney moves from its normal bed of fat but does not produce symptoms described in this case.
    2 Hardening of the kidney does not present the symptoms described.
    3 Collection of urine in the kidney does not present the symptoms described.

369. Application, planning, environment (a)
    2 Straining urine allows observation of passage of the stone(s).
    1 On the contrary, fluid should be encouraged to flush out the stone(s).
    3, 4 These are not medically necessary.

370. Application, implementation, environment (a)
    4 2 mg per 1 ml (cc); desired is 5 mg; have 2 mg per 1 ml; dose is 2.5 ml.
    1, 3 This is too low a dose.
    2 This is too high a dose.

371. Comprehension, evaluation, environment (b)
    2 Peristalsis is activation of wavelike motion that assists in forcing food through the digestive tract.
    1 There has not been not sufficient time for the digestive process to begin working.
    3 There could be insufficient time for the digestive process to begin working or the IV could be maintained long after the digestive process has been restored.
    4 There is no direct relationship.

372. Knowledge, planning, health (a)
    2 These foods are high in calcium.
    1 These foods are high in protein.
    3, 4 These foods are most noted for their vitamin and fiber content.

373. Comprehension, evaluation, health (b)
    2 This combination of foods contains very little calcium.
    1 Cheese and green salad are high sources of calcium.
    3 Yogurt and broccoli are high sources of calcium.
    4 Spinach and skimmed milk are high sources of calcium.

374. Knowledge, assessment, environment (b)
    3 Painless hematuria is the most common early symptom of cancer of the bladder.
    1 Suprapubic pain may be present in cancer of the bladder, but it is not the most common early symptom.
    2 Elevation of temperature is usually a symptom of an infection or inflammatory disease; it is not necessarily an early sign of cancer of the bladder.
    4 Dysuria may be a symptom of cancer of the bladder, but painless hematuria is the earliest symptom.

375. Comprehension, assessment, physiologic (b)
    4 Urinary retention due to enlargement of the prostate is a classic symptom of benign prostatic hypertrophy (BPH).
    1, 2, 3 Bleeding and pain usually do not occur with BPH unless there is an infection present.

376. Application, implementation, physiological (a)
    2 To obtain the urinary output, subtract the amount of solution from the total urinary drainage in the bag.

$$\begin{array}{r} 3800 \text{ ml} \\ - 2000 \text{ ml} \\ \hline 1800 \text{ ml} \end{array}$$

    1 This amount is too much.
    3, 4 These amounts are too little.

377. Application, implementation, environment (b)
    3 Assessing for urinary retention resulting from blockage would be the priority initial intervention at this time.
    1 Mild spasms are normal. A feeling of having to void could indicate urinary blockage and must be assessed further.
    2 This is not to be done if the bladder is already full.
    4 Assessment of the bladder must be done first and findings reported to the team leader.

378. Comprehension, planning, environment (b)
    4 Kegel exercises can strengthen the perineal muscles and help control bladder function.
    1, 2, 3 These will not promote urinary control.

379. Comprehension, assessment, physiological (a)
    3 Because of blockage as a result of the neoplasm, the patient has had increasing problems with urine passing through the urethra.
    1 Incorrect response; urine is not creating the urgent need to void.
    2 Incorrect response; urine is not able to pass, so the patient is not voiding frequently.
    4 Incorrect response; there is not much chance of burning sensation when blockage is the problem.

380. Knowledge, planning, physiological (b)
    2 This condition is a common occurrence with the over-55 male group.
    1 Recurrent infection is not a predisposing factor.
    3 Sitting on the job is not a contributory factor.
    4 Sexual inactivity is not a predisposing factor.

381. Comprehension, planning, environment (a)
    4 Incision is made through the abdomen; the bladder is opened and the gland is removed from above.
    1 This is a perineal prostatectomy.
    2 This is a transurethral prostatectomy.
    3 This is a retropubic prostatectomy.

382. Application, implementation, environment (b)
    3 It is important to observe for bleeding, clots, concentration of the urine, and for satisfactory amount of urine output.
    1 This is important, but it is not a major consideration.
    2 Incorrect response; increased fluid intake is important to not only hydrate the patient but to flush the system.
    4 This may be indicated, but it is not a major consideration.

383. Application, implementation, environment (b)
    1 This is an indication that the tubing is not patent and that there may be blockage preventing flow of urine.
    2 As long as the urine is flowing there is no need for irrigation.
    3 Inappropriate response; judgment must be based on clinical indications.
    4 Pain is not always an indicator of problems with urinary flow.

384. Application, implementation, health (b)
    2 It is important to use sterile techniques with the presence of urine to avoid infection and skin irritation.
    1 Incorrect response; the sterile technique must be followed.
    3 Inappropriate response; appropriate care of the wound and skin needs to be maintained.
    4 Inappropriate response; the analgesic will not decrease or stop spasm or urine flow.

385. Application, implementation, physiologic (b)
    3 Bowel sounds should be present in all four abdominal quadrants before the patient is given food.
    1 Food may be given when bowel sounds are present. Food intake may help the patient expel flatus.
    2 This is not necessarily true.
    4 IV fluids are usually continued until the patient is able to retain at least a clear liquid diet.

386. Knowledge, planning, environment (a)
    3 Ice cream does not come from a clear liquid and is therefore not included in the diet.
    1 Tea and coffee without milk or cream is permitted.
    2 Popsicles and gelatin come from clear liquids.
    4 Chicken and beef broth or bullion are clear liquids.

387. Application, implementation, physiological (b)
    1 Under normal circumstances, Mr. Bell should be able to stand beside the bed to void. This facilitates bladder emptying for men.
    2 Applying pressure over the bladder is contraindicated for a herniorrhaphy.
    3 Noninvasive interventions should be tried before catheterization is done.
    4 Notify the physician if noninvasive measures have not been successful. The physician usually orders a catheterization prn.

388. Application, implementation, health (b)
    3 After a herniorrhaphy, the patient should avoid lifting or straining for 6 weeks. Using a book as an example gives the patient a reference weight.
    1 After a herniorrhaphy most patients can return to work as soon as they feel they are able, as long as they understand that they may not lift or strain.
    2 A soft diet is not necessary. Roughage should be increased to avoid constipation and straining.
    4 A shower is the best method of bathing because running water keeps the incision clean. Tub bathing is not the best method of bathing.

389. Comprehension, assessment, physiological (b)
    4 Because of the retention of waste products, including sodium, hypertension is an expected result of acute renal failure.
    1, 2, 3 These are not signs of acute renal failure.

390. Application, implementation, environment (c)
    3 Elevating the head of the bed to high-Fowler's position would be the first nursing action for a patient who is experiencing dyspnea.
    1, 2 No. 3 would be done before these.
    4 No. 3 would be done before this. In any case this may not be appropriate, depending on the cause.

391. Comprehension, assessment, physiological (b)
    4 Hearing a bruit indicates that blood is rushing through the shunt and the shunt is functioning properly.
    1, 2, 3 It is not conclusive that the shunt is patent.

392. Comprehension, evaluation, health (b)
    3 Applesauce and raisins contain no protein.
    1 Custard is made with milk and eggs, which contain protein.
    2 Yogurt is made with milk.
    4 Gelatin contains protein and cream also has a small amount of protein.

393. Application, implementation, environment (a)
    4 Diagnosis is confirmed by a gram-stained smear of the discharge from the penis.
    1 A blood test is used to diagnosis syphilis, not gonorrhea.
    2 Cervical cultures are usually inadequate in diagnosing the disease in women; it is necessary that cultures from a variety of areas be taken (cervix, urethra, throat, and anus).
    3 See response to No. 2.

394. Knowledge, implementation, environment (a)
    2 Lying on her back with thighs flexed on the abdomen allows for easier accessibility to the perineal area; position also allows for easier visualization of the reproductive organs.
    1 Lying on her side with a knee drawn up does not allow for easy access to the perineal area.
    3 Lowering the head with feet elevated does not allow for easy access to the perineal area.
    4 Lying down with moderately flexed, outward rotated extremities does not provide easy access to the perineal area.

395. Comprehension, implementation, health (a)
    2 Her age category places her at high risk for cervical cancer, so early detection is imperative.
    1 Incorrect response; irregular periods are caused by a variety of reasons.
    3, 4 Incorrect response; she is in a high-risk category, and early detection is imperative.

396. Knowledge, planning, environment (a)
    1 This allows for comfort, safety, visualization of the uterus, and a decrease in pressure caused by a full bladder that lies just behind the uterus.
    2 This has no direct relationship to the examination.
    3 It is unnecessary to restrict fluid because there is no direct relationship to the examination.
    4 An increased amount of urine in the bladder affects comfort, safety, and visualization of the uterus.

397. Knowledge, planning, environment (a)
    4 Scrapings of secretions and cells from the cervix are analyzed for the presence of cancer cells.
    1 Blood tests are used to determine ovarian function.
    2 There is no test available to do so; the length of the cervix is not really important.
    3 The pH of vaginal secretions is determined by use of nitrazine sticks.

398. Knowledge, assessment, physiological (a)
    2 Menorrhagia is defined as abnormally heavy or long menstrual periods that occur occasionally during most women's reproductive years.
    1 This is the absence of menstruation.
    3 This is uterine bleeding other than that caused by menstruation.
    4 This is painful menstruation.

399. Application, implementation, psychosocial (b)
    3 This response indicates recognition and understanding by the nurse and allows the patient the opportunity to discuss her feelings in greater detail.
    1 With this response the nurse does not recognize the patient's concern and assumes too much specific to the relationship between the patient and her husband.
    2 This response, although a possibility, does not offer recognition or understanding by the nurse.
    4 This response by the nurse does not address the patient's concern nor does it indicate understanding of the patient's feelings at this time.

400. Comprehension, planning, health (b)
     3 A physical activity that does not cause strain is swimming, which is often helpful for both physical and emotional well-being.
     1 Resuming sexual activities is permitted within 4 to 6 weeks following surgery; 2 weeks is too soon.
     2 Strenuous activities such as jogging, dancing and fast walking cause congestion of blood in the pelvis; avoid such activity for several months.
     4 Heavy lifting and strenuous physical activity should be avoided for several months.
401. Knowledge, planning, environment (b)
     2 This is an abnormal condition characterized by ectopic growth and function of endometrial tissue.
     1 This is an inflammatory condition of the endometrium, usually caused by bacterial infection.
     3 This is an inflammatory condition of the internal eye, in which the eye becomes red, swollen, painful, and sometimes, filled with pus.
     4 This is an infection of the intestine or liver by a species of pathogenic amebas.
402. Application, implementation, physiological (b)
     1 Maintaining the patient in a low-Fowler's position or flat in bed will prevent increased intraabdominal pressure strain on the suture line.
     2 A laxative and several enemas are given 24 hours before surgery to ensure a relatively empty bowel. Clear fluids are given 24 hours before surgery to reduce the contents of the bowel. For 5 days after surgery only liquids are permitted by mouth.
     3 Camphorated tincture of opium (paregoric) is administered to further inhibit bowel function.
     4 Enemas to relieve flatus and cleanse the bowel are withheld for at least 1 week following surgery.
403. Application, implementation, environment (a)
     3 Treatment of choice for stage I cervical cancer is a radical hysterectomy with pelvic lymph node dissection.
     1 This is stage II of cervical cancer; it does not involve the lower third of vagina.
     2 This is stage 0 of cervical cancer.
     4 Cervical cancer stage IV is all-inclusive; the cancer extends outside the cervix, involving the pelvic wall, the lower third of the vagina, bladder and rectum. Metastatic spread may also be indicated.
404. Comprehension, planning, physiological (c)
     3 A decrease in the systolic pressure causes cessation of glomerular filtration. The body at this point is unable to rid itself of fluid and nitrogenous wastes. Treatment for shock usually is done by fluid replacement and vasoactive drugs. Response to treatment assists urinary output to return to normal.
     1 Activity tolerance is an expected outcome; pulse increase should be no more than 20 per minute.
     2 This is an expected outcome, but not necessarily for toxic shock syndrome.
     4 This is an expected outcome, but it is not a greater priority than No. 3.

405. Knowledge, assessment, physiological (b)
     3 The vaginal discharge is as described and in most instances the vulva are inflamed, edematous and often excoriated as a result of scratching. Similar white and curdlike patches seen in the newborn are known as thrush.
     1 A white vaginal discharge normally occurs in varying amounts and consistency during the course of the menstrual cycle and is not indicative of disease.
     2 This describes the vaginal discharge from a patient with bacterial vaginosis.
     4 This describes the vaginal discharge from a patient with trichomoniasis.
406. Application, implementation, health (b)
     4 Nurses are vital in the role as patient educators; for this patient the nurse's teaching includes aspects of self-care, prevention, transmission and ways to prevent recurrence of the disease.
     1 This is not the most appropriate response. The patient is 18 years of age and not usually concerned about infertility. No. 4 is priority in the prevention of infertility.
     2 It is strongly recommended that both the patient and all sexual partners are treated individually. Sharing would reduce effectiveness of the treatment and could possibly lead to unwanted complications (an allergic response to the medication).
     3 The condition in and of itself is not life-threatening.
407. Application, implementation, health (a)
     3 Breast self-examinations done on a regular basis are the most accessible tool to detect early breast lesions. Although statistics indicate that 90% of all breast cancers are discovered by self-examinations, many detections are not reported immediately because of fears of mutilation and of death.
     1 This is currently being evaluated for use in detecting lesions in dense breasts of younger women. Its value as a diagnostic tool for breast cancer is still being determined.
     2 Annual mammography is recommended for all women over 50 years of age, according to the American Cancer Society.
     4 This is an important aspect of prevention; however, this does not replace the necessity of doing regular breast self-examinations.
408. Application, implementation, environment (a)
     4 A sign should be made indicating that blood pressure checks, injections and blood tests are not to be done on the affected side because these would increase potential for impairment of circulation and infection. Lymph edema is a very real concern for this patient.
     1 This may be so, but it is not the most appropriate response.
     2 Although a quiet and comfortable environment is a goal, patient observation is an absolute must. A dimly lit room may not be the best environment, especially immediately following surgery.
     3 This is true, but it is not the most appropriate response.

409. Comprehension, assessment, environment (b)
    4 Bleeding from a mastectomy can trickle down the side to the back of the patient. Turning the patient and feeling her side will detect such bleeding.
    1 This would miss bleeding on the side. Dressings are usually removed by the physician immediately after surgery.
    2 Every 4 hours would be too long to wait to check the patient.
    3 This is unnecessary and could lead to the development of infection. Dressings are usually removed by the physician initially after surgery.

410. Application, implementation, environment (b)
    3 This position elevates the extremity high enough to prevent lymphademia.
    1, 2 Abduction and adduction of the affected arm is contraindicated after a mastectomy. The arm should not be suspended.
    4 The patient's arm is not elevated high enough in this position.

411. Application, implementation, psychosocial (a)
    4 This statement reflects on the patient's feelings, allowing for open communication.
    1 This is giving advice, closing communication between nurse and patient.
    2 Silence would not be an appropriate method of fostering communication at this time.
    3 Commenting on how everyone else feels does not help the way the patient feels; this blocks communication.

412. Application, implementation, environment (b)
    3 To prevent damages to the lymphatic circulation, this is most important for the patient to understand.
    1 The diet should be high in protein and vitamin C to ensure wound healing.
    2 Exercises should be performed at least three to four times a day; once is not enough.
    4 Although important, No. 3 is more important.

413. Comprehension, evaluation, health (b)
    1 This step is important to assess for symmetry of the breast.
    2 The pillow should be under the right shoulder when examining the right breast.
    3 The patient must be in a flat supine position when examining the breasts.
    4 To flatten breast tissue, her right arm must be over her head when examining her right breast.

414. Application, assessment, physiological (c)
    2 18% for the chest, 4.5% for one inner arm and 4.5% for the other inner arm.
    1, 3, 4 These are incorrect totals.

415. Comprehension, planning, physiological (b)
    1 Fluid replacement is based on the combination of body surface burned and body weight.
    2 The patient's usual intake has no relationship to fluid lost from the burned surface.
    3 The standard requirement does not take into consideration body surface burned and weight.
    4 This is part of the formula to determine the amount of fluid replacement, but the patient's weight is needed as well.

416. Comprehension, planning, physiological (a)
    4 This monitors renal functioning on an hourly basis.
    1 The bedpan is difficult and painful to use, and it decreases the chance of accurate measuring of output.
    2 This is not a significant factor.
    3 This has no relationship to caring for burned patients.

417. Comprehension, implementation, environment (b)
    4 Burn patients are highly susceptible to transmitted infection.
    1 This is the purpose of isolation precautions.
    2 Isolation precautions are taken to protect hospital personnel.
    3 Protects the patient from microorganisms being transmitted to him by visitors.

418. Knowledge, assessment, environment (a)
    3 Protective or reverse isolation is used for burn patients because they are more susceptible to infections.
    1 Enteric precaution is for illnesses that transmit microorganisms through excreta.
    2 Drainage or discharge precaution is for illnesses that transmit microorganisms through the drainage or discharge from a wound.
    4 Respiratory isolation is for illnesses that transmit microorganisms through the respiratory tract.

419. Knowledge, assessment, physiological (a)
    3 A homograft is done primarily to help prevent fluid loss from the burn site and to prevent infection.
    1 Pain is only decreased through narcotic or analgesics in first- and second-degree burns.
    2 A homograft will aid in improving circulation at the burn sites, but it is used primarily to prevent fluid loss and infection.
    4 The patient's diet will assist the body in healing itself and in rebuilding lost tissue.

420. Knowledge, assessment, health (a)
    4 There is pain associated with first- and second-degree burns, and a narcotic is given.
    1 Meperidine hydrochloride (Demerol) is given preoperatively to allay anxiety; it is given in this situation for pain.
    2 Meperidine hydrochloride does not prevent nausea, which is an adverse effect of this drug.
    3 Meperidine hydrochloride is not used to promote sleep, but dizziness and drowsiness are adverse effects of this drug.

421. Application, planning, health (c)
    1 Cheese and nuts are high in protein content. A diet rich in protein helps to rebuild tissue destroyed by burns.
    2 Cheese spread contains protein but the potato chips contain little or no protein.
    3 Jello with cream contains little or no protein. Milk is a complete protein.
    4 Popcorn and pretzels contain little or no protein.

422. Comprehension, implementation, physiological (b)
    2 Exposed skin area and burned skin increase the incidence for infection significantly.
    1 This may be secondary, depending on the patient's past health history and heart condition.
    3 Close monitoring of urinary output decreases the incidence of this being a causative factor.
    4 Inappropriate response.

423. Comprehension, evaluation, health (b)
    1 The condition of the burns and her total well-being are major factors.
    2 This is included in her total well-being.
    3 Self-care is included in her total well-being.
    4 This is important, but the patient is the primary factor.

424. Application, planning, physiological (a)
    3 The otoscope is the instrument used to visualize the internal structures of the ear.
    1 The ophthalmoscope is used to examine the eye.
    2 The laryngeal mirror is used to examine the throat.
    4 The Pomeroy syringe is used to irrigate the ears.

425. Application, planning, physiological (a)
    2 The laryngeal mirror is used to visualize the throat.
    1 The Schioetz tonometer is used to measure intraocular pressure.
    3 The ophthalmoscope is used to visualize the internal structures of the eye.
    4 The otoscope is used to examine the ear.

426. Comprehension, assessment, physiological (a)
    4 A characteristic symptom of a developing cataract is progressive blurring of vision that seems like a film over the eye. This is a result of partial or complete opacity of the crystalline lens or its capsule. There is an eventual loss of vision.
    1 Refractive errors indicate a condition in which the light rays do not appropriately focus on the retina.
    2 Glaucoma is a result of increased intraocular pressure.
    3 Retinal detachment occurs when the retina is dislodged and the usual symptoms are spots and bright flashes of light.

427. Application, planning, environment (a)
    1 The ophthamologist is a medical physician who specializes in diagnosis, treatment, and surgery of the eyes. The physician may also prescribe corrective lens if necessary.
    2 The optometrist prescribes corrective lenses for refractive errors. This person does not diagnose disease, prescribe medication, or treat disease of the eyes.
    3 The optician fills prescriptions for corrective lenses and makes adjustments of glasses for proper fitting.
    4 The neurologist specializes in the diseases and treatment of the nervous system.

428. Knowledge, assessment, physiological (b)
    1 Trauma, infection, or disease process is the most likely cause of a cataract developing in a person under the age of 40.
    2 It is common for cataracts to develop as a result of the aging process, but this is not the correct answer for this question.
    3 Weight is not a factor that leads to the development of a cataract.
    4 Cataracts are not related to any occupational factor or how much the eyes may be used in working or reading.

429. Knowledge, assessment, environment (a)
    4 Spots (floaters) and flashes of light are indicative of retinal detachment.
    1 This is not indicative of retinal detachment, but it could be an adverse reaction to medication.
    2 This is not indicative of retinal detachment or other complications related to cataract extraction.
    3 Myopia (nearsightedness) and purulent drainage are not appropriate responses. Myopia is a refractive error and purulent drainage could be infection.

430. Comprehension, assessment, physiological (a)
    2 There is a gradual opacification of the lens as a result of the aging process.
    1 This is a symptom of glaucoma.
    3 Incorrect response.
    4 This is a separation of the retina from the choroid in the posterior area of the eye.

431. Comprehension, planning, environment (a)
    3 It is important to ensure the proper technique of handwashing, administration of the medication, and application of the eye patch.
    1 There is no need for lengthy bed rest.
    2 This is not needed, except in the bright sunlight.
    4 This is an inappropriate response.

432. Application, implementation, psychosocial (b)
    4 This response allows the patient to talk about her feelings and raises questions that need to be addressed.
    1 This response cuts the patient off and does not allow her to state what is really bothering her.
    2 This gives false reassurance.
    3 This response doesn't address the patient's concerns.

433. Comprehension, implementation, physiological (a)
    1 These symptoms indicate complications such as internal bleeding, increased fluid, or internal pressure in the eye.
    2 This is a common occurrence with retinal detachment.
    3 This is an inappropriate response.
    4 This is not the best response; blurred vision is to be expected.

434. Knowledge, assessment, environment (a)
    2 It is not necessary to speak in a louder voice because the patient does not have a hearing problem.
    1 Orientation to the room is particularly important to this patient.
    3 It is important to encourage the patient to express his needs.
    4 This is important for all patient admissions.

435. Application, planning, physiological (b)
    3 It is important to medicate the patient promptly if nausea occurs because vomiting may place undue pressure on his eyes.
    1 Coughing and deep breathing may cause pressure on the patient's eyes and should not be done.
    2 Mr. Charles should be able to move freely. He will need some ambulation assistance initially to regain his sense of balance.
    4 There is no reason why Mr. Charles cannot have visitors.

436. Application, implementation, environment (a)
    4 The nurse should orient the patient to where the food is located on his plate. Using the clock position as an example is very helpful.
    1 Assuming that he will need to be fed will hurt his sense of self-esteem.
    2 There is no reason to chop the food into small pieces. It may be helpful to ask if he would like any of his food cut up.
    3 The patient will need some assistance. Managing the meal by himself may be frustrating.

437. Knowledge, assessment, environment (a)
    3 Tonometry involves indirect measurement of intraocular pressure. The patient with glaucoma has an increased intraocular pressure.
    1, 2, 4 These tests are not specific for glaucoma.

438. Knowledge, assessment, physiological (a)
    4 The tonometer is used to measure intraocular pressure.
    1 The ophthalmoscope is used to visualize the internal structures of the eye.
    2 The Snellen chart is used to check refraction errors.
    3 The otoscope is used to examine the ear.

439. Comprehension, assessment, physiological (a)
    2 Increased intraocular pressure is a result of a blockage of the aqueous humor fluid in the anterior chamber of the eye.
    1 The vitreous humor is in the posterior chamber of the eye.
    3 An increase, not a decrease, of aqueous fluid is what causes glaucoma.
    4 In glaucoma there is an increase, not a decrease, in the intraocular pressure.

440. Knowledge, assessment, physiological (b)
     3 Acute glaucoma and closed-angle glaucoma are the same. The symptoms are sudden and require immediate attention.
     1 This refers to chronic glaucoma.
     2 This term indicates increased ocular pressure without symptoms.
     4 Chronic glaucoma symptoms are slow and progressive. Often the patient is not aware of damage until vision is lost.
441. Knowledge, assessment, health (a)
     4 The incidence of glaucoma increases over the age of 40.
     1, 2, 3 These are not related to the incidence of glaucoma.
442. Comprehension, assessment, physiological (b)
     2 Loss of peripheral vision is a sign of open-angle glaucoma.
     1 This could be a sign of infection, not glaucoma.
     3 Pain is not a symptom of open-angle glaucoma; it is a sign of closed-angle glaucoma.
     4 A reddened eye is a sign of closed-angle glaucoma, not open-angle.
443. Comprehension, evaluation, environment (a)
     4 Timoptic is a beta blocker that directly reduces the production of aqueous humor.
     1 There is no action on the pupil.
     2 Timoptic decreases the production of aqueous humor.
     3 There is no effect on the muscles of the eye.
444. Comprehension, assessment, physiological (c)
     1 Timolol (timoptic) could cause hypotension, so blood pressure readings are important before administering the drug. Acetazolamide (diamox) is a diuretic and could cause a loss of potassium; therefore, it is important to assess electrolyte balance.
     2 Timolol could cause bradycardia, but blood levels of these drugs are not significant.
     3 Blood pressure readings are important; urinalysis is not necessary.
     4 These readings would not be effected by timolol or acetazolamide.
445. Comprehension, planning, environment (b)
     1 Antihistamines could contain atropine, which increases intraocular pressure.
     2 Patching the eye is not necessary.
     3 This would be dangerous because visual activity is affected.
     4 Medications for glaucoma must be taken for life.
446. Knowledge, assessment, physiological (b)
     2 Flashes of light are a symptom of a detached retina.
     1 Detached retina is painless.
     3 This could be a symptom of cataracts or glaucoma, not detached retina.
     4 This is a symptom of acute open-angle glaucoma, not detached retina.
447. Comprehension, planning, environment (a)
     1 Bed rest is indicated preoperatively to prevent further tearing and bleeding of the retina.
     2 Coughing is contraindicated because it increases intraocular pressure and could cause further bleeding.
     3 Irrigation is not necessary in detached retina.
     4 Both eyes are patched to prevent ocular movements.

448. Comprehension, assessment, physiological (a)
     1 These are symptoms of Meniere's disease. Usually only one ear is affected. The patient experiences recurrent episodes of vertigo with associated nausea and tinnitus and sometimes hearing loss. During these attacks vomiting, diaphoresis and nystagmus may occur. Sudden movements aggravate symptoms.
     2 Meniere's disease is a *chronic* disease of the middle ear in which there is an increase in endolymph fluid either from increased production or decreased absorption. Although there is no specific therapy for this disease, fluid restriction, diuretics and a low-salt diet are usually prescribed in an attempt to decrease fluid pressure.
     3 This is most common in women between the ages of 50 and 60.
     4 The diagnostic testing includes an audiological tuning fork which shows a sensorineural deficit. Vestibular testing reveals lack of balance.
449. Comprehension, assessment, physiological (b)
     4 In heat stroke the body becomes overheated, but the cooling mechanism of perspiration does not operate, causing the body to store excessive heat.
     1 These are symptoms of food poisoning.
     2 These are symptoms of *heat exhaustion*.
     3 These are symptoms of frostbite.
450. Comprehension, planning, physiological (a)
     3 Establishing and maintaining an airway is a priority nursing intervention. It is important to cool the person as quickly as possible.
     1 This is the intervention for frostbite.
     2 This is the intervention for insulin reaction.
     4 This is the intervention for *heat exhaustion*.
451. Comprehension, planning, environment (b)
     2 This is a vasodilator that increases blood circulation and relieves bronchospasms in respiratory distress.
     1 This drug is for hypotensive conditions not associated with respiratory distress.
     3 Neosynephrine produces local vasoconstriction; it comes in drops or spray form.
     4 This is a slower-acting bronchodilator that is given by mouth.
452. Knowledge, evaluation, environment (b)
     4 A sudden release of histamines decreases the amount of blood available for circulation, thereby causing capillary hyperpermeability.
     1 This is the reaction of the nervous system to an emotional stimulus.
     2 Neurogenic shock is the result of failure of the nervous system to maintain normal contractions of the blood vessels.
     3 Anaphylatic shock is the result of poor heart function caused by various cardiovascular abnormalities.
453. Comprehension, assessment, physiological (b)
     1 This indicates a systemic reaction to increased histamine, which decreases the amount of blood for circulation.
     2 These are not symptoms presented with increased histamine in body. Pulse increases and blood pressure decreases.
     3 Cold and clammy skin accompanies shock.
     4 Lowered respiratory symptoms occur.

454. Comprehension, assessment, health (b)
    2 Patients often use denial and attribute the pain to something like indigestion. They will commonly use some form of home remedy before they realize the seriousness of their situation.
    1 Calling for help immediately is usually not the first action.
    3 Calling the physician is not usually the first action.
    4 Most patients will first try some form of remedy.

455. Application, assessment, health (a)
    4 The first rescuer should ascertain the presence of breathing and pulse. If it is not necessary to start cardiopulmonary resuscitation (CPR) immediately, the rescuer should call for help.
    1 The patient should not walk; he should lie down wherever he is.
    2 CPR is never initiated when the patient is still breathing and has a pulse.
    3 In the event of a heart attack, the rescuer should call for help rather than driving the victim to the hospital because there is no other assistance in the vehicle if it is needed for CPR.

456. Comprehension, implementation, environment (b)
    1 Airway patency commands primary consideration. If the airway is not patent, all ventilatory attempts will be futile and vital organs will quickly become oxygen-deprived.
    2 Breathing is definitely imperative, but as above, if the airway is not patent, oxygen/carbon dioxide exchange cannot occur.
    3 Promotion of circulation is another important consideration. However, it will be ineffective if the circulating blood is not properly oxygenated.
    4 Definitive therapy follows once the arrest state has been corrected.

457. Comprehension, assessment, physiological (c)
    3 Sinus tachycardia is a regular rhythm with a P wave for every QRS complex and a rate of 100 to 160 beats/min.
    1 Complete heart block indicates no impulses from the atria being conducted to the ventricles; the atria and ventricles contract independently of one another.
    2 Atrial fibrillation is characterized by a total disorganization of atrial electrical activity without effective atrial contraction. The atrial rate may be as high as 300 to 400 beats/min, while the ventricular rate is 100 to 160 beats/min.
    4 Sinus bradycardia is a regular rhythm with a P wave to every QRS complex and a rate of 40 to 60 beats/min.

458. Knowledge, planning, physiological (b)
    4 *Elective* cardioversion is a procedure in which electrical voltage is emitted via defibrillator paddles to restore normal electrical activity of the heart and thus eliminate rapid rhythms.
    1 *Elective* cardioversion is not the choice when ventricular conduction is in disharmony. This situation calls for *immediate* action, not elective.
    2 Cardioversion does not directly affect the pump action of the right ventricle, or for that matter, of any of the other chambers of the heart.
    3 Heart block is typically characterized by a disruption of electrical impulses through the atria and ventricles. Cardioversion may make the disturbance worse.

459. Knowledge, implementation, environment (c)
    2 Immediate defibrillation is the first choice to correct ventricular fibrillation.
    1 From a cardiac perspective, atropine's main action is to increase the heart rate; therefore it would be contraindicated in the treatment of ventricular fibrillation.
    3 Endotracheal intubation does not affect the electrical activity of the heart. However, the situation may warrant intubation once the fibrillatory state is corrected.
    4 Cardioversion is used for terminating rapid, less lethal dysrhythmia, not ventricular fibrillation.

460. Knowledge, planning, physiological (b)
    3 An electrocardiogram is a graphic measurement of electric currents generated by the conduction within the heart.
    1, 2 Echocardiography is a noninvasive technique that evaluates the internal structures and motions of the heart and great vessels. It shows internal dimensions of the chambers, size and motion of the intraventricular septum and posterior left ventricular wall; valve motion and anatomy; and direction of blood flow.
    4 Arterial blood gas studies provide information on the diffusion of gas across the alveolar capillary membrane and the adequacy of oxygenation of tissues.

461. Application, assessment, psychosocial (c)
    2 Anxiety and fear of dying is not unusual when a person has suffered a heart attack.
    1 The nurse is not giving Mr. Yates reassurance.
    3 This feeling is not typical.
    4 The heart attack does not necessarily affect the mind.

462. Knowledge, assessment, physiological (c)
    1 Oxygenated blood flows from the ascending aorta to nourish the heart muscles.
    2 The left subclavian artery carries blood to the upper left extremities.
    3 The carotid arteries carry blood to the head.
    4 Intercostal arteries carry blood to the chest wall.

463. Comprehension, assessment, physiological (b)
    2 These enzymes are mainly found in the heart muscle and released into the blood stream when there is injury to the myocardium.
    1 This is not applicable in damage to the myocardium.
    3 These are signs/symptoms of other conditions.
    4 Enzymes would be increased, not decreased.

464. Knowledge, planning, health (a)
    2 Legally, the nurse should obtain an account in her own words.
    1 Legally, this is not a requirement. The patient may feel more safe and secure if the nurse stays with her.
    3 Legally, this is not a requirement. In addition, the patient may not prefer to be alone.
    4 This would be preferable for the patient; however, it is not a legal requirement.

465. Knowledge, assessment, environment (a)
    4 It is important to prevent the transmission of venereal disease by early diagnosis and treatment.
    1 Painful urination may occur; however, a urinalysis is needed.
    2 Dysmenorrhea is painful menstruation; it is not a key reason for a physical examination.
    3 A pregnancy would be too early to detect. A prophylaxis can be given if a method of contraception is not already in use.

466. Knowledge, implementation, environment (a)
    2 Accountability is defined as being answerable for one's own actions.
    1 Responsibility refers to the carrying out of duties within the practice of nursing.
    3 Autonomy is acting independently within the boundaries of practice; it allows patients to make decisions about their care.
    4 Advocacy is a relationship between the nurse and the patient in which the nurse supports and promotes the patient's well-being.

467. Application, implementation, environment (c)
    4 Autonomy is acting independently within the boundaries of practice.
    1 Independence means being free from the influence or control of others; however, the professional term for this concept is autonomy.
    2 Accountability is defined as being answerable for one's own actions.
    3 Responsibility refers to the carrying out of duties within the practice of nursing.

468. Knowledge, assessment, health (b)
    3 The goal is to help the nurse reenter nursing in a systematic, planned and safe way. This may include restriction on narcotics for a period of time.
    1 If a colleague is suspected, it is important to notify the supervisor, who will often notify the state nursing association or board of nursing.
    2 Before peer assistance programs, often nurses would be fired or be free to move to other facilities where the abuse could continue.
    4 The basis of peer assistance programs is one nurse helping another nurse.

469. Knowledge, implementation, environment (a)
    1 The major need is personal and body functioning.
    2 This is an inappropriate response; they need to have a purpose in life.
    3 Isolation with only some group contact is unacceptable. It causes a mere state of existence rather than as full a life as possible.
    4 This is an unacceptable approach. These residents should be involved in making as many decisions as possible to maintian a sense of self-worth.

470. Knowledge, planning, health (a)
    3 Studies and evidence do not support this idea; creativity and intelligence do not change with age.
    1 This statement is true.
    2 This statement is true, although elderly people generally do not limit their ability to manage their households.
    4 The majority of elderly people have at least one weekly contact with family and a network of friends.

471. Knowledge, assessment, health (a)
    2 The myth is that most older people *are* isolated and alone. The majority of elderly people have at least weekly contact with family, and many have developed a network of friends who provide support and relationships.
    1 This is a myth because in reality, studies and evidence indicate the decline is not inevitable. Creativity and intelligence do not appear to decline. Serious decline in mental capabilities is generally the result of a disease process, not age.
    3 This is a myth because only 5% of the elderly reside in hospitals or nursing homes. The majority own and live in their own homes.
    4 This is a myth. Although most elderly people have at least one chronic condition, these conditions generally do not limit their ability to manage their households and activities on a day-to-day basis.

472. Comprehension, planning, environment (c)
    3 MDS clearly identifies areas that need to be addressed in planning resident care.
    1 This is not true. It is a valuable tool in planning care.
    2 This is incorrect. It is comprehensive information pertinent to the resident as a total person and his needs.
    4 This is not necessarily true. Some states have been given permission to use an alternate version.

473. Comprehension, planning, environment (c)
    4 RAPs are a tool that identifies problems and specific interventions to address in care plans.
    1 This is untrue because it is a valuable tool in planning care and possible changes as needs change.
    2 This is incorrect because this tool generates comprehensive information pertinent to the resident as a total person and his needs.
    3 This is incorrect because this tool provides the specific care needs.

474. Comprehension, assessment, health (c)
    1 U.S. Congress sought federal approval to ensure quality of care.
    2, 3, 4 These are incorrect because these requirements are for both Medicare and Medicaid.

475. Comprehension, assessment, health (c)
    3 Assessments must be conducted or coordinated by RNs along with appropriate participation of other health-care professionals.
    1, 2, 4 All health care personnel can participate, but the RN is the designated coordinator.

476. Comprehension, assessment, psychosocial (b)
    3 Adjusting to changes in one's health, family relationships and such problems as the loss of a job are normal characteristics for a middle-aged adult.
    1 Although the patient may be having trouble adjusting to the hospital, help from a social worker is premature at this time.
    2 If the patient has always provided for his wife, this is not an abnormal reaction to his illness.
    4 It is important to recognize that growing older is difficult for some, and adjusting to a loss of children and possibly a job is frightening to anyone, whether ill or not.

477. Knowledge, implementation, environment (a)
     1 Narrative charting describes events in sequence throughout the course of a nursing shift.
     2 SOAP charting is problem-oriented in nature; the S stands for subjective data; the O for objective data; A addresses the assessment or analysis of the problem; and the P relates to the plan.
     3 Focus charting is a modification of the SOAP charting method and uses a DAR format; the D stands for data; A represents action; and R is response.
     4 PIE is a problem-oriented form of charting; PIE is the acronym for problem, intervention, and evaluation.

478. Knowledge, implementation, environment (a)
     2 The "S" in SOAP charting is representative of what the patient states.
     1, 2, 4 These are examples of objective data.

479. Knowledge, implementation, environment (a)
     4 A Kardex is not a permanent part of the record and is altered frequently; therefore, using a pencil is appropriate.
     1 The flow sheet is part of the permanent record and the use of a pen is legally required for making entries.
     2 The discharge summary is a permanent part of the chart and therefore requires the use of a pen.
     3 The medication record is part of the permanent record, and the use of a pen is required.

480. Application, implementation, environment (c)
     4 This documentation provides specific objective information about the patient's neuromuscular status.
     1 "Limited" response is neither objective not specific.
     2 "Decreased" strength is broad and subjective.
     3 "At intervals" and "most of the time" are subjective assessments since they are nonspecific.

481. Comprehension, implementation, environment (c)
     2 The use of reassuring clichés is a barrier to therapeutic communication because these responses tend to convey to the patient that the nurse feels the patient is worrying needlessly or that the nurse does not understand the problem.
     1 The nontherapeutic technique of disagreeing with the patient implies that what the patient said is not acceptable. Disagreeing may serve to threaten the patient.
     3 By belittling the patient's feelings, the nurse devalues them by implying they are commonplace and insignificant. Belittling serves to lower the patient's self-esteem.
     4 The technique of giving approval creates a block by shifting the focus to the nurse's values. The nurse now becomes judgmental.

482. Knowledge, implementation, environment (b)
     1 The use of direct eye contact is one of the characteristics of attentive listening, conveying an attitude of caring and interest.
     2 The overuse of personal experiences focuses on the nurse and not the patient.
     3 The misuse of social graces implies that the nurse is not attentively listening.
     4 Providing privacy is an appropriate action to the situation; however, the use of direct eye contact *best* indicates that the nurse is interested in what the patient is saying.

483. Comprehension, implementation, environment (b)
     3 Denial is subconscious blocking of anxiety-producing events. Reality is distorted or transformed.
     1 Rationalization is a defense mechanism that transfers the self-responsibility to a person or an object.
     2 Regression is defined as a coping strategy that produces behaviors associated with an earlier developmental stage.
     4 Compensation as a defense mechanism means making up for a deficiency in one aspect of self-image by focusing on a feature that is considered to be an asset.

484. Comprehension, implementation, environment (c)
     1 Patients with an expressive aphasia have difficulty in speaking and writing. Associating words or providing pictures of physical objects assists the patient in communicating his needs.
     2 The patient with expressive aphasia can communicate, but he will need assistance.
     3 To best help the patient with expressive aphasia, the nurse should not supply the correct word immediately. The patient should have a longer time in which to respond.
     4 The patient should be encouraged and stimulated to talk.

485. Comprehension, assessment, environment (b)
     1 The cholecystogram is diagnostic for gallbladder disease.
     2 The gastroscopy procedure involves the use of an illuminated scope to visualize the stomach and surrounding structures.
     3 The fluorsocopy is an x-ray examination of the stomach that could reveal pathology.
     4 Gastric analysis examines gastric secretions to determine the presence of malignant cells.

486. Knowledge, assessment, physiological (a)
     1 Blood urea nitrogen (BUN) is one of the significant tests done to measure kidney function; it is elevated in renal disease.
     2 Inaccurate response; BUN is elevated in renal disease.
     3 The BUN is directly related to kidney disease.
     4 This is one of the most significant tests for determining renal function, particularly when correlated with blood creatinine levels.

487. Knowledge, assessment, physiological (c)
     3 CK-MB, isoenzymes LDH_1 and LDH_2 specifically measure the amount of myocardial tissue damage (necrosis).
     1 Although SGOT and SGPT may elevate in cardiac necrosis, these enzyme tests are more specific for liver dysfunction.
     2 CPK enzyme elevation may occur in cardiac necrosis; however, it may also elevate in musculoskeletal and/or cerebral injury. Therefore it is not specific for measuring cardiac damage. SGPT is more specific for determining liver dysfunction.
     4 Neither of these exist as a laboratory enzyme study.

488. Application, implementation, environment (b)
     2 When a 24-hour specimen is disrupted, a new container should be obtained and the collection should be restarted. Documentation of the reason for starting again and the time the new collection was started should be made in the nurses notes.
     1 The specimen collection could be inaccurate if all the urine for 24 hours was not collected.
     3 Adding to the urine already collected would result in some of the specimen being over 24 hours old, which could give false readings.
     4 There is no justification for waiting until the next morning unless the physician prefers to wait.

489. Comprehension, assessment, physiological (a)
     4 Once food is digested, gastric juices needed for digestion have no more food to work on; they irrigate stomach lining, forming ulcerations.
     1 Symptoms do not occur when food is in the stomach.
     2 Symptoms are less severe or absent when food is in the stomach.
     3 Gastric juices are stimulated by introduction of food.

490. Comprehension, implementation, environment (b)
     3 Having the patient take deep breaths will relax the external sphincter, allowing for easier passage of the catheter.
     1 Coughing would constrict the urinary meatus and sphincter.
     2 This technique would contaminate the catheter and increase the risk of introducing microorganisms into the bladder.
     4 This approach also increases the risk of contamination of the urinary tract.

491. Knowledge, assessment, physiologic (a)
     2 Residual urine is defined as the urine that remains in the bladder after urination.
     1 Reflex incontinence is an involuntary loss of urine occurring at predictable intervals when a specific urinary volume is reached.
     3 Urge incontinence is an involuntary passage of urine after a strong sense of urgency to void.
     4 Retention is an accumulation of urine in the bladder because the bladder is unable to empty.

492. Knowledge, assessment, physiologic (a)
     3 Residual urine measures the amount of urine left in the bladder after the patient voids.
     1 This methodology only measures urine output in an 8-hour period.
     2 This procedure does not relate to any urine testing method.
     4 This is not an appropriate method to test for residual urine. However, it may be used in urine glucose testing.

493. Knowledge, implementation, environment (a)
     2 It is suggested that 50 to 100 ml of urine be sent to the laboratory if possible, so that a thorough assessment can be performed.
     1 The size of the container has nothing to do with the suggested amount of urine to be collected.
     3 Water is contraindicated because it may dilute and/or contaminate the specimen.
     4 A routine urinalysis does not require the use of a sterile container; however, urine for culture and sensitivity does.

494. Comprehension, implementation, physiological (a)
     2 Reporting potential complication symptoms is an accountable nursing action. The vital signs are imperative for baseline assessment data.
     1 This is appropriate, but the patient needs first-priority assessment.
     3 This selection indicates poor clinical judgment, for it does not address the immediate potentially complicating symptoms.
     4 This could be done simultaneously in the assessment phase; however, selection No. 2 is the more complete nursing action, given the situation.

495. Application, implementation, physiological (c)
     2 This noninvasive method of a tight face mask will produce a range of 40% to 65% O_2 within the mask with the flow rate at 6 to 12 L/min.
     1 The nasal cannula will produce an oxygen range of 24% to 40% and will not usually be adequate for anesthesia recovery. The rate of 1 to 4 L/min is also inadequate.
     3 This method produces only varying amounts of O_2 to the patient.
     4 Rebreathing CO_2 in a paper bag will not provide O_2 levels to support increased tissue perfusion.

496. Application, implementation, physiologic (b)
     1 Removing as much mucus as possible allows more air to reach the smaller air passages.
     2 If the patient breathes as rapidly as possible, he may feel dizzy and hyperventilate.
     3 The patient should sit up as much as possible to allow for better use of the diaphragm.
     4 Some postoperative patients may not want to try the spirometer because of fear or postoperative discomfort; they must be encouraged.

497. Application, implementation, physiological (c)
     2 Clean gloves are permissable to remove the dressing, which should be removed one layer at a time to avoid dislodging the penrose drain.
     1 Removing the dressing all at once may dislodge or pull out the Penrose drain.
     3 The entire dressing should be changed.
     4 It is normally necessary to touch the clean gauze during a dressing change; therefore, clean, nonsterile gloves may be used to remove the old dressing and sterile gloves may be used to apply a clean dressing.

498. Application, assessment, physiological (b)
     3 Redness and swelling are common signs of a wound infection after surgery.
     1 An oral temperature of 101° F (38.3° C) is more indicative of an infection.
     2 A small amount of clear yellow drainage may be a normal part of the healing process. Cloudy, yellow/green drainage is not normal.
     4 A sudden drop in blood pressure on the day of surgery is more indicative of hemorrhage.

499. Application, assessment, physiological (b)
     3 Dorsiflexing the patient's foot is a good postoperative nursing action for the possible complication of an emboli. The nurse should report any complaints of pain (Homans' sign.)
     1 Patients ambulate or do passive exercises as soon as possible after surgery to prevent the formation of emboli.
     2 If used, elastic stockings should be worn constantly. They may be removed for a bath.
     4 The patient's legs should never be rubbed. This can stimulate the movement of a clot forming in the leg.

500. Knowledge, implementation, environment (a)
     3 100° F (37.7° F) to 105° F (40.5° C) is warm to the body.
     1, 2 These options are cooler than body temperature and will defeat the goal of warmth to the perineum.
     4 This temperature is hot enough to endanger skin integrity.

501. Application, implementation, environment (a)
     2 Of the four choices, this is the most important safety measure.
     1 To maintain the bed in low position is appropriate, but it is not the highest priority in this situation.
     3 Removing the pillow may be warranted; however, it is more a comfort measure than a safety measure.
     4 This is an important factor in safety principles, but it is not the highest priority in this situation.

502. Application, implementation, physiological (b)

2 A low blood pressure in one arm can be misleading, especially if the patient feels well and has no symptoms. The nurse should always compare the pressure in both arms before other interventions are initiated.

1 The physician may suggest that the pressure also be assessed in the other arm; two phone calls will have to be made instead of one.

3 It is safe practice to verify an abnormal reading with another nurse, but only after the assigned nurse has assessed the situation thoroughly.

4 This blood pressure warrants further investigation and this procedure alone would be unsafe.

503. Application, implementation, psychosocial (b)

4 Explaining that the protection is for him as well as the nurse would lessen his fear of being "dirty."

1 Just because it is hospital policy does not make the procedure any less threatening to the patient. This explanation does not offer enough support to the patient.

2 The nurse seems defensive in this response and needs to realize that the patient does not understand hospital policy.

3 This is a negative response that may imply that the nurse does not want to deal with any patient.

504. Comprehension, implementation, environment (b)

4 The urine in the Foley bag should never be allowed to flow back into the bladder. Urine in the bag could harbor microorganisms that could cause a urinary infection.

1 The overbed table is designated for eating and would probably be above the bladder.

2 In the patient's lap, the urine could flow back into the bladder.

4 The Foley catheter should be maintained as a closed system and does not need to be disrupted for this reason.

505. Application, assessment, physiologic (b)

1 The problem may simply be a result of the patient turning, causing kinks and blockage in the tubing.

2 The nurse should assess for other problems before alerting the physician.

3 The patient may feel fine even though the Foley is not draining well. This action may yield little help in solving the problem.

4 This should not be done first of all unless an order is obtained. Secondly, an increase in fluids may produce severe discomfort for the patient if the Foley is not working properly.

506. Comprehension, implementation, environment (c)

1 It is recommended to instill no more than 5 ml of irrigating solution into the ureters because of their small diameter and the close proximity to the kidney; more would allow for a greater risk of infection.

2, 3 This is too large an amount. It may flow directly into the kidneys, thus increasing the risk for infection.

4 This is not a sufficient amount of fluid for irrigation.

507. Knowledge, assessment, physiological (a)

4 Immobility promotes urinary stasis, lending itself to stone formation.

1 Increased fluid intake would decrease the formation of urinary stones.

2 Fat and protein metabolites are not known to be associated with urinary calculi.

3 Exercise may decrease stone formation, but it is not a significant preventive measure.

508. Knowledge, implementation, physiological (b)

3 Nitroglycerin is the primary drug of choice in the treatment of angina; it promotes coronary vasodilation.

1 Demerol, a narcotic analgesic, is used in the treatment of moderate to moderately severe pain and does not directly elicit coronary artery dilation.

2 In recent years, aspirin has been linked with decreasing the incidence of myocardial ischemia; it is thought that aspirin "thins" the blood and thus decreases the likelihood of clot formation. However, it has *no* effect on coronary dilation.

4 Although morphine sulfate induces a smooth muscle dilation, it is not the first drug of choice in treating angina because of its potency and potentially addictive properties.

509. Knowledge, implementation, physiological (a)

4 Perineal exercises strengthen the muscles of the perineum that support the urinary bladder; this helps reduce incontinence.

1 Perineal exercises do not effect the formation or amount of residual.

2 Urinary retention is not relieved by perineal exercises.

3 Dysuria usually indicates a bladder infection; perineal exercises may not be prescribed.

510. Knowledge, implementation, physiological (a)

3 Massage increases circulation to the affected area, thereby supplying nutrients to promote tissue health.

1 Alcohol causes drying, and rubbing the area may promote tissue destruction.

2 A semi-Fowler's position would cause direct pressure to the coccyx region.

4 Heating increases vasodilation; this measure is suggested when dealing with an open wound.

511. Comprehension, assessment, health (b)

3 Risk behavior is defined as any behavior or practice that increases a patient's susceptibility to accident or illness.

1, 2, 4 These selections promote wellness; therefore, they are not risk factors.

512. Comprehension, assessment, environment (a)

3 Assessment involves gathering, verifying and communicating data about a patient, which is the first phase of the nursing process.

1 The implementation process includes the nurse's performing or assisting in the achievement of patient-centered outcome. However, this is step No. 3 in the overall process.

2 The evaluation component measures the patient's response to outcomes. In this process, the nurse may need to alter the plan of care.

4 Nursing diagnosis follows the assessment phase and is the responsibility of the registered nurse.

513. Knowledge, assessment, physiologic (a)

2 A reduction in the volume of packed red blood cells per 100 ml of blood or in hemoglobin or in the number of circulating red blood cells may indicate an anemic condition.

1 This is the term used to designate a malignant neoplasm of blood-forming organs.

3 Hemolysis designates the breaking down or destruction of red blood cells.

4 Leukocytosis refers to an abnormally high white blood cell count (leukocytes).

514. Knowledge, assessment, physiologic (a)

3 Edema of the fingers is indicative of Na^+ retention.

1 Heartburn is not a symptom of fluid imbalance.

2 Skin rash is not a symptom of fluid imbalance.

4 Excessive tearing, when not related to crying, is usually indicative of a disorder of the lacrimal glands.

515. Comprehension, assessment, health (a)
    3 An illness that develops from an invasion of microorganisms is termed an infection.
    1 Inflammation is the body's reaction to injury or irritation, not to an invasion of pathogenic microorganisms.
    2 Allergy is an antigen-antibody reaction of the body to a substance, causing the body to be hypersensitive to that substance.
    4 Immunity is the body's ability to have a resistance to a specific disease. Resistance is the result of either active or passive immunity.

516. Comprehension, assessment, physiological (b)
    3 The heart's pumping mechanism fails, resulting in an insufficient amount of blood to meet the body's demand.
    1 Sudden spasms are not directly related to congestive heart failure.
    2 Clots are not present in the heart chambers.
    4 The problem is with the pumping action, not the structure.

517. Knowledge, assessment, physiological (a)
    4 The term syndrome designates a group of symptoms, which may be subjective or objective, as in a nephrotic syndrome, which is another name for nephrosis.
    1 This is the type of symptom that the patient describes to the nurse.
    2 This is the type of symptom that the nurse observes.
    3 A sign is a term that detects objective evidence. An example of an objective sign would be the "finding" following use of an instrument such as a percussion hammer, or blood pressure cuff.

518. Knowledge, assessment, physiological (a)
    3 A sign is objective evidence that is obvious and definitive as well as separate from the patient's impression (e.g., blood pressure reading).
    1 This is the type of symptom that the patient expresses to the nurse.
    2 This is the type of symptom that the nurse observes.
    4 The term syndrome designates a group of symptoms, such as in a nephrotic syndrome.

519. Knowledge, assessment, environment (a)
    2 Nausea is a subjective experience reported by the patient.
    1 Temperature is measurable; therefore it is an objective finding.
    3 Blood pressure results are an objective finding.
    4 Rapid shallow respirations are a visual quantitative finding.

520. Knowledge, assessment, environment (a)
    4 Temperature measurement is an objective finding that is obtained by the nurse.
    1 Loss of appetite is a subjective experience determined by the patient.
    2 Pain is a subjective experience reported by the patient. It may also include objective findings.
    3 Nausea is a subjective sensation reported by the patient.

521. Comprehension, assessment, environment (b)
    4 As the patient inhales and exhales, the nurse should observe a rise and fall of water level.
    1 Over 50 ml/hr of drainage is considered excessive.
    2 Excessive bubbling in the water-seal chamber may indicate an air leak.
    3 This would mean the suction apparatus is off or not working.

522. Comprehension, assessment, physiologic (b)
    3 In this way the nurse will transmit the organisms from her hands to her eyes.
    1, 2 Coming in contact with the person is not enough to transmit the disease.
    4 Transmission will not occur through a third person.

523. Application, implementation, environment (a)
    3 This follows universal precaution guidelines to decrease the possibility of needlestick injury.
    1 This action is a violation of the Centers for Disease Control (CDC) guidelines for universal precautions.
    2 This maneuver is in violation of CDC standards and has been linked to an increased incidence of needlestick injury.
    4 This action is not recommended and is not regarded as safe practice.

524. Knowledge, planning, environment (b)
    3 The vaccine provides resistance to and decreases the severity of the disease if it is contracted.
    1 The vaccine is to provide resistance to the organism before the possibility of contracting the disease.
    2 Human blood plasma is not used; it does not spread the disease.
    4 This is an incorrect response because different organisms cause the disease and vaccines are organism-specific.

525. Knowledge, planning, health (a)
    4 Cranberry juice acidifies the urine.
    1, 2, 3 These do not cause the urine to become acidic.

526. Comprehension, assessment, physiological (b)
    3 Suggested oral intake is approximately 1500 ml/24 hours; 800 to 1000 ml would be a moderate restriction given no further directions.
    1, 2 These amounts are not restrictive in nature.
    4 200 to 400 ml could lead to cellular dehydration and is rarely recommended.

527. Application, implementation, environment (b)
    3 Mouth care will relieve thirst and provide comfort to a patient who is NPO and who has a nasogastric tube to suction.
    1 The patient is NPO; he cannot have sips of water.
    2, 4 These will not relieve thirst.

528. Knowledge, planning, health (a)
    3 A high-fiber diet promotes regular defecation patterns.
    1 Low-fiber diets decrease peristalsis, which could possibly result in constipation.
    2 Low-fat diets are usually recommended for cardiovascular diseases.
    4 High-fat diets are contraindicated in health-promoting teaching.

529. Knowledge, planning, health (b)
    4 Puddings are usually made with whole or skim milk.
    1 Fresh pineapple's main nutrient value is a high vitamin C content.
    2 Fish is high in protein and low in fat.
    3 Potatoes are high in vitamin B and carbohydrates.

530. Knowledge, implementation, health (a)
    1 Sherbet is made without milk and can be included on a clear-liquid diet.
    2 This contains milk. It may be included on a full-liquid diet.
    3 Oatmeal is considered a soft food, not a clear liquid.
    4 Skim milk makes this a full liquid.

531. Knowledge, planning, environment (b)
    4 This intervention will prepare the patient for the painful dressing change.
    1, 2 These measures promote comfort, but the use of pain medication before the procedure is the more appropriate nursing measure.
    3 Diversion therapy is an appropriate nursing measure but does not take priority in alleviating the pain.

532. Comprehension, assessment, physiological (a)
    4 Pain is a subjective experience. It is helpful if the patient can freely describe his perception of the pain.
    1 Leaving the patient unattended may elevate anxiety and increase pain perception.
    2 This is nontherapeutic; it challenges his perception of the pain.
    3 This selection is supportive but does not address the nature of the pain.

533. Knowledge, planning, health (b)
    4 Although other selections may be true, this selection enables the nurse to design a plan that will ultimately promote the change to a healthful behavior.
    1 This fact could be incorporated in the patient teaching; however, it is not the prime consideration in promoting healthy behaviors.
    2 This is inappropriate because it challenges the patient's sense of being and does not promote a therapeutic relationship.
    3 This fact should be included in promoting healthful behaviors, but it is not the correct answer given the other selections.

534. Comprehension, planning, health (c)
    4 Before teaching is begun, the patient must realize he has a problem. Then he must work with the nurse to set his own goals for behavior change.
    1, 2 These will be done later.
    3 Both the patient and his wife must be involved in this.

535. Knowledge, implementation, psychosocial (a)
    1 Attentive listening promotes emotional well-being.
    2 This measure does not necessarily promote emotional well-being.
    3 This procedure may only be promoting physical well-being.
    4 The promotion of emotional well-being usually implies some contact between the patient and the nurse; avoidance behavior may not necessarily do this.

536. Knowledge, assessment, physiological (a)
    1 This is one of the most common side effects of narcotic analagesics and a common problem for the terminally ill patient. Other contributing factors are poor dietary intake and inactivity.
    2 Anorexia may be caused by nausea, vomiting, constipation, dysphagia, stomatitis, and infections.
    3 Nausea can be caused by narcotic analgesics; however, this is not the most commonly reported cause. Anxiety and constipation can also be causes.
    4 This is not a reported side effect.

537. Comprehension, implementation, environment (b)
    1 The licensed practical nurse or licensed vocational nurse works under the supervision of a physician and registered nurse. Bedside nursing interventions appropriate to the terminally ill are provided.
    2 This is the responsibility of the primary nurse who is usually a licensed registered nurse. The primary nurse evaluates the patient's response to treatment and is an advocate between patient, family, physician, and an interdisciplinary team.
    3 The hospice volunteer usually assumes these duties. The volunteer has completed volunteer training of at least 24 hours and continues support throughout the bereavement period.
    4 These functions are through the primary pastor who supports the patient and family in coping with their fears and uncertainties.

538. Knowledge, assessment, environment (a)
    4 Palliative care is alleviating or controlling symptoms, but it does not produce a cure.
    1 Although support to the patient is provided, this is not the definition of palliative care.
    2 Palliative care is *not* curative in nature, nor is it centered in curative measures.
    3 Palliative care is just one part of holistic care. The holistic care approach focuses on numerous aspects that may include physical, psychosocial, and spiritual issues using the disciplinary team.

539. Comprehension, planning, psychosocial (b)
    1 According to the Patient Bill of Rights, the patient has autonomy in the course of his care whenever possible.
    2 According to the Patient Bill of Rights, the patient has the right to informed consent or to refuse treatment. The physician can only act independently in emergency situations or when the patient is unable to respond.
    3 The nurse is regarded as the patient advocate and thus facilitates the wishes of the patient.
    4 A relative is only able to make minor decisions regarding treatment or care when the patient is unable to do so.

540. Comprehension, implementation, psychosocial (c)
    4 A recently enacted law requires residents to have a legally designated person to make decisions about his health care in the event that he is not able to do so.
    1 This does not have to do with financial decisions.
    2 This is not intended to take away the decision-making power from residents who are able to make such decisions.
    3 This does not have to do with health-care financing.

541. Comprehension, implementation, psychosocial (c)
    2 These are all aspects related to his physical and mental health while a resident is in the nursing home.
    1 This does not have to do with personal finances.
    3, 4 These do not have to do with responsibilities after death.

542. Application, planning, environment (b)
    2 Pain medication needs to be given early in the cycle so it will reach its peak effectiveness as the pain begins to worsen. If she has not been relieved of pain for the interval between medication, this information should be reported.
    1 If she has no pain she does not need to inform the nurse, nor would the nurse wish to promote scheduled drug administration without need.
    3 If pain is already severe, medication may not be as effective.
    4 The nurse wants patients to inform her if their pain medication is not having a long enough duration. The nurse may need to replan.

543. Application, implementation, environment (b)
    2 If blood is aspirated, a new needle and syringe should be prepared, and an alternative site used.
    1 The nurse should never proceed, because there is danger of injecting the medication directly into the blood stream.
    3 The nurse should never inject, because of the danger of giving medication directly into the bloodstream.
    4 The needle and syringe are contaminated and need to be changed before injecting in an alternative site.

544. Comprehension, planning, environment (c)
   3 Decreased metabolism and excretion of drugs occur in the aged; therefore it is prudent to give smaller doses, farther apart.
   1 Smaller doses may not achieve a desired effect, and because metabolism is decreased in the aged, there is a risk for the accumulation if doses are given too close together.
   2 Larger doses closer together are never given, as metabolism and excretion are decreased in the normal aging process.
   4 Larger doses could potentially lead to toxicity because metabolism and excretion are slowed in the aged.

545. Comprehension, implementation, physiological (b)
   2 Pulling the tissue taut reduces resistance to the needles entry through the skin.
   1 This is for disinfection.
   3 This is a safety measure to prevent intravenous administration.
   4 Medication should be injected slowly to decrease tissue discomfort.

546. Knowledge, implementation, physiological (a)
   2 Medication labels should be checked when retrieving the medication from the shelf or drawer, before pouring, and when replacing the container or discarding.
   1 Checking the order is to be sure it was transcribed correctly.
   3 The medication should be checked before it is poured, not after.
   4 The medication has already been given. The right drug should have already been verified.

547. Application, implementation, environment (b)
   4 Immunizations should be stored inside the refrigerator and maintained at 35° to 46° F and may become toxic or ineffective if frozen or they become too warm.
   1 This is unsafe; the pharmacy may not check on the agents until the refrigerator has cooled down again and the vaccines may mistakenly be used by others.
   2 This is unsafe; another employee may not notice the defect and use the vaccine.
   3 Agents should never be used once warmed to 80° F. Some of the agents may become virulent or inactive.

548. Application, implementation, environment (c)
   2 Unless witnessed, a nurse should refuse to sign any record concerning scheduled drugs. She could be held liable in a court of law.
   1 Although nurses may trust each other, the nurse is legally accountable for anything signed.
   3 Forgetting the incident does not correct the situation; this could present a problem later.
   4 Initials are as legally binding as a signature.

549. Application, implementaton, environment (b)
   4 The nurse should be consistent with the practice of the patient at home to ensure delivery of the same dose of insulin. Using an air-lock allows all the medication to clear the needle shaft. Lack of an air-lock may allow some of the medication to remain in the needle.
   1 Although use of an air-lock may or may not be taught with a subcutaneous injection, the nurses' preference is not the best answer in this situation.
   2 The length of the needle or the size of the patient does not change the use of an air-lock for subcutaneous injections.
   3 Neither frequency of administration nor age influences the decision to use an air-lock.

550. Comprehension, implementation, environment (a)
   4 The abdomen is the preferred site for a heparin injection because of the large amount of fat tissue.
   1, 2, 3 These are not sites for subcutaneous administration of heparin.

551. Knowledge, implementation, environment (a)
   1 The wrist band check is the most accurate means of patient verification.
   2 Calling the patient by name is not a method to ensure accuracy, because the patient may respond to any name.
   3 Bed cards may not be updated; this method does not ensure accuracy.
   4 Patients are frequently moved from room to room, and their medication record may not reflect this occurrence.

552. Application, implementation, physiological (b)
   4 This is the correct dosage. The nurse would use the formula $\dfrac{\text{Desire}}{\text{Have}} \times \dfrac{\text{Milliliter}}{1}$

$$\text{Example:} \quad \frac{250,000 \text{ U}}{100,000 \text{ U}} \times \frac{1 \text{ ml}}{1} = 2.5 \text{ ml}$$

   1, 2, 3, These amounts would be less than what the doctor orders.

553. Application, implementation, environment (a)
   3 $\dfrac{\text{Desire}}{\text{Have}} \times \dfrac{\text{Milliliter}}{1}$

$$\text{Example:} \quad \frac{500 \text{ mg}}{125 \text{ mg}} \times \frac{5 \text{ ml}}{1} = 20 \text{ ml}$$

   1, 2 These doses are too low.
   4 This dose is too high.

554. Application, implementation, physiological (a)
   1 $\dfrac{D}{H} \times \dfrac{5000}{10,000} = 0.5 \times 1 \text{ ml} = 0.5 \text{ ml}$
   2 3, 4 Incorrect calculations

555. Application, implementation, physiological (a)
   3 60 mg = 1 gr
     1½ gr = 90 mg, or 1½ tablets
   1 ½ tablet = ½ gr or 30 mg
   2 1 tablet = 60 mg or 1 gr
   4 2 tablets = 120 mg or 2 gr

556. Application, implementation, environment (b)
   3 $15 \times \dfrac{6 \text{ ml}}{100\text{U}} = \dfrac{15 \times 6}{100} = \dfrac{90}{100} = 0.9 \text{ ml}$
   1, 2 These dosages are too low.
   4 This dosage is too high.

557. Comprehension, implementation, physiological (a)
   1 100 : 2 ml = 75 : X ml
     100 X = 150 ml
     X = 1.5 ml
   2, 3, 4 These are not a sufficient amount.

558. Application, implementaton, environment (a)
   4 $\dfrac{1000 \times 1\cancel{0}}{8 \times 6\cancel{0}} = \dfrac{1000}{48} = 20.8 = 21 \text{ gtt}$
   Drops are always rounded to the nearest whole number
   1, 2 These calculations are incorrect.
   3 This calculation is rounded incorrectly.

559. Application, implementation, environment (b)
    4 Patients may refuse medication, but nurses who are responsible for the patient's safety, the plan of care, and the legal status of their license will provide and document the teaching provided to the patient regarding the actions of the drug and reasons for its use.
    1 The response discounts the patient's rights to participate in and decline treatment if desired.
    2 This answer is true, but it is less complete than answer No. 4.
    3 This response does not allow the patient to make her decision now; it is bargaining with the patient to avoid a problem.

560. Comprehension, planning, physiologic (b)
    3 Stool softeners are more gentle to the gastrointestinal tract and promote regularity.
    1 Oil retention enemas are usually used for a fecal impaction.
    2 Strong laxatives are not routinely administered to relieve constipation, and they are not given on a regular basis.
    4 Saline enemas are only occasionally used to relieve constipation because there is the risk of inducing an electrolyte imbalance.

561. Application, implementation, physiological (b)
    4 Standard protocol for management of anginal pain is to use sublingual nitroglycerin at 5-minute intervals to total no more than 3 to 5 doses. The patient should seek emergency care if pain continues.
    1 This answer is nontherapeutic and ineffective.
    2 This answer is incorrect; the medication may be used more frequently.
    3 A decrease in severity of pain usually occurs within 1 to 3 minutes; this may require as many as 3 tablets.

562. Comprehension, planning, physiological (b)
    3 The Maalox would be given 1 hour pc and not at the same time as the digitalis.
    1 An antacid and digitalis preparation should not be given together because of interference with absorption.
    2 The time of the Maalox does not comply with the order.
    4 Although this would probably be acceptable in most agencies because it is given within 30 minutes before or after the specified time, it is still close to the administration of digitalis and could result in interference.

563. Comprehension, implementation, environment (c)
    3 The order for the Fiorinal, which contains aspirin, should be changed to a pain medication without aspirin.
    1 This could result in unsafe practice; another nurse may not see the note or notice the combination of drugs.
    2 This would be appropriate only if the patient had no complaints of pain. This is not implied.
    4 Heparin and aspirin should not be given together.

564. Comprehension, assessment, environment (c)
    2 The laboratory work could have been drawn after the 9 AM dose and given a false high reading. Checking this first could save time.
    1 The physician should be notified if the results are truly correct. All other areas of concern should be monitored first.
    3 The vitamin K will be required if bleeding occurs, but this is not the first step.
    4 Protamine sulfate is the antidote for heparin.

565. Comprehension, assessment, health (c)
    3 This stimulates diruresis by preventing the antidiuretic from functioning.
    1, 2, 4 These are incorrect responses.

566. Application, implementation, physiological (b)
    1 This indicates decrease in myocardium contraction and buildup of fluid in the lungs.
    2 This is not indicative of holding the medication.
    3 This is a positive sign that is sought.
    4 This is not indicative of a problem by itself.

567. Application, implementation, environment (b)
    3 This order is incomplete, and the medication should not be given until clarified. The order should not have been transcribed onto the medication record sheet as written.
    1 Nurses should never assume if and when medications are involved.
    2 The nurse is taking the legal responsibility for the dosage given.
    4 The dosage could be different from the standard two tablets and should be clarified first. See No. 3 for the correct rationale.

568. Comprehension, evaluation, physiological (b)
    2 Wheezing would signify that the bronchioles are constricted and that the medication is ineffective.
    1 Bronchodilators dilate the bronchiole and do not change fremitus.
    3 Crackles could be present even if the bronchodilator is effective.
    4 The characteristics of the sputum may not change because of the bronchodilator.

569. Knowledge, planning, health (a)
    3 Antibiotics, especially tetracyclines, lower the effectiveness of oral contraceptives. Patients often need to use other forms of contraception in addition to pills while on tetracycline products.
    1 Birth control pills do not interact with antithyroid medications.
    2, 4 These medications do not interfere with oral contraceptives.

570. Knowledge, planning, health (a)
    3 Body temperature is the measurement for determining ovulation when using the rhythm method of birth control.
    1 Weight does not directly affect ovulation.
    2, 4 These are not altered during ovulation.

571. Application, implementation, environment (a)
    1 All medications should be clarified with the physician if the method of administration must change.
    2 Medication should not be held without notifying the RN or physician.
    3 Enterically coated medication should not be crushed because it will lose its ability to protect the stomach, resulting in delayed absorption.
    4 Swallowing tablets with a nasogastric (NG) tube in place can endanger the airway and may conflict with the reason the NG tube was originally placed.

572. Comprehension, assessment, environment (a)
    2 Allergies to medication are common and many drugs such as cephalosporins may have cross allergies with penicillin products.
    1, 3, 4 All of the other facts are good to assess; however, this was a lower priority than allergies.

573. Comprehension, assessment, health (b)
    3 Most frequently there is a loss of appetite. Newer *therapeutic* implications are associated with marijuana. THC has been used to combat nausea and vomiting associated with cancer chemotherapy. Current scientific studies are being completed.
    1, 2, 4 In addition to these symptoms, she may also experience diarrhea and sleep disturbances.

574. Application, implementation, physiologic (b)
    3 Diuretics given after 5 PM may work effectively but may keep the patient up all night. Scheduling the drugs early in the morning would allow the action to occur during waking hours.
    1 The action of diuretics is to decrease sodium reabsorption.
    2 Osmotics are used to decrease intraocular pressure.
    4 Carbonic anhydrase inhibitors are weak and infrequently used today.
575. Comprehension, evaluation, environment (a)
    1 A soft toothbrush will not injure the gums and will therefore prevent bleeding.
    2 Green leafy vegetables contain vitamin K, which interferes with the action of warfarin (Coumadin).
    3 Aspirin interferes with clotting time and will increase bleeding tendencies.
    4 This is not necessary.
576. Comprehension, planning, health (a)
    2 Vitamin K is the antidote for an overdose of warfarin (Coumadin).
    1 This is an antidote for heparin.
    3, 4 These are not antidotes for warfarin.
577. Knowledge, planning, physiological (a)
    3 Antiemetics act upon the trigger zone located in the medulla, controlling nausea/vomiting responses.
    1 Antispasmodics decrease vagal stimulation and motility; they are not related to the control of nausea and vomiting.
    2 Anticholinergics affect the parasympathetic nervous system by blocking the action of acetycholine; this leads to decreased gastrointestinal secretions and peristalsis.
    4 Cathartics increase peristalsis and water content of the feces, promoting elimination.
578. Knowledge, implementation, physiological (a)
    2 Antipyretics are agents that reduce the body temperature.
    1 Antibiotics are used when an infection is identified.
    3 Antiemetics are used to control nausea and vomiting.
    4 Antihistamines are used to control symptoms of allergy.
579. Application, implementation, physiological (b)
    3 A diuretic is usually given in the morning so the patient can urinate while awake.
    1 A diuretic given at 6 PM would require the patient to urinate frequently during the night.
    2 Any medication, including diuretics, that are ordered daily are usually given in the morning hours.
    4 A diuretic given at 4 PM would interfere with visitation and sleep.
580. Knowledge, implementation, physiological (a)
    2 Spironolactone (Aldactone) is a potassium-sparing diuretic.
    1 Furosemide (Lasix) is a potassium-eliminating diuretic.
    3 Sulfisoxazole (Gantrisin) is classified as an antiinfective.
    4 Methenamine (Mandelamine) is classified as a urinary antiseptic.
581. Knowledge, evaluation, knowledge (a)
    1 Heparin is an anticoagulant and therefore may increase bleeding potential.
    2 The side effects of heparin do not include numbness.
    3, 4 The side effects of heparin do not involve the central nervous system.

582. Comprehension, assessment, physiological (a)
    3 Cimetidine (Tagamet) specifically inhibits the production of hydrochloric acid by blocking the histamine receptor sites.
    1 Cimetidine does not have a direct healing effect on the ulcer site.
    2 Tagamet is not a neutralizing agent.
    4 Tagamet does not affect peristalsis.
583. Knowledge, assessment, environment (a)
    3 Cocaine is usually sniffed by inhalation through the nostrils; this is likely to cause red, irritated nostrils.
    1, 2, 4 These are not signs of cocaine use.
584. Application, implementation, environment (c)
    3 This is the best answer because these measures are helpful in overcoming thirst and a dry mouth.
    1 Untrue; this is a common side effect.
    2 Sucking on hard candies will increase thirst and predispose the patient to dental caries.
    4 Rinsing the mouth with plain water may be beneficial. This should *not* include salt water because many elders also have conditions such as congestive heart failure or kidney disease which would cause fluid retention.
585. Comprehension, assessment, health (c)
    2 Anticoagulants such as heparin or warfarin (Coumadin) are given to reduce chances of clotting; analgesic drugs such as morphine are given to control pain; and antidysrhythmics such as lidocaine (Xylocaine) IV is used to treat ventricular dysrhythmias.
    1 These are frequently used medications for rheumatoid arthritis.
    3 These are medication therapy for congestive heart failure.
    4 These are medications for pheripheral artery disease.
586. Application, implementation, environment (b)
    4 The amount, route, place and reason are all listed in this description.
    1 Although the description of the discomfort is good, the notes do not state where it was given.
    2 This charting does not indicate that the injection was given Z- track.
    3 This charting does not designate on which side the injection was given.
587. Knowledge, planning, environment (a)
    4 Flurazepam (Dalmane) is a sedative/hypnotic of the benzodiazepine group.
    1 Nalbuphine (Nubain) is a narcotic analgesic.
    2 Magaltrate (hydroxymagnesium aluminate) is an antacid.
    3 Indomethacin (Indameth) is a nonsteroidal antiinflammatory agent.
588. Knowledge, planning, environment (a)
    3 Acetazolamide (Diamox) is a carbonic anhydrase inhibitor and as such promotes diuresis.
    1 Acetazolamide has no effect on light sensation.
    2 Acetazolamide has no effect on sugar levels.
    4 Acetazolamide has no cardiac effects.

589. Application, planning, environment (b)
    3 The patient has a fresh open line to the central venous system and is beginning immunosuppressive medication; there is an increased risk for infection.
    1 She has no communicable disease process requiring isolation.
    2 The site will only need daily care.
    4 If stomatitis occurs, this would be true. At this time the nurse must optimize the patient's nutritional intake in an effort to prevent skin breakdown.

590. Application, assessment, environment (b)
    4 Patients receiving corticosteroids often retain fluid and have a blood pressure elevation as the therapeutic levels are attained. Nurses must monitor and report these changes.
    1 Although bone demineralization may occur with long-term steroid use, this is not a routine nursing assessment.
    2 Steroids may cause insomnia, but this is a lower priority than fluid and electrolyte balance.
    3 Steroid use may redistribute fat stores, but this can be visually observed and is not as high a concern as fluid retention and hypertension.

591. Comprehension, implementation, environment (b)
    1 Preoperatively, atropine is primarily used for its anticholinergic effects to decrease peristalsis and suppress GI secretions.
    2 The atropine may slightly effect an increase in heart rate, but it is not given for this reason. Atropine IV is used to increase the cardiac rate.
    3 Atropine has no effect on pain or anxiety.
    4 Atropine has no effect on the anaesthetic.

592. Application, implementation, environment (a)
    3 All medication orders in question should be clarified with the physician as soon as possible, especially orders that need to be given immediately.
    1 The vocational/practical nurse does not have authority to prescribe and therefore may not independently alter a physician's order.
    2 If the medication is out of the therapeutic dose range, the nurse is responsible to ensure the safety of her patient by clarifying the order and not giving a potentially dangerous dose.
    4 Holding a "now" order of medication until the physician makes rounds may have deleterious effects on the patient and is personal nursing judgment.

593. Application, planning, environment (b)
    2 Stat orders, especially if the order is for cardiac-related medication, should always receive high priority. Control for strong pain is also a high priority. Most institutions have a time range in which routine medication can be safely given.
    1 A routine antibiotic is not as high a priority as a stat order for nitrates, which can be life-sustaining.
    3 Pain control, although highly important, is in this case a prn order that is lower priority than a stat order, which indicates *immediately*.
    4 This places the stat order in lowest priority and could cause a worsening of a potentially dangerous disorder.

594. Knowledge, implementation, physiological (a)
    1 Morphine is given to patients with chest pains that are a result of coronary occlusion.
    2 Morphine does not relieve nausea.
    3 Morphine does not relieve vomiting.
    4 Morphine helps to relax and improve breathing, but this is not its primary use in this case.

595. Knowledge, implementation, physiological (c)
    3 Warfarin (Coumadin) is an anticoagulant. *Anti* means against; coagulation refers to blood clotting.
    1 An anticoagulant used in excess would cause bleeding.
    2 Warfarin is used for blood infection.
    3 This is not applicable.

596. Comprehension, planning, physiological (a)
    1 This interferes with the transmission of impulses from the thalamus to the cortex of the brain, causing sedation.
    2 An antiepileptic (anticonvulsant) drug such as phenytoin (Dilantin) decreases convulsions/seizures.
    3 An antidepressant is a substance such as amitryptyline that decreases depression.
    4 A tranquilizer is a substance used to calm anxious or agitated people without decreasing consciousness.

597. Comprehension, planning, psychosocial (b)
    1 Tranquilizers depress the central nervous system for antianxiety effects.
    2, 3 Major tranquilizers such as derivatives of phenothiazine, bulyrophenone and thioxanthene are generally used in the treatment of acute and chronic psychoses.
    4 Epilepsy is treated by use of anticonvulsant drugs such as phenytoin (Dilantin).

598. Application, implementation, physiological (b)
    3 The first priority is to keep the patient safe from harm.
    1 A seizure is controlled by medications, ordered by the physician.
    2 The patient is never restrained; fractures may occur if he or she is restrained.
    4 Oxygen may be ordered to increase circulation to the brain, but the first priority is to protect the patient.

599. Knowledge, evaluation, psychosocial (a)
    3 The action of this drug would be to relieve the apprehension, thus inducing sleep.
    1 This is the action of an antitussive.
    2 This is the action of an analgesic.
    4 This result, along with a decrease in respirations, is an adverse reaction to this medication.

600. Knowledge, planning, environment (a)
    2 This is a schedule II drug, a synthetic narcotic analgesic that is less potent than morphine.
    1 This is hydromorphine, a potent synthetic compound that maximizes analgesic effects and minimizes some of the common side effects of morphine.
    3 This is the trade name for the anticonvulsant phenytoin.
    4 This is an anticoagulant prescribed for prophylaxis and treatment of thrombosis and embolism.

Maternal/Child Health Nursing

1. Knowledge, planning, health (a)
   1 Improved quality and availability of prenatal care have had greater impact on reducing maternal and infant morbidity and mortality than other options listed.
   2, 3, 4 This is important, yet recognition of prenatal care as vital and essential has proved to be more beneficial than other options listed.

2. Comprehension, planning, health (b)
   1 Old programs such as WIC and Head Start have limited funds available and are still functioning; these programs offer prenatal and preschool assistance to families.
   2 There have been no new programs initiated since 1976.
   3 This is not so; there were no new programs to dismantle.
   4 No former programs have been relegated to the states; some states are struggling to maintain the programs they do sponsor.

3. Knowledge, planning, health (a)
   3 This is the "true" female pelvis.
   1 This is the male pelvis.
   2 This type resembles the pelvis of anthropoid apes.
   4 This is the type classified as a flat pelvis.

4. Knowledge, implementation, health (a)
   3 In the fifth month of growth and development the fetus is fully developed and the fetal heart rate is heard by the examiner using a fetoscope.
   1, 2 Too early.
   4 From the sixth through the ninth months the fetus grows in size and weight.

5. Comprehension, planning, health (b)
   4 In normal pregnancy, some clotting factors including fibrinogen are increased.
   1 The RBC count increases, but later in the pregnancy, and is less than plasma volume.
   2 Hemoglobin values are decreased because of an increase in the ratio of plasma to red cells.
   3 A decreased white blood cell count could indicate compensation in bone marrow function; this is not a normal occurrence.

6. Knowledge, implementation, health (b)
   2 Fetal lungs do not function as organs of respiration. Oxygenated blood enters fetal circulation through the umbilical vein.
   1 Arterial blood is brought to the fetal liver via the umbilical vein.
   3 The fetal brain receives oxygenated blood via the ascending aorta.
   4 The fetal kidneys receive oxygenated blood via the abdominal aorta. Small amounts of urine are being secreted by week 12.

7. Knowledge, implementation, health (a)
   3 The umbilical vein carries oxygenated blood and nutrients to the fetus; the two umbilical arteries carry metabolic wastes to the maternal circulation.
   1, 2 A single umbilical artery is associated with congenital anomalies.
   4 There is only one umbilical vein.

8. Application, implementation, health (a)
   3 Demonstration and explanation is the most appropriate response.
   1, 2 Showing a picture of these with no explanation does not answer the patient's question in a satisfactory manner.
   4 Use of a chart is recommended, but the information is incorrect.

9. Knowledge, implementation, health (a)
   4 Fertilization of the ovum can only occur while the ovum is in the distal third of the fallopian tube.
   1 The ovum matures within the ovary and is released into the fallopian tube where fertilization occurs.
   2 The fertilized ovum normally implants in the upper third of the anterior uterine wall.
   3 After being deposited in the vagina, sperm rapidly move into the cervix, then to the uterus and into the fallopian tube where fertilization takes place.

10. Knowledge, implementation, health (a)
    2 Volume of amniotic fluid increases at the rate of 25 ml/week during the first trimester, 50 ml/week during the second trimester and reaches a total of about 1000 ml at full term; it is replaced every 3 hours.
    1 This amount is low for a full-term pregnancy and is bordering on being an abnormal amount.
    3 2000 ml or more would be considered abnormal and is called hydramnios, which is often associated with diabetic or cardiac conditions in the mother; it can also be indicative of fetal abnormalities such as cardiac defects.
    4 300 ml or less is considered abnormal and is called oligohydramnios. It is usually associated with fetal anomalies or disease.

11. Knowledge, implementation, health (a)
    2 Milk and cheese products, especially hard cheeses such as cheddar, are excellent sources of calcium.
    1 Liver and organ meats are excellent sources of iron, not calcium.
    3 Dark yellow vegetables supply vitamin A.
    4 Enrichment usually provides nutrients such as B complex vitamins, not calcium.

12. Knowledge, planning, health (a)
    4 Powdered milk contains all the nutrients the milk from which it is made contained and is the least expensive form of milk.
    1 This is more expensive than powdered milk, but it does contain all the nutrients.
    2 This is low in calcium and vitamins as compared to whole milk.
    3 This is lower in vitamins and more expensive.

13. Knowledge, implementation, health (a)
    3 Raw fruits and vegetables with their high fiber content stimulate peristalsis.
    1 Milk and dairy products are low-residue foods that do not stimulate peristalsis; in some instances, cheese has been known to cause constipation.
    2 The process of refining cereals tends to lessen the amount of bulk or cellulose; this in turn decreases peristalsis.
    4 Nonfibrous meats tend to decrease peristalsis; this in turn leads to constipation.

14. Knowledge, planning, health (a)
    4 Increased protein is important for the growth of baby, placenta, maternal tissues and circulating blood; increased calcium is needed for bones and teeth of the fetus.
    1 Intake of sodium should be maintained at present levels; an increase may predispose the patient to fluid retention and probability of additional complications.
    2 Calories should be maintained or somewhat increased to meet increased energy demands; sodium intake should be maintained, not decreased.
    3 Increases of protein are important for tissue building in mother and fetus; carbohydrates for increased energy demands.

15. Knowledge, implementation, psychosocial (b)
    2 WIC is a federally subsidized supplementary food program providing food for mothers as well as for infants and children under 5 years of age. Those in the program must meet certain criteria to be eligible.
    1 The patient asked for supplemental foods.
    3 W.I.C. is not a full food program.
    4 The patient did not request information about welfare.
16. Comprehension, planning, physiological (b)
    1 The calcium requirement is higher in adolescent girls than in adult women.
    2 The need for calcium is not lower; bones have not finished growing.
    3 The adult's need decreases because full growth is achieved.
    4 The calcium need is not always met; adolescents frequently eat junk food and fast food.
17. Comprehension, planning, physiological (a)
    2 Proteins build and repair body tissue.
    1 Iron combines with protein to produce blood.
    3 Vitamin K is given to infants following delivery to prevent bleeding.
    4 Calcium supplements are given to mothers to aid in building bones and teeth in the fetus.
18. Knowledge, planning, physiological (a)
    2 During gestation the fetus stores the iron necessary for the first 5 or 6 months of life, a time in which the infant's diet is lacking in iron because the principal food, milk, is lacking in iron.
    1 Prenatal iron reserves last longer than 3 months.
    3 Iron reserves are only sufficient for 5 or 6 months; a supplemental vitamin or food source of iron is needed after this time.
    4 Iron reserves sustain the infant for only the first 5 or 6 months of life.
19. Knowledge, implementation, health (a)
    3 Because it contains all essential amino acids, cheese is considered a complete protein; crackers are a source of carbohydrates.
    1 Cereal is a source of carbohydrates.
    2 Peanuts, although they contain protein, are considered to be an incomplete protein food.
    4 Although peanut butter contains protein, it is an incomplete protein food; an apple is a source of carbohydrates.
20. Comprehension, implementation, health (a)
    4 These are a good source of low-cost protein.
    1 Red meats and fish, although high in protein, are also expensive.
    2 These are a good source of vitamins, especially vitamin A and vitamin C, but not protein.
    3 These contain carbohydrates and B-complex vitamins, but not protein.
21. Comprehension, planning, health (a)
    2 Abdominal ultrasound is not a routinely ordered examination. It may be used to confirm suspected pregnancy at an early date, to evaluate fetal development, or to evaluate placental placement.
    1, 3, 4 These are routinely done on the initial prenatal visit.
22. Comprehension, implementation, psychosocial (b)
    2 A conductive oil or gel is spread on the skin to reduce friction from the transducer as it is moved across the abdomen.
    1 Ultrasound is a noninvasive procedure using ultrasound waves rather than dyes or radiation.
    3 The patient is positioned on her back.
    4 This is an explanation for amniocentesis.

23. Comprehension, planning, health (b)
    2 The presence of antibodies to rubella indicates that Ms. Paul has had a rubella infection sometime in the past.
    1 An elevated titer can only indicate rubella in the past, not *when* in the past.
    3 Rubella titer drawn on the mother cannot indicate anything about the fetus.
    4 Only rubella vaccination can protect a patient.
24. Comprehension, implementation, health (b)
    2 Most obstetricians do this as a routine for patients over 35 years of age; it helps to identify high-risk mothers and possible fetal problems.
    1 This would not be evident during early stages of pregnancy.
    3 Nothing in her medical history would necessitate doing this test; heterozygote testing is for unrecognized genetic problems.
    4 This test is usually done during the last trimester.
25. Comprehension, assessment, environment (a)
    1 This is the most complete response; the original reason for these tests was to prevent pregnancy-induced hypertension.
    2 This is true, but it does not answer precise reasons for the tests.
    3 Urinalysis may be indicative of further testing for diabetes; however, this response does not include other complications that an increased blood pressure and weight gain would indicate.
    4 These tests would not be sufficient in detecting congenital anomalies.
26. Knowledge, implementation, physiological (a)
    3 Fetal heart tones heard by an examiner are a positive sign of pregnancy; other options listed are probable or presumptive signs.
    1, 2, 4 See response to No. 3.
27. Comprehension, assessment, environment (b)
    3 Presumptive signs of pregnancy include amenorrhea, fatigue, and urinary frequency. Chadwick's sign and positive pregnancy tests are probable signs of pregnancy. Fetal movements felt by anyone other than the mother are a positive sign of pregnancy.
    1 See above; quickening is a subjective symptom of presumptive signs that, combined with probable signs, strongly suggest pregnancy.
    2 See above; nausea and vomiting in and of itself can have other causes; however, morning sickness is considered a subjective symptom of presumptive signs of pregnancy.
    4 See above; breast changes can also be considered subjective symptoms of presumptive signs of pregnancy.
28. Knowledge, planning, health (b)
    4 "Morning sickness" is a frequent problem for patients during the first few months of pregnancy. Receiving adequate rest and increasing carbohydrates in the diet helps reduce this problem.
    1 This would not be a routine solution to the problem.
    2, 3 These would not resolve or reduce the problem.

29. Knowledge, planning, health (a)

3 This is seen as a danger signal in pregnancy and should be reported immediately to the physician; other danger signals include visual disturbances, vaginal bleeding, constant headaches, dizziness, and constant vomiting. All are signs of impending danger, ranging from possible eclampsia to premature separation of the placenta. These danger signals should be reported to the physician immediately.

1 Sexual intercourse is permissible as long as it is not uncomfortable and the cervix is closed; however, if a patient has had numerous miscarriages the physician might suggest that the patient refrain from intercourse during the first 3 months to lessen the danger of a miscarriage.

2 The recommended weight gain is about 25 lb; a weight gain slightly over that would not be considered excessive. It depends on the patient and what her weight was at the start of the pregnancy.

4 Childbirth preparation classes are encouraged but not mandatory; this is not the best answer.

30. Comprehension, implementation, physiological (b)

4 The primary benefit would be to allow the mother to assist, if so desired, in as much of the birthing process as possible and to decrease the amount of actual medication used during labor.

1 This may be true in some cases; rapidity of delivery and pain threshold varies with each individual.

2 This may be true in some cases; pain threshold varies with each individual; small doses of medication are given and may actually facilitate the birthing process.

3 This too may also be true, but it is not considered to be the prime benefit of the classes.

31. Knowledge, planning, environment (a)

1 The estimated date of confinement (EDC) is the estimated delivery date and is calculated by Nägele's rule.

2 This is an incorrect response, as indicated above.

3 This is some of the information necessary in using Nägele's rule.

4 This is an incorrect response, as indicated above; it has no real significance.

32. Knowledge, implementation, health (a)

1 Prima means first; gravida means pregnant.

2 A multipara is a woman who has delivered two or more babies.

3 A primapara is a woman who has delivered her first baby.

4 A multigravida is a woman during her second and subsequent pregnancies.

33. Comprehension, planning, environment (a)

2 This ensures optimal care of mother and baby.

1 Lightening occurs before labor; late to ensure optimal care.

3 Morning sickness varies in time; late to ensure optimal care.

4 This usually occurs between 4 and 5 months of gestation; late to ensure optimal care.

34. Knowledge, assessment, health (a)

2 Colostrum is the thin, watery secretion from the breast that occurs during latter stages of pregnancy and after delivery.

1 Lochia is the vaginal discharge that occurs following delivery.

3 Chloasma is the pigmentary discoloration primarily found on the face during pregnancy.

4 Chorion is a fetal membrane.

35. Application, assessment, health (a)

2 German measles can cause deformities in the fetus, especially during the first trimester.

1, 3 These do not cause deformities.

4 Gonorrhea is a transmitted disease that can cause ophthalmic neonatorium in infants.

36. Knowledge, implementation, health (a)

2 During pregnancy, progesterone is responsible for securing implantation, development of the placenta, and inhibiting uterine contractility.

1 During pregnancy, estrogen is responsible for uterine growth, elasticity and contractility, breast growth, and enlargement of external genitalia.

3 Leutinizing hormone is responsible for the maturing of the graafian follicle and its release from the ovary (ovulation) during the menstrual cycle.

4 Follicle-stimulating hormone stimulates the growth and development of ovarian follicles from about days 4 to 14 of the menstrual cycle.

37. Application, implementation, health (b)

1 This is a normal occurrence as the pregnancy nears term; lightening occurs when the presenting part descends into the pelvis, accounting for greater pressure on the bladder.

2 The patient did not indicate burning or other symptoms more commonly associated with a urinary tract infection.

3 Restriction of fluids is not recommended and would not resolve the problem of urinary frequency.

4 All complaints made by patients should be reported to the physician, but this one, as given in the situation, does not need immediate attention by the physician.

38. Knowledge, implementation, health (a)

4 In the fourth month of antepartal growth and development, muscles are developed and movements of the fetus may be felt by the mother.

1, 2 Movement is usual and expected during these months.

3 It is too early to feel movements during this month.

39. Knowledge, planning, health (a)

3 Most physicians recommend a weight gain of 20 to 25 lb for an entire pregnancy; greater gains are thought to contribute to problems, however, dieting to achieve weight loss during pregnancy may be harmful to fetal development.

1, 2, 4 The average is as stated above; the amount of weight gain can be individualized accordingly.

40. Knowledge, assessment, health (a)

3 Enlargement and tenderness of the breasts, amenorrhea, and frequency are all signs and symptoms of pregnancy that the nurse can assess.

1 The physician usually assesses enlargement of the uterus during the physical examination.

2 This requires an internal examination and is not the responsibility of the nurse.

4 These signs and symptoms of pregnancy are usually not apparent during an initial prenatal visit, which most often occurs during the second or third month of pregnancy; fetal movements are usually felt by the mother during the fourth month, when quickening occurs.

41. Comprehension, implementation, health (a)

3 This is the best explanation and advice.

1 Wearing high heels during pregnancy should be discouraged for both health and safety reasons.

2 Wearing lower heels may help, but this does not prevent varicose veins.

4 This is good advice, but it does not explain consequences.

42. Application, implementation, environment (a)
    4 Dependent edema occurs with decreased circulatory return and is relieved by elevating the legs.
    1 Dependent edema, which resolves after a night's sleep, does not require complete bed rest.
    2 Pregnancy-induced hypertension is characterized by hypertension, proteinuria, and edema.
    3 Sodium intake is not restricted for dependent edema. Reducing excessive sodium is encouraged for all.

43. Application, implementation, health (a)
    3 Questions should be answered honestly by giving information on the child's level of understanding.
    1 Putting off his questions may affect the way he relates to the new baby.
    2 Stork tales do not deal with reality.
    4 Avoidance and putting him off on his father does not give him satisfaction, nor does it guarantee the father will give him the answer.

44. Application, implementation, health (a)
    2 It is helpful to give the correct explanation using the word "uterus" instead of stomach, which connotes something being eaten.
    1 This is false information; eating is not the cause of growth.
    3 This is false information; the baby is not growing in the stomach.
    4 Emphasis on baby can cause negative feelings.

45. Application, implementation, psychosocial (a)
    4 Involving him in the process gives him more positive attention.
    1 Avoidance doesn't solve the problem.
    2 This is false assurance.
    3 This is negative reinforcement.

46. Application, implementation, health (c)
    1 Various hormonal changes tend to promote resistance to insulin, thus increasing the need for insulin.
    2 There is nothing to indicate a change in activity level.
    3 Prevention of urinary tract infections relies on frequent urine cultures, careful hygiene, and strict control of serum glucose levels.
    4 The fetus produces its own insulin.

47. Application, implementation, health (a)
    3 Flushing out the urinary tract reduces the amount of bacteria present.
    1 Fluid intake should be at least eight 8-oz glasses of fluid per day.
    2 Excessive carbohydrate and sugar intake may result in glycosuria, which promotes bacterial growth.
    4 Cotton underwear better absorbs moisture.

48. Knowledge, planning, physiological (a)
    3 Persistent, excessive vomiting accompanied by weight loss and fluid and electrolyte imbalance.
    1,4 This is a condition of pregnancy characterized by hypertension, edema, and proteinuria.
    2 This is nausea and vomiting in pregnancy, usually subsiding by the twelfth week of gestation.

49. Knowledge, assessment, health (a)
    4 Untreated, this condition will cause death as a result of electrolyte, metabolic, and nutritional imbalances.
    1 This is not likely because the embryo or fetus would die as a result of severe starvation, resulting in hypoproteinemia and hypovitaminosis. Bleeding from mucosal surfaces occurs as a result of vitamin C and B complex deficiency and hypothrombinemia.
    2 This is completely unrelated.
    3 See response to No. 1.

50. Comprehension, evaluation, environment (c)
    3 Magnesium sulfate will reduce edema on the brain, thus reducing central nervous system symptoms. The plan of care should always include observing patient response to treatment.
    1 This has nothing to do with pulse rate; this drug is used to prevent seizures and can also be used as a cathartic.
    2 This drug is not an oxytocic.
    4 Any such outcome would be detrimental to the patient; this drug is not used for relief of epigastric pain.

51. Application, assessment, health (a)
    2 Elevated blood pressure (over 140/90) is a hallmark sign of preeclampsia.
    1 Fundal height is not affected by preeclampsia.
    3 Urine sugar and acetone are not affected.
    4 FHT will only be abnormal if the fetus is compromised, which is uncommon with the onset of preeclampsia.

52. Application, implementation, physiological (b)
    2 Bed rest reduces the effect of gravitational pull and reduces uterine activity.
    1 No routine salt restrictions are indicated.
    3 Good nutrition should be maintained.
    4 There is no indication to reduce fluids.

53. Knowledge, assessment, environment (b)
    3 True labor starts when uterine contractions occur regularly. There is complete effacement of cervical canal, and the cervix dilates.
    1 Expelling the plug is a sign that labor is about to start.
    2 Membranes rupture before or after labor starts.
    4 Usually the fetus drops into the pelvis brim a week or two before delivery.

54. Comprehension, planning, environment (a)
    4 Providing for a clean delivery reduces the possibility of an infection.
    1 An enema does not prevent constipation during labor.
    2 An enema does not provide relief of pressure in case of episiotomy.
    3 This definitely does not ease contractions.

55. Application, planning, environment (a)
    2 Vaginal examinations should be done under conditions of strict cleanliness. Wash vulva well, examiner should use sterile gloves.
    1, 2, 3 These are not necessary to do a vaginal examination.

56. Comprehension, assessment, environment (b)
    4 This is a below-normal rate, which indicates fetal distress.
    1 Meconium is a potential problem; the nurse should check fetal heart tones frequently to determine fetal distress. This is not the best answer.
    2 Fetal inactivity itself is not a cause for alarm.
    3 This does not necessarily indicate danger; the nurse should note the time, amount, color, and odor.

57. Comprehension, implementation, environment (a)
    4 This is the most common area to begin finding fetal heart tones.
    1, 3 These are correct but not precise.
    2 This is incorrect for the vertex position.

58. Comprehension, implementation, environment (b)
    2 These are the correct instructions and posture for bearing down.
    1 Head back is the wrong position.
    3 The patient must hold her breath and push, or slowly let the breath out while pushing.
    4 Bearing down and pushing are impossible with this kind of instruction.

59. Comprehension, planning, environment (b)

3 The physician is referring to the degree of dilation (opening) of the cervix as expressed in centimeters; the term "cephalic" refers to the part of the fetus, in this case the head, that is against the cervical opening and will be delivered first.

1 The term denoting the thickness of the cervix is "effacement"; the term denoting the height of the presenting part in relation to ischial spines is "station."

2 Although the fetal head may be against the cervix, there is no indication that the physician has determined effacement or thinning of the cervix.

4 There is no indication that the physician has determined the station.

60. Comprehension, assessment, environment (b)

2 The normal range for fetal heart tones is 120 to 160 per minute; rates higher or lower may indicate fetal distress.

1, 3 A rate of 150 is within the normal range; it is not considered high.

4 A rate of 150 is within the normal range; the situation did not indicate if patient was having a contraction at the time the fetal heart rate was determined.

61. Application, implementation, environment (b)

3 A prepared father or other support person should be allowed to assist in the mother's care; the nurse is responsible for monitoring the fetal heart tones and validating the pattern of contractions.

1 In this option the nurse avoids nursing responsibilities.

2 In this option the nurse assumes her responsibilities but can also increase the father's anxiety level.

4 This option may be interpreted as discounting the father's preparation for the event.

62. Application, assessment, environment (a)

3 The cord may have been compressed as the fluid left the uterus and the fetus settled into the pelvis. The fetal heart rate changes as a result of fetal distress.

1 Nitrazine testing is done to confirm the presence of amniotic fluid.

2 This is a part of assessment during labor, but it is not the priority after rupture of the membranes.

4 Rupture of the membranes may result in fetal distress, not maternal distress.

63. Comprehension, assessment, environment (b)

3 During the first stage of labor, in both the latent and active phase with the exception of transition, breathing techniques promote relaxation of abdominal muscles. This relaxation increases the size of the abdominal cavity that in turn decreases friction between the uterus and abdominal walls, thus decreasing discomfort.

1 The presenting part is at the ischial spines; the patient would not have an irresistible urge to push.

2 The patient would be too self-focused at this point in her labor to inquire about what is going to happen during delivery.

4 Patients will not generally fall asleep during contractions once such are firmly established (active labor).

64. Comprehension, planning, environment (b)

2 In the early latent phase of the first stage of labor, the cervix dilates from 0 cm to 4 cm.

1 False labor is characterized by irregular contractions that may stop with walking; there is little change in dilation or effacement of cervix.

3 True labor is characterized by regular contractions, increasing in duration and intensity, spontaneous rupture of membranes, and bloody show; transition is the last phase of the first stage of labor.

4 In the active phase of the first stage, the cervix dilates from 5 cm to 10 cm; the third stage is from delivery of the fetus to delivery of the placenta.

65. Comprehension, evaluation, environment (b)

2 Pudendal anesthesia blocks the pudendal nerve, providing pain relief in the lower two thirds of the vagina and perineum.

1, 3, 4 There is no blockage of nerves to these areas.

66. Application, implementation, environment (a)

3 An enema may further enhance labor. In a multipara with a history of rapid labors, assessment of mother and fetus has priority.

1 An external fetal monitor will not further stimulate labor; it will aid in fetal assessment.

2, 4 These will not further stimulate labor; they will be of use in maternal assessment.

67. Comprehension, implementation, psychosocial (a)

1 This indicates recognition by the nurse that anyone the mother chooses can play a supportive role during labor.

2 This ignores the patient's anxiety, which may be caused by her feeling "alone."

3 This response ignores the feelings of this individual patient.

4 Saying nothing in this situation excludes possibilities for reducing anxiety.

68. Knowledge, planning, environment (a)

1 This is true for most women delivering their first child; for subsequent pregnancies, the time is usually shorter.

2, 3 Labor varies, yet the average is 14 to 16 hours.

4 Labor varies; it is doubtful that the physician would permit a patient to be in really active labor for this period of time before evaluating for possible complications.

69. Comprehension, planning, environment (b)

3 The lower part of the spinal canal (L4-5) is injected.

1 A pudendal block results in pain relief and relaxation of the perineum.

2 Local infiltration is used to inject anesthetic to the perineum.

4 Injecting an anesthetic agent into the uterine cervix is known as a paracervical block.

70. Knowledge, implementation, environment (b)

1 The length of a contraction from beginning to end is called duration.

2 The degree of hardness/firmness of the uterus is called intensity.

3 Frequency is how often contractions occur, in minutes or seconds.

4 The interval is the time from the beginning of one contraction to the beginning of the next.

71. Application, implementation, physiological (b)

2 The strongest muscular contractions can be felt on the fundus, or top, of the uterus.

1 This area is too low.

3 This is not a suitable area.

4 Not applicable.

72. Comprehension, application, psychosocial (c)

4 This stage is usually the most difficult. The patient may display irritability and unwillingness to be touched.

1 Stage two is the expulsion of the infant.

2 Stage three is the delivery of the placenta.

3 This is the beginning of labor.

73. Comprehension, evaluation, physiological (b)
    2 Oxytocic drugs are given to help strengthen contractions of the uterus and prevent excessive bleeding.
    1 The drug is not used for this purpose.
    3 The drug does not hasten this process.
    4 The drug does not prevent uterine inversion.

74. Comprehension, assessment, environment (b)
    3 The third stage of labor is complete with the delivery of the placenta.
    1 This is usually noted as completion of the second stage of labor.
    2 This is usually done immediately following the birth of the baby.
    4 This is a dangerous complication in which the uterus is turned inside out so that the fundus intrudes into the cervix or vagina; it is caused by a too-vigorous removal of the placenta before it detaches from the uterine wall via the natural process of labor.

75. Knowledge, implementation, environment (b)
    4 This is the correct response; the letters mean "vaginal birth after cesarean."
    1 There is no such organization.
    2 There is no such surgical procedure.
    3 There is no such carrier.

76. Application, implementation, physiological (b)
    2 Shaking and chills are normal in the first hour after delivery; warmed blankets will provide comfort.
    1 An actual elevation of temperature is best identified by checking temperature after the chill has subsided.
    3 Shaking and chills are not indications for oxygen administration.
    4 The presence of a fever has not been assessed.

77. Application, implementation, environment (b)
    4 A soft (boggy) uterus must be massaged immediately to prevent postpartum hemorrhage; other options lose time and may allow for greater blood loss.
    1, 2, 3 Loss of time; may allow for greater blood loss.

78. Comprehension, implementation, physiological (b)
    1 Magnesium sulfate is a central nervous system depressant. It decreases nerve impulses from the brain to the muscles.
    2 This drug is not an analgesic.
    3 The drug does not increase blood pressure.
    4 The drug is not used for induction of labor.

79. Application, evaluation, environment (c)
    2 Respirations of less than 14, a decrease or absence of patellar reflexes, and urine output of less than 25 ml/hr are signs of magnesium sulfate toxicity.
    1 The nurse should record and monitor information, but she should also call the physician.
    3 The drug is discontinued immediately.
    4 This is not a normal result.

80. Application, implementation, environment (c)
    4 It takes about 72 hours for the danger of seizures to pass.
    1, 2, 3 The possibility of seizures lasts longer, about 72 hours.

81. Comprehension, implementation, environment (b)
    4 Maintaining the patient in this position for at least 8 hours is recommended as a means of preventing a spinal headache, which occurs as a result of loss of cerebrospinal fluid from the subarachnoid space and results in traction of the meninges on the pressure-sensitive intracranial structures.
    1 The fundus is palpated as with a normal vaginal delivery because hemorrhage is a very real possibility. This type of patient is really two patients in one, a surgical patient and an obstetrical patient, neither of which should be overlooked.
    2 This may not be necessary because these patients are not usually given general anesthesia in addition to the spinal anesthesia.
    3 This is not necessary because the patient will usually have an indwelling catheter in place following the surgery.

82. Comprehension, evaluation, environment (b)
    1 The epidural block is safer for both mother and baby; it has minimum after-effects.
    2 A general anesthetic predisposes the infant to respiratory depression.
    3 The pudendal block is a regional anesthetic.
    4 Bier's block is a regional anesthetic; it has no effects on the abdomen.

83. Application, planning, psychosocial (a)
    2 A cesarean delivery is not a contraindication for breast-feeding. Assistance from staff will decrease some anxiety and promote self-assurance for the mother.
    1 Encouragement will assist the patient in her decision to breast-feed.
    3 This is not necessary unless there is a physical problem.
    4 This response might discourage her; she needs a "listener."

84. Application, implementation, environment (c)
    4 The risk of intrauterine infection associated with premature rupture of the membranes (PROM) is assessed by a close monitoring of maternal vital signs.
    1, 3 These are not a priority in assessment of PROM.
    2 Monitoring for a developing infection takes priority.

85. Comprehension, assessment, physiological (a)
    4 As the low-lying placenta separates during dilation or effacement, blood flows from the vagina.
    1 This is associated with the concealed bleeding present with abruptio placentae.
    2 This is associated with the bleeding occurring in abruptio placentae.
    3 Bleeding associated with placenta previa generally occurs before labor begins. Because the blood flows out the vagina, the uterus does not become hard.

86. Comprehension, assessment, environment (b)
    3 Abruptio placentae is the premature separation of a normally implanted placenta before birth.
    1 This is a pregnancy outside the uterus, usually in the fallopian tubes.
    2 Placenta previa is an abnormal implantation of a normal placenta.
    4 A complete abortion occurs when all of the products of conception are expelled.

87. Application, implementation, psychosocial (b)
    2 Mrs. Johnson needs information to help relieve her anxiety and to help her to understand treatment and procedures.
    1 The nurse should do this only after assessment, providing information, and treatments—if the Johnsons so desire.
    3 Emergencies such as maternal shock and fetal distress can occur at any moment. The patient is not left alone.
    4 Everything may not be alright.
88. Comprehension, implementation, environment (b)
    4 Pitocin, an oxytocin, is a strong uterine contractor and must be regulated so there are desirable intervals between contractions; titanic contractions (very strong continual contractions) could jeopardize both the mother and the fetus.
    1, 2, 3 This may be so, but it is not the best answer.
89. Knowledge, planning, physiological (c)
    3 The cocaine will, however, have an effect on the newborn.
    1, 2 Cocaine addiction does not affect labor.
    4 Because labor is not affected, the need for sedation is no different than for a nonaddicted mother; if withdrawal symptoms occur, the patient may have to be evaluated for relief or control.
90. Comprehension, assessment, physiological (b)
    3 The classic signs of preeclampsia are elevated blood pressure, proteinuria, and edema.
    1 Not necessarily.
    2 This is not an indication.
    4 This is not related to the situation.
91. Knowledge, planning, environment (a)
    3 Rubber gloves are worn and the hands are washed after each contact with the patient; care should be taken to prevent transfer of virus from vesicles to other skin or mucous membranes of the patient or any other individual.
    1 The condition does not warrant complete or strict isolation.
    2 This should be exercised at all times, not only when preparing the patient for delivery.
    4 This should also be done, but it is not the only consideration of the nurse, as noted in the rationale for the correct response.
92. Knowledge, planning, health (b)
    2 Lactation produces an increased need for maternal energy, protein, minerals and vitamins; these aid secretion of milk, provide nourishment for the infant via the mother's milk, and protect the mother's stores of nutrients. A well-balanced diet with an extra 640 calories and extra fluids (as much as 3000 ml) is required for the breast-feeding mother.
    1 This is not sufficient fluid intake for a breast-feeding mother; see above.
    3 As long as the mother follows a well-balanced diet, there is no real need for supplements.
    4 See response to No. 3; milk can be considered part of the 3000 ml of fluids.
93. Comprehension, implementation, physiological (b)
    4 The nursing mother may have some breast engorgement as her milk comes in; nursing the newborn will often help relieve or reduce this congestion.
    1 This will not resolve the situation for the mother.
    2 This will not resolve the situation for the mother unless additional signs and symptoms of an infection are present.
    3 This action is taken only when the patient is known to be bottle feeding, not breast feeding, her infant.

94. Knowledge, planning, physiological (a)
    3 Demand feeding is popular and allows the newborn to be fed at the time and in the amount desired.
    1 Crying does not always indicate hunger.
    2, 4 These are not considered part of the demand feeding method.
95. Application, implementation, psychosocial (a)
    3 This is the most appropriate response because the nurse fully responds to both concerns in a correct manner.
    1 This response is inadequate because it offers no reassurance to the patient in any way; this is information the nurse should know.
    2 The first part of the response is correct; the second part of the response offers incorrect information.
    4 This is true, but it is not the most appropriate response because it does not respond fully to the patient's concerns.
96. Comprehension, implementation, psychosocial (a)
    4 Rooming-in allows mothers and new babies to share accommodations rather than being separated; ideally the maternity unit is designed so that the crib can be at the mother's bedside or in a nursery conveniently adjacent to the mother's room.
    1 The father may be present in the room, but this is not the true definition of the term "rooming-in."
    2, 3 These options are not applicable to the "rooming-in" situation.
97. Knowledge, implementation, physiological (a)
    2 The warm water in a sitz bath promotes vasodilatation, leading to increased comfort.
    1 Increased ambulation may cause additional discomfort because of increased engorgement and pressure.
    3 This technique serves no physiological purpose in this situation.
    4 While this might be an appropriate intervention, non-medication therapy should be considered first.
98. Comprehension, implementation, health (b)
    2 Normal elimination patterns may be reestablished and constipation relieved by a well-balanced diet and ambulation.
    1, 4 These are irrelevant to the situation.
    3 These measures would not facilitate return to normal elimination patterns if used on a continual basis.
99. Application, implementation, physiological (a)
    3 From eating little, there may be little bulk to stimulate bowel movement; fluids keep the stool moist and easier to pass.
    1 Ambulation is to be encouraged; an enema should be administered by the third day if the mother has not responded to the other measures.
    2, 4 Fecal impaction takes more than 2 days to develop.
100. Knowledge, planning, physiological (b)
    4 Bromocriptine mesylate (Parlodel) is a lactation inhibitor.
    1 Ibuprofen (Motrin) is an analgesic/antiinflammatory drug.
    2 Docusate sodium (Colace) is a fecal softener.
    3 Pitocin is an oxytocic drug.
101. Comprehension, planning, health (b)
    3 This amount provides necessary intake of nutrients and fluid within a 24-hour period.
    1 There is no set routine established to ensure adequate intake.
    2 This is an adequate intake of nutrients and fluid.
    4 This is generally too much fluid for a 9-lb baby to tolerate.

102. Application, assessment, environment (b)
    1 Some bleeding can happen later, but most postpartum hemorrhage occurs during the first hour as a result of atony of uterus or vaginal lacerations.
    2, 3 Bleeding is usually a result of retention of placental tissue.
    4 Not usually; most bleeding will occur within the first hour following delivery; see No. 1.

103. Knowledge, assessment, environment (a)
    4 When quick saturation and clots are involved, it is considered heavy.
    1 Moderate bleeding does saturate pads.
    2 This term is not used to describe lochia.
    3 This is the normal preferred amount of discharge after 24 to 48 hours.

104. Comprehension, implementation, physiological (a)
    4 Lochia rubra is bright or dark red, lasting 2 to 3 days.
    1 Lochia serosa is pinkish to brownish, lasting 2 to 5 days.
    2 Lochia alba is creamy and yellowish, lasting 5 to 10 days.
    3 This is not normal.

105. Knowledge, assessment, physiological (a)
    1 Lochia rubra occurs in the first few days postpartum; it is bright red and may have small clots.
    2 This follows the lochia rubra stage.
    3 This follows the lochia serosa stage.
    4 No such term used to describe lochia; puerpera is defined as "of or pertaining to a woman who has just given birth to an infant."

106. Comprehension, assessment, physiological (a)
    2 A full bladder causes the uterus to lie to either side instead of being centrally located.
    1 Stomach distention does not cause this.
    3 The uterus should be centrally located in the abdomen.
    4 Not applicable.

107. Comprehension, planning, environment (a)
    3 An overdistended bladder leads to atony of the bladder wall, resulting in urinary distention, which provides an environment favorable to infection.
    1 A hematoma develops as a result of hemorrhage under the vaginal mucosa or in the connective tissue of the vulva; development of a hematoma is not related to an overdistended bladder.
    2, 4 These are not related to bladder distention.

108. Comprehension, planning, psychosocial (c)
    4 Because sibling jealousy is related to competition for parents' love, Betsy will need special attention and time alone with her parents.
    1 Sibling jealousy relates to time, attention, and love rather than to material things.
    2 Betsy will need help to deal with her jealousy rather than help in loving the new baby.
    3 Knowing that she is a big girl will not help in relieving Betsy's jealousy.

109. Knowledge, assessment, physiological (a)
    1 Para indicates the number of live births.
    2 Gravida indicates the number of pregnancies.
    3, 4 Incorrect number.

110. Application, implementation, psychosocial (b)
    4 Siblings need to be a part of the care and attention given to the new baby.
    1, 2 Isolation keeps them apart from the care and attention given the baby.
    3 This response gives false assurance.

111. Comprehension, planning, environment (c)
    1 As a result of the overdistention of the uterus with two fetuses, the uterus may not contract sufficiently to control bleeding.
    2 Multiple gestation is not a risk factor for mastitis.
    3, 4 Multiple gestation is not a risk factor in these postpartum complications. Cesarean delivery greatly increases the risk of these complications.

112. Comprehension, implementation, psychosocial (a)
    3 Knowing this is a normal response often decreases anxiety and encourages the patient to talk.
    1 This situation requires a nursing response.
    2 This response neglects an opportunity to teach the patient the normalcy of her feelings.
    4 Psychiatric intervention is not required at this point because postpartum blues are a normal response.

113. Application, implementation, psychosocial (b)
    3 It is important to find out the patient's plans or ideas and explore possibilities with her.
    1 This reveals a judgmental attitude, which serves no purpose.
    2 The mother might not want to discuss the father.
    4 This would make her feel dependent, with no choices.

114. Comprehension, planning, physiological (b)
    3 Clearing the airway of mucus will prevent aspiration.
    1, 4 This is usually done after breathing is established.
    2 This is usually done at 1 minute and 5 minutes after delivery.

115. Application, planning, environment (c)
    3 Vastus lateralis is the best-developed muscle in infants and is therefore the safest for intramuscular injections.
    1, 4 These are not suitable sites for injection.
    2 This might cause injury to the sciatic nerve.

116. Knowledge, implementation, physiological (b)
    4 Vitamin K given IM soon after birth reduces likelihood of hemorrhage. Vitamin K is not normally manufactured in the intestinal tract until the second week of life.
    1 Vitamin K does not start peristalsis.
    2 Vitamin K does not increase the calcium level.
    3 This choice is not applicable.

117. Comprehension, evaluation, physiological (b)
    2 Ten (10) is the highest score an infant can attain. Each area evaluated is scored as 0, 1, or 2. The evaluation is ordinarily done 1 minute and 5 minutes after delivery.
    1 This score is not high enough to be the best.
    3, 4 These scores are not applicable; the highest attainable score is 10.

118. Knowledge, implementation, physiological (b)
    4 Muscle tone is the fifth item in the scoring system.
    1 Although this is done, it is not included in the Apgar score.
    2, 3 These are not included in Apgar scoring.

119. Comprehension, planning, physiological (a)
    2 If the newborn's body temperature drops, respiratory depression will develop.
    1 Weight can wait; every effort is taken to make sure the infant is breathing well and is stable.
    3 A bath will usually drop the newborn's temperature.
    4 This is done before discharge, not at birth; not all newborn males are circumcised.

120. Knowledge, planning, health (a)
    3 Silver nitrate effectively kills the gonococcal organism.
    1, 2 These do not cause blindness.
    4 Blindness is caused by high concentrations of oxygen.

121. Application, implementation, environment (b)
  3 Wrapping the foot chosen for the heel stick in a warm wet cloth for 5 minutes and elevating the head of the crib to increase circulation to the extremity is the appropriate action.
  1 Not so; see response to #3.
  2 Elevating the foot of the crib will decrease, not increase, circulation to the area.
  4 Saline solution would not affect circulation to the area and "soaking" would be difficult to accomplish with a newborn; there is no need to involve both feet.
122. Knowledge, implementation, environment (a)
  4 Identification is legally validated in most states or areas by recording the infant's footprints and the mother's fingerprint.
  1 This is usual hospital policy and procedure and can be considered routine.
  2 This is not usual practice.
  3 This has nothing to do with legal identification of the infant; it is routine practice.
123. Knowledge, implementation, health (a)
  4 In 1975 the American Academy of Pediatrics found no medical indication for routine newborn circumcision. For personal reasons, parents choose circumcision.
  1 Careful daily bathing provides adequate hygiene.
  2, 3 There is no scientific evidence to support this statement.
124. Comprehension, planning, physiological (b)
  1 Petroleum keeps the area from scabbing over and sticking to the diaper and thus prevents bleeding.
  2 Complications do not occur often because circumcision is a relatively minor procedure.
  3 Voiding is not frequently affected.
  4 Healing usually occurs quickly.
125. Comprehension, assessment, physiological (b)
  1 Vital signs are not stable in the newborn. Respirations can fluctuate from 30 to 60 per minute.
  2 This response can instill fear in the mother.
  3 The message to the mother is that she is not knowledgeable.
  4 Incomplete information being offered.
126. Knowledge, assessment, psychosocial (b)
  2 This is acccurate information and the best nursing response.
  1 This response assumes that the information was covered in prenatal classes.
  3 This response gives false assurance.
  4 This response does not allay her fears.
127. Knowledge, assessment, physiological (b)
  1 This is accurate information and the best nursing response.
  2 This response incorrectly accuses the mother.
  3 This response gives false information.
  4 This response can instill fear in the mother, and it is not within scope of nursing practice to make such a decision.
128. Knowledge, assessment, physiological (b)
  3 Physiologic jaundice between 48 and 72 hours of life is usually a result of the immature liver being unable to conjugate indirect bilirubin, the newborn's high red blood cell count, and hemolysis of fetal red blood cells.
  1 Pathologic jaundice associated with Rh incompatibility occurs within the first 24 hours of life.
  2 Pathologic jaundice associated with ABO incompatibility occurs with the first 24 hours of life.
  4 Biliary atresia is the obstruction of or absence of a portion of the bile duct. Jaundice is the earliest evidence of a problem. It may be apparent at birth, but it is not usually apparent until the child is 2 to 3 weeks of age.

129. Knowledge, assessment, physiological (a)
  1 This is the correct definition of the rooting reflex.
  2 This is a normal reflex noted in a young infant. It is elicited by a sudden loud noise that results in flexion of the legs, an embracing position of the arms, and a brief cry.
  3 It is a normal response in newborns to extend the arm and the leg on the side of the body to which the head is quickly turned while the infant is in the supine position, and to flex the limbs of the opposite side.
  4 This is the involuntary sucking movement of the circumoral area in newborns in response to stimulation; reflex continues throughout infancy and often occurs without stimulation, even during sleep.
130. Comprehension, assessment, environment (b)
  2 This is peripheral cyanosis, a blue color of hands and feet in most infants at birth that may persist for 7 to 10 days.
  1, 3 These conditions even in adults are usually noted in the hands. These options were too general even though warming, in adults, induces vasodilation, and the blue discoloration becomes mottled with red.
  4 The most probable substance with which a newborn may be covered is vernix caseosa, which is a white cheesy substance that is not usually confined to the extremities.
131. Comprehension, assessment, physiological (a)
  4 Respirations in the newborn may be irregular and range from 32 to 48 per minute. Respiratory distress evidenced by abnormal rate, cyanosis, substernal retractions, and flaring of the nares should be reported immediately.
  1 Respirations are often irregular; 36 is within normal range, but 24 is too low and would be evidence of respiratory distress.
  2 True respirations would probably be irregular; 40 is within the normal range, but 58 is too fast and would be evidence of respiratory distress.
  3 Respirations would most likely be irregular; 30 to 44 per minute falls within the normal range.
132. Knowledge, planning, environment (a)
  1 Air swallowed during feeding most frequently causes regurgitation; therefore it is wise to burp the infant frequently during and following completion of the feeding.
  2, 3 These are inappropriate responses.
  4 This condition does not exist.
133. Application, implementation, environment (b)
  3 The eyes of the newborn may initially be puffy and red as a result of the delivery and instillation of silver nitrate solution. Gentle cleansing of exudate is sufficient intervention at this time; purulent or odoriferous drainage should be reported.
  1, 2, 4 These are not appropriate at this time.
134. Knowledge, assessment, environment (a)
  2 The first stool of a newborn is known as "meconium" and is blackish-greenish and tarry.
  1, 3, 4 This does not describe the first stool of the newborn; changes are noted in color and consistency of stool as the infant begins to take formula or be put to breast.

135. Knowledge, assessment, physiological (a)
    2 (a)   8.0 lb (3600 g) (b)   16.0 oz
               ×10%   × 0.8
                0.8 lb   12.8 oz weight loss
    (c) 7 lb 16.0 oz − 7 lb 12.8 oz = 7 lb 3 oz (3200 g)
    1, 3, 4 Incorrect calculations.
136. Comprehension, implementation, environment (a)
    4 The condition will disappear by itself.
    1 This will cause damage and may cause infection.
    2 Binders are used for engorged mothers.
    3 Hot packs are used by breast-feeding mothers.
137. Knowledge, assessment, physiological (a)
    1 Discharge is normal because of maternal hormonal transfer across the placenta. At the time of delivery a greater exchange of hormones may occur, which causes a temporary increase of the infant's hormone level.
    2 Birth trauma does not usually occur in this area.
    3 The infant has not produced the increased hormonal level; see rationale No. 1.
    4 There is no such thing.
138. Comprehension, assessment, physiological (a)
    3 Physiological jaundice occurs because the newborn destroys red blood cells (RBCs) no longer needed; RBCs cause bilirubin levels to rise and jaundice appears in 72 hours.
    1 Jaundice appearing in the first 24 hours of life is pathological.
    2 It is more likely to be 3 days (72 hours) because of the timing factor in breakdown of the RBCs.
    4 After 5 days jaundice is likely to have another cause.
139. Comprehension, planning, environment (b)
    4 Infection control is mandatory until all blood, amniotic fluid, and vernix are removed.
    1 Bath depends on temperature control, not PO intake.
    2 The nurse should begin with eyes and wash entire body.
    3 Cord care follows the bath.
140. Application, implementation, environment (b)
    4 A syringe against the interior aspect of the cheek will administer the medication far enough back to avoid spitting and will help to avoid choking.
    1 The results of mixing medication with formula are unpredictable; the newborn may not drink all the formula.
    2 Newborns have a protrusion reflex of the tongue that makes spoon-fed foods unreliable.
    3 As in Nos. 1 and 2, newborns will probably spit amounts of cereal out because of protrusion of the tongue. Giving cereal is not appropriate for the age of the baby.
141. Knowledge, assessment, physiological (a)
    1 A normal neonate's pulse rate usually ranges between 120 and 160 beats/min; therefore, this neonate's pulse rate falls within the normal parameter.
    2 Infarction is defined as the death of tissue. The pulse rate is not directly related to such an occurrence.
    3 While the pulse rate may be an indicator of heart disease, this neonate's range is within normal limits.
    4 With respiratory distress syndrome, the neonate's pulse rate will not be within normal limits of 120 to 160 beats/min; it would more likely be increased.

142. Knowledge, assessment, physiological (a)
    1 Respiratory rate is fairly slow; would be irregular; not regular.
    2 Breathing is quiet, irregular, and 35 to 50 per minute.
    3 Respiratory rate is too high; would be irregular; not regular.
    4 Breathing is quiet but not shallow.
143. Comprehension, assessment, environment (b)
    4 This promotes safety and provides injury control.
    1 In this nursing response, there is no learning for the mother or safety for the baby.
    2, 3 In these responses by the nurse, there is no learning for the mother.
144. Application, evaluation, psychosocial (c)
    4 This response communicates findings of data collected.
    1, 2, 3 These nursing attitudes lack insight into the behavior exhibited.
145. Comprehension, evaluation, environment (b)
    1 Watery green stools result from extra bilirubin being excreted because of the phototherapy.
    2 This is the stool commonly noted in a baby that is being breast fed.
    3 Meconium is formed during fetal life and is passed within the first 24 hours after birth in normal infants.
    4 This is the stool commonly noted in a baby that is being bottle fed.
146. Comprehension, planning, physiological (c)
    4 ABO incompatibility involves type A or type B infants born to type O mothers.
    1 Physiologic jaundice occurs after the first 24 hours.
    2 Rh incompatibility occurs with an Rh-negative mother and an Rh-positive father.
    3 Jaundice in the infant with hepatitis B occurs after the fourth week of life.
147. Application, implementation, environment (c)
    4 The newborn's temperature may rise when exposed to the heat produced by the phototherapy bulb.
    1 The infant's eyes are securely covered with patches.
    2 Fluids are encouraged to aid in excretion of bilirubin.
    3 The diaper is left on to protect genitalia.
148. Comprehension, planning, physiological (c)
    2 A combination of A negative with A positive can produce A positive; if the infant is positive, the mother produces antibodies that cross the placenta barrier and damage the infant's red blood cells.
    1 Two Rh-negatives do not create an Rh-positive.
    3 This combination should not present any difficulties.
    4 Two Rh-positives do not create an Rh-negative.
149. Knowledge, assessment, health (a)
    3 This is infection of the newborn's eyes and is caused by gonococci.
    1, 2 These are not correct.
    4 Syphilis can cause congenital deformities.
150. Comprehension, assessment, physiological (b)
    1 Within the first week of life, the newborn with congenital syphilis may develop a rash over the face, palms, and soles of the feet, as well as a purulent nasal discharge.
    2 These are not associated with congenital syphilis.
    3 These are signs of central nervous system damage associated with congenital syphilis that appears later in life.
    4 These are not associated with congenital syphilis.

151. Application, implementation, environment (b)
    3 Implementation of the universal precaution protocol is recommended in all health-care facilities when dealing with aids or HIV-positive patients.
    1 While this is still a procedure in the nursery, universal precautions are being used in health-care facilities when caring for AIDS or HIV-positive patients. In fact, whether or not an infant or its mother is tested for the virus, most health-care facilities recommend that nurses wear gloves during initial care of the newborn.
    2 It is not the responsibility of the nurse to report to the Center For Disease Control; the nurse is responsible to his or her supervisor, whose duty it is to report such cases.
    4 The mask, gown, and gloves at all times are not really necessary because most HIV-positive patients are not necessarily ill with the signs and symptoms of active AIDS. Use of masks, gowns and gloves is for the patient whose immune system places him at risk.
152. Comprehension, evaluation, physiological (c)
    1 Because the newborn has been receiving cocaine on a continual basis throughout the pregnancy, it has become addicted to the drug and will undergo withdrawal symptoms if the drug is not resupplied.
    2 Prolonged use of drugs before conception may affect both the mother and the unborn child; prolonged use of the drug throughout the pregnancy will definitely lead to addiction in the newborn.
    3 Cocaine is dangerous; mixing it with other drugs could lead to problems of drug incompatability; the statement that the infant would be doubly addicted is incorrect.
    4 Cocaine does impair uterine growth, but it does not in and of itself give rise to RDS (respiratory distress syndrome).
153. Comprehension, planning, psychosocial (c)
    2 Punishment should follow wrong-doing.
    1 This should not affect the consequence of wrong-doing.
    3 Punishment should not be used as an outlet for parent's feelings.
    4 Punishment is not appropriate.
154. Knowledge, implementation, health (a)
    4 A positive environment contributes to good eating habits.
    1 Forcing them can ultimately turn them off to certain foods.
    2 This is not an important consideration with children.
    3 The child's selection may not always be the best; also, it does not allow for food preparation ahead of time.
155. Knowledge, assessment, psychosocial (a)
    4 The time period to develop trust is the infancy period, birth to 1 year of age; Psychosocial need, trust vs. mistrust (Erikson).
    1 This is the adolescence period, 12 to 19 years of age; Psychosocial need, identity vs. role confusion (Erikson).
    2 This is the preschool period, 3 to 6 years of age; Psychosocial need, initiative vs. guilt (Erikson).
    3 This is the school-age period, 6 to 12 years of age; Psychosocial need, industry vs. inferiority (Erikson).
156. Comprehension, assessment, physiological (b)
    4 At one month the infant can turn its head from side to side when placed on its abdomen.
    1 Between 3 and 4 months of age the infant can roll from back to side.
    2 At 4 months the infant can smile and laugh aloud when talked to.
    3 At 2 months the infant can hold a rattle for a brief period of time.
157. Knowledge, assessment, physiological (a)
    2 At 4 months the infant is mastering these developmental tasks.
    1 At 2 months the infant cannot hold its head erect when in a sitting position.
    3, 4 At these ages the infant has mastered these developmental tasks and is trying to master other tasks appropriate for those developmental levels.
158. Knowledge, assessment, physiological (a)
    4 The anterior fontanel closes between 15 and 18 months of age.
    1 The posterior fontanel closes between 2 and 3 months of age.
    2, 3 The posterior fontanel should have closed, but the anterior fontanel has not.
159. Knowledge, planning, health (a)
    1 Basic simple language is easily learned and understood.
    2 Many words are too new and not easy to understand.
    3 This prevents growth.
    4 This communication is beyond the child's level of comprehension.
160. Knowledge, implementation, physiological (a)
    4 Physiological development of the anal muscles and readiness for toilet training occurs at 2 years of age.
    1 The toddler can feed himself/herself with a spoon by 15 months of age.
    2 Walking with assistance occurs between 11 and 12 months.
    3 Manipulating building blocks occurs between 15 and 18 months. The toddler can build a tower of 2 blocks.
161. Comprehension, planning, psychosocial (a)
    3 Training pants are much like regular pants, but they have the absorbency in case he does wet accidentally.
    1 These are difficult to get off, and they do not provide a chance for developmental progress.
    2 The message is that it is okay to wet his diaper or pants.
    4 Overalls are difficult to get off quickly.
162. Comprehension, planning, health (b)
    2 This allows release of extra energy and gives the child a healthy outlook.
    1, 3 Giving in reinforces the idea that tantrums get you what you want, so it's good to continue to have them.
    4 He is not at a level where such comprehension is possible.
163. Comprehension, planning, environment (b)
    4 Toddlers are curious and continue to search out by feeling and tasting.
    1 Toddlers are too young to realize the concept of fear.
    2 Swallowing objects is not a usual means for this age group of getting attention.
    3 Easy access, while a possible factor, is not the main motivating factor for children to act on their need to explore.
164. Comprehension, implementation, psychosocial (b)
    4 The child has no comprehension of sharing at this age; they also "parallel play," a form of play among a group of children, usually toddlers, in which each play independently, yet together, and are not influenced by one another or share their toys/playthings.
    1 The child would not benefit from this.
    2 This is a very inappropriate answer.
    3 The mother should not encourage or push the child.
165. Knowledge, implementation, psychosocial (c)
    2 The child realizes some measure of control over his surroundings and begins to test the extent of his power.
    1 This is Erickson's stage for school-age children.
    3 This is Erickson's stage for infants.
    4 This is Erickson's stage for preschoolers.

166. Knowledge, assessment, physiological (a)
    1 Gross motor coordination involves the use of large muscles in the body, as in running and walking.
    2 Tying represents fine-motor coordination.
    3 Writing uses muscles in hands and fingers, which is fine-muscle coordination.
    4 Sewing represents fine-muscle coordination and manual dexterity.

167. Knowledge, assessment, environment (a)
    2 90 to 100 beats/min for 2 to 6 years of age.
    1 76 to 90 beats/min for children over 10 years of age.
    3 110 to 140 beats/min for an infant, 1 month to 1 year of age.
    4 120 to 150 beats/min for a neonate, birth to 1 month of age.

168. Comprehension, implementation, psychosocial (c)
    3 Playing with other children the same age and giving and sharing are important to the socialization process.
    1 This will not necessarily change.
    2 This may not have a direct relationship.
    4 This may be an outlet but is not the focus.

169. Knowledge, assessment, psychosocial (a)
    2 Industry occurs during the school age period, 6 to 12 years of age. Psychosocial need, industry vs. inferiority. Learning to win recognition by producing things (Erickson).
    1 This is the toddler period, 1 to 3 years of age. Psychosocial need, autonomy vs. shame. Trying out own (self) powers of speech (Erickson).
    3 Preschool period, 3 to 6 years of age. Psychosocial need, initiative vs. guilt. Questioning and exploring own body and development (Erickson).
    4 This is the young adulthood period, 20 to 40 years of age. Psychosocial need, intimacy vs. isolation (Erickson).

170. Knowledge, assessment, psychosocial (c)
    2 During the middle childhood period, 7 to 11 years of age, children engage in concrete operations. Reasoning is logical but limited to personal experience (Piaget).
    1 This is the period of "formal operations," a time during which the child, 11 to 16 years of age, acquires the ability to develop abstract concepts; becomes oriented to problem solving (Piaget).
    3, 4 The Preoperational Phase of cognitive development extends from age 2 to age 7 and is divided into two phases: the preconceptual phase, ages 2 to 4, during which the child is able to form general concepts but is not yet capable of reasoning; and the phase of intuitive thought, ages 4 to 7, a time during which perceptual thinking occurs and the child is capable of some reasoning but can concentrate on only one aspect of a situation at a time (Piaget).

171. Knowledge, assessment, physiological (a)
    3 Females usually complete puberty by 14 years of age.
    1 Females are slightly ahead of males in physical development.
    2 Males usually begin pubertal changes at 14 years of age.
    4 Females experience puberty slightly ahead of males.

172. Knowledge, assessment, psychosocial (a)
    2 Although strong in our society, adolescent rebellion need not be inevitable. There is little evidence that a full-blown rebellion characterizes most relationships between teenagers and their parents.
    1 True. Many conflicts between parents and teens focus on sexuality and many adolescents have difficulty discussing sexual matters with their parents.
    3 True. Four out of 10 of today's 14-year-old girls will become pregnant in their teens if trends continue.
    4 True. There has been a steady trend by society in general toward acceptance of more sexual activity in more situations.

173. Comprehension, evaluation, psychosocial (b)
    2 Seclusiveness and moodiness are behavior characteristics of the 13-year-old.
    1 Hormonal influences and uncertainty about self-identity make for very unpredictable behavior.
    3 The adolescent is usually not very accepting of parent's ideals; can be rebellious.
    4 The goal of the adolescent is to move from dependency to self-reliance, increasing autonomy.

174. Comprehension, planning, psychosocial (b)
    4 Adolescents, age 12 to 18, are at the stage in which they are searching for their own identity.
    1 This is the stage of school-age children, ages 6 to 12.
    2 This is the stage of infants, birth to 1 year of age.
    3 This is the stage of the child, 3 to 6 years of age.

175. Comprehension, planning, psychosocial (b)
    2 The adolescent is trying to become independent of parents and family.
    1, 3, 4 These are major developmental tasks during this period.

176. Knowledge, planning, health (a)
    2 A baby has a total of 20 deciduous teeth.
    1 This is too few.
    3, 4 These are too many.

177. Comprehension, planning, health (c)
    2 This is the recommended schedule published in the Morbidity and Mortality Weekly Report by the US Department of Health and Human Services.
    1, 3, 4 These are not the recommended schedule.

178. Comprehension, evaluation, health (c)
    2 Immunizations have decreased the incidence of many communicable diseases, but some children are not receiving immunizations. This accounts for the fact that communicable diseases are still a major problem in children.
    1 Not all children have been immunized.
    3 Some communicable diseases are necessary to build up natural immunity.
    4 Some conditions are serious, and no immunization is available.

179. Knowledge, implementation, health (a)
    3 Diphtheria, pertussis, tetanus (DPT) and trivalent oral polio vaccine (TOPV) are the first immunizations given according to schedule at the age of 2 months.
    1 Rubella is not given until the age of 15 months.
    2 DPT is given at the age of 2 months, along with TOPV.
    4 Measles and mumps not given until the age of 15 months.

180. Knowledge, planning, health (b)
    4 The MMR should not be given until the child is 15 months of age because of the presence of maternal antibodies in the child.
    1, 2, 3 This is too early.

181. Knowledge, planning, health (a)
    1 A banana would be considered more nutritious, and it does not contain sodium.
    2 A candy bar would not be considered nutritious; it may contain some sodium.
    3 A ham sandwich would be omitted because ham contains sodium.
    4 Tuna salad would be omitted because tuna is found in salt water.

182. Knowledge, implementation, health (a)
    1 To avoid food allergies, the mother should introduce one food at a time.
    2, 3 This is important, but the concern of allergic reactions takes priority.
    4 Formula feedings are also supplemented with vitamins and iron.

183. Knowledge, implementation, health (a)
    3 Cereal is suggested at 5 months.
    1, 2 Breast milk or formula are suggested at these ages.
    4 Strained fruits, meats, and finger food are suggested at 7 to 8 months.

184. Knowledge, implementation, health (a)
    2 The complete proteins contain the eight essential amino acids required for growth and development.
    1, 3, 4 These foods provide incomplete protein.

185. Knowledge, implementation, health (a)
    4 This is the recommended procedure to prevent contamination of the vulvar area from organisms around the anal area. It is also recommended after bowel movements to avoid fecal contamination of the vulvar area.
    1 This may prove helpful for a time, but it is not sufficient to avoid further contamination over a period of time.
    2 The situation does not indicate antibiotics were administered. In any case such advice is incorrect because antibiotics must be taken as ordered over a specified period of time, even after symptoms have subsided.
    3 Cranberry juice has no direct effect on bacteria. In any case, drinking only cranberry juice would not be a likely order.

186. Application, implementation, physiological (c)
    1 Although cardiac catheterization usually has no complications, there can be some danger. The nurse should assess the catheter insertion site for bleeding or hematoma.
    2 The patient's peripheral pulses are checked every 15 minutes for an hour after the test and frequently after that for several hours. Monitor more frequently than every 2 hours.
    3 Some physicians keep the patient in bed for the rest of the day. Place the child in a reclining position for several hours after the cardiac catheterization to avoid a drop in blood pressure and bleeding at the catheter insertion site.
    4 This should have been done preoperatively. The patient has returned to his room and requires postoperative assessment.

187. Application, implementation, environment (c)
    4 $\dfrac{60}{60} \times \dfrac{20}{1} = \dfrac{1}{1} \times \dfrac{20}{1} = 20$ drops/min
    1, 2, 3 Incorrect calculations

188. Knowledge, assessment, physiological (b)
    4 The clinical signs and symptoms given indicate patent ductus arterious.
    1 Aortic stenosis is rarely symptomatic during infancy. In severe cases the infant will have decreased cardiac output. Older children will have chest pain, shortness of breath, and dyspnea.
    2 In pulmonary stenosis, the child is generally asymptomatic but may have decreased exercise tolerance and dyspnea and cyanosis with severe obstruction.
    3 In childhood, coarctation of the aorta is usually asymptomatic, and growth and development are normal.

189. Knowledge, assessment, physiological (b)
    3 Patent ductus arteriosus (PDA) is an opening between the pulmonary artery and the aorta caused by failure of the fetal ductus arteriosus to close after birth.
    1 Atrial septal defect (ASD) is an abnormal opening in the septum between the left atrium and right atrium.
    2 Ventricular septal defect (VSD) is an abnormal opening in the septum between the right and left ventricles.
    4 This is anomalous venous return, in which oxygenated blood returning from the lungs is carried abnormally to the right side of the heart by one or more pulmonary veins into the right atrium.

190. Comprehension, planning, physiological (c)
    1 In leukemia, the bone marrow is characterized by being hypercellular, lacking fat globules, and containing an increased number of immature white cells.
    2 Gastric analysis helps to determine some stomach conditions; it is not diagnostic for leukemia.
    3 ABGs determine oxygen needs and acid base balance; they are not diagnostic for leukemia.
    4 The cardiac echogram helps diagnose heart conditions; it is not diagnostic for leukemia.

191. Knowledge, planning, environment (a)
    3 Painful joints are a common symptom often relieved by bed rest. Exacerbated joint pain may be severe, especially in advanced stages.
    1 There is no cyanosis present.
    2, 4 These are not related to the situation.

192. Comprehension, assessment, physiological (c)
    3 As leukemia progresses, membranes of the anal area tend to ulcerate and bleed.
    1 This is not applicable.
    2 Leukemia patients' skin is usually pale lemon-yellow.
    4 This is seen more commonly in heart or respiratory disease.

193. Knowledge, planning, physiological (c)
    2 The combination of drugs helps induce remissions that may last for weeks, months, or even years.
    1 These drugs do not have analgesic actions.
    3 These are not antibiotics.
    4 This is not applicable.

194. Application, evaluation, psychosocial (a)
    2 The nurse is allowing the child to express her feelings about dying. This response opens a line of communication.
    1 This response cuts the patient off from discussing her feelings.
    3 With this response, the child might think the nurse doesn't care.
    4 It is best not to avoid the issue; this response discourages the child from ventilating feelings.

195. Knowledge, planning, physiological (b)
    4 These, including lethargy and fever, are all symptoms of the disease.
    1, 2 The white blood count is elevated in acute leukemia.
    3 Hemoglobin is decreased in acute leukemia.

196. Comprehension, assessment, physiological (b)
    1 Petechiae, fever, weight loss, pallor, hemorrhages, and bone and joint pain are also symptoms due to accumulation of white cells in the bone marrow.
    2 Bleeding is not within the GI tract; it is more so under the skin. Nausea and vomiting are not usual symptoms.
    3 Fever does occur but there is usually no accompanying rash or itchy skin.
    4 There is bleeding under the skin but not in the gastrointestinal tract. There is no rash.

197. Comprehension, planning, environment (a)
    3 The disease is considered a malignant neoplasm of the blood-forming organs; it is characterized by diffuse replacement of bone marrow with proliferating leukocyte precursors, and abnormal numbers and forms of immature white cells in circulation.
    1 Red blood cells and platelets are decreased; patients receive blood transfusions as part of their treatment.
    2 The opposite is true; weight loss, pallor and fatigue are characteristic of the disease.
    4 The opposite is true; immature white blood cells are in circulation.

198. Comprehension, planning, health (b)
    4 These provide infection control and blood replacement for lost red blood cells and platelets.
    1 Once diagnosis is made and treatment is started, weight loss will stabilize.
    2 Weight loss is not a result of edema.
    3 Home care is not really necessary because the child is not home-bound in the early stages.

199. Application, implementation, psychosocial (b)
    1 It is important for the nurse to be honest and truthful, and to explain procedures and answer questions as they come up.
    2, 3 These concerns may occur and be handled better if her coping ability is developed.
    4 Important but not priority at this time; not best response.

200. Knowledge, assessment, physiological (b)
    4 The pathology of rheumatic fever is not clearly understood, but the disease tends to follow a recent infection with the beta-hemolytic *Streptococcus.*
    1 Virus is not a cause.
    2, 3 These are not applicable.

201. Comprehension, planning, environment (a)
    4 During the acute stage, the patient is on complete bed rest and must be turned.
    1 He needs a bed bath, not a shower.
    2 He should not be allowed to walk.
    3 This is not applicable to situation.

202. Comprehension, planning, physiological (b)
    3 Aspirin is used for rheumatic fever primarily to relieve joint pain, inflammation, and fever.
    1 If carditis develops, corticosteroids are added to drug therapy.
    2 Aspirin is not used for this condition.
    4 Aspirin is not an antiemetic.

203. Comprehension, evaluation, environment (c)
    2 Valvular heart damage, especially mitral valve disease, is common following rheumatic fever.
    1, 3 These do not usually occur.
    4 There is no paralysis with this condition.

204. Application, planning, health (c)
    4 Exercise such as sports requires increased glucose. Without a snack of a high-carbohydrate food, he may become hypoglycemic.
    1 Exercise requires more glucose. Administering extra insulin will make him more hypoglycemic.
    2 Jimmy needs an extra snack. Skipping a meal will make him more inclined to hypoglycemia.
    3 There is no reason to stop playing as long as he knows to eat an extra snack.

205. Comprehension, planning, health (b)
    3 Exchange lists for fast-food restaurants are available and enable the adolescent to be like his peers when eating out.
    1 This is an unrealistic expectation because adolescents do not want to be noticeably different from their peers. Lettuce-and-tomato salads should also be counted on the diabetic exchange list.
    2 A stable blood glucose level is desired. Varied fluctuations can lead to complications.
    4 Eating anything and ignoring the effects on blood glucose levels can lead to complications.

206. Application, planning, health (c)
    2 Jimmy should have a snack with him when he is driving in case he begins to feel hypoglycemic. This is a safety measure.
    1 If Jimmy understands that he needs to have a snack with him, there is no reason why he cannot drive.
    3 There is no reason to have another driver with him.
    4 The department of public safety will issue a driver's license; however, Jimmy's diabetes should be noted on the back of the license.

207. Knowledge, implementation, health (b)
    2 The anterior pituitary gland produces the growth hormone, thyroid-stimulating hormone, adrenocorticotropic hormone, melanocyte-stimulating hormone, follicle-stimulating hormone, luteinizing hormone, interstitial cell–stimulating hormone, and prolactin.
    1 The thyroid gland produces thyroxin, triiodothyronine, and thyrocalcitonin.
    3 The posterior pituitary gland produces oxytocin and the antidiuretic hormone.
    4 The adrenal medulla produces adrenaline (epinephrine) and aldosterone.

208. Knowledge, planning, physiological (b)
    1 The pituitary gland is also called the hypophysis; therefore, the term for removal of the pituitary gland is hypophysectomy.
    2 This is the term for removal of the thyroid gland.
    3 This is the term for removal of the parathyroid glands.
    4 This is the term for removal of the adrenal gland.

209. Comprehension, assessment, physiological (c)
    1 These are complications with removal of the anterior pituitary gland because of the other hormones produced by the gland.
    2 These complications should be observed with a thyroidectomy.
    3 These are complications that occur in diabetes mellitus.
    4 These are complications that occur with an adrenalectomy.

210. Comprehension, implementation, health (b)
    1 This syndrome is a metabolic defect precipitated by the ingestion of rye or wheat gluten.
    2, 3, 4 Lean meats, vegetables and fruits are not contraindicated.

211. Knowledge, assessment, health (a)
    3 A soft diet of low-fiber, low-residue, bland foods that have a high protein and caloric content is ordered for patients with Crohn's disease.
    1 A full-liquid diet consists of only liquids and foods that liquefy at body temperature. There is no residue or fiber in this diet, which is usually ordered for patients unable to consume soft or semifluid foods after surgery.
    2 A clear liquid diet supplies fluids and provides minimal residue. The diet is nutritionally inadequate and is usually prescribed for a limited amount of time, such as 1 day, following surgery. Proteins are needed more than potassium.
    4 A soft diet is okay, but high-fiber foods are not permitted.

212. Comprehension, assessment, physiological (b)
 1 Edema is the prime symptom of nephrosis. It may be so severe that the child gains twice his normal weight.
 2 Proteinuria, not hematuria, is present.
 3 Petechial rash is not associated with this disease.
 4 This is not a prime symptom.

213. Comprehension, assessment, physiological (b)
 2 The urine reveals large amounts of proteinuria with blood not usually present.
 1 No hematuria is revealed.
 3 This is not significant in this case.
 4 Albuminuria is abnormal in this case.

214. Comprehension, planning, physiological (c)
 4 Protein is usually limited in kidney disorders, but it is needed for replacement of urinary protein loss.
 1 Sodium and increased fluids tend to retain fluids in tissues.
 2 Protein is needed to maintain blood albumin levels.
 3 These are not relative to the situation.

215. Knowledge, assessment, environment (b)
 3 Eczema occurs more commonly in winter months and tends to run in families.
 1 Impetigo is an infectious disease of the superficial layers of the skin; it is seen in infants and is caused by staphylococci.
 2 This is an abnormal chronic inflammatory disease of the sebaceous glands and hair follicles. It affects 90% of all adolescents in varying degrees.
 4 Dysplasia is an abnormal development of tissue.

216. Application, implementation, physiological (a)
 3 Keeping the skin clean and dry aids in the prevention of infection.
 1 The child's position should be changed frequently to avoid constant pressure to one area as well as severe itching.
 2 To reduce itching and subsequent scratching a minimum amount of clothing is recommended.
 4 Warm, moist dressings would increase the itching; cool moist dressings should be used.

217. Knowledge, assessment, health (a)
 1 Ringworm is caused by a fungus and can occur on the scalp (tinea capitis), body (tinea corporis), or feet (tinea pedis).
 2 Pediculosis is an infestation of lice.
 3 Herpes is caused by a virus.
 4 Uticaria is more commonly known as hives, often caused by allergies to foods and animal furs.

218. Knowledge, assessment, physiological (a)
 4 *Microsporum audouinii* is the major fungal pathogen that causes tinea capitis (ringworm of the scalp).
 1 A virus is a minute microorganism that can only replicate within a cell of a living plant or animal; it is not a fungus.
 2 This is a genus of aerobic, gram-positive, spore-producing bacteria in the family Bacillaceae; it is not a fungus.
 3 Bacteria are any of the small unicellular microorganisms of the class Schizomycetes; bacteria are not a fungus.

219. Comprehension, implementation, environment (a)
 2 To administer 20 mg of meperidine (Demerol) elixir, the nurse would convert teaspoon measurement to milliliters and give 2 ml.
 1 Incorrect dose; too little.
 3, 4 Incorrect doses; too much.

220. Comprehension, planning, physiological (b)
 2 Immobilization of the recipient site prevents the possibility of dislodging the graft and destroying the tissue-building process.
 1, 3, 4 These actions do not necessarily facilitate acceptance of the graft.

221. Comprehension, planning, environment (b)
 1 During long periods of immobilization, calcium from bones and other tissues enters the circulatory system to be filtered and excreted by the kidneys; increased levels of calcium and urinary stasis in the renal pelvis predispose the child to renal calculi.
 2, 3, 4 These are inappropriate responses; these are not relevant to the situation.

222. Knowledge, planning, physiological (a)
 1 This is the definition of the term; scoliosis of the spine occurs because of rapid growth and is most often noted in girls.
 2 This is a disease of the kidneys, causing edema and proteinuria.
 3 This is a concave curvature of the spine, commonly known as swayback.
 4 This is a convex curvature of the spine, commonly known as hunchback.

223. Comprehension, evaluation, physiological (b)
 4 The child attempts to maintain balance and an erect posture, resulting in a compensatory curve.
 1 Pain is rare in children with scoliosis, although some children experience chronic discomfort from continually sitting on their buttocks.
 2 If the deformity is uncorrected, it will result in respiratory compromise.
 3 Detection is simple by visual examination of the spine as the child bends from the waist.

224. Comprehension, implementation, environment (a)
 1 Swelling and edema of the injured limb may increase after application of a cast; tightness of the cast should be determined to ensure that pressure areas that may constrict circulation are not present.
 2, 3, 4 These are definitely inappropriate statements and nursing actions.

225. Comprehension, evaluation, psychosocial (b)
 4 This response informs the grandmother that bed-wetting is normal in children Will's age and that hospitalized children frequently regress into some behaviors that would not normally be seen at home.
 1, 2, 3 These are inappropriate nursing responses.

226. Knowledge, planning, environment (b)
 1 The nurse should be knowledgable of the type and purpose of traction to plan nursing care.
 2 The nurse must know more than function only.
 3 The nurse needs more information than this alone.
 4 The age of the patient is important to know in providing appropriate care.

227. Application, implementation, environment (a)
 2 Ropes, pulleys, and weights are equally important in maintaining correct traction.
 1 Weights set on the floor will defeat the purpose of pulling or tension.
 3 Not applicable.
 4 The nurse should adjust the bed as necessary but should also maintain proper alignment and weight.

228. Application, implementation, physiological (b)
 1 The nurse should check the skin condition for breakdown resulting from complete bed rest and limited movement.
 2 The nurse might check the left leg, but the right leg is affected.
 3 The child should have some kind of activity in bed to prevent complications.
 4 Although important, the mother's reaction is not included in the assessment.

229. Application, planning, physiological (b)
   4 The nurse should encourage activity in bed to prevent complications such as calcification and atrophy during bed rest.
   1 The nurse should encourage activity; see No. 4.
   2 The nurse does not do this routinely or without an order.
   3 Not necessarily every 2 hours.
230. Knowledge, planning, environment (a)
   4 Alignment and immobilization allow the limb to heal.
   1 The fracture does not heal immediately.
   2 It is difficult to keep a child in bed without a reason.
   3 This is not necessarily true.
231. Knowledge, planning, physiological (a)
   2 Cerebral palsy is trauma to the motor centers of the brain.
   1 It is not caused by premature birth alone; a variety of prenatal, perinatal, and postnatal factors contribute to the cause of this condition.
   3 Genetics play no part in cerebral damage.
   4 Erythroblastosis fetalis is a type of hemolytic anemia that occurs in newborns as a result of maternal-fetal blood group incompatibility, specifically involving the Rh factor and the ABO blood groups.
232. Comprehension, planning, environment (b)
   1 Seizures for whatever reason are a major nursing concern and occur whenever there is damage to the motor centers of the brain.
   2, 3 Muscle tone can either be increased or decreased, depending on the nature and distribution of neuromuscular dysfunction.
   4 While sensory impairments, hearing loss, and/or abnormalities of vision are important, they are not life-threatening.
233. Application, implementation, environment (b)
   3 The flow of formula should be well-paced with no pressure and with a water flush to prevent clogging.
   1 Forced pressure can cause damage.
   2 Discarding the formula decreases the amount of nourishment and fluid needed.
   4 Gastrostomy tubes are permanently in place.
234. Comprehension, planning, health (b)
   1 These programs will ensure that educational and social needs will be met, including emotional aspects related to those needs.
   2 This is not a specific enough response.
   3 This is not the most inclusive plan for overall management of care.
   4 The focus needs to be goal-oriented.
235. Comprehension, evaluation, psychosocial (c)
   2 The goal is to allow him to be as independent as possible in those areas in which it can be achieved.
   1 This does not allow for individuality and growth.
   3 Inappropriate response; a study does not assist in the development of family relationships.
   4 This does not encourage him to grow and develop to his full potential; as such may hinder move to become independent.
236. Knowledge, planning, environment (a)
   1 Down's syndrome is a chromosomal abnormality characterized by varying degrees of mental retardation and multiple defects. It is also known as trisomy 21, mongolism, trisomy G syndrome or mongoloid idiocy.
   2, 3 The condition is congenital and is not caused by an infection.
   4 Varying degrees of mental retardation are apparent in Down's syndrome. This is directly related to the chromosomal abnormality and is not a result of oxygen deprivation at birth.

237. Knowledge, planning, physiological (b)
   4 Phenytoin, more commonly known as Dilantin, is classified as an anticonvulsant.
   1 Cimetidine (Tagamet) is used in treatment of gastritis. It is the trade name for a histamine H_2 receptor antagonist (cimetidine).
   2 Hydroxyzine is a short-acting central nervous system depressant. It is a minor tranquilizer known as vistaril.
   3 Compazine is a tradename for a phenothiazine, prochlorperazine, used as an antiemetic and antipsychotic.
238. Application, implementation, psychosocial (b)
   2 Assuming a sitting position beside the father communicates concern and a willingness to help the person in emotional crisis.
   1, 3 These responses do not communicate concern; they create a closed situation.
   4 This action will discourage, not encourage, communication.
239. Comprehension, implementation, psychosocial (b)
   1 When responding to someone in crisis, it is better to respond to the questions and provide only the information asked for by the individual.
   2, 3 These are not appropriate at this time.
   4 This is an inappropriate nursing intervention; it shows lack of both concern and willingness to help. The individual must face the situation and find ways to cope.
240. Comprehension, assessment, physiological (b)
   1 A complication of myelomeningocele is neurologic dysfunction at and below the site of the spina bifida; the parasympathetic and sympathetic nerve damage results in atonia of the bladder and the bowel.
   2, 3, 4 These are not relevant to the situation.
241. Comprehension, assessment, physiological (a)
   1 Before, and especially after, surgery, the infant is observed for movement in the extremities and functioning of bowel and bladder to determine the extent of neurologic dysfunction.
   2, 3, 4 These are not relevant to the situation.
242. Comprehension, implementation, psychosocial (a)
   3 Parent-child bonding can be impeded by separation of the ill neonate from the parents. The bonding process can be encouraged by allowing the parents to touch, hold, and talk to their infant. The infant receiving proper stimulation will thrive more quickly than one deprived of such stimulation.
   1 There is also the need to touch and hold as stated above.
   2 The nurse should explain the process, but the parents should start as soon as possible.
   4 This is an inappropriate nursing action; allowing parents to verbalize feelings will facilitate the parent-child relationship.
243. Comprehension, implementation, physiological (b)
   1 Projectile vomiting is the result of increased intracranial pressure; the infant should be fed small frequent meals to decrease the possibility of aspiration of the feeding. The hydrocephalic head must be supported to prevent trauma to the neck from the weight of the head.
   2, 3 These are inappropriate means of feeding this infant.
   4 This is not usually necessary.
244. Comprehension, planning, physiological (b)
   3 The postoperative position of the head is on the non-operative side to prevent fluid and brain shift, which would traumatize the operative area of the brain.
   1 Incorrect position; this would traumatize the operative area of the brain.
   2, 4 These are not appropriate for the situation.

245. Application, implementation, psychosocial (b)
    3 The head circumference provides data to determine change over a period of time.
    1, 2 These responses may cause great concern for the mother.
    4 This is an inappropriate and nasty response by the nurse.

246. Application, implementation, environment (b)
    3 The young child is placed in a sitting position with the neck flexed to separate the spinous processes and thus ease insertion of the needle. While in this position the child must be observed for breathing difficulties from poor lung expansion.
    1, 4 Inappropriate nursing actions; incorrect position.
    2 Inappropriate nursing action; not a routine part of the procedure.

247. Knowledge, planning, environment (b)
    3 This is the correct definition of an omphalocele.
    1 This is a displacement of some of the abdominal organs through an opening in the diaphragm into the chest cavity.
    2 This is a displacement of part of the intestine through an incomplete closure at the fetal end of the umbilical cord.
    4 This defines a condition in which the esophagus ends in a blind pouch and the lower end of the esophagus attaches to the trachea.

248. Comprehension, planning, physiological (b)
    1 These are the most common symptoms of the disease, including severe headache and pain.
    2 Dyspnea and high blood pressure are not common to the disease.
    3, 4 Red, raised rash is not common to the disease.

249. Application, implementation, environment (b)
    4 Time and description of the seizure are important.
    1 This is true, but only after the seizure has passed.
    2 Protection is important, but restraint could lead to severe injury.
    3 This could lead to injury of the child's mouth, especially after the seizure has started; this action is no longer recommended.

250. Application, implementation, psychosocial (b)
    2 After the tantrum is over, the mother will be able to deal with Jody in a calm and more controlled manner.
    1 This is a bribe; it is not recommended because it will only facilitate rather than inhibit episodes of tantrums.
    3 This action does not get at the cause of the matter.
    4 Finding out what the problem may be is good advice, but not while the child is out of control. It would be impossible to deal effectively with Jody during a tantrum.

251. Application, implementation, environment (a)
    4 Direct pressure applied for one to two minutes will control the bleeding.
    1 This is not an immediate action.
    2, 3 These are not relevant to the situation.

252. Comprehension, planning, environment (b)
    2 Bacterial infections treated with antibiotics for 24 hours are not considered communicable.
    1, 4 These are incorrect, not necessary; see response No. 2.
    3 This is only one of the primary concerns.

253. Comprehension, assessment, physiological (b)
    3 Periodic comparative observations are made to note differences in vital signs, neurologic status and renal function; accurate intake and output measurements are essential to determine fluid replacement needs and to detect cerebral edema.
    1 These are general observations that are routine when caring for an infant with an IV infusion.
    2, 4 These are abnormal signs and should be reported; however, these are not specific only to the care of this infant.

254. Application, implementation, environment, (a)
    1 Maintenance and care of the IV site are of primary importance in caring for the child with meningitis who receives medication intravenously. The long-term fluid and antibiotic therapy increases the child's susceptibility to phlebitis and fluid infiltration at the site.
    2 This is an incorrect procedure; see above response.
    3, 4 These are not necessary.

255. Comprehension, assessment, physiological (c)
    4 The traumatic episode produces psychotic-type behavior.
    1 It is a misconception that mental illness occurs.
    2 This is a violent jarring or shaking of the brain caused by a sudden change in momentum of the head.
    3 Negative symptomatology *is* related to the extent of organic damage.

256. Comprehension, planning, physiological (b)
    1 Elevating the head of the bed 45 degrees or helping the patient to sit up usually remedies the situation automatically.
    2, 3, 4 These actions would not resolve the situation.

257. Knowledge, planning, health (a)
    1 Cranberry juice promotes acidic urine and cuts down on stone formation.
    2, 3 These can possibly lead to stone formation as a result of acids found in these foods.
    4 Milk can possibly lead to stone formation as a result of calcium found in this food.

258. Comprehension, assessment, physiological (b)
    2 Changes in motion or sensation in the extremities are the most reliable determination of the presence of edema of the spinal cord; edema causes trauma to motor and sensory nerves.
    1, 3, 4 These are symptoms of autonomic dysreflexia.

259. Knowledge, implementation, physiological (a)
    2 Decadron prevents and alleviates spinal cord edema. It is administered by local injection, and it has a rapid onset and long duration.
    1 This drug is a systemic corticosteroid.
    3, 4 These drugs are diuretics.

260. Comprehension, planning, environment (b)
    2 Addiction to narcotics can develop in a short time. Other measures must be found to alleviate pain caused by long-term problems.
    1, 3, 4 These are not relevant to the question asked.

261. Comprehension, planning, physiological (b)
    3 The head of the bed should be elevated, not kept flat, to facilitate breathing.
    1, 2, 4 These are common in the management and care of a child with asthma.

262. Knowledge, assessment, physiological (a)
    2 This is a classical symptom of asthma and is caused by the trapping of air in the alveoli.
    1 Noisy and hoarse inspirations are commonly seen in croup.
    3, 4 These are not common symptoms of asthma.

263. Application, planning, physiological (b)
    2 Asthma is an obstructed airway disease caused by hypersensitivity to such agents as foods, animal fur, and pollens.
    1 Pneumonia is an acute inflammation of the lungs.
    3 Cystic fibrosis is a hereditary disease that affects the mucus-producing glands of the body.
    4 This is hay fever; it does not affect the bronchial tubes.
264. Application, implementation, environment (b)
    3 DD = 40 mg
    DH = 160 mg
    V = 1 tsp (5 ml)
    $\dfrac{DD}{DH} = \dfrac{40}{160} \times 5 \text{ ml} = \frac{1}{4} \times 5 \text{ ml} = 1.25 \text{ ml} = \frac{1}{4} \text{ tsp}$
    1, 2, 4 These are not the correct dose.
265. Application, implementation, physiological (c)
    1 This is done to prevent trauma to membranes as a result of suction from catheter.
    2 Only the inner cannula is removed.
    3 The nurse should withdraw the catheter in a circular motion, rotating the catheter between thumb and forefinger to prevent unnecessary hypoxia.
    4 To prevent accidental dislodgment of tracheostomy, remove ties while someone holds it in place. Ties are only removed when cleansing, not when suctioning.
266. Comprehension, assessment, physiological (b)
    3 Intrinsic factors would be from internal causes, often triggered by respiratory infections.
    1 Injury to the nose is extrinsic, caused by external factors.
    2 Pollen from flowers is extrinsic, caused by external factors.
    4 Allergens in the environment are extrinsic, caused by external factors.
267. Knowledge, implementation, physiological (a)
    1 Adrenalin relieves most cases of acute bronchospasm.
    2 Adrenalin acts as a bronchodilator.
    3 Adrenalin increases cardiac output.
    4 Adrenalin does not stimulate constriction of the respiratory muscles.
268. Application, implementation, environment (c)
    3 A 25-gauge, ⅝-inch needle is used for subcutaneous injections.
    1 A 19-gauge, 1-inch needle is used for blood infusions.
    2 A 22-gauge, 1-inch needle is used for infants and children for intramuscular injections.
    4 A 27-gauge, ½-inch needle is used for insulin injections.
269. Comprehension, planning, physiological (b)
    4 Cool humidified air helps to relieve the respiratory distress; syrup of ipecac may be ordered to induce vomiting, which often produces some relief of respiratory distress.
    1 Antibiotics are not used for croup; this disease is usually of viral origin; cool humidified air is used.
    2 Sedatives may produce increased respiratory distress.
    3 Antiemetics are not ordered for croup.
270. Comprehension, assessment, environment (c)
    1 Exocrine glands become obstructed as a result of thick mucoprotein.
    2 Fetal lungs usually develop normally but are later damaged by the thick tenacious secretions.
    3 Untreated upper respiratory infections do not lead to cystic fibrosis. This disease is genetically inherited.
    4 Cystic fibrosis is not caused by the use of antibiotics or the suppression of the immune system.

271. Application, assessment, physiological (c)
    2 Children with cystic fibrosis do not absorb the fat-soluble vitamins A, D, E, and K. The failure to absorb vitamin K leads to easily acquired bruises.
    1 There is no connection between a neurological deficit and cystic fibrosis.
    3 There is no indication that Sheila has inadequate play supervision.
    4 Most children do not normally fall down and bruise easily.
272. Comprehension, assessment, physiological (c)
    4 With cystic fibrosis there is a decreased amount of pancreatic enzymes; therefore the intestines cannot absorb fats or proteins well.
    1 They should be able to eat all kinds of foods.
    2 Large, foul-smelling stools are a symptom of cystic fibrosis but are not a result of antibiotic intake.
    3 Continual vomiting is not a common symptom of cystic fibrosis.
273. Application, implementation, physiological (c)
    1 Pancreatic enzymes are best taken before or with meals and snacks to promote the absorption of fats and other nutrients.
    2, 3, 4 These are incorrect methods of administration; medication will not be effective.
274. Knowledge, implementation, physiological (a)
    3 Undigested food, mainly unabsorbed fats and proteins, is excreted as a result of the lack of the digestive enzymes trypsin, chymotrypsin, amylase, and lipase. The lack of these enzymes is caused by obstruction of the pancreatic ducts.
    2 The disease process causes marked impairment in the digestion and absorption of nutrients, mainly fats and proteins and to a lesser degree carbohydrates; this is not the best answer.
    1 The chloride channel defect in the sweat glands prevents reabsorption of sodium and chloride; this does not affect stools.
    4 The impaired ability to absorb fats results in a deficiency of the fat-soluble vitamins A, D, E, and K; anemia is common; this does not affect stools.
275. Comprehension, assessment, physiological (b)
    4 In infants and children the eustachian tube is relatively short and straight, allowing pathogens easy access from the pharynx to the middle ear.
    1 This is true only if a blow to the ear is severe enough to rupture the tympanic membrane, allowing microbes to enter the middle ear.
    2 The intact tympanic membrane keeps pathogens in the external ear from entering the middle ear.
    3 A myringotomy is a surgical incision of the tympanic membrane; the surgery is performed to relieve pressure caused by otitis media.
276. Comprehension, planning, physiological (c)
    2 The principal complication is loss of hearing from a variety of reasons (negative middle ear pressure, effusion in the middle ear, structural damage to the tympanic membrane); the most dreaded result of the hearing loss is the effect this loss has on speech and language development as well as on cognitive abilities.
    1 This is not a complication of this condition.
    3 This is not relevant to the situation; mastoiditis, infection of the mastoid sinus, is rare but possible.
    4 Not relevant to this situation.

277. Comprehension, implementation, environment (a)
    2 Lying on the affected side facilitates drainage of the exudate, thus decreasing pressure buildup and promoting comfort.
    1, 3 These are not the preferred positions; see above response.
    4 Positioning on the unaffected side will not facilitate drainage; discomfort is likely to increase as a result of buildup of pressure.

278. Knowledge, planning, environment (a)
    3 Pinkeye is also known as conjunctivitis; it is caused by bacterial or viral infection, allergy, or environmental factors.
    1 Degeneration does not occur.
    2 Pinkeye does not involve the lacrimal sac.
    4 This is a cataract.

279. Knowledge, implementation, physiological (b)
    4 Choice of treatment depends on the causative agent, which may include antibacterial agents, antibiotics, or corticosteroids.
    1 This has no effect on conjunctiva; it constricts pupils.
    2 This has no effect on conjunctiva; it burns localized tears.
    3 This has no effects on conjunctivitis.

280. Comprehension, implementation, health (b)
    1 The nurse should clear away the crusting from the inner aspect of the eye outward so as not to cross-contaminate the eye with the infection.
    2 This method cross-contaminates the eye with the infected material on the cotton ball.
    3 Removal of the crusted material is necessary for the maximum effect of the antibiotic.
    4 Hydrogen peroxide should not be used in the eyes.

281. Application, implementation, health (b)
    4 Follow orders given by the physician and 5 days thereafter to ensure that there is no further bacterial infection.
    1, 2 These options give no consideration to the effect of the medication on the infection.
    3 This response gives no guidance to the mother.

282. Comprehension, planning, physiological (c)
    4 Alcohol addiction is preventable; nurses can be instrumental in recognizing the symptoms and planning effective counseling for mothers and babies in these situations.
    1 "Failure to thrive" babies are not usually hyperactive and have a starved look about them—sunken eyes, large head and very thin body (they lack body fat).
    2 Genetic or hereditary defects are identifiable by chromosomal and/or genetic workup and are usually identifiable through laboratory analysis and counseling.
    3 Symptoms are the same as in No. 4, except that one would not find the altered facial feature.

283. Comprehension, assessment, physiological (c)
    2 Clinical signs of severe dehydration include tachycardia (rapid, thready pulse), dry skin/mucous membranes, sunken fontanel, delayed capillary filling time, poor skin elasticity, and coolness and mottling of extremities (signs of circulatory collapse).
    1 Blood pressure is low, not elevated, in severe dehydration; see response to No. 2.
    3 Pulse is rapid and thready, not slow; see response to No. 2.
    4 As the body's compensatory mechanisms take over to adjust to fluid losses, circulation is compromised and blood pressure falls, eventually resulting in the development of metabolic acidosis. The body attempts to compensate via the respiratory system; therefore, respirations are deep and rapid (Kussmaul breathing). See response to No. 2.

284. Knowledge, evaluation, health (b)
    1 Chicken pox involves no serious complications. Some lesions, if scratched, may become infected.
    2 Hearing is not impaired.
    3 Eyesight is not affected.
    4 The muscular system is not involved in chicken pox.

285. Knowledge, evaluation, health (c)
    1 The exact contagious stage is not completely defined, but mumps is considered contagious until all swelling is gone.
    2 No rash is involved.
    3 The temperature will subside before swelling does.
    4 Mumps is considered contagious from 1 to 2 days before onset of symptoms until swelling completely disappears.

286. Comprehension, planning, environment (a)
    1 Orchitis is an inflammation of one or both of the testes, characterized by swelling and pain, often caused by mumps, syphilis or tuberculosis; it is the most common complication of mumps in teenage and adult males.
    2 Meningitis is an infection or inflammation of the membranes covering the brain and spinal cord; this is not a common complication of mumps.
    3 Myositis is an inflammation of muscle tissue, usually of the voluntary muscles, caused by infection, trauma or infestation by parasites; this is not a common complication of mumps.
    4 Pyelonephritis is a diffuse pyogenic (pus-producing) infection of the pelvis and parenchyma of the kidney; this is not a common complication of mumps.

287. Knowledge, assessment, health (b)
    2 This is a true statement.
    1 Child abuse includes both physical and emotional abuse.
    3 Child abuse has been noted on all socioeconomic levels, yet studies do indicate that it is more common in the lower socioeconomic class.
    4 Studies indicate that many times, but not always, the abused child has congenital deformities, a chronic illness, or other problems that in general are more difficult for the parents to manage.

288. Knowledge, planning, environment (a)
    2 HIV or human immunodeficiency virus type I is the official name for the virus.
    1 CMV is a member of a group of large species-specific herpes-type viruses which produce a wide variety of disease effects.
    3 This is a virus that is the cause of common warts of the hands and feet, as well as lesions of the mucous membranes of the oral, anal, and genital cavities.
    4 Any of the five related viruses including herpes simplex type I and type 2, varicella zoster virus, Epstein-Barr virus, and cytomegalovirus.

289. Knowledge, implementation, environment (a)
    3 This is the safest and most accurate method of taking a temperature in a 2-year-old child.
    1 The rectal temperature is the method of choice, although the axillary method can be used if the rectal route cannot be used; this is not the best answer.
    2 An oral temperature should never be taken in a child of this age; rectal temperature is the method of choice; this option is inappropriate because it includes an incorrect method.
    4 The temperature could be taken by this method, but it is not the most accurate and should not be used unless the rectal route is contraindicated.

290. Comprehension, assessment, physiological (b)
   1 The nurse would need to know the average respiratory rate for age to determine abnormalities.
   2 The child's developmental level is important for the nurse to know, but the nurse can monitor the respiratory rate without this knowledge.
   3 This is very important, but no bronchodilator has been ordered.
   4 This will be important for the nurse to know if the child is given this drug to avoid theophylline toxicity.

291. Application, implementation, environment (a)
   1 To adhere and to seal properly, the self-adhesive plastic bag must be applied to a clean and dry area.
   2, 3, 4 These are incorrect procedures for obtaining a urine specimen from an infant.

292. Knowledge, assessment, environment (a)
   2 By definition, vesicles are small, thin-walled, raised skin lesions containing clear fluid; a blister.
   1 Macules are usually less than 1 cm in diameter; they are circumscribed alterations with elevations or depressions.
   3 These are macules that become slightly raised.
   4 Papules are less than 1 cm in diameter; they are solid elevations with no visible fluid.

293. Comprehension, assessment, environment (a)
   3 Minor movements such as twitching of eyelids or face, lip smacking and slight hand movements are commonly observed in absence seizures (petit mal).
   1 This is common to the tonic phase of the tonic-clonic seizure (grand mal).
   2 This is common to the clonic phase of the tonic-clonic seizure (grand mal).
   4 This can occur during the clonic phase of the tonic-clonic seizure (grand mal) as a result of muscle relaxation; there may also be incontinence of feces.

294. Application, implementation, environment (a)
   4 During seizure activity the patient is never restrained because injury may occur; the bed or crib sides are padded to protect the child from injury.
   1, 2 These are not advisable; see response to No. 4.
   3 This action would serve no particular purpose.

295. Comprehension, implementation, health (b)
   4 Using the actual equipment or a replica can eliminate anxiety and help the child understand what will happen. This can help the child become familiar with the equipment.
   1 A 5-year-old child is capable of some reasoning but can only concentrate on one aspect of a situation at a time.
   2 This should be done, but the child may not be ready for complex situations or materials.
   3 This can be done, but in this situation the child may not be knowledgeable at all of this treatment.

296. Knowledge, planning, environment (b)
   4 The site is basically free of major blood vessels and nerves; this is a large muscle with well-defined landmarks for safe administration. It is easily accessible from a variety of positions.
   1 The deltoid muscle can be used for small amounts of fluid; it is a small muscle close to axillary and radial nerves; it is not a preferred site.
   2 This site can be used, but it is not preferred because it is composed of thick subcutaneous fat and thus increases the possibility of injecting into subcutaneous tissue rather than into muscle. In this way it can also increase danger of sciatic nerve injury.
   3 This is the preferred intramuscular site for infants.

297. Knowledge, implementation, environment (a)
   4 In infancy, this muscle is developed and is large enough to ensure a good intramuscular site.
   1 Deltoid muscles should never be used for injection sites in infancy.
   2 The ventrogluteal muscle is not often developed enough in infants to ensure a deep intramuscular injection.
   3 The dorsogluteal muscle often does not gain size until after children start walking.

298. Comprehension, planning, environment (b)
   1 Patient safety is always a high priority. The child must be still for an injection; a second person will ensure this safety measure.
   2 Antibiotic ointment on injection sites, although not harmful, is not necessary.
   3 A toy may help focus an infant's attention for a very brief period, but when the child is touched and prepared for the injection, the toy will not distract him.
   4 The name on the identification device is generally all that is required in the patient check.

299. Application, implementation, environment (a)
   2 gr 5 = 300 mg; 1 tablet is the correct dose.
   1 This dose is too low.
   3, 4 These doses are too high.

300. Application, implementation, environment (b)
   3 $\dfrac{\text{Weight in pounds (75)} \times \text{adult dose (300 mg)}}{150}$

   $75 \times 300 = \dfrac{22,500}{150} = 150 \text{ mg}$

   1, 2 These doses are too low.
   4 This dose is too high.

301. Application, implementation, environment (a)
   1 $\dfrac{\text{Child's age (8)}}{\text{Age (8)} + 12} \times \text{average adult dose (500 mg)}$

   $\dfrac{8}{20} \times 500 \text{ mg} = \dfrac{2}{5} \times 500 \text{ mg} = 200 \text{ mg}$

   2, 3, 4 These doses are too high.

Psychiatric/Mental Health Nursing

1. Knowledge, planning, health (a)
   2 A complex interaction between body and mind influences the health of the individual.
   1 The individual's role in his world may influence his well-being, but this does not describe the concept of holism.
   3 Although this may be a valid point of view, it is not the concept of holism.
   4 The collective life of the community does not describe the concept of holism as it pertains to individual health.

2. Comprehension, planning, health (c)
   4 In keeping with the concept of holism, these are the dimensions considered in planning care for an individual.
   1 These are management considerations, but they do not necessarily guide nursing-care planning.
   2 These may also be management considerations, but they are not aspects of nursing care planning.
   3 These are treatment modalities that may be considered in the plan of care.

3. Comprehension, assessment, environment (c)
   3 The context of the specific behavior is as important as the behavior itself in making the determination of mental health or mental illness.
   1 Those closest to the individual are not always objective observers.
   2 Intelligence and education are not necessarily determinants of mental well-being.
   4 Healthy behavior is often pleasing to others, but it does not have to be pleasing to be considered healthy.

4. Comprehension, assessment, environment (a)
   2 Behaviors of the mentally ill differ in the degree of response to a situation rather than the kind of response made.
   1 A degree of conformity is expected, yet it is possible for a person to be mentally healthy without conforming entirely.
   3 The more severely disturbed the individual, the more difficult the behavior is to understand; however, the behavior can be understood.
   4 This is a common misconception. Behaviors are the result of a complex interplay of biological, psychological and social influences.

5. Knowledge, assessment, health (b)
   3 This is the best definition. It suggests flexibility and the ability to cope with life's changes.
   1, 2 These may be important characteristics of mental health, yet these are not the fullest definition.
   4 Although mentally healthy individuals possess positive characteristics that one hopes to find in leaders, winning power over others is not necessarily a feature of mental health.

6. Knowledge, assessment, environment (a)
   2 The nursing process is the same with mentally ill individuals as with physically ill individuals and begins with assessment.
   1 Although it is useful to let the patient know what is expected of him, the nurse must first assess his problems.
   3 This is a very important element of building rapport with the patient so that the nurse can assess his problems.
   4 This may be important to some patients, but it is not assessment.

7. Comprehension, planning, environment (a)
   3 This describes essential personal characteristics of the nurse who is successful in working with people.
   1 This is a commonly held misconception. The nurse's role does not include holding the patient to the nurse's personal value system.
   2 Another misconception. Although personal problems can interfere with one's work while they are acute, seeking professional help and working through personal problems increases one's skill in helping others.
   4 Enforcement of societal rules is not the role of the nurse, although successful mental health care will often render many patients more capable of living productively in society.

8. Knowledge, implementation, environment (a)
   2 This is the best answer. Successful communication results in a negotiated understanding between two or more people.
   1, 3 These may be aspects of communication, but they are not a complete definition.
   4 This is true of the communication process, but there is more to the definition of communication.

9. Comprehension, assessment, psychosocial (a)
   2 This is the correct observation to make about this interchange.
   1 Although this may be true, this requires the nurse to interpret the communication in a way that may not be accurate.
   3 The nurse is not able to assess this on the basis of this limited communication. The nurse may have misinterpreted her.
   4 The nurse needs more information from Linda before she can make this interpretation.

10. Application, intervention, psychosocial (c)
    2 This identifies a feeling and allows the patient opportunity to express herself.
    1 Although this conveys interest, questions that begin with "Why" often invite people to become defensive.
    3 This question may sound hostile to Amy.
    4 This response invalidates the patient's experience and may damage the nurse's therapeutic relationship with her.

11. Application, intervention, psychosocial (a)
    1 This response invites Amy to talk about her feelings.
    2, 3 These responses are judgmental and nontherapeutic.
    4 This is nontherapeutic because it does not acknowledge Amy's feelings.

12. Application, intervention, psychosocial (b)
    3 The nurse is seeking clarification. Once communication is clarified, the nurse has a basis for understanding.
    1 This sounds angry. Even if Dee Ann is annoying in her agitated state, the nurse does not want to sound angry with her.
    2 Dee Ann may be angry, but the nurse cannot determine this until Dee Ann can express herself.
    4 This response belittles the patient and is nontherapeutic.

13. Application, intervention, psychosocial (a)
    2 This invites Pat to talk about her perceptions and beliefs.
    1 This cuts off her communication with the nurse.
    3 This can make Pat feel as if the nurse is invalidating her and taking sides with the other individual.
    4 This suggests to Pat that she is falsely accusing.

14. Knowledge, assessment, psychosocial (a)

3 The key to this is goal-directedness. The nurse is in a therapeutic relationship with the patient to facilitate the improvement of his well-being.

1 There may indeed be a feeling of warmth in the nurse-patient relationship, but the statement implies a social rather than a therapeutic relationship.

2 It is certainly possible that the nurse and the patient may enjoy and appreciate one another, yet this is not the purpose of a therapeutic relationship.

4 In a therapeutic relationship, the nurse promotes the patient's capacity for independence.

15. Application, intervention, environment (b)

2 This olfactory hallucination is common in patients experiencing tumors of the frontal lobe. The nurse's observations of clinical symptoms aid the diagnostic process.

1 It is appropriate to present reality to the patient, but the nurse must first verbally acknowledge what he has said.

3 This is not relevant.

4 This is optional and entirely dependent on the patient's preference; it is not the priority.

16. Comprehension, planning, environment (b)

1 This provides a means of developing trust.

2 These come from within the patient and cannot be communicated.

3 This is an ineffective approach to care.

4 The patient is not always able to verbalize his or her difficulties.

17. Comprehension, implementation, environment (b)

4 Promises are never made to patients. The information may be important to the safety or health of the patient or other patients. The patient must decide whether or not to share information after being informed that the nurse cannot make promises.

1, 2, 3 These are inappropriate, nontherapeutic responses.

18. Comprehension, intervention, environment (b)

2 The time the nurse has contracted with Mr. Jay is his time. Adhering to the contract with Mr. Jay indicates that the nurse views the session as important and that she means what she says.

1 This is contracted time with Mr. Jay only. Inviting Mrs. Lane to remain indicates to Mr. Jay that the nurse does not view her time with him as important. It also indicates that the nurse didn't mean what she said when she contracted with him. This action will affect Mr. Jay's ability to trust the nurse.

3 No patient should be rejected. The interruption can be handled without rejecting Mrs. Lane.

4 This response is inappropriate because it places Mr. Jay in an uncomfortable position and violates the nurse's contract with him.

19. Application, intervention, environment (c)

4 Sometimes patients will open up dynamic topics just as the interview time is up. Frequently this is done to manipulate or test the nurse. The nurse should, without rejecting the patient, adhere to the terms of the contract.

1, 3 The nurse should not extend the contracted interaction time. Adhering to the contract illustrates that the nurse means what she says, and this fosters trust.

2 Same as No. 1; also, rudeness is never appropriate.

20. Comprehension, planning, environment (b)

3 This lets the patient know that the nurse does not want harm to come to him, and that the situation is serious and must be shared with other staff.

1 The nurse is reacting by feeling responsible for talking the patient out of it; this is inappropriate.

2 This is inappropriate and could be interpreted by the patient as approval of his plan.

4 Although necessary, this is not the priority action.

21. Application, implementation, health (b)

3 Acceptance of the patient is important, but setting a limit on inappropriate behaviors is also necessary.

1 The chances of manipulation are increased if all staff interacts with the patient.

2 The patient must understand that getting hurt is a possibility but not a reason to avoid others.

4 The patient must have the chance to observe healthier behaviors and role models.

22. Comprehension, planning, health (b)

3 Depending upon where, with what populations, and under what kinds of supervision the nurse practices, her role can involve many different aspects of mental health care.

1 This is not necessarily the case, especially in the role of the practical nurse.

2 Physicians and social workers may provide many types of service; however, they do not control nursing practice, which is defined by legal parameters.

4 This setting can be stressful, but nursing practice is always legally defined.

23. Knowledge, assessment, health (b)

4 These would not necessarily impact on an inpatient client, but they could influence a vulnerable client attempting to function in the community.

1, 2, 3 The nurse on the inpatient unit should always assess these factors to give appropriate care.

24. Application, assessment, environment (b)

3 All of these observations relate to the patient's affect.

1 None of these observations can accurately reveal the patient's feelings.

2 None of these observations can accurately reveal the patient's thoughts.

4 None of these observations can assess whether the patient is oriented.

25. Comprehension, assessment, environment (c)

4 Her distraction, confusion, and difficulty paying attention all indicate a change in level of consciousness.

1 There is not enough information to indicate this.

2 There is no indication that she is frightened.

3 There is no indication that she is cognitively impaired.

26. Application, assessment, environment (c)

3 She would not be able to perform the tasks described if her coordination were impaired.

1, 2, 4 These assessments cannot be made from this information.

27. Application, assessment, environment (c)

1 The patient's ability to give this information correctly tells the nurse that her ability to think is intact.

2 There is no indication of her emotional status.

3 There is no indication of what her usual style of communicating would be.

4 There is no indication that would reveal her coping style.

28. Application, implementation, psychosocial (a)

    4 This response acknowledges the patient's feelings and provides the opportunity for him to ventilate them.

    1 This statement does not acknowledge the patient's feelings. The focus should be on the patient, not the nurse.

    2 This will likely make the patient angrier, and it does not encourage him to verbalize his anger.

    3 This does not acknowledge the patient's feelings or encourage verbalization of his anger.

29. Application, implementation, psychosocial (b)

    4 Taking the time to sit with her indicates care and concern for her as an individual.

    1 This is the nurse's need; it demonstrates that the nurse is uncomfortable with the patient's behavior.

    2 This fails to acknowledge the patient's feelings and her ability to make her own decisions.

    3 In some circumstances, this might be appropriate, but it is not supportive.

30. Application, implementation, psychosocial (a)

    4 Use of reflection will help the patient identify her feelings and encourage verbalization of them.

    1, 2, 3 These responses are nontherapeutic; they do not acknowledge the patient's feelings.

31. Application, implementation, psychosocial (b)

    2 Using a broad opening acknowledges what the patient has said and encourages her to discuss her feelings.

    1, 4 Giving reassurance blocks communication because it is not based on truth or factual information. Also, it blocks the patient's opportunity to discuss her feelings.

    3 Challenging the patient will put her on the defensive and block communication.

32. Application, implementation, psychosocial (a)

    3 Making a broad opening statement is an effective communication strategy for encouraging the patient to verbalize her feelings.

    1 Giving reassurance is inappropriate because it is not based on fact, and it blocks the patient's opportunity to discuss her feelings. Stereotypical comments communicate that the nurse does not understand the patient's feelings.

    2 Giving reassurance blocks communication.

    4 The competency of the physician is not the issue requiring focus. The patient's feelings need to be acknowledged by the nurse.

33. Application, implementation, psychosocial (b)

    2 Stating observations encourages the patient to identify and discuss his thoughts and feelings; this is therapeutic.

    1 This reinforces the patient's perceived symptoms and is nontherapeutic.

    3 This gives false reassurance and is nontherapeutic.

    4 Changing the subject diverts the communication at an important point. It also indicates that the nurse is unable or unwilling to listen to the patient.

34. Application, implementation, environment (c)

    4 The pacing and the yelling indicate that he could benefit from prn medication at this time before he becomes more out of control.

    1 This has a threatening quality that is inappropriate.

    2, 3 Patients should never be threatened.

35. Application, implementation, psychosocial (c)

    3 Stating observations will encourage Mrs. McCreary to further identify her feelings and thoughts.

    1 Giving directions thwarts Mrs. McCreary's ability to think through her feelings.

    2 Judgmental statements block communication.

    4 "Guilty" is an emotionally charged word that may cause Mrs. McCreary to withdraw. At this point, the nurse should encourage Mrs. McCreary to verbalize her feelings and thoughts.

36. Knowledge, assessment, psychosocial (b)

    4 This is the definition of personality.

    1 This would include orientation to time, place, and person, as well as affect, mood, thought processes, thought content, memory, and judgment.

    2 This is similar to mental status.

    3 Behaviors, thoughts and feelings are influenced by education, but this is not a complete answer.

37. Knowledge, planning, psychosocial (a)

    1 Understanding this basic theory will support the nurse's understanding of human behavior.

    2 This is an important part of Freud's theory, but this pertains to consciousness, not personality.

    3 This is Berne's theory. It is similar to Freud's theory, but it offers more modern explanations.

    4 These are developmental phases that are integral to building personality.

38. Knowledge, planning, psychosocial (c)

    3 This is Berne's twentieth-century version of Freud's classic nineteenth-century theory.

    1, 2 These terms belong to Freud.

    4 These are Freud's developmental phases.

39. Knowledge, planning, psychosocial (c)

    4 The animal drives of the id/child give us the energy, motivation and passion to live.

    1 This is a function of the superego/parent.

    2, 3 These are functions of the busy ego/adult.

40. Comprehension, assessment, psychosocial (c)

    2 The ego/adult makes the rational decisions. This function integrates the needs and wishes of the id/child with the responsibilities held by the superego/parent.

    1 The id/child may be interested in having fun but may not be able to make the most responsible decisions.

    3 The superego/parent may forget how important it is to have fun.

    4 The unconscious has an influence on the personality.

41. Knowledge, planning, psychosocial (c)

    2 This is the valuable work of the superego/parent.

    1 This occurs from the cooperation between the id/child and the ego/adult.

    3 This is the work of the ego/adult.

    4 This is the work of the id/child.

42. Comprehension, assessment, psychosocial (a)

    2 This ability demonstrates coping behavior as child becomes independent.

    1 Mental illness is unrelated.

    3 This ability is not a dysfunction.

    4 This ability does not indicate autism because autistic children usually have learning problems.

43. Comprehension, implementation, psychosocial (b)

    3 Ego ideal is one's perception of how one should be, compared to how one perceives oneself to actually be.

    1 Body image is part of identity.

    2 Role is a description of how one fits into the society, whereas body image is one's perception of one's body.

    4 See above explanations.

44. Knowledge, assessment, psychosocial (c)

    4 This is focused on interpersonal relationships.

    1 This is the theory of Otto Rank.

    2 This is the theory of J. L. Morena.

    3 This is the theory of Karen Horney.

45. Knowledge, implementation, psychosocial (c)

    1 Roger's focus was on client-centered therapy.

    2 Sullivan's focus was on interpersonal relationships.

    3 Berne's focus was on transactional analysis.

    4 Erikson's focus was on the eight stages of development.

46. Comprehension, assessment, psychosocial (a)

    2 The use of defense mechanisms becomes a problem when they prove ineffective in helping the individual implement his or her roles and responsibilities.

    1, 3, 4 Defense mechanisms protect the individual against painful experiences; these would not be criteria of defense mechanism use.

47. Comprehension, assessment, psychosocial (a)

    4 The consciousness is protected from painful memories by repression. This frees the individual to function in daily life. The defense does not always work, and eventually the painful memories must be dealt with therapeutically so that healing can occur.

    1 Denial is the refusal to recognize reality.

    2 Rationalization is offering an apparently logical or socially acceptable explanation for unacceptable behaviors.

    3 Projection is falsely attributing one's own thoughts, feelings, and impulses to another person.

48. Comprehension, assessment, psychosocial (c)

    2 This is a functional defense that may occur on a conscious or an unconscious level.

    1 Denial is the refusal to recognize reality.

    3 Repression is the involuntary exclusion from consciousness of painful feelings, ideas or situations.

    4 Rationalization is offering an apparently logical or socially acceptable explanation for unacceptable behaviors.

49. Comprehension, assessment, environment (a)

    4 Tom unconsciously projects his guilt onto Carol.

    1 There is always a small measure of denial of one's own feelings when these feelings are projected onto others.

    2 Repression is the involuntary exclusion from consciousness of painful feelings, ideas, or situations.

    3 Rationalization is offering an apparent logic explanation or socially acceptable explanation for unacceptable behavior.

50. Comprehension, assessment, environment (c)

    3 Rob is displaying an extreme discrepancy between the functioning of his superego/parent and that of his id/child.

    1 The defense of reaction formation always contains a measure of denial, just as in the defense mechanism of projection.

    2 Rob may have repressed some of his feelings; however, this is not being displayed in this description.

    4 He has not necessarily regressed to an earlier level of functioning.

51. Comprehension, assessment, environment (a)

    1 Kathryn is coping with the stress of her move by returning to an earlier developmental stage.

    2 This situation does not describe denial. A young child can use denial, however. Her true feelings may be expressed in her play.

    3 A young child who is using repression as a defense will behave more like a brave little soldier.

    4 This situation does not describe reaction formation. A young child using reaction formation may behave as though she is older than she really is. This pseudomaturity is a sign of stress in a child.

52. Comprehension, assessment, psychosocial (c)

    3 Barbara is using her intellectual abilities to process what is occurring in her life. This will work well for her. When she is ready, she will deal effectively with her feelings.

    1 There is a rational quality to Barbara's behavior. She is using her intellect to help her cope with her experience.

    2 Denial of her feelings is a part of her intellectualization.

    4 The use of fantasy creatively employs the imagination. Children use this especially well.

53. Comprehension, assessment, psychosocial (a)

    2 Identification is a healthy process by which children begin to adopt ego/adult functions.

    1 This is not a description of denial.

    3 There are no intellectual defenses in evidence here.

    4 The child is developmentally moving forward, not backward.

54. Comprehension, assessment, psychosocial (a)

    2 Her anger is displaced on the unfortunate cat.

    1 This situation does not involve identification.

    3 This situation does not involve introjection. Introjection occurs in grief work. Someone may take on the values and behaviors of a lost loved one.

    4 This situation does not involve reaction formation.

55. Comprehension, assessment, psychosocial (c)

    1 Fantasy is a thinking process that involves wishful thinking, employs the creative use of imagery, and helps the individual manage painful feelings.

    2 Denial of painful feelings may be involved to some degree when a person is employing fantasy. Like fantasy, denial is a healthy defense against pain that enables the individual to cope with life. It only becomes unhealthy when it gets in the way of effective coping.

    3 Fantasy, repression, and denial are similar in that they free the person to cope with life. This situation correctly describes fantasy because of the creative use of imagery.

    4 Descriptions of defensive behaviors often overlap. This does not offer the best description of reaction formation.

56. Comprehension, assessment, psychosocial (a)

    4 Regression is reversion to an earlier development level. One can expect Tommy to be toilet trained at age 5; he is demonstrating developmental achievement loss.

    1 Compensation is an unconscious making up for a perceived limitation.

    2 Denial is avoiding reality by refusing to recognize it.

    3 Projection is attributing to another person one's own unacceptable or objectionable impulses or thoughts.

57. Application, assessment, psychosocial (c)

    2 Denial is a defense mechanism in which unpleasant realities are denied and repressed from conscious awareness.

    1 Projection is an unconscious defense mechanism in which a person attributes his or her own unacceptable traits or impulses to another.

    3 Withdrawal is a term given to a person who responds to severe physical danger or stress by retreating, being apathetic, lethargic, or depressed.

    4 Compensation is a complex defense mechanism that allows a person to avoid unpleasant or painful feelings of inadequacy. This person may engage in extraordinary efforts to replace the painful feeling(s), such as becoming a perfectionist to replace weakness or failure.

58. Comprehension, assessment, psychosocial (a)

    1 Mr. McCreary is clearly ignoring normal feelings about major surgery.

    2 Compensation is an exaggerated presentation in an effort to protect oneself from acknowledging one's limitations.

    3 Repression is excluding from awareness unacceptable thoughts, desires, behaviors, or wishes.

    4 Suppression is conscious exclusion of specific feelings or thoughts suppression may also occur on an unconscious level.

59. Knowledge, assessment, psychosocial (b)
    2 There is evidence to suggest that Sandra is in a relationship in which she is able to have her emotional needs met. Her partner is likely to be an important support for her.
    1 Homosexuality is now viewed as a healthy alternative lifestyle. Individuals may be well adjusted or poorly adjusted in their personal relationships, just as heterosexuals may be.
    3 This is a myth which has no place in a therapeutic relationship.
    4 This is another myth that is not useful for a health-care provider.

60. Application, implementation, environment (a)
    2 This is the best answer. The patient requires further assessment by the physician for this concern.
    1 Although this may be true, it is not helpful to suggest this until the patient is more fully assessed.
    3 This may be true; one would naturally want to allay his anxiety. It is best to encourage him to seek further physical assessment.
    4 This is true, but the nurse should still encourage him to see his physician.

61. Knowledge, assessment, psychosocial (b)
    2 These symptoms are indicators that the anxiety has progressed beyond the functional level of alertness. Focused intellectual performance becomes more difficult.
    1 At the alertness level, there may be perception of some threat; however, there is no decrease in organization.
    3 Severe anxiety is more pronounced and includes a sense of imminent disaster. Focused intellectual performance becomes even more difficult.
    4 The panic level of anxiety is extremely uncomfortable. Actions and behavior are extremely disorganized.

62. Knowledge, assessment, environment (a)
    3 The presence of a specific, definable threat differentiates fear from anxiety.
    1 Fear and anxiety are physiologically similar.
    2 Behavioral responses of fear and anxiety may be similar or they may differ in that in a state of fear, a person may attempt to deal with the perceived threat.
    4 Emotional responses in states of fear and anxiety may be similar.

63. Comprehension, assessment, environment (b)
    4 Panic-level anxiety in an individual who is not psychotic is differentiated by severely restricted perception and impairment of logical thought processes.
    1 In the alertness level, there is no evidence of distorted and disconnected thoughts.
    2 Apprehension does not bring about disconnected thoughts.
    3 Severe anxiety, although quite uncomfortable and distracting, does not cause distorted and disconnected thoughts.

64. Comprehension, assessment, environment (a)
    3 Anxiety is a common experience around the turning points in one's life. It has many physiological manifestations.
    1 Phobias are irrational fears; there's nothing in the situation that indicates Laura's symptoms are a result of irrationality.
    2 Anxiety and depression are often seen together. If she is depressed, she will express sadness and hopelessness in addition to the symptoms she has already presented.
    4 As in anxiety, fear is experienced both psychologically and physiologically. Fear occurs in response to a known stressor.

65. Comprehension, assessment, environment (b)
    3 The level of anxiety Edward is experiencing is related to garnering the energy necessary to completing the project.
    1 His anxiety as presented will not interfere with the completion of his project.
    2 There is no evidence that he has something else on his mind.
    4 There is no evidence that his anxiety level will escalate.

66. Knowledge, planning, environment (a)
    1 Mild anxiety helps one to garner the energy to focus attention and interest on the material to be learned.
    2 Learning is more difficult at this higher level of anxiety because it becomes more difficult to focus one's attention.
    3 With increasing anxiety, the individual is experiencing increasing distress. This is uncomfortable and distracts the individual from learning.
    4 Panic is extremely uncomfortable and is experienced in a similar way to severe pain. Learning becomes nearly impossible.

67. Knowledge, assessment, environment (b)
    4 This patient's panic-level anxiety must be identified quickly so that intervention can be provided. He is in acute distress.
    1 Louis' symptoms are beyond the alertness level.
    2 Louis is experiencing a degree of anxiety greater than that of apprehension.
    3 Even at the severe anxiety level, one might expect the individual to follow simple instructions.

68. Application, implementation, psychosocial (b)
    4 While being supportive, the nurse should try to get her to relax.
    1 This inappropriately supports the described symptoms.
    2 Identifying the anxiety and past experiences are not therapeutic in this situation.
    3 This is an unacceptable response as the patient may interpret this to indicate that she is having a heart attack now.

69. Application, planning, psychosocial (c)
    1 A concrete, short-term solution may resolve the crisis.
    2, 3, 4 As long-term solutions, these are not indicated in a crisis situation.

70. Comprehension, assessment, psychosocial (c)
    2 This is an unacceptable drive pressing for conscious discharge from within.
    1 It is fear that originates from a specific source; fear is contained through reasoned action.
    3 A phobia directly relates to a specific danger.
    4 Situations are not always known on the conscious level.

71. Application, evaluation, psychosocial (c)
    3 Antianxiety drugs decrease physiological manifestations of anxiety such as elevated levels of blood pressure, pulse, and respiration.
    1 These are signs of anxiety.
    2 These are paradoxical reactions that would not support evidence of positive effects of drug therapy.
    4 These are signs of anxiety.

72. Comprehension, assessment, environment (b)
    3 The patient's purposeless activity, intense somatic complaint, absorption with self, and focus on his unattended apartment are all characteristics of severe anxiety.
    1 Pacing indicates more than mild tension-relieving behavior.
    2 Although pacing and somatic complaints are characteristic of moderate anxiety, the patient's *inability to concentrate* places him in the severe category.
    4 Panic-level characteristics are not described in the situation.

73. Knowledge, evaluation, environment (a)
    1 Drowsiness is the only CNS side effect listed.
    2 Dry mouth is a gastrointestinal side effect.
    3 Dizziness is a cardiovascular side effect.
    4 Urine retention is a genitourinary side effect.
74. Comprehension, assessment, psychosocial (b)
    2 Rituals around food and exercise are typical ways in which these patients attempt to control overwhelming anxiety.
    1 Patients with anorexia do not believe they are sick.
    3 Anorexic individuals exercise compulsively to increase calorie output.
    4 This is partly true, but it is not the primary reason.
75. Application, implementation, environment (b)
    4 Patients with anorexia must be reminded of the consequences of extreme weight loss, because they do not believe themselves to be doing anything harmful.
    1 This kind of statement is threatening to these patients because it confronts them with loss of control.
    2 These patients do not believe extreme thinness to be unattractive.
    3 A patient with anorexia will never take this seriously.
76. Comprehension, assessment, psychosocial (b)
    4 Patients experiencing mild anxiety are alert and able to perceive connections between situations.
    1 This indicates panic-level anxiety.
    2, 3 These indicate moderate anxiety.
77. Comprehension, assessment, health (a)
    3 Motivation is defined as the gathering of personal resources to perform a task or reach a goal. It may be derived from perceived reward or threat of punishment. It is influenced by self-esteem and hope. Motivation is a key factor in recovery from any major illness.
    1 Frustration with the sick role and perception of the opportunity to live more productively may positively influence rehabilitative efforts. Excessive frustration tends to inhibit recovery.
    2 Anxiety is one of several factors that influence recovery from illness. Alertness level can positively influence recovery while higher levels of mild activity may inhibit recovery.
    4 Just as in the previous factors, optimal levels of stress tend to increase motivation. Excessive stress, however, leads to exhaustion.
78. Knowledge, assessment, psychosocial (c)
    2 The general adaptation syndrome, also known as GAS, is a group of similar symptoms or phenomena that occur in response to a variety of physiological or emotional stressors.
    1 Alternative lifestyle reflects a pattern of choices based on a complex set of personal interests and resources.
    3 Management of frustration is a necessary skill in everyday life. Excessive levels of frustration promote stress.
    4 Management of anxiety is also a skill necessary to one's everyday functioning. Excessive anxiety, however, brings about excessive levels of stress.
79. Knowledge, assessment, environment (b)
    2 A perceptual experience that occurs in the absence of external stimulus is a hallucination.
    1 Ingestion of toxic chemicals such as street drugs can cause sufficient disruption of brain chemistry to produce the type of hallucinations that are caused by mental illness.
    3 Conflict does not cause hallucinations. Conflict may be manifested in the content of some hallucinations. For example, a psychotic person who has low self-esteem may hear a voice telling him he is worthless.
    4 Similar to conflict, frustration does not cause hallucinations. Frustration may be symbolically manifested in the content of hallucinations.
80. Knowledge, assessment, environment (a)
    3 A fixed false belief is a delusion.
    1 Steve may experience severe anxiety or panic, which he may attribute to the delusion he believes to be true.
    2 This is too extreme to be a manifestation of stress alone.
    4 There is no evidence here of perceptual experiences.
81. Application, intervention, environment (a)
    3 Linda is in increasing distress; thus the likelihood of her responding to her command hallucinations is quite high. She requires immediate high-level suicide precautions. The psychiatrist will be able to order a medication that can diminish her distress.
    1 Linda's level of distress has become too high for her to benefit from group activities that are ordinarily helpful. Her safety is now the nurse's most pressing concern.
    2 This intervention is helpful, but it takes time and much repetition. The priority is patient safety.
    4 The priority is patient safety.
82. Application, implementation, environment (b)
    2 Edna's visual hallucinations are symptomatic of disturbance in brain physiology. This disturbance may be the result of electrolyte imbalance or beginning infection. The physician and/or charge nurse needs this information immediately.
    1 This is an excellent intervention. Visual hallucinations are diminished in a well-lit room. This is an important comfort measure. The nurse would most certainly do this. The *priority* is notifying the physician and/or charge nurse.
    3 This is important, too. The nurse will most certainly want to do this after notifying the physician and attending to her needs for comfort.
    4 This is of no particular importance at this time.
83. Application, intervention, environment (a)
    2 The nurse will not be able to change the patient's delusion, but she can change the focus of his thoughts to lessen preoccupation with delusional thoughts.
    1 The nurse should not argue about the content of delusions; she should acknowledge the patient's feelings and present reality.
    3 Although the nurse cannot change the patient's delusion, she will need to build a rapport by beginning to communicate respect and concern for him.
    4 Sharing humor with patients is important at times. This is not appropriate, however, when patients are experiencing sensory perception alterations.

84. Comprehension, assessment, environment (b)

    3 Delusions of guilt or sin are common in depression. The individual may feel like a truly bad person, although this may not be true. Low self-esteem is also common in depression. Delusions of guilt and sin are similar to low self-esteem, but they are more severe.

    1 Delusions of grandeur involve the individual's perception that he is extremely important, privileged or gifted. This kind of delusion is most likely to occur in a manic episode.

    2 Delusions of persecution include one's belief that a conspiracy exists to thwart or to kill the individual. This kind of delusion is often associated with delusions of grandeur. It is most likely to be seen in patients experiencing manic or paranoid episodes.

    4 Flight of ideas is seen in manic or highly agitated patients. The individual's thoughts move rapidly though logically from one subject to another. There is a quality of distractability often associated with euphoria.

85. Knowledge, assessment, psychosocial (a)

    3 The vision is a false sensory perception.

    1 Delusion is not a fixed false belief.

    2 In this situation there is no sensory perception that is distorted or mistaken.

    4 The defense mechanism regression is a return to an earlier developmental level.

86. Comprehension, planning, psychosocial (b)

    3 Schizophrenic individuals have difficulty making choices; therefore, choices should be simple.

    1 This choice violates the understanding of the nature of schizophrenia.

    2 Because he is paranoid, such a discussion might be easily misunderstood.

    4 There are times when a second staff member may be required. Psychiatric attendants are equally trained, and it is descriminatory to request gender-specific assistance. If you need help, you state only that you need help.

87. Comprehension, assessment, psychosocial (a)

    2 The patient is not oriented in time because he thinks it is 1886.

    1 The patient is not oriented in time.

    3 Although confused, "not oriented" better describes John's state.

    4 The patient may or may not be dishonest, but this is not relevant to the situation.

88. Comprehension, assessment, psychosocial (b)

    1 Scattered thoughts are indicated by rapid and frequent topic changes.

    2 Rapid speech may or may not indicate a scattered thought process.

    3, 4 These are only general indicators.

89. Comprehension, assessment, psychosocial (b)

    3 In schizophrenia the thought process is distorted; there is nonreality in thinking.

    1 He is not minimizing or avoiding anxiety.

    2 He is not exhibiting "highs" and "lows" in behavior.

    4 He is not exhibiting suspicious or distrustful behavior.

90. Application, implementation, psychosocial (c)

    2 This allows him to describe what he sees so that the nurse can further discuss what he is experiencing.

    1 Denying what he sees does not help him deal with what he believes he sees.

    3 The nurse should introduce conversation gently, but there's no indication in the situation that simple statements need to be used.

    4 Changing the subject is not therapeutic.

91. Comprehension, planning, psychosocial (b)

    3 Monoamine oxidase inhibitors are antidepressants that provide the enzyme crucial in cognitive and language difficulties.

    1, 2, 4 These provide neither the symptomatic control nor the replacement of amino acids, which are low.

92. Application, evaluation, environment (c)

    1 These antidepressants mainly affect the central nervous system.

    2, 4 These are side effects of the tricyclic antidepressant drugs.

    3 This is a side effect of trazadone hydrochloride antidepressant drugs.

93. Comprehension, implementation, environment (b)

    4 Tyramine stimulates release of the catecholamines epinephrine and norepinephrine. Foods to be avoided are aged cheeses and meats, bananas, yeast-containing products, and alcoholic beverages.

    1 Histamine is a compound found in all cells; it is released in allergic, inflammatory reactions and causes dilation of capillaries, decreased blood pressure, increased secretion of gastric juice, and constriction of smooth muscles of the bronchi and uterus.

    2 Phenylalanine is an essential amino acid necessary for normal growth and development of infants and children and for normal protein metabolism throughout life.

    3 Lysine is an essential amino acid necessary for proper growth in infants and for maintenance of nitrogen balance in adults.

94. Application, evaluation, psychosocial (c)

    4 Antipsychotic drugs are used to remove psychotic symptoms (auditory hallucinations) or reduce their intensity. Reduction in loudness of voices Mrs. Edwards hears indicates a decrease in intensity.

    1 This statement indicates no change in psychotic symptoms.

    2 The fact that the patient is not hearing voices at the moment in no way indicates an absence of auditory hallucinations.

    3 Again, the statement indicates that the patient continues to hear voices.

95. Comprehension, implementation, physiological (b)

    3 Foods in their own containers, such as milk or juice in cartons, hard-boiled eggs, or oranges, are more likely to be eaten by this type of patient.

    1 This reinforces the delusion; it is nontherapeutic.

    2 This is unsafe; it places the patient at risk nutritionally.

    4 This is threatening and definitely nontherapeutic.

96. Application, implementation, psychosocial (b)

    1 This response presents reality, acknowledges the patient's statement, and casts doubt on the patient's altered thought process, all of which are therapeutic.

    2, 3 This challenges the patient's thought process, which he may be compelled to defend; therefore, this would be nontherapeutic.

    4 This reinforces the patient's hallucination and is thus nontherapeutic.

97. Knowledge, planning, health (a)

    2 Cottage and cream cheeses are the only cheeses allowed on a tyramine-restricted diet.

    1, 3 These are high in tyramine.

    4 Summer sausage and unrefrigerated fermented sausages are high in tyramine.

98. Knowledge, planning, psychosocial (a)
    2 Chlorpromazine is the only antipsychotic listed. It is the prototype antipsychotic drug and the least potent of the antipsychotics.
    1 This is an antianxiety agent.
    3 This drug is a mood stabilizer.
    4 This is an antidepressant.
99. Comprehension, evaluation, environment (b)
    4 Syncope is the only central nervous system side effect listed.
    1 This is a gastrointestinal side effect.
    2 This is a respiratory system side effect.
    3 This is a cardiovascular system side effect.
100. Knowledge, implementation, environment (b)
    2 This is exactly the effect that this medication has, although the exact way in which this works is still unknown.
    1 This is untrue; antipsychotic drugs work on the neurotransmitter system in the brain.
    3 This is also untrue. Reality is unchanged; it is the decrease in unwanted stimuli that allows the patient to function.
    4 This is untrue; these medications act on dopamine synthesis.
101. Knowledge, assessment, psychosocial (a)
    2 Auditory hallucinations are quite common in schizophrenia. Thought processes are highly symbolic. It is difficult to follow the logic of the patient's thoughts, which the patients often describe as racing.
    1 Unstable moods are sometimes associated with schizophrenia, but this symptom is less prominent than the racing thoughts and auditory hallucinations. Delusions of grandeur may occur, but this is more commonly associated with mania.
    3 Depressive thoughts are not necessarily indicative of schizophrenia. Many patients become depressed as a result of their awareness of the impact the illness has on their lives.
    4 Many schizophrenic patients retain good judgment. Complicated legal problems are commonly associated with the antisocial personality.
102. Application, implementation, psychosocial (b)
    1 Simple structured tasks involving interaction with only one person at a time are best for Dave while he is exhibiting psychotic symptoms.
    2 Group activity is too complex for Dave to handle while he is actively psychotic. He will feel confused and lost.
    3 Although it is true that activity and human interaction are important for him, he is unable to apply this knowledge. He needs to be led to simple interactions while he is psychotic.
    4 A nurse should never feed into the patient's hallucinations; such actions are nontherapeutic.
103. Application, implementation, psychosocial (c)
    1 A simple structured plan will be easiest for him to understand. He can follow only simple instructions and may need reminders.
    2 This is not a good time for him to begin the emotion-filled work of exploring his feelings; he is actively psychotic.
    3 The nurse will want to observe Dave closely while he is actively psychotic. A structured schedule will help keep him in contact with reality.
    4 There's no indication in the situation that mechanical restraints are required.
104. Application, implementation, psychosocial (b)
    4 Dry mouth and blurred vision are the most common side effects of all major tranquilizers. Informing the patient of this and helping him cope with the side effects can bring about improved compliance with the medication regimen.
    1 These side effects are not commonly reported with major tranquilizers.
    2 These are not common side effects. They may indicate a hypersensitivity to the medication. Should this occur, the nurse would report it to the psychiatrist and record it in the chart.
    3 Endocrine system side effects include moderate breast enlargement and loss of libido.
105. Comprehension, evaluation, environment (c)
    2 Extrapyramidal reactions are common side effects of major tranquilizers. Although they are not life-threatening, they are acutely uncomfortable for the patient. They require rapid intervention with medications such as diphenhydramine (Benadryl), benztropine (Cogentin), or trihexyphenidyl (Artane).
    1 Many patients believe this experience represents an allergic reaction. This is not the case.
    3 Sometimes the patient's pacing and odd movements are mistaken for a worsening of his psychosis. This can be an unfortunate error and can lead to the patient's being improperly treated.
    4 Rare side effects include agranulocytosis, cholestatic jaundice, and the occasionally fatal neuroleptic malignant syndrome.
106. Knowledge, implementation, physiological (a)
    3 Cogentin is commonly used to treat extrapyramidal reactions to major tranquilizers.
    1 Aspirin is not effective for the extrapyramidal symptoms associated with major tranquilizers.
    2 Ativan is a minor tranquilizer used to treat anxiety.
    4 Lithium is used to treat both mania and depression. It is of no benefit in treating extrapyramidal reactions.
107. Comprehension, assessment, psychosocial (b)
    3 Delusions of this type are associated with paranoid schizophrenia.
    1 Catatonic schizophrenia typically causes the individual to appear immobile though he may have periods of extreme excitability.
    2 Geoff's delusions, though unrealistic, are organized. This does not occur in disorganized schizophrenia.
    4 Fixed delusions are not a feature of undifferentiated schizophrenia.
108. Application, implementation, psychosocial (c)
    2 Immediate action is required to prevent this patient from leaving the hospital. Command hallucinations are extremely dangerous in this patient. There is a risk he will kill someone.
    1 Safety of the patient and the community is the priority.
    3 Although the nurse will always want to establish a rapport with a patient, the safety issue takes precedence.
    4 The patient is not in a frame of mind at this time to comprehend this kind of concept. He is likely to believe he has a moral imperative to kill someone. Again, safety is the priority.

109. Application, implementation, psychosocial (b)
   3 It is important to be specific and straightforward when giving medication information. This will help build trust and decrease the patient's suspicion.
   2 This is likely to increase the patient's suspicion and foster distrust. The patient is calling about his medication; this is the issue to be addressed. Further assessment should take place after the issue of concern to the patient is given attention.
   1 Many psychotropic medications have the potential for abuse and are frequently used in suicide attempts. These medications are usually prescribed in small amounts so the patient has to return often to have the prescription refilled.
   4 Degrading a patient is never appropriate.
110. Comprehension, evaluation, health (b)
   4 Phototoxicity is a common side effect of chlorpromazine (Thorazine). Patients should be taught to apply a strong sunscreen when in the sun. Clothes and hats that cover the skin are also recommended.
   1 Nasal congestion is a common side effect. A nasal decongestant spray and an increase in fluid intake generally reduce this.
   2 Gastrointestinal distress can be relieved if the medication is taken with food.
   3 Antipsychotic drugs increase the appetite, resulting in weight gain. Patients should monitor their nutritional intake to avoid gaining unnecessary pounds.
111. Comprehension, assessment, psychosocial (c)
   2 Because delusions are a protection, they can only be abandoned when the patient feels safe and secure.
   1 The patient's delusions are not funny. Joking about delusions makes the patient feel unimportant.
   3 Patients can gain insight into their delusions, but that doesn't mean they are able to alter them.
   4 Patient and nurse do not have to like each other for the nurse-patient interaction to be therapeutic.
112. Comprehension, planning, environment (b)
   3 There is conflict between Jack's right to personal freedom and the obligation of health-care providers to protect his life.
   1 Restriction of Jack's freedom, without a clear clinical reason, could be viewed as illegal incarceration.
   2, 4 There is moral obligation to protect his life.
113. Application, implementation, health (c)
   4 This gives a point of understanding from which to proceed in dealing with the behavior.
   1 This comes after understanding underlying cause of behavior.
   2 Not an issue in this situation.
   3 Inappropriate response; rules have no meaning at this point.
114. Comprehension, assessment, psychosocial (b)
   4 Pressured is the word used to describe rapid speech patterns.
   1 The speech pattern is not unintelligible; he was understood.
   2 Disorganized may be true but irrelevant.
   3 Variable would not be true; the speech is described as rapid.

115. Comprehension, assessment, psychosocial (b)
   3 This statement is typical of the self-focus and careless attitude of the patient in the manic phase of bipolar illness.
   1 This is an unlikely answer. She would not express worry or this level of reasoning in this stage of her illness.
   2 This expression of guilt is more typical of depression, not mania.
   4 This is a very rational, appropriate statement, not typical of an individual who is manic.
116. Application, implementation, environment (b)
   1 Individuals who are manic need food they can eat while walking around or engaging in activity so they can maintain calorie intake.
   2 Manic individuals will not spend the time to eat a large meal.
   3 Manic individuals will not respond to a quiet environment; restlessness will not allow them to eat.
   4 Extra vitamins will not be sufficient to make up for the calorie deficit from mania.
117. Application, assessment, health (b)
   3 This would be an indication that her status is normalizing.
   1 Her appetite is not an adequate indicator.
   2 Eating at scheduled times does not ensure her intake is adequate.
   4 This is not a reliable indicator because she may not be eating very much anyway.
118. Comprehension, assessment, psychosocial (b)
   3 This is mood instability, as seen in her mood swing from pleasantness to rage.
   1 Flight of ideas is not indicated in her behavior.
   2 Ideas of reference are not demonstrated.
   4 Looseness of association is not indicated in this behavior.
119. Application, implementation, environment (b)
   1 It is important to set a limit on the patient but also to offer the support of the nurse while setting that limit.
   2 The other patient's behavior is not the issue.
   3 This is likely to cause her to escalate her behavior and to become angrier.
   4 A manic patient cannot accept this type of redirection.
120. Knowledge, planning, psychosocial (b)
   3 The patient's unstable mood/affect makes him prone to sudden violence until he has recovered sufficiently to think before acting.
   1 There is no evidence his family is not coping.
   2 There might be anxiety, but it is because of the threat of violence, not necessarily their inability to cope.
   4 There is potential for injury but not to self.
121. Application, implementation, health (c)
   2 This sets a limit without providing additional stimulus to cause further escalation of behavior.
   1 Yelling for someone can have the effect of escalating his behavior.
   3 This is false reassurance; if he is out of control enough, he will most likely attempt to hurt her.
   4 This is an overreaction and will escalate the problem needlessly without correcting it.
122. Knowledge, assessment, environment (b)
   4 This level is very high; the patient should be assessed immediately.
   1 This level is above therapeutic range.
   2 This level is toxic range.
   3 See No. 4, above.

123. Application, implementation, environment (c)
    3 These are all symptoms of lithium toxicity.
    1 She is not experiencing a dystonic reaction.
    2 These are not signs of potassium depletion.
    4 These are signs, not side effects, of toxicity.
124. Application, assessment, environment (b)
    3 Flight of ideas is the rapid change from one idea to another without connections; commonly seen in mania.
    1 Confabulation is the term that describes an attempt to fill gaps in memory with "made up" information, most commonly seen in dementia.
    2 Primary process refers to a type of thinking in which everything that happens refers to that particular individual, even when there is no connection.
    4 Neologisms are "made up" words, usually seen in schizophrenia.
125. Application, implementation, psychosocial (c)
    2 Because of her distractibility, she will benefit from the nurse's calm presence. It is helpful for the nurse to talk soothingly to her and to show her some relaxation exercises.
    1 Her condition renders her unable to follow these instructions.
    3 This may have to be the nurse's second choice if the nurse is unable to calm her.
    4 She cannot benefit from the stimulation of the other patient's activity. This may tend to excite her further.
126. Knowledge, implementation, psychosocial (b)
    1 Haldol will provide sedation that will enable the patient to rest. It will also promote more organized thought processes.
    2 Over-medication with haloperidol (Haldol) will tend to over-sedate the patient and render her inactive. This has been referred to as chemical restraint.
    3 The medication does not stimulate the appetite. The side effect of dry mouth will sometimes cause the patient to crave sweets. This can lead to weight gain.
    4 The medication will alleviate anxiety, but this is not its primary purpose for a patient with this diagnosis.
127. Knowledge, implementation, psychosocial (b)
    2 Fine tremors are common side effects of lithium carbonate.
    1 Food cravings are a common side effect of drugs that have anticholinergic properties, such as antidepressants and antipsychotics.
    3 This has not been reported as a side effect of lithium.
    4 Individuals taking lithium are sensitive to the effects of heat and must be careful of their fluid intake in hot weather. Thorazine is a drug that produces sensitivity to sunlight.
128. Application, planning, psychosocial (b)
    3 Lithium levels should be drawn 8 to 14 hours after the last dose. This would be in the morning before the first dose, when the medication is ordered tid.
    1, 2 Twelve to 14 hours should elapse after the last administered dose before obtaining a serum lithium level.
    4 Toxicity usually appears at serum levels higher than 1.5 mEq/L. The purpose of monitoring lithium levels is to maintain the therapeutic serum range.
129. Comprehension, evaluation, environment (c)
    4 Muscular weakness is the only side effect of lithium carbonate listed.
    1 This is a side effect of antidepressant medications.
    2, 3 Blurred vision is considered a toxic effect of serum concentrations above 1.5 mEq/L.

130. Comprehension, implementation, psychosocial (b)
    2 This is the most appropriate and safe response regarding lithium therapy.
    1 The nurse should be able to respond to the concern being raised by the patient's husband.
    3 Although the combination of lithium and a neuroleptic drug is often used and does achieve more rapid results, it is not within the practice of nursing to suggest this.
    4 Although this is true, it does not address the issue being raised by the patient's husband.
131. Application, implementation, environment (c)
    4 Vital signs should be taken and reported to the physician along with other assessment data.
    1 There is no indication in the situation that a code should be called at this point in time.
    2 Desired maintenance blood levels are 0.6 to 1.2 mEq/L; moderate to severe reactions occur at levels 2 to 2.5 mEq/L; lethargy and nonresponsiveness are characteristic of toxic drug levels; the priority action is to take vital signs and notify physician.
    3 On the basis of the situation data, vital signs should be taken and reported to the physician, along with a description of the patient's level of consciousness.
132. Comprehension, evaluation, environment (b)
    4 This response indicates the patient understands the importance of taking her medication as prescribed.
    1 Patients should be informed never to double up on dosages if they miss a dose. The nurse should explain the dangers of increased serum concentrations and give clear directions to the patient on how and when to take medications.
    2 The physician will order appropriate laboratory work.
    3 Above normal sodium intake will raise excretion, reducing the drug's effectiveness. The patient should be cautioned to maintain a normal sodium intake and understand that any dietary modifications should be ordered by the physician.
133. Comprehension, assessment, psychosocial (b)
    4 Lithium is a mood stabilizer effective in treating bipolar mood disorders. Cyclothymia, schizophrenia, and schizoaffective disorders have also been treated with some success with lithium.
    1 The patient is in a manic state.
    2 Lithium does not affect one's sex drive. Female manic patients tend to demonstrate flirtations and seductive behavior as evidence of their bipolar disorder.
    3 Lithium is classified as a mood stabilizer prescribed to achieve equilibrium of mood. The patient is currently in a manic phase; it would be dangerous to increase her manic state.
134. Comprehension, planning, environment (c)
    2 Carbamazepine can cause aplastic anemia, leukopenia, and thrombocytopenia, all of which are life-threatening reactions. It is imperative that complete blood count results be monitored.
    1 Blood sugar levels are not adversely affected by carbamazepine.
    3 Although there is the possibility of gastrointestinal side effects, a gastric analysis would not be indicated for a patient receiving carbamazepine.
    4 Urine for C & S is not a laboratory test related to carbamazepine therapy.
135. Comprehension, planning, environment (b)
    3 Patient safety is always the priority.
    1, 2, 4 These are appropriate diagnoses, but the priority is dealing with the potential for violence.

136. Application, planning, psychosocial (c)
    2 Manic patients are unable to establish limits and frequently are unaware of their impaired abilities. The nurse should evaluate how much responsibility the patient can tolerate.
    1 The patient's ability to deal with stimuli is impaired and the attention span is too short to assist in planning unit activities.
    3 The patient's ability to deal with others is impaired, making this option inappropriate.
    4 The patient's attention span is short, rendering this response inappropriate.
137. Application, implementation, psychosocial (a)
    3 The patient should be informed in a nonthreatening but firm manner that her behavior is unacceptable; she should be directed toward activities that encourage more appropriate behavior. This will help her attain control.
    1, 4 These are inappropriate because it is the nurse's responsibility to protect other patients from the impact of negative behavior.
    2 It is never appropriate to threaten a patient.
138. Knowledge, assessment, environment (a)
    4 Tactile hallucinations are common in alcohol withdrawal. The nurse should be sure to observe, report, and record this important clinical symptom.
    1 Olfactory hallucinations or those involving the sense of smell can occur in alcohol withdrawal, but they are more commonly associated with tumors on the brain and some seizure disorders.
    2 Jacob is quite likely to experience visual hallucinations in addition to the tackle hallucinations he is currently experiencing.
    3 Some individuals experience auditory hallucinations during alcohol withdrawal; however, these hallucinations are most commonly seen in schizophrenia.
139. Comprehension, planning, environment (c)
    4 This therapy is designed to help regressed and disoriented patients become more aware of present reality.
    1 This is more for self-help, without a designated leader.
    2 This helps in changing problematic aspects of behavior and is not applicable for him.
    3 Not applicable; this is for learning and practicing relaxation techniques.
140. Comprehension, assessment, environment (c)
    1 Poor work records are characteristics because they indicate a lack of responsibility.
    2 This is characteristic of borderline personality disorder.
    3 This is characteristic of histrionic personality disorders.
    4 This is characteristic of passive-aggressive personality disorders.
141. Comprehension, planning, environment (b)
    2 Manipulative patients want limits set on their behavior. The extent should always be that which is necessary to protect the patient and others.
    1 It is inappropriate and not necessary to set limits on all behavior, because all behavior is not manipulative.
    3 The patient should not independently set limits on his behavior but rather do so with the assistance of the nurse.
    4 It is not the role of the community to set limits on patient behavior. This is the staff's responsibility.

142. Comprehension, planning, environment (b)
    3 Realistic consequences should always be addressed at the time limits are set. It is important that the patient know what consequences have been established so he has the opportunity to discuss his reactions and feelings.
    1 As a motivation to change his behavior, the patient should know the consequences at the time the limit is set.
    2 Again, consequences should be preestablished to be consistently enforced by all staff members.
    4 Manipulative patient behavior can be quite frustrating to staff members. Manipulative behaviors should be immediately identified, and consequences enforced to motivate the patient to change his behavior.
143. Application, implementation, psychosocial (c)
    4 This is a fundamental skill that these patients lack and is at the root of many of their other problems.
    1, 2 These might not be possible until other issues are resolved.
    3 This is important but is part of the primary goal; see No. 4.
144. Comprehension, assessment, psychosocial (b)
    1 Manipulation is a characteristic style of relating in individuals with personality disorders.
    2 Projection is used by these individuals as a way of expressing unacceptable feelings.
    3, 4 These are not commonly used mechanisms by those with personality disorders.
145. Knowledge, assessment, psychosocial (b)
    3 The most reliable evidence is that personality disorders begin at the stage of separation/individuation from the mother and that the family of origin is usually dysfunctional in some way.
    1 There is no evidence at present to suggest biochemical imbalance is involved in personality disorder.
    2 There is no evidence of a gene for personality disorder.
    4 Birth complications do not cause personality disorders.
146. Application, planning, environment (c)
    4 Individuals with personality disorders have persistent and severe difficulties in personal relationships.
    1 The patient may or may not have problems with this.
    2 If the patient is a substance abuser, this may or may not be problematic, depending on how severe and how recent substance use has been.
    3 This patient may have difficulty with rules, but this will not be the primary problem.
147. Knowledge, planning, environment (a)
    4 Some substances produce no physiologic dependence but do cause powerful psychologic dependence in the user.
    1, 2 These are each only one symptom of addiction.
    3 Not all substances that are addictive produce both of these symptoms.
148. Knowledge, assessment, environment (b)
    2 Alcoholic cardiomyopathy, hypertension, and atherosclerotic changes are only a few of the consequences of long-term alcohol abuse.
    1 Changes in the function of the pituitary and thyroid glands can also occur, but these changes are less common and not as serious.
    3 Poor nutrition and increased alcohol intake can cause loss of calcium from bones and can contribute to muscle atrophy, but cardiac changes are still more serious.
    4 Sterility and erectile dysfunction also are common with long-term alcohol abuse.

149. Application, implementation, health (c)
    3 Role modeling by the nurse is the best way to teach him how to maximize his mother's strengths and cope with her deficits until she improves.
    1 This gives false reassurance; it may take much longer, and there is no way to predict how much she will recover.
    2 This would deprive her of the comfort of his visits and denies him the opportunity to monitor her progress.
    4 This will not necessarily answer his questions any more completely or give him any more reassurance than talking with the nurse.

150. Comprehension, assessment, psychosocial (c)
    1 Maladaptation in interpersonal and social relationships is consistently a feature of personality disorders.
    2 Some individuals who have personality disorders often have the capacity to irritate others, yet others may be overly anxious to please everyone.
    3 This self-centeredness and inflexibility may be a part of a personality disorder, yet this description is less complete.
    4 The individual who is attention-seeking and overly anxious to entertain may represent a type of personality disorder. Similarly, the individual who is overly serious or withdrawn may represent another type of personality disorder.

151. Knowledge, assessment, psychosocial (b)
    3 Antisocial personality disorder is manifested by little respect for the law as well as little respect for the rights and needs of others.
    1 Avoidant personality disorder is manifested by a lack of interpersonal skills but a real desire to relate to others.
    2 Schizotypal personality disorder is manifested by a lack of genuine interest in relating to others.
    4 Impulsive personality disorder is manifested by an inability to control impulses, which leads to poor judgment.

152. Comprehension, assessment, psychosocial (c)
    3 It is useful to assess the patient's coping style. The understanding the nurse gains from this will facilitate her understanding of the patient's health education needs.
    1 A disruptive life-style is not an illness, but it does not promote health.
    2 A disruptive life-style may contribute to the development of a perceptual or affective disorder.
    4 Genetically inherited personality traits have some influence on personality and life-style.

153. Comprehension, planning, psychosocial (c)
    3 Personality disorders are resistant to change. Long-term therapy is needed.
    1 Medication is not helpful, but is usually used on a short-term basis to manage specific symptoms.
    2 Group therapy is helpful but generally not highly successful.
    4 He is not likely to be having very much anxiety. He is more likely to cause anxiety in others.

154. Comprehension, assessment, psychosocial (c)
    2 The nurse may expect Chip to display restricted affects. He interprets teasing from others in a concrete and paranoid way. The nurse may need to protect him from teasing from other patients or his family.
    1 Paranoid personalities feel misjudged and mistreated by others and display jealousy, not sentimentality.
    3 He will not be self-indulgent. He is likely to be very disciplined in his drive for self-achievement.
    4 This is characteristic of histrionic personalities.

155. Application, implementation, psychosocial (b)
    1 He will appreciate the nurse's honesty. It is very difficult for him to trust anyone.
    2 He needs to maintain social interactions. Isolation leads to further distortions of reality.
    3 Making decisions for him will invite his distrust and is nontherapeutic.
    4 He needs to be kept well involved in his treatment plan.

156. Knowledge, health, implementation (b)
    2 Pinpoint pupils are easily identified in someone who has taken any drug of the opiate class. Euphoria is common, and respiratory depression occurs with larger doses.
    1 These symptoms occur when an addicted person begins to experience withdrawal symptoms.
    3 Dilated pupils, drowsiness and visual hallucinations occur as a result of drugs that have anticholinergic properties. Phencyclidine (PCP) and marijuana have these properties.
    4 These are the effects of ingestion of amphetamines.

157. Comprehension, assessment, environment (c)
    2 Ray has ingested PCP. His skin is flushed and dry because the anticholinergic properties of the drug will not allow his body to perspire. The clinical picture is similar to that of cocaine ingestion.
    1 Heroin would have caused Ray to have pinpoint or constricted pupils. He would not be hallucinating nor would he be violent.
    3 Barbiturates would produce drowsiness in addition to the dilated pupils.
    4 Marijuana produces dilated pupils, and sometimes sedation. There may be hallucinations, but they are less vivid. There is a low incidence of violent behavior with marijuana use.

158. Knowledge, assessment, environment (b)
    3 A level of .10 mg/dl is most commonly accepted as the legal standard for intoxication.
    1 At this level, the individual is almost always quite obviously intoxicated. If he is not intoxicated, then he has excessive alcohol tolerance.
    2 This is a toxic level. Expect to see respiratory depression and coma. The individual requires intensive care and may not survive.
    4 This is lower than the legal level of intoxication. This level occurs when someone has had a drink several hours before the blood sample is taken.

159. Knowledge, assessment, environment (a)
    4 Symptoms are usually quite unpleasant. They include headache, gastritis, fatigue, malaise, and irritability.
    1 Blood alcohol level may remain elevated in someone who has impaired liver function as a result of chronic alcoholism. This does not describe hangover.
    2 Hangover is accompanied by hypoglycemia and an increase of lactic acid in the blood.
    3 A sense of euphoria may occur after alcohol is ingested. It does not persist.

160. Knowledge, assessment, environment (b)
    3 Blackouts occur for the period of time during which the person is intoxicated. Many individuals deny that they have lost memory of the events.
    1 Social impairment occurs with alcoholism as a result of progressive brain damage.
    2 Wernicke's syndrome is a type of dementia that occurs as a result of the toxic effects of alcohol on the brain.
    4 Certainly one might want to forget events that occurred during a binge; however, this individual has not willfully forgotten. The toxic effects of alcohol have impaired his brain's ability to remember recent events.

161. Knowledge, assessment, environment (a)
    4 Sedatives and barbiturates are the second most commonly abused class of drugs. Many people believe that these drugs are not addictive because they are prescribed by physicians. A pattern in increasing tolerance that leads to increased use of the drugs tends to promote addiction. Use of even small quantities of alcohol in combination with these drugs greatly increases the likelihood of addiction.
    1 Amphetamines are less commonly used than sedatives.
    2 Cocaine is less commonly used than sedatives and is classified as a narcotic.
    3 Narcotics are less commonly used than sedatives.
162. Comprehension, evaluation, environment (c)
    2 Alcohol and diazepam (Valium) are cross-tolerant and therefore cross-addicting. The combination of the alcohol and diazepam have a cumulative effect on Margaret's addiction. In addition to the discomfort associated with the withdrawal, Margaret may still be experiencing the anxiety for which she had previously required diazepam.
    1 Her motivation cannot be fairly judged. She is undergoing an acutely uncomfortable experience.
    3 It makes no difference that one was a prescription drug and the other is not. They are still cross-addicting.
    4 This is not true. She will need to consider herself a recovering alcoholic/addict. Remaining involved in a Twelve Step or AA program will facilitate her recovery.
163. Comprehension, assessment, environment (c)
    2 The withdrawal syndrome produces effects that are opposite to the effects of the medication. If not medically managed, withdrawal from Valium can produce seizures.
    1 The nurse would not expect to find stupor. She would expect the patient to be overstimulated. It is possible for the patient to become confused and disoriented during the course of the withdrawal.
    3 Margaret will not be gregarious. She will be irritable and will need to limit her contact with others. She will not be euphoric.
    4 Unmanaged withdrawal can lead to seizures, coma, and death. Since Margaret is hospitalized, it is likely that these complications will be prevented.
164. Application, implementation, physiological (b)
    1 Monitoring vital signs is essential because of the nature of the physiologic stress that patients experience. They require support and encouragement because of discomfort.
    2 Attendance at group therapy sessions may be overstimulating during the withdrawal process. Group therapy becomes extremely important after the withdrawal is complete.
    3 Adherence to mental health unit rules is helpful in that it promotes safety and involvement in treatment. The staff will need to decide which rules must be enforced and which rules require flexibility.
    4 It is not productive to explore feelings in an effort to develop insight during the withdrawal period. This kind of work is an essential part of the recovery process once the withdrawal is complete.

165. Knowledge, assessment, environment (c)
    4 Mild paranoia and irritability are associated with amphetamine drug use.
    1 Her drug use interferes with her disposition and her attitude toward compliance.
    2 The history does not indicate that her drug use and anorexia have progressed to the point that she would become disoriented and her appearance disheveled. With continued untreated drug use and the accompanying malnutrition, she could experience sufficient damage to her brain to produce these effects.
    3 As above. Without medical care, she could progress to become psychotic and delusional.
166. Knowledge, assessment, environment (c)
    4 Depression, fatigue and lethargy are common to the syndrome of withdrawal from amphetamine drugs.
    1 Chest pain, diaphoresis, and palpitations are not part of the expected withdrawal syndrome. The patient is at risk for the development of complications such as bleeding ulcer and cardiac problems. The nurse would observe, report, and record these symptoms *immediately*.
    2 The nurse would expect the patient to experience the opposite of these symptoms.
    3 These symptoms are common to withdrawal from opiate drugs.
167. Knowledge, assessment, environment (b)
    4 Profound depression that can last for some months or years is the most likely effect. This requires ongoing therapy with good medical and psychiatric management if she is to be successful in giving up the drug.
    1 This symptom is common to withdrawal from opiate drugs.
    2 Common to intoxication with amphetamine drugs or PCP.
    3 Euphoria is not common to withdrawal syndrome.
168. Knowledge, assessment, environment (b)
    3 He will exhibit pinpoint pupils for several hours after his last use of heroin.
    1 Dilated pupils indicate the onset of the withdrawal syndrome. If the nurse does not see these symptoms but continues to see pinpoint pupils, she suspects that this patient has managed to acquire drugs while in the hospital.
    2 If this patient exhibits hostility, it is not a result of heroin intoxication. It may be a result of his psychological response to his arrest or it may be an indication of other psychological problems.
    4 It is unlikely that this patient would experience profound depression at this time.
169. Knowledge, assessment, environment (b)
    1 Dilated pupils is a common symptom of withdrawal from heroin and other opiates.
    2 Hostility may occur, but it is not the direct result of the withdrawal syndrome.
    3 Pinpoint pupils lead the nurse to suspect that the patient has found a way to acquire more heroin while in the hospital.
    4 This patient is unlikely to experience profound depression at this time.

170. Comprehension, planning, physiological (c)
    3 Hypomagnesemia is a common problem during alcohol withdrawal; serum magnesium levels should be monitored every 1 to 3 days.
    1 Antabuse interferes with alcohol metabolism; one must be alcohol-free for a minimum of 12 hours before therapy with Antabuse is initiated.
    2 Intravenous calcium is used to treat hypermagnesemia.
    4 Morphine sulfate is a narcotic analgesic. Many drug users take a variety of drugs simultaneously. It would be inappropriate to substitute one substance for another.

171. Application, implementation, environment (a)
    3 Vital signs should be closely monitored as delirium tremens is a life-threatening situation. Also, the need for medication will depend on blood pressure measurements.
    1 This is inappropriate when the patient is experiencing the discomfort of withdrawal.
    2 To prevent exhaustion and reduce agitation, sedation should be established and maintained.
    4 Although the nurse should monitor output, vital signs are the priority.

172. Application, implementation, psychosocial (c)
    1 Silence gives the patient time to collect his thoughts and reflect on what has been said. When used effectively, it encourages the patient to communicate. The patient should be the one to break the silence.
    2, 3 These actions do not encourage the patient to communicate about his problem.
    4 The patient will speak when he's ready.

173. Knowledge, assessment, psychosocial (b)
    2 Memory losses are the most common symptom of the first stage of this disease.
    1 Gradual loss of motor function is characteristic of stage II of the disease.
    3 Loss of gross motor coordination is seen in stage II.
    4 Loss of fine motor coordination is seen in stage II.

174. Comprehension, assessment, environment (c)
    4 This will elicit information about his feelings, especially because depression is a common secondary symptom of Alzheimer's disease.
    1, 2 These are important, but they do not address emotional changes.
    3 This is important, but it addresses judgment.

175. Application, planning, environment (c)
    3 This acknowledges that the patient is probably tired and may be frightened as a result of his mental deficits. It gives him the opportunity to feel some control in the process of being evaluated and makes the nurse an ally, not an enemy.
    1 This is true, but there is nothing to be gained and it needlessly aggravates the patient to continue to question him when he is obviously unwilling to continue at this time.
    2 There is no reason to doubt the truth of what the patient says he is feeling. Doubting him may make him angry and argumentative.
    4 This might also be true, but his family's wishes are not the priority at this time.

176. Application, implementation, environment (c)
    4 This removes him from the distraction and stimulation of the general waiting area, increasing the likelihood that he will be compliant and have his scan done.
    1 He may never feel ready and may actually opt to leave.
    2 This will not decrease his anxiety or confusion; it may actually make it worse.
    3 This will not increase the likelihood that he will cooperate; it may make him angry.

177. Application, planning, health (c)
    4 This is the most accurate answer. Alzheimer's disease progresses at a different rate in different patients, although the end result is always the same.
    1 This is untrue. He will not recover from his deficits.
    2 This is true, although it does not really explain anything to his family.
    3 This is not necessarily true because the nurse has only seen him under stress. This can make his deficits appear more pronounced than they are.

178. Comprehension, evaluation, environment (b)
    2 Audrey's short-term memory is too impaired to allow her to stick with the task of feeding herself.
    1 This is unlikely.
    3 There is no indication that Audrey is delusional.
    4 Audrey is at risk for becoming depressed, which is characteristic of Stage I of Alzheimer's disease. Depression is probably not the cause of her not eating.

179. Application, implementation, physiological (b)
    3 She needs support and encouragement to feed herself. The nurse should help her to maintain her independence as much as possible.
    1 This is indicated only if Audrey is physically weak or impaired.
    2 The nutritionist will be helpful, but this measure is not the priority.
    4 This will not address Audrey's difficulty in feeding herself.

180. Application, implementation, environment (c)
    4 A well-lit room will help her to remain oriented when she awakens in the night.
    1 Any sleeping medication will further compromise her brain functioning. If she receives any medication such as a benzodiazepine or a barbiturate, she will be significantly more disoriented for several days. It takes much longer for an older person to clear these drugs from the body.
    2 This is a good intervention for a younger person. It is not especially effective in an older person.
    3 Even if she had been markedly agitated during the night, she may not recall it.

181. Knowledge, assessment, psychosocial (a)
    4 Conversion reactions usually follow an event that triggers psychological conflict. The primary gain is relief; the secondary gains are sympathy and increased attention from others.
    1 This is suppression.
    2 This is rationalization.
    3 This is projection.

182. Comprehension, planning, environment (a)
    4 Taking measures to reduce threats to her physical well-being caused by her ritual is the most appropriate nursing intervention.
    1 Preventing the ritual will increase the patient's anxiety.
    2 The patient already knows the ritual is silly; it is not appropriate to call attention to the ritual.
    3 Rushing the patient will increase her anxiety, which will increase her need to perform the ritual.

183. Comprehension, evaluation, psychosocial (b)
    2 This indicates anxiety has been reduced and adaptive substitutes have been acquired.
    1, 3, 4 These are symptoms of obsessive-compulsive disorder.

184. Comprehension, assessment, environment (c)
    4 The symptoms of posttraumatic stress disorder (PTSD) usually begin several months or years after the traumatic event. Symptoms include nightmares, depression, and anxiety.
    1 These are not symptoms of PTSD.
    2 These symptoms can occur, but they are not the primary symptoms of PTSD.
    3 These are symptoms of schizophrenia, catatonic type.

185. Comprehension, assessment, psychosocial (b)
    4 Compulsive personalities are preoccupied with rules, details, and conformity. Work and productivity are their priorities; perfectionism and superiority negatively affect their interpersonal relationships.
    1 This is characteristic of histrionic personalities.
    2 This is seen in borderline personalities.
    3 This describes schizotypal personalities.

186. Comprehension, assessment, psychosocial (b)
    1 Perfectionism is a feature of the compulsive personality disorder. There is a tendency to see things as either all bad or all good, all right or all wrong.
    2 Decisiveness, or the ability to make decisions, is impaired by the need to make perfect decisions.
    3 Empathy is impaired by the person's tendency to be wrapped up in his own needs.
    4 The capacity to cooperate is impaired by the need to be in control and to have things done one's own way.

187. Application, implementation, psychosocial (c)
    3 Contracting with the patient to take control of some of the compulsive behavior will help the patient become more conscious of the behavior. This will eventually help the patient to make other choices.
    1 This can be very helpful to most patients, but it is not the *most* appropriate nursing intervention.
    2 The nurse might discuss the patient's compulsive behavior after the patient has become more conscious of the behavior.
    4 Building assertiveness skills is helpful to most patients, but it is not the *most* appropriate response.

188. Comprehension, planning, psychosocial (c)
    1 Individuals with anorexia worry about being liked and wanted by those around them. They believe that being as thin as possible will help to achieve this goal.
    2 This is not true. Individuals with anorexia tend anyway to be high achievers in intellectual tasks.
    3 They worry about control over themselves, not others.
    4 Individuals with anorexia never feel safe from the threat of potential weight gain.

189. Comprehension, assessment, environment (c)
    2 Valerie is suffering from bulimia. Self-induced vomiting and physical attractiveness are the cues.
    1 In anorexia nervosa, the individual simply avoids eating.
    3 Agoraphobia is the fear of open spaces.
    4 The narcissistic personality disorder is sometimes associated with eating disorders. There is no indication that Audrey has a personality disorder.

190. Comprehension, assessment, environment (b)
    3 Anorexic individuals fear becoming obese even though they are underweight.
    1 This is characteristic of binge eating.
    2 The thought of eating usually disgusts the anorexic.
    4 Anorexic individuals experience a loss of appetite or they use denial as a defense mechanism.

191. Comprehension, assessment, psychosocial (b)
    2 Anorexic individuals have a disturbance in the way they experience their body shapes, size or weight. Ann clearly states her disturbance over the size of her hands and feet.
    1, 3, 4 This is an appropriate nursing diagnosis for the patient with anorexia nervosa. The situation, however, does not indicate this as a priority diagnosis for Ann.

192. Comprehension, assessment, psychosocial (b)
    2 The parents of anorexics are characteristically rigid and overprotective.
    1, 4 These are characteristics of anorexia nervosa.
    3 These are characteristics of bulimia.

193. Comprehension, implementation, psychosocial (a)
    1 This is an appropriate goal.
    2 False reassurance is not helpful.
    3 Secluding the patient is not helpful.
    4 Future planning may only depress the patient more.

194. Comprehension, evaluation, environment (b)
    2 Goals should be stated in behavioral terms.
    1, 3 It is difficult to know if the goal is achievable because there is no criteria for performance.
    4 It is not a behavioral goal; it does not meet nursing process criteria for an expected outcome (goal).

195. Knowledge, planning, psychosocial (a)
    1 The theory is that patients fare better when they return to the community quickly with their support systems maintained.
    2 Although mental health of the community is a goal, it is impossible to ensure that a whole community is healthy.
    3 This is opposite of the theory, above.
    4 Although some restructuring may occur, this is not the main goal.

196. Comprehension, implementation, environment (b)
    2 Goal-oriented activity is needed to provide structure.
    1 This is ineffective because it allows patients to lead the group.
    3 This is ineffective because the patient's functioning may be disturbed, disoriented, or disorganized.
    4 This is ineffective because repression does not allow feelings to be expressed.

197. Application, intervention, psychosocial (a)
    2 Listening allows the patient to experience himself more freely and fully and encourages him to work through his feelings.
    1, 3 These responses ignore the patient's need to express his feelings to the nurse.
    4 This insensitively ignores the patient's feelings and blocks communication.

198. Comprehension, planning, psychosocial (c)
    4 Contracts emphasize patient responsibilities and level of participation.
    1 Contracts emphasize what the nurse will do *with* the patient rather than *for* the patient.
    2, 3 Emphasis is always on the patient's strengths, responsibility, and participation, not on what the nurse will not do.

199. Comprehension, planning, health (a)
    2 Liquid medications are ordered for hospitalized patients with a history of noncompliance and for patients that the staff suspects may be "cheeking" or hoarding. The oral route of administration is always the preferred route. To counter noncompliance tendencies in outpatients, long-acting depot injections are recommended. Patients have the right to refuse treatment, and this includes medications.
    1, 3 Not recommended for noncompliant patients; too easy to "cheek" and hoard.
    4 In a psychiatric emergency only medications can be given without consent to prevent harm to the patient or to others. The parenteral route should be used only if it is clear that without the medication, the patient poses a danger to himself and/or others.

200. Application, evaluation, health (c)
    4 Her grieving will not begin to be resolved until she is able to verbalize her feelings about her miscarriage instead of acting them out by becoming dysfunctional.
    1 This addresses her lack of appropriate employment, but not her grieving.
    2 This could potentially address any unresolved feelings she has about his leaving her, but it does not address her grief over the loss of the baby.
    3 This may not be a good idea at this time; she may need the support of her parents as she begins to verbalize her feelings of grief and loss.

201. Application, planning, health (c)
    2 Taking medications on a regular basis is the most important thing she can do to prevent a recurrence of her symptoms.
    1 These are important, but they are not the nurse's first priority.
    3 This is important for social skills, but it is not the first priority.
    4 This may not be realistic as a goal for this patient.

202. Application, implementation, health (c)
    2 This is an opportunity to explore how her family will or will not participate in her recovery.
    1 This is true, but it does not address what her mother is asking.
    3 This is also true, but it does not address the question of the important part played by her family.
    4 This is not the case. Attendance is strongly suggested, but no program can make it a mandatory condition of discharge.

203. Comprehension, assessment, environment (b)
    4 Patient safety is always the priority. The patient's statement that there is nothing left to be taken from her is the cue.
    1, 2, 3 These nursing diagnoses are all appropriate for the depressed patient, but the situation does not indicate that any of these problems are of immediate concern.

204. Knowledge, implementation, psychosocial (a)
    4 This is the only accurate information and therefore the *most appropriate* response.
    1 This statement is inaccurate and does not answer the patient's question.
    2 This is an inaccurate statement and would certainly increase the patient's anxiety
    3 The actual shock generally takes only a few seconds, but each treatment lasts approximately 15 minutes from beginning to end.

205. Application, planning, health (c)
    3 After 2 years of grieving, verbalizing on a daily basis, even if only for a few minutes, is realistic and necessary.
    1 She will need to verbalize or she will not be able to be discharged.
    2 This does not provide enough opportunity to resolve such a lengthy period of dysfunction.
    4 A weekly visit might have been sufficient earlier in this problem, but not at this point. Also, she will need more contact than this to build trust.

206. Comprehension, planning, health (b)
    1 Family support has been shown to be an important reason why patients remain compliant with treatment.
    2 Education does not guarantee that families will always cooperate with treatment.
    3 The goal of teaching is for patients and families to understand that taking medications must be the responsibility of the patient.
    4 Teaching does not ensure the approval of the family. The family's *support* is sought, not their approval.

207. Knowledge, evaluation, environment (b)
    2 Akathesia is the sensation of not being able to sit still.
    1 Dystonia is abnormal muscle spasms of the upper body.
    3 Tardive dyskinesia is abnormal movements of the face, lips, tongue, and lower extremities.
    4 Pseudoparkinsonism is abnormal stiffness of movement and facial expression.

208. Knowledge, implementation, environment (b)
    4 The ordered dose is questionable, as the initial dose is usually 2 to 5 mg. The daily dosage range is 1 to 30 mg.
    1 This is incorrect.
    2 Haloperidol (Haldol) is available in both oral and IM form.
    3 Haloperidol is a short-acting antipsychotic drug that is often given to control acute psychotic symptoms.

209. Knowledge, implementation, environment (b)
    2 Benztropine (Cogentin) is prescribed specifically to counteract the side effect of dystonia, which is what this patient is experiencing.
    1, 4 These are antianxiety drugs and will not be of help.
    3 Chlorpromazine (Thorazine) is another antipsychotic drug that will worsen the reaction that he is having.

210. Comprehension, planning, environment (b)
    3 It is important that the nursing staff be consistent and support one another in the care of this patient. It is neither possible nor wise to enforce all of the rules. The team must decide which rules are in the patient's best interest.
    1 This kind of behavior causes staff splitting. If the patient is allowed to choose favorites, staff cohesion is undermined and the staff is less effective in working together.
    2 Betty needs to have limits set on her behavior so that she can benefit from treatment.
    4 The staff has the responsibility of enforcing rules to bring about an effective treatment environment for the patient community.

211. Comprehension, assessment, environment (b)
    4 Peggy can experience a normal grief reaction. Her emotional experience of grief may be complicated if she has been overly dependent on her mother or if she has difficulty expressing herself.
    1 This is not true. Mentally retarded people are capable of forming close, warm, satisfying relationships.
    2 There is no indication that she will abuse alcohol.
    3 It is not likely that she will become psychotically depressed.

212. Knowledge, assessment, psychosocial (a)
    1 Shock and denial are common reactions to this kind of news. Denial is a useful defense mechanism in that it protects the person from emotional pain and thus frees him to deal with his affairs. Denial can become a dysfunctional defense if it interferes with his perception of reality or if it interferes with his seeking appropriate medical care.
    2 Anger that one has a fatal illness usually occurs after shock and denial.
    3 The degree to which one becomes depressed about a terminal illness varies with the individual.
    4 Acceptance is something one may or may not reach in the grieving process. It is healthier if one can achieve some acceptance. Emotional support from loved ones facilitates this.

213. Knowledge, assessment, environment (c)
    2 Mary is developing awareness of the impact the loss of her husband will have on her life. This is a very difficult period in her life. Grief is quite demanding physically. Mary is predisposed to the development of illnesses as a result of the effect grief has on the body.
    1 She has moved beyond the stage of shock and denial.
    3 During the phase of restitution, Mary will cope with her loss and begin to develop new ways of living a fulfilling life.
    4 Normal grieving is very distressing. There is no reason to suspect her grief reaction will be distorted.

214. Comprehension, assessment, physiological (c)
    2 NMS is characterized by these symptoms.
    1 These are symptoms of encephalitis. Symptoms resemble those of meningitis, but their onset is more gradual.
    3 These are classic symptoms of meningococcal meningitis (bacterial meningitis).
    4 These are symptoms of gram-negative bacteremia.

215. Comprehension, evaluation, health (c)
    2 Salad dressings that do not contain MSG or cheese are allowed on a tyramine-restricted diet.
    1, 3, 4 Cheese pizza, sauerkraut, and sherry are forbidden foods on a tyramine-restricted diet.

216. Comprehension, planning, environment (b)
    3 Crisis intervention therapy, being short term, is usually from 1 to 6 weeks. A crisis is usually resolved within a 4- to 6-week period and focuses on the current problem only.
    1, 2, 4 Crisis intervention therapy is short-term and lasts 1 to 6 weeks.

217. Knowledge, assessment, environment (a)
    3 Child abusers have a history of emotional deprivation, abuse, or neglect as a child.
    1 Child abuse occurs in all socioeconomic groups.
    2 Abusive parents tend to look to the child to fill their need for acceptance and love; these are unrealistic expectations of a child.
    4 Abusive parents are described as suspicious of others and have minimal, if any, social interaction.

218. Comprehension, assessment, environment (b)
    1 Abused children become visibly uncomfortable when they hear other children cry.
    2 Habit disorders are characteristics of emotional abuse.
    3 Poor peer relationship is indicative of sexual abuse.
    4 Emotional or mental lag is associated with emotional abuse.

219. Comprehension, planning, environment (a)
    3 Expressive therapy such as art or play therapy enables the child to communicate painful emotions nonverbally. Verbalization of feelings is more threatening.
    1 Group therapy requires verbal sharing, which is more threatening than nonverbal types of therapy.
    2 Hypnosis is helpful in identifying a source of anxiety. In this situation, sexual abuse is already the known source.
    4 This type of therapy is effective for phobic patients.

220. Knowledge, assessment, environment (b)
    2 Violence and abuse against women most often occurs for the first time or increases in frequency and severity during pregnancy.
    1 Battered women in most cases do not present themselves for treatment related to abuse.
    3 Battered women do not usually seek mental health services as a result of being abused.
    4 Only a small percentage of battered women seek or receive legal assistance in dealing with their abusers.

221. Knowledge, assessment, psychosocial (b)
    2 Women from middle and upper socioeconomic status (SES) groups have more access to private physicians who will not reveal their patients are being abused. Women from lower SES groups have to rely more on public clinics and emergency departments for treatment.
    1 Battering and abuse of women is a cross-class issue. One socioeconomic group is no more likely to encounter abuse from their partners than any other.
    3 The reverse is often true; the police are less likely to seriously respond to complaints from poor and lower SES women.
    4 There is no evidence to support this; men of all classes abuse women.

222. Application, implementation, health (c)
    4 Men who batter their partners have learned to use violence as a way of expressing their feelings; they can be taught to behave differently.
    1 This is not necessarily true. Some men who have battered their partners in the past have stopped doing so with the appropriate interventions.
    2 This is not necessarily true, either. She may have sound reasons to hope that he can be different, and the nurse should explore those with her.
    3 This is judgmental and casts her in the role of victim, which will inhibit any chance of change taking place in the relationship.

223. Application, planning, health (c)
    2 Use of alcohol lowers inhibitions and increases the possibility that a person who would use violence will do so.
    1 This is not true. If he is a person who uses violence as a means of expression, he will do so even if not drinking.
    3 This is not true. Alcohol use decreases inhibitions and makes inappropriate behavior more likely to occur.
    4 This also is untrue. The causes of battering are many; drinking can only increase the likelihood that abuse will occur at a particular time.

224. Knowledge, planning, environment (b)
    1 This is an absolutely fundamental need for the nurse to address before anything else.
    2 This is important, but it comes only after her safety is ensured.
    3 This may or may not be an issue at this time, but it is not the nurse's first priority with her.
    4 She will probably do this if she feels safe and trusting.

225. Knowledge, planning, psychosocial (b)
    3 Ego ideal is one's perception of how one should be, compared to how one perceives oneself to actually be.
    1 Body image is one part of identity.
    2 Role is a description of how one fits into the society, while body image is one's perception of one's body.
    4 See above descriptions.
226. Comprehension, implementation, environment (b)
    4 Although the time period varies from state to state, written notice to be discharged is required of voluntary psychiatric admissions.
    1, 3 Informal admissions (no formal or written application for admission) may leave a psychiatric facility by signing against medical advice (AMA).
    2 Voluntary admissions do not require court-ordered releases.
227. Application, implementation, physiological (a)
    2 Restating and repeating the main idea is a technique that enhances communication.
    1 This challenges the patient, places the patient on the defensive, and blocks attempts to discuss unmet needs.
    3 Requesting an explanation can be intimidating to the patient, and it can block communication.
    4 Giving advice is not the role of the psychiatric nurse, nor is it therapeutic. It implies that the nurse knows best, and this fosters dependence.
228. Comprehension, implementation, psychosocial (b)
    1 This encourages the patient to use her own resources, which will minimize feelings of dependency and hopelessness associated with depression.
    2, 4 This ignores the patient's need and blocks communication.
    3 The nurse should not act for the patient unless absolutely necessary.
229. Application, implementation, health (c)
    1 Learning their symptoms can help patients to obtain rapid treatment and perhaps avoid hospitalization.
    2 This will not affect her vulnerability to depression.
    3 Decreasing stressors is constructive, but this does not affect the physiologic processes of depression.
    4 This does not guarantee that she will not become ill.
230. Application, implementation, psychosocial (b)
    2 This is not the kind of information that the nurse can keep confidential. The patient who voices suicidal ideation may indeed take her own life. The nurse needs the support of the nursing team to intervene on the patient's behalf.
    1 The nurse is obligated to reveal the patient's suicidal ideation because this is life-threatening. Concern for her safety takes precedence over maintaining confidentiality.
    3 Because the nurse has an established rapport with Una, the nurse will discuss suicide with her at some point. The nurse's immediate concern, however, is to see that appropriate limits are set so that Una may survive to have that discussion.
    4 The nurse should not bring this up in group therapy. Group members assume the active role in group psychotherapy. The therapist acts as a facilitator of the group process.
231. Comprehension, planning, environment (b)
    2 Constipation is a common side effect of tricyclic antidepressant drugs. Severe constipation requires immediate medical attention.
    1, 4 These are not common side effects of Pamelor.
    3 The change in her mood will be gradual over a period of 1 to 3 weeks.

231. Comprehension, planning, environment (b)
    2 Constipation is a common side effect of tricyclic antidepressant drugs. Severe constipation requires immediate medical attention.
    1, 4 These are not common side effects of Pamelor.
    3 The change in her mood will be gradual over a period of 1 to 3 weeks.
232. Application, implementation, psychosocial (a)
    3 It is very pleasant to work with patients who improve and who appreciate the nurse's contribution to that improvement. Nevertheless, the nurse must maintain professional boundaries. It is not appropriate to meet the patient for lunch after she has been discharged.
    1, 4 It is not appropriate to agree to meet the patient for lunch. See No. 3.
    2 This is true, but the patient needs to be given an explanation so as not to feel rejected.
233. Knowledge, planning, psychosocial (c)
    3 Play therapy is the most common treatment for depression in a child. Children have the capacity to express deep feelings through symbols they choose in their play.
    1 Cognitive therapy is used for adults. This therapy emphasizes healthy ways of thinking about oneself and one's circumstances.
    2 Insight-oriented psychotherapy is used for adults. It is a deeper exploration of the self.
    4 Work therapy is used for adolescents and adults. It emphasizes building self-esteem through meaningful work.
234. Application, implementation, psychosocial (b)
    2 This is a broad opening statement that encourages the patient to verbalize.
    1 False reassurance and stereotypical comments block communication.
    3 Giving directions denies the patient independence with problem-solving and is nontherapeutic.
    4 Questions of this nature make the patient feel defensive and create a stressful situation for the patient.
235. Application, assessment, psychosocial (b)
    4 Patient has five high-risk factors: sex, age, drinking, job loss, and family history of suicide.
    1, 2, 3 There are too many factors in this case for the patient to have a low risk.
236. Comprehension, planning, psychosocial (b)
    2 A suicidal patient may not perceive possible options, and he may need to learn new strategies for dealing with problems.
    1 It is difficult to separate gestures from realistic attempts at suicide.
    3 There is no specific requirement.
    4 Asking for reasons is not helpful.
237. Comprehension, planning, environment (b)
    3 Confusion is one of the major side effects. Frequent orientation is necessary during the treatment course.
    1 Electroconvulsive therapy (ECT) is not a permanent cure for depression. Maintenance treatment decreases the relapse rate.
    2 An individual who has received ECT usually completely recovers from memory loss.
    4 A decrease in symptoms of depression usually occurs after 1 to 3 weeks of treatment.
238. Comprehension, evaluation, psychosocial (b)
    4 The patient is threatening to harm herself. Keeping her safe is the nurse's highest priority.
    1, 2 These are correct, but they are not the highest priority.
    3 This may or may not be true.

239. Knowledge, planning, health (b)
3 All community mental health centers are required by law to have in place a fully developed suicide risk detection and prevention program for all age groups.
1 Most community mental health centers have these, but they are not legally required.
2 Some community mental health centers offer these programs, but they are not required.
4 These are not required to be provided by these centers.

240. Knowledge, assessment, psychosocial (b)
2 This is the highest risk. This statement shows that the person has made a clear plan, has the means to commit the act, and has selected a time.
1 Of all the statements, this indicates the lowest risk. If the chronic frustration continues, the risk may increase.
3 This statement may indicate the second highest risk. It suggests the individual may make a suicide gesture in an effort to manipulate or control the girlfriend. A suicide gesture done in an effort to manipulate can be lethal.
4 This statement suggests relatively low immediate risk. It also suggests that the individual requires observation for an increase in suicidal intent.

241. Application, implementation, environment (c)
2 The nurse must evaluate his suicidal intent. It may be that this suicide gesture has resolved nothing for him. He may leave the hospital only to make a more lethal gesture later.
1 Provoking guilt in the patient will not promote his mental health.
3 This is an accusational remark and will damage the nurse's relationship with the patient.
4 As above. This kind of remark inhibits building professional rapport with the patient.

242. Comprehension, implementation, environment (c)
2 One-to-one observation should begin immediately so the patient is in full view at all times.
1 Patients who do not respond to limit-setting may need to be restrained. Restraints should be employed only when all other safety measures have failed. This is not, however, the first nursing action.
3 Seclusion is used only when all other safety measures have failed; it would not be the first nursing action.
4 Removing dangerous possessions is a priority and should be done by the staff member assigned to one-to-one observation.

243. Application, implementation, environment (a)
3 Sharp items should be removed.
1, 2 There is no need to deny the patient these items.
4 Shoe laces should be removed from the shoes. There is no need to deny the patient her shoes.

244. Application, implementation, health (b)
2 Many times an entire family feels traumatized by an act of violence toward a loved one. Professional counseling can be useful for the entire family.
1 This is a correct statement, but it is not the best answer.
3 Sometimes the family may feel it is better to let the person work things out for herself. This usually results from their feeling of helplessness. Glenna and her family can help one another through the guidance of a professional.
4 Although this may sometimes be true, it does not sufficiently answer the mother's question.

245. Comprehension, assessment, psychosocial (c)
4 Numbness is a characteristic of posttraumatic stress disorder, as evidenced by Marge's lack of affect when speaking of the event.
1, 2 These may be part of the syndrome, but they are not shown in this situation.
3 Reliving is not described in this situation.

246. Application, planning, health (b)
3 Before anything is done, the rape victim must be informed of her options in regard to reporting the rape and her rights as a victim.
1 She should not have anything done until she is informed of her rights and options.
2 She should not shower until a decision has been made about whether physical evidence will be gathered.
4 This should not be done until she is informed of her rights and options.

247. Comprehension, planning, environment (a)
1 The patient will be confused following the treatment and will need assistance with reorientation to his surroundings.
2 Memory loss can persist for weeks following the course of treatment. Although this is important for the patient to know, immediately after treatment when the patient is confused is not the appropriate time for this intervention.
3 Seizure precautions are implemented during the treatment. After the shock is administered, the patient experiences a grand mal seizure.
4 The patient is npo the morning of the treatment and voids just before treatment. Until the patient is fairly alert following the treatment, fluids would not be offered. It is appropriate to note the first voiding after treatment, but it is not necessary to monitor intake.

248. Knowledge, assessment, environment (a)
3 Patients who are severely depressed and who cannot take or have not responded to medication therapy are appropriate candidates for electroconvulsive therapy (ECT). ECT has also been used for manic patients not receiving lithium and for highly suicidal patients for whom the antidepressant therapy effectiveness waiting period cannot be risked.
1, 2, 4 Individuals with these disorders are not candidates for ECT because other more appropriate treatments are available.

249. Comprehension, planning, environment (b)
3 In an individual in the alcoholic state, vital signs are usually elevated. Autonomic overactivity occurs, which would account for the profuse sweating.
1 Pupils would be dilated; temperature and pulse elevated.
2 These are psychological, not physiological, manifestations.
4 Tachycardia and diaphoresis are correct, but the blood pressure is usually elevated.

250. Knowledge, evaluation, psychosocial (a)
1 This is privileged communication.
2 This refers to release from hospital, not to any relationship.
3 There are no special malpractice laws.
4 This is not related to the situation; this term refers to a temporary substitute for a physician who is away from the practice.

CHAPTER 7

Answers and Rationales for Comprehensive Examinations

All questions have been classified by cognitive level, nursing process, patient need, and level of difficulty. These classifications are provided following the question number.

The first word signifies the cognitive level of the questions: knowledge, comprehension, or application. The second word indicates the phase of the nursing process: assessment, planning, implementation, or evaluation. The third word indicates the type of patient need and is abbreviated as follows: environment = safe, effective care environment; physiological = physiological integrity; psychosocial = psychosocial integrity; health = health promotion/maintenance.

The letters in parentheses indicate the difficulty of the question. The letter *a* signifies that more than 75% of students should answer the question correctly; *b* signifies that between 50% and 75% should answer correctly; and *c* signifies that between 25% and 50% should answer correctly.

Rationales for all four answer choices for each question are provided. The rationale for the correct answer is listed first, followed by the rationales for the incorrect answer choices.

COMPREHENSIVE EXAMINATION ONE: PART 1

1. Comprehension, assessment, physiological (a)
   2 Homans' sign (calf pain with dorsiflexion of the foot) is indicative of a probable thrombus in the leg veins.
   1 In adults the Babinski reflex is supposed to be negative.
   3 Although borderline high, this blood pressure could be a result of anxiety, pain, or various other factors.
   4 Ankle swelling is significant for many disorders, but it does not strongly point to any specific disorder. If it is in both legs, then it may be dependent edema that is caused by many factors.
2. Application, evaluation, environment (a)
   4 Intramuscular injections should be avoided in patients receiving anticoagulants.
   1 Warfarin (coumadin) is affected by food, so it should be given before meals.
   2 Prothrombin time levels are collected daily at the onset of therapy and weekly thereafter to monitor therapeutic levels at the desired prothrombin time.
   3 If the patient is near discharge, the nurse would begin to ambulate to ensure his activity at home would be safe. After 7 to 14 days the thrombus would dissolve and the patient would need to resume activity to prevent further thrombus.

3. Application, planning, physiological (b)
   3 This patient is at risk for seizures, delusions, and neurological impairment.
   1 Intake and output is not a factor of high priority; reporting it every 2 hours would only be significant if it were markedly abnormal.
   2 Neurologic checks every hour would waste time on nonessential tasks and take away from the quiet restful environment this patient needs.
   4 Sedation is a medical order that is physician-dependent. Although sedation is likely, it is not an independent nursing action.
4. Comprehension, evaluation, environment (b)
   2 Orinase frequently interacts with many other medications and must be mentioned every time a new drug is prescribed.
   1 Many factors influence blood sugar; one drug cannot keep levels stable at all times.
   3 This drug should be taken before breakfast; if it causes gastrointestinal upset, it should be taken with meals.
   4 Although nausea may be a side effect, it is not normal to frequently feel nauseated. This sensation should be reported to the patient's physician.
5. Application, implementation, health (b)
   3 This is a reassuring statement. It correctly informs the patient that the stoma has no nerve endings in the inner luminal lining and therefore the patient cannot perceive pain in that location.
   1 This is reassuring, but it does not inform the patient that the stoma has no pain receptors.
   2 Dressing or pouch changes should not cause the patient pain.
   4 This response ignores the patient's concern and instead focuses on the nurse.
6. Application, implementation, psychosocial (b)
   3 By asking Mr. Sam if he would like to see the stoma, the nurse can evaluate his readiness to begin learning about his care.
   1 Showing Mr. Sam the stoma if he is not ready to see it does not provide care appropriate to his stage of grieving.
   2 This action ignores Mr. Sam's feelings and does not help him move through the grieving process.
   4 Discussing home care is inappropriate when the patient is not ready to learn.

7. Application, implementation, health (b)
   4 This response helps the patient view the situation from his wife's point of view. The discussion should take place between the spouses.
   1 Moving to another room or another bed may cause emotional distancing from the spouse.
   2 This response closes the discussion with the patient.
   3 It is the nurse's responsibility to help family members learn about home care, not to try to work out emotional problems between spouses.

8. Application, evaluation, health (b)
   2 Foods such as cabbage, cucumbers, and radishes produce more gas, causing more odor from the colostomy.
   1 Citrus fruits are helpful in the healing process. Acetic acid is vitamin C.
   3 Foods high in iron help in the healing process. Oatmeal and cream of wheat help keep the stool soft, which is normal for a transverse colostomy.
   4 Juices such as apple and cranberry help keep the stool soft and reduce the amount of odor from the stool.

9. Application, implementation, psychosocial (b)
   3 This response acknowledges the patient's feelings and leads to further discussion.
   1 This response does not adequately acknowledge the patient's feelings and closes the discussion.
   2 This response ignores the patient's feelings and leads her to believe that something was wrong with the fetus.
   4 Physiologically, this response is correct, but it ignores the patient's feeling of loss in this pregnancy.

10. Application, implementation, psychosocial (b)
    2 Babies with Down's syndrome may appear hypotonic (floppy). This may lead the mother to believe that the baby does not like to be held or cuddled. The nurse should role-model mothering and assist the mother to hold the baby.
    1 To promote mother-infant bonding, the baby should not be kept in the nursery unless absolutely necessary.
    3 Leaving the mother and baby alone does not facilitate bonding or grieving.
    4 The infant does not need to be in Isolette unless there are additional physical problems. Mrs. Jenkins should be allowed to handle the baby's care, if possible.

11. Knowledge, evaluation, environment (a)
    3 After the age of 35, a mother has an increased risk (1 in 400) of having a baby with Down's syndrome.
    1 Pitocin is not related to the development of Down's syndrome. Down's syndrome is a genetic anomaly.
    2 A prolonged labor, even with possible fetal anoxia, does not cause Down's syndrome.
    4 Multiparity by itself does not cause a genetic anomaly.

12. Comprehension, assessment, physiological (c)
    3 Hallucinogens have a profound psychological effect on people, often described as a process of amplification. This effect is called a "trip." A negative experience is referred to as a "bad trip," during which the individual feels the reaction to the drug will never end and a panic reaction ensues.
    1 These are symptoms or effects of central nervous system depressants.
    2 These are physical effects of marijuana.
    4 These are symptoms of withdrawal from inhalants.

13. Knowledge, planning, physiological (a)
    1 Silver nitrate might prevent gonorrheal infection of the eyes, which can lead to blindness.
    2 Syphilis can cause deformities in the fetus.
    3 Oxygen pressure (PO_2) of arterial blood is measured. If PO_2 is greater than 100 mm Hg, retrolental fibroplasia, which results in blindness, occurs.
    4 This is not an occurrence.

14. Knowledge, planning, physiological (c)
    1 Menstruation does not usually occur but ovulation may; thus pregnancy is possible.
    2 Ovulation may occur.
    3 She does not have to stop breast-feeding.
    4 The uterus still returns to normal in 3 to 4 weeks.

15. Comprehension, assessment, environment (c)
    2 Hallucinogens primarily affect changes in thought content, perception and subjective emotional experience. Other hallucinogens include mescaline, psilocybin and psilocin, and morning glory seeds (heavenly blue, pearly gates, flying saucers).
    1 Bennies and speed are amphetamines; hash is marijuana.
    3 These refer to heroin, which is a narcotic.
    4 Rainbows are barbiturates, and M refers to morphine.

16. Application, implementation, environment (a)
    3 Foul odor may indicate an infection requiring some antibiotics.
    1 Foul odor is not normal.
    2 This is not likely, unless the physician specifically orders it.
    4 Counting pads does not take care of the problem.

17. Application, implementation, physiological (c)
    1 Morphine is an opiate receptor that affects the central nervous system, causing more relaxed respirations.
    2 The causative factor is not removed when administering oxygen.
    3 The causative factor is not removed when talking to her alone.
    4 This is contraindicated because it increases circulating blood to heart and lungs, which can increase the respiratory rate.

18. Comprehension, implementation, health (c)
    3 In addition, a person may experience flashbacks (the spontaneous recurrence of the drug experience without using the drug). There may be changes in thought content, perception, subjective emotional experience, and judgment. Physically, there may be increased pulse rate, sweating, and tremors.
    1 LSD is not physically addictive.
    2 These are withdrawal signs of barbiturates; there are not any specific withdrawal symptoms for LSD.
    4 These are characteristics of amphetamine intoxication.

19. Application, implementation, environment (c)
    2 This is a truthful statement and does not make a judgment. It lets the patient know the nurse understands where he is.
    1 This gives false assurance.
    3 With this response the nurse is making a moral judgement.
    4 This is too technical and may be misinterpreted.

20. Knowledge, evaluation, environment (b)
    1 There are no scientific studies that prove that LSD increases creativity.
    2, 3, 4 These are common side effects of LSD.

21. Application, implementation, environment (a)
    3 $150 \text{ mg} \times \dfrac{5 \text{ ml}}{25 \text{ mg}} = 6$
    1, 2 These are incorrect calculations; doses are too low.
    4 Incorrect calculation; dose is too high.

22. Application, planning, environment (b)
    3 The antibiotic must be maintained at a therapeutic blood level and should be taken as ordered every 6 hours, without skipping a dose, until completed.
    1 Even though the child may begin to feel better and the signs and symptoms decrease, the antibiotic should be continued for the prescribed time.
    2 A therapeutic blood level cannot be reached with long periods between doses.
    4 The antibiotic may aid in reducing the temperature before the pneumonia/bronchitis is completely resolved.
23. Application, planning, health (b)
    4 The injection should be made up after the child is no longer ill. The measles, mumps, rubella (MMR) can be given after 15 months of age.
    1 The MMR should not be administered during times of illness or fever.
    2 Reye's syndrome could occur as a result of aspirin administration given during febrile conditions.
    3 Injections can be postponed but should never be entirely skipped. A second MMR is now required for entry into school.
24. Knowledge, evaluation, health (b)
    2 Malaise, soreness, and a raised red area at the site of infection is common after most immunizations. Instruct the mother that this may remain for several days.
    1 Two of these symptoms are severe and would warrant referral to the physician.
    3 These symptoms are not common and would warrant referral to the physician.
    4 Although immunizations can cause low-grade fever and malaise, whelps and high-grade fever are unexpected reactions and require further assessment.
25. Comprehension, planning, environment (b)
    4 Aerosolization is the normal route for the spread of the Mycobacterium tuberculosis.
    1 Repeated close contact is usually needed for transmission of tuberculosis.
    2 Feces is not the route of transmission for tuberculosis.
    3 These common tests do not transmit tuberculosis.
26. Comprehension, assessment, physiological (c)
    1 A positive response is the development of an indurated area measuring 10 mm or more around the intradermal injection site on the forearm.
    2 A rash on both forearms indicates another clinical problem.
    3 The test is administered on the inner aspect of the forearm, not the deltoid muscle.
    4 A productive cough is usually present with tuberculosis, but it is not made worse by testing.
27. Application, planning, environment (c)•
    1 Isolation is needed with respiratory precautions. The nurse should wear a mask and wash her hands carefully.
    2 Isolation is needed. The nurse need normally wear only a mask. Only if there is a possibility of gross contamination of the nurse's clothing are a gown and gloves necessary.
    3, 4 Isolation is necessary with the patient remaining in her room. The nurse should wear a mask.
28. Application, implementation, health (b)
    2 Most patients with tuberculosis have anorexia, nausea, and weight loss accompanying the disease. Good nutrition is essential to healing.
    1 There is no reason why the patient cannot cook at home.
    3 If the patient prefers "fast foods," these will need to be included to an extent in the diet instruction. This statement is an assumption.
    4 The medication needed for treatment will most likely make her anorexia, nausea, and weight loss worse.

29. Application, planning, health (c)
    1 After beginning the medication therapy, compliant patients are not contagious after about 3 weeks and may return to work. Followup therapy is necessary for one year.
    2 While therapy may be completed at home, it is not necessary to remain away from work for the entire year.
    3 Patients are no longer sent to a tuberculosis hospital or sanitorium.
    4 Patients are contagious during the first 3 weeks of therapy and should remain away from work no matter how they feel.
30. Comprehension, assessment, environment (c)
    3 The laboratory results are lower than normal. The average range is: hematocrit, adult female, 38% to 47%; hemoglobin, adult female, 12 to 16 g/dl.
    1 The values are not higher than normal.
    2 The values are not within the normal range.
    4 While the values are below the normal range, they are not considered life-threatening. Tissue perfusion can still occur.
31. Application, planning, environment (b)
    3 Patients with low hematocrit and hemoglobin values may become light-headed and faint during ambulation.
    1 Ability to take oral fluids normally should not be affected.
    2 Adequate medication for pain control should be administered.
    4 Laboratory values are not low enough to grossly interfere with renal function. The patient should be able to void.
32. Application, evaluation, health (b)
    3 Iron preparations such as ferrous sulfate are often taken with meals to prevent gastric irritation.
    1 Iron preparations taken on an empty stomach may be more completely absorbed but can cause gastric irritation and distress.
    2 Laxatives may promote inadequate absorption of nutrients. If the patient becomes constipated, the nurse should recommend an increase in the amount of roughage in the diet.
    4 Liquids will not provide the bulk needed to prevent gastric distress.
33. Application, implementation, health (a)
    4 Because of the patient's hematocrit and hemoglobin levels, the nurse should emphasize leafy green vegetables as a good source of iron.
    1 Citrus fruits are excellent sources of vitamin C and should be included in the diet, but in this situation the sources of nutritional iron should be emphasized.
    2, 3 These foods are not good sources of iron.
34. Application, implementation, physiologic (b)
    1 The secretions are scant because the patient has been NPO and the peristaltic action is diminished from the surgery and anesthetic.
    2 Physicians should be called immediately only in emergency situations.
    3 While patency is an important consideration, irrigation is implemented with caution in gastric surgeries; if implemented, this is done only in small amounts of solution and by physician's orders.
    4 High suction is always contraindicated in any situation unless specifically ordered by a physician.

35. Comprehension, assessment, environment (c)
    4 Vitamin B$_{12}$ stimulates the intrinsic factor, which is needed for red blood cell formation.
    1 Vitamin B$_{12}$ does not relieve distention.
    2 Vitamin B$_{12}$ aids in blood cell formation and neural function.
    3 Vitamin B$_{12}$ does not directly stimulate appetite.
36. Knowledge, planning, physiological (a)
    3 Ulcerative colitis is the inflammation and ulceration of the colon and rectum.
    1, 2 These are incorrect definitions.
    4 Constipation does not usually occur in ulcerative colitis.
37. Knowledge, assessment, physiological (a)
    1 A change in bowel patterns is the earliest warning of cancer of the large intestine.
    2 Although weight loss does accompany cancerous processes of the gastrointestinal system, it is not always the earliest sign.
    3 Clay-colored stools usually accompany problems of the biliary system.
    4 Flatulence can be a symptom of many GI disorders, not specifically cancer.
38. Application, implementation, environment (c)
    4 Unless the tray was also contaminated, the drape can be replaced easily and the tray can still be used.
    1 Sterile trays are quite expensive and unless contaminated, the tray should be saved.
    2 This is unsafe and could result in contamination to the patient.
    3 The physician should be informed of the contamination, but starting over may not be necessary; see No. 4 response.
39. Knowledge, implementation, environment (a)
    3 Good handwashing is the single most effective way to help prevent the spread of infections and should be practiced before and after all contact with a patient.
    1 Sterile gloves are not always needed for procedures and treatment.
    2 Isolation gowns are an effective way to decrease contamination, but they are not always necessary.
    4 Unless providing wound care or a special procedure, the family should not need nonsterile gloves.
40. Application, implementation, environment (a)
    2 Gown and gloves would be necessary if the nurse is coming in contact with soiled or infective materials. Until a more definite diagnosis is determined, all dressings would be potential contaminants.
    1 Respiratory isolation frequently calls for a mask and gloves.
    3 Use of a mask and gown without gloves is unlikely.
    4 Strict isolation or reverse isolation may call for each of these items.
41. Application, implementation, psychosocial (b)
    1 The family may need the time with the deceased family member so they can cope with the death.
    2 The grieving process may not begin until the realization that the death of their loved one really has occurred. This may require a viewing of the body.
    3 Waiting may only increase the grieving and create suspicion in the family that something is being hidden.
    4 Friends may be helpful during a crisis, but often families need private time with the deceased.
42. Application, planning, environment (b)
    4 Because of his age and medical conditions, epinephrine would not be recommended because it can increase the blood pressure and raise the blood sugar.
    1 Benzalkonium (zephiran) is used before surgery on unbroken skin.
    2 Benzoin spray is a demulcent and protectant.
    3 Epinephrine is combined with lidocaine to slow the absorption and prolong the effect of the local anesthetic. A prolonged increase in blood pressure would not be suggested for this patient; see No. 4 response.
43. Knowledge, assessment, environment (a)
    1 By definition, mental illness may be exhibited by behavior that is conspicuous, threatening, and disruptive of relationships or that deviates significantly from behavior that is considered socially acceptable.
    2, 3, 4 These are signs of mentally *healthy* individuals.
44. Comprehension, assessment, physiological (b)
    2 By definition, stress is a specific response by the body to a stimulus that disturbs normal functioning.
    1 This defines defense mechanisms.
    3 This is the definition of anxiety.
    4 This describes frustration.
45. Comprehension, implementation, health (b)
    4 Stress is individualized. How stress is perceived by an individual determines whether the stress produces anxiety in the individual.
    1 Health factors do affect individual stress.
    2 The nurse should help patients develop *adaptive* patterns.
    3 Any type of changes in situations or events can contribute to stress.
46. Knowledge, assessment, psychosocial (c)
    4 With rationalization, the person denies actual thoughts and justifies his actions by giving untrue, but seemingly acceptable, reasons for his behavior.
    1 Reaction formation takes place when the conscious behavior is completely opposite to the unconscious process.
    2 Compensation is when an individual makes up for a "deficiency" in one area by excelling in or emphasizing another area.
    3 In conversion, emotional conflicts are turned into a physical symptom, which provides the individual with some sort of benefit (secondary gain).
47. Knowledge, assessment, physiological (a)
    3 Breech presentation could be buttocks, feet, or knees first.
    1 The long axis of the body indicates a transverse lie, which means that the fetus is lying crosswise in the uterus; normal delivery is impossible.
    2 In the shoulder position, the scapula is presenting.
    4 The vertex position is a cephalic (head) presentation.
48. Comprehension, planning, physiological (c)
    1 Presentations other than cephalic or those in which the presenting part is not fully engaged, predispose the patient to the complication of a prolapsed cord.
    2 No hemorrhage is usually involved with rupture of the membranes.
    3 This is a very rapid delivery, usually without sterile preparation.
    4 A nuchal cord is an abnormal but common condition in which the umbilical cord is wrapped around the neck of the fetus in utero or of the baby as it is delivered.

49. Comprehension, evaluation, physiological (a)

    3 This is considered a normal range. A 30 beat/min deviation from the baseline may be used to determine conditions.

    1, 2 Below 120 beats/min is considered to be bradycardia.

    4 Above 160 beats/min is considered to be tachycardia.

50. Knowledge, evaluation, physiological (b)

    4 This occurs with dilation of the cervix.

    1 This refers to the relation of the presenting part to the mother's birth canal.

    2 This is not applicable.

    3 This describes Braxton-Hicks contractions.

51. Comprehension, evaluation, physiological (c)

    1 The pH of amniotic fluid is 7.5, or alkaline.

    2 The pH of amniotic fluid is always alkaline, never acid.

    3, 4 These do not verify rupture of membranes.

52. Application, implementation, health (b)

    3 Skipping doses can alter the therapeutic blood level necessary to keep the patient free of seizures.

    1 This response does not emphasize the need to avoid skipping doses.

    2 This response is not inappropriate, it should, however, be followed with instruction on the proper way to take the medication as prescribed.

    4 Organizing the medication by each day does not stress the need not to miss a dose.

53. Knowledge, assessment, physiological (a)

    2 Other symptoms may include anorexia, irritability, and an occasional cough.

    1 These are symptoms of gastroenteritis.

    3 These are symptoms of acute otitis media.

    4 These are symptoms of intussusception.

54. Application, implementation, environment (b)

    3 The nurse's initial concern is the patient. To control the environment, the nurse should remove him from the room and have the oxygen discontinued.

    1 The fire alarm may not be necessary at this time. The nurse should further assess the situation.

    2 The supervisor should be notified, but only after the patient is safely out of the room.

    4 This is an acceptable response but only after the patient is safe.

55. Knowledge, assessment, physiological (a)

    3 Amphetamines are drugs that stimulate the central nervous system (CNS) stimulants and result in insomnia, tremors, and excitability.

    1 Alcohol, a CNS depressant, produces sleep and sedation.

    2 Antihistamines usually produce drowsiness, although they can produce CNS excitation in children. They usually do not produce tremors.

    4 Sympathomimetic drugs can produce anxiety, but they lessen fatigue.

56. Knowledge, planning, environment (a)

    2 Sympathomimetic drugs include Adrenalin, which is usually given in cases of allergic reaction.

    1 Ganglionic agents are usually recommended in antihypertensive crisis.

    3 Parasympathetic blocking agents include mydriatic, cycloplegic, and antispasmodic drugs.

    4 Neuromuscular blocking agents are used for relaxation of muscles and spasms.

57. Application, implementation, physiological (b)

    1 The decreased peristalsis could show signs of improvement in the diarrhea, but the medication could lead to constipation and dehydration. A physician's assessment of the medication is necessary.

    2 Increasing the fluids could lessen the concern for dehydration; however, the nurse does not have the authority to lessen the dose to one quarter.

    3 Again, the nurse does not have the authority to change a dose without a physician's order; also, decreasing fluids could enhance dehydration.

    4 This is not the safest option for the patient. If bowel sounds are hypoactive, chances are they will be the same or there will be further decrease in activity after another dose. In addition, assessment of the stools is necessary.

58. Comprehension, assessment, health (b)

    3 A breast-feeding mother should always check with the physician concerning medications that may be passed to the infant through the breastmilk.

    1 The medicine may be detrimental to the infant the first time it is taken; the side effects for the infant could be severe.

    2 Even half of an adult dose could be harmful to the infant.

    4 Although textbooks state pregnancy classifications for drugs, there is no guarantee that a drug will not affect the infant.

59. Application, planning, health (b)

    4 Use of oral contraceptives and antibiotics together may cause the contraceptives to be ineffective in preventing pregnancy. The patient should use additional protection.

    1 Antibiotics should always be taken until completed, unless otherwise instructed by the physician.

    2 Erythromycin can be irritating to the stomach and is better tolerated with food.

    3 Erythromycin is a relatively safe drug. Allergies should always be assessed; however, any questionable allergy warrants further investigation.

60. Application, planning, physiological (b)

    2 The relaxation of skeletal muscles from these agents could result in severe respiratory depression, even apnea leading to death if respirations are not assisted.

    1 The central nervous system is not altered; the patient should be aware of surroundings.

    3 Although prolonged lack of oxygen because of respiratory difficulty could result in this diagnosis, the priority choice is altered respiratory function.

    4 These drugs do not produce sedation or loss of consciousness; the patient still feels pain.

61. Application, evaluation, health (b)

    2 The patient should be weighing himself every day at about the same time, in the same type of clothing, and on the same scale set at zero every morning. Assessment of accurate weighing could determine a false weight gain.

    1 Unless other signs and symptoms of distress are apparent, the 10-lb weight gain may be managed by adjusting the medication and may not require hospitalization.

    3 Seeing the physician would be sound advice if other signs and symptoms were present. The first step, however, would be to assess that the 10-lb weight gain is accurate.

    4 A decrease in fluids without accurate assessment of the weight gain could lead to serious problems.

62. Application, implementation, psychosocial (a)
    1 This response acknowledges the patient's fears and keeps the discussion open.
    2 This statement negates the patient's feeling of fear.
    3 This statement concurs with the patient's fear.
    4 This statement changes the topic and ignores the patient's fear.

63. Knowledge, implementation, physiological (b)
    3 The apical pulse should be taken for one full minute and the medication withheld if the rate is below 60.
    1 A cardiac monitor is not usually needed for the stable patient.
    2 The radial pulse is not accurate because there may be a pulse deficit.
    4 Because Mr. Watson is oriented, there is no need to check his mouth.

64. Application, implementation, physiological (c)
    1 This response is appropriate to clarify the situation and assess the potential for violence. The nurse should ask, "Are you thinking of hurting yourself now?" If the answer is yes, the nurse should ask, "How are you going to hurt yourself?" Following a response, the nurse should ask "Can you agree not to hurt yourself for _____ (a specific period of time) without talking with me first?" If the patient will *not* commit to not acting, the nurse should stay with her while appropriate alternative care is sought.
    2 Avoiding the subject is unwise; it is best to investigate.
    3 It is not necessary to describe other patients who have had similar feelings.
    4 It is premature to outline alternative measures.

65. Application, evaluation, physiological (b)
    3 Patients who have planned a time with little chance of discovery, use lethal methods, and act on that plan are very serious about their identified solution of suicide.
    1 The patient's suicide plan could not be analyzed with the information given.
    2 She planned a time when her husband was away; therefore she did not intend to be rescued.
    4 Sleeping pills are a lethal tool and are often used because they are considered painless.

66. Comprehension, evaluation, environment (b)
    1 ECT creates a neurologic response like a grand mal (tonic-clonic) seizure and often causes short-term memory loss and somnolence.
    2 ECT should not cause any permanent damage to the brain.
    3 Somnolence immediately after the procedure and short-term memory loss are normal side effects.
    4 Memory loss should not be permanent following the procedure.

67. Comprehension, assessment, psychosocial (b)
    2 Rationalization is logically explaining away unacceptable thoughts or acts.
    1 Suppression is consciously removing a thought from awareness.
    3 Displacement is substitution of a socially acceptable feeling for an unacceptable one.
    4 In conversion, an individual converts a psychologic problem to a physical symptom.

68. Knowledge, implementation, environment (c)
    2 This is the correct procedure for Leopold's maneuver.
    1 Homans' sign is pain in the calf with dorsiflexion of the foot; indicative of thrombophlebitis or thrombosis.
    3 Chadwick's sign is a bluish coloration of the vagina in early pregnancy.
    4 Ritgen's maneuver assists in delivery of the fetal head.

69. Application, assessment, physiological (b)
    3 It is important to establish a baseline so changes may be assessed.
    1 This is true, but it is not the primary reason.
    2 It is a policy in some institutions, but this is not the primary reason.
    4 The care plan is important, but to evaluate patient needs, the baseline is necessary.

70. Knowledge, planning, physiological (a)
    1 A magnesium preparation is the treatment of choice for convulsions in pregnancy. This controls convulsions by blocking neuromuscular transmission.
    2 A low potassium level could result in similar symptoms, but potassium is not the recommended electrolyte for these conditions.
    3 Sodium would increase the fluid retention that usually occurs in eclampsia.
    4 Calcium may be needed for replacement in pregnancy, but it will not aid in eclampsia.

71. Knowledge, assessment, physiological (b)
    1 The sodium and chloride content of sweat is increased five times above average when cystic fibrosis is present.
    2 This is usually a normal finding.
    3 This is expected among preschool children.
    4 This may be a normal finding among preschool children.

72. Application, assessment, physiological (c)
    3 The presence of large, bulky, foul-smelling stools is another symptom of cystic fibrosis.
    1 This is not related to the child's problem.
    2 This is not priority information.
    4 This is important, but it is not a priority at this time.

73. Application, evaluation, physiological (c)
    3 Pulmonary therapy should not be done immediately before or after meals because of the fatigue and loss of appetite that may occur.
    1 Therapy done before meals may make Tara too tired to eat, or she may lose her appetite from coughing up the thick secretions.
    2 Therapy should be done routinely as a pulmonary prophylaxis.
    4 Therapy must be done on a routine basis.

74. Comprehension, assessment, environment (b)
    1 Fractures occurring during infancy or toddlerhood are commonly a result of abuse or trauma. Fractures are not normally sustained by the infant while in a crib.
    2 Whether Melissa is crying or not, at 18 months of age it would be difficult to get accurate information from her in the emergency room.
    3 This is not a priority at this time.
    4 This is not a priority at this time. If her immunizations are up-to-date, a tetanus immunization is not needed.

75. Application, implementation, health (b)
    2 Child protection services must be notified. This is required by the Federal Child Abuse Prevention and Treatment Act of 1974.
    1 This may be done; however, the priority is notification of child protection services.
    3 This may be recommended by child protection services or the court.
    4 This is not appropriate at this time; however, the mother should be told that child protection services will be notified.

76. Application, implementation, psychosocial (b)
    4 It is important to set limits and present reality to support this patient as she deals with the emotional stress, powerlessness, and physical illness that may be precipitating her manic episode.
    1 Emphasizing the diet plan supports the exaggerated thoughts.
    2 This requires a physician's intervention.
    3 It is unrealistic to expect a manic patient to remain in bed.

77. Application, assessment, psychosocial (c)
    1 Poor impulse control may be demonstrated through drinking, overeating, and substance abuse. Other characteristics include attempts to manipulate others, periodic over-dependency on others, and inappropriate behavior for the situation.
    2 Characteristics include severe anxiety, physical manifestations of anxiety, and attacks occurring suddenly and without reason. Onset is frequently in the late twenties.
    3 This disorder is known as schizophrenia and is characterized by inappropriate emotional responses, displays of incoherent, bizarre behavior, and trouble relating to others.
    4 Mood swings with one or more manic episodes, possibly alternating with episodes of depression, are characteristic.

78. Comprehension, implementation, psychosocial (a)
    3 Obtaining drugs and taking them is a full-time job for an addict. The person needs to learn new skills and interests.
    1, 2, 4 It may be true the addict fears authorities, avoids family and friends, and possibly has a false sense of security, but these are not the main reasons a new lifestyle is necessary.

79. Application, implementation, environment (b)
    3 Potassium often burns at the infusion site and is not tolerated at fast rates. A slower rate may be tolerated better, but an order from the physician would be needed.
    1 The IV site may not be irritated yet and the IV may not need to be restarted.
    2 This option does not provide adequate protection for the nurse, and it requires a physician's order.
    4 High concentrations of potassium can lead to thrombophlebitis and can cause extreme discomfort if administered too fast.

80. Application, implementation, physiological (b)
    3 Trendelenburg's position places the head lower than the feet. Increasing the intravenous fluids could raise the blood pressure until the physician is notified.
    1 Low-Fowler's position requires the head to be raised about 20 inches and could drop the blood pressure further.
    2 Semi-Fowler's position requires the head to be raised 45 degrees and could increase both blood pressure and dizziness.
    4 Reverse Trendelenburg's position is placing the feet lower than the head with the bed flat; this position could lower the blood pressure.

81. Comprehension, assessment, physiological (b)
    3 Any time there is concern about a pulse counted in 15 seconds, the nurse should check the apical pulse for one full minute. The apical pulse is more accurate than a radial pulse.
    1 Even for one full minute, the radial pulse can be misleading if ectopic beats or an irregular rhythm exist.
    2 An apical pulse taken for 15 seconds is not as accurate as a pulse taken for a full minute.
    4 The radial pulse could be erroneous in both arms if the rhythm is irregular or the pulse is weak.

82. Knowledge, implementation, physiological (a)
    3 Fatigue is an approved NANDA nursing diagnosis treatable by the licensed nurse.
    1, 2, 4 These are regarded as medical diagnoses warranting collaborative interventions.

83. Comprehension, implementation, physiological (c)
    2 With a myocardial infarction, there is a decrease in the amount of available oxygen for tissue perfusion; therefore, oxygen is given.
    1 Chest pain is treated by medication administration.
    3 Anxiety may be treated by medication, explanations, or control of the environment.
    4 Alterations in heart rate is monitored by electrocardiograms and medication.

84. Comprehension, planning, environment (a)
    2 This statement is correct; the outcome is patient-centered and measureable, and it includes a time frame.
    1 This statement is incorrect; it is neither patient-centered nor measureable.
    3, 4 These choices are inappropriate; they do not contain outcome terminology.

85. Comprehension, implementation, environment (a)
    1 The primary function of advocacy is to inform and support; by informing the surgeon, the nurse supports the patient's right to choose his own health care.
    2 This option disregards the patient's primary concern.
    3 This response ignores the patient's wishes.
    4 This selection overlooks the patient's major request to forego the surgery.

86. Comprehension, implementation, psychosocial (b)
    4 The current goal of community treatment is to return the individual to the home environment as soon as possible and to provide a support system within the community. This facilitates treatment and return to as near-normal functioning as possible.
    1 The goal is to return the patient home as quickly as possible. The development of support systems and change of attitude are *not* the most recent changes.
    2, 3 These are not recent developments; they were used in very early treatment of mental illness.

87. Comprehension, assessment, psychosocial (c)
    4 An individual with an antisocial personality has a history of difficulties with personal relationships. This person does not profit from experience or punishment; he has no real loyalties to any individuals, groups or codes; and he uses the defense mechanism of rationalization. Those with personality disorders have difficulty handling change.
    1, 2, 3 These are other types of personality disorders.

88. Application, planning, environment (c)
    4 Depressed patients are difficult to relate to because of their feelings of hopelessness and apathy. The lack of success by the nursing assistants may lead to withdrawal or feelings of anger toward the patient.
    1 Depressed patients are not necessarily lazy.
    2 Poor personal grooming may be a factor; however, this can be easily managed.
    3 Depressed patients are typically dependent on others.

89. Comprehension, assessment, environment (c)
    2 Elavil is an antidepressant with sedative effects. It usually takes 2 to 4 weeks to achieve favorable results.
    1, 3, 4 These are incorrect. Although the sedative effect may be apparent before the antidepressant effect is noted, an adequate therapeutic effect may take as long as 30 days to develop.

90. Application, implementation, environment (a)
    3 Postoperatively the patient should lie flat or in low-Fowler's position on the unoperated side to avoid undue strain on the operative area.
    1 Turning and deep-breathing may be permitted, but coughing is contraindicated because of the danger of complications such as bleeding or retinal detachment.
    2, 4 These positions are contraindicated immediately following surgery.
91. Comprehension, planning, physiological (b)
    3 Retinal detachment is a serious complication that may occur as a result of the intricate surgery of a cataract extraction.
    1 Refractive errors are not a complication of cataract extraction and may even be corrected by this type of surgery.
    2 This is an inflammation of the conjunctiva and would not be a complication of cataract extraction.
    4 Optic atrophy relates to atrophy of the optic nerve; it is unrelated to complications of cataract surgery.
92. Comprehension, planning, physiological (b)
    3 Edema occurs following trauma and immediately following cast application. Elevation of the extremity best controls the situation. Controlling edema also helps alleviate neurovascular compromise.
    1 Following cast application, there is some swelling. Cast application to an extremity is done primarily for immobilization.
    2 Medication therapy is not considered the most effective way to control edema.
    4 Heat should not be applied to the cast because damage may result.
93. Knowledge, implementation, physiological (a)
    4 The drying of the cast is a gradual process. Keeping the cast uncovered will facilitate the process; covering the cast prolongs the drying process. The patient should also be repositioned (unless restricted) so that all sides of the cast are exposed to the air.
    1 The cast should dry naturally. Application of heat (lamps, fans) can cause the cast to dry unevenly. The strength of the cast will be affected.
    2 The cast should be handled with the palms of the hands. Fingertips could leave an indentation and could create a pressure area.
    3 Casts are "windowed" only in emergency situations.
94. Comprehension, assessment, physiological (b)
    2 Pain, pallor, or paresthesia are indicative of possible neurovascular complications. Early recognition of impairment can result in reversal; however, if symptoms are not observed and reported, permanent damage to the extremity can result.
    1, 3, 4 Odor, drainage, and temperature usually indicate infection. Findings should be recorded and reported.
95. Knowledge, implementation, environment (a)
    4 To maintain effective traction, the weights should hang free. The weights should not rest on the floor or touch the bed. The ropes holding the weights should also hang free of any obstruction.
    1 The patient should be encouraged to move and continue ROM exercises of the unaffected joints as permitted. The patient can use the trapeze to help himself. Immobilization can lead to skin breakdown.
    2 The amount of weight ordered is to be maintained for the traction to be effective. The weights hold the fractured bone in place.
    3 Skeletal traction is applied by the physician. The nurse should have a baseline measurement of the amount of protrusion of the pin. If there is a change, the nurse should notify the physician.

96. Application, assessment, environment (b)
    3 Previous injuries may be documented in older medical records or x-ray examinations.
    1 This action is not necessary.
    2 This action is not usually necessary and may frighten the child.
    4 This is not an appropriate action.
97. Comprehension, planning, physiological (a)
    4 Respiratory difficulties are life-threatening and therefore take the highest priority in responding to a neonate's needs.
    1 Skin eruptions may be normal or abnormal, but they are not life-threatening.
    2 Frequent crying may indicate an underlying problem, but given the selections, respiratory difficulties take priority.
    3 Cyanotic hands and feet are expected in the neonate because the circulation of the blood in the baby at birth is not at the same development throughout the body.
98. Knowledge, assessment, physiological (a)
    2 Milia are plugged sebaceous glands usually found on the nose and cheeks of neonates.
    1 Vernix caseosa is a grayish-white, cheeselike body of creamy substance found on the infant at birth; it protects the skin of the fetus in the uterus.
    3 Lanugo is soft fine hair found on the baby at birth.
    4 Mongolian spots are darkened pigmented areas found on the lower back or buttocks; usually found on dark-complexioned neonates.
99. Comprehension, assessment, environment (b)
    4 The human immunodeficiency virus (HIV) test is used to detect the HIV virus, which is the virus that causes acquired immunodeficiency syndrome (AIDS). A positive HIV test documents the exposure of the patient to the HIV.
    1 The test indicates exposure to the HIV virus.
    2 AIDS-related complex (ARC) is a series of clinical findings that are suggestive of immunodeficiency related to HIV exposure; they do not "match" the CDC guidelines for AIDS.
    3 The definite diagnosis of AIDS is inclusive of the whole syndrome and usually indicates the presence of opportunistic diseases.
100. Knowledge, evaluation, environment (a)
    3 Kaposi's sarcoma is a malignant opportunistic cancer occurring in AIDS. The lesions may have the appearance of bruises or moles and are often described as purplish-red or dark purple.
    1 Tuberculosis is a bacterial infection commonly occurring in the lungs.
    2 Herpes simplex is a skin disease producing small blisters.
    4 *Pneumocystis carinii* pneumonia is respiratory disease and is seen in many patients with AIDS. The infection is usually fatal without treatment.
101. Comprehension, evaluation, environment (b)
    3 The Centers for Disease Control (CDC) recommends that blood and body fluid precautions (universal precautions) be consistently used for *all* patients.
    1, 2, 4 These options do not reflect CDC recommendations.
102. Application, assessment, environment (b)
    4 The mother's perception of the need for harsh discipline may indicate abusive methods.
    1 This question is not directly related to the situation.
    2 This is not a priority or necessary question.
    3 This is not necessary information at this time.

103. Application, assessment, physiological (c)
    3 The peak action of NPH (intermediate-acting) insulin is 10 to 16 hours after administration.
    1, 2, 4 These are incorrect times for peak action of intermediate-acting insulin.
104. Knowledge, implementation, health (a)
    2 These are the signs and symptoms of mononucleosis.
    1 These are symptoms of AIDS.
    3 These are symptoms of juvenile-onset diabetes mellitus.
    4 These are potential signs of substance abuse.
105. Application, assessment, environment (b)
    2 Diarrhea is the frequent passage of loose liquid stools. It indicates a disturbance in intestinal motility and absorption that could interfere with fluid and electrolyte balance.
    1 The frequency varies; although the color is usually green, foods can affect the color.
    3 Amounts vary with individuals; the color can be affected by foods.
    4 Frequency and amounts vary with individuals.
106. Comprehension, planning, psychosocial (a)
    3 This selection focuses on the specific needs (love and belonging) of a toddler who has a new sibling.
    1 This suggestion is unrealistic and impractical.
    2 Ignoring jealous behavior will *not* diminish this normal response and in fact may exacerbate the jealous reactions.
    4 The children need to be together to develop a bond that leads to a healthy relationship.
107. Knowledge, implementation, health (a)
    1 A neonate instinctively knows his own hunger needs. The neonate will eventually establish a pattern of regularity on the basis of his need.
    2, 3 These options violate the accepted standard of demand feeding.
    4 This selection does not allow for the infant's need of hunger.
108. Knowledge, planning, physiological (a)
    2 At birth, the clamping procedure eliminates blood and oxygen supply to the cord area; because of this procedure, the umbilical cord normally falls off between the seventh and tenth day.
    1 At days three and four, the cord is still firmly attached at the umbilicus.
    3, 4 If the cord is still attached after 10 days, the area should be assessed for moisture and/or infection. If these are present, the mother should be instructed to notify the physician.
109. Comprehension, planning, environment (b)
    2 Most causes of acute diarrhea are considered infectious; to rest the bowel, nothing is offered by mouth.
    1 This may be offered *after* frequency of stools has decreased.
    3 This is the intervention for pyloric stenosis.
    4 This is the intervention for hyperthermia.
110. Comprehension, assessment, environment (a)
    1 With the sudden change in the frequency and character of the stool, there is a rapid loss of fluid that results in acid-base imbalance and dehydration.
    2, 3, 4 These are not usually findings in diarrhea.
111. Comprehension, implementation, physiological (b)
    3 A pacifier satisfies a baby's sucking needs.
    1, 2 These may help, but they won't satisfy the baby's sucking needs.
    4 Infants with diarrhea are usually kept in isolation initially because they may have a communicable disease.

112. Application, implementation, environment (b)
    3 Increased fluids are needed because there is a potential fluid volume deficit related to decreased oral intake and because it is necessary to liquify secretions and aid in their expectoration. A cool-air humidifier helps to moisten mucous membranes and prevent further irritation. Adequate rest and nutrition are primary measures to encourage healing.
    1 This is intervention for otitis media.
    2 This is intervention for meningitis.
    4 This is intervention for asthma.
113. Comprehension, assessment, environment (b)
    3 Hypertension is one of the primary causes of renal failure.
    1, 2, 4 Based on the patient's history, these are not related to the problem. By themselves they are not viewed as causes of renal failure.
114. Application, planning, psychosocial (b)
    4 This provides an opportunity for the patient to express his concerns and frustrations and helps reduce feelings of loneliness.
    1 This does not address immediate problems; it ignores his feelings and actual behavior (crying).
    2, 3 These measures ignore feelings and actual behavior.
115. Application, evaluation, health (c)
    1 The patient is at increased risk for infections; therefore he should have someone else clean the cat's litter pan.
    2, 3 This is not appropriate teaching.
    4 AIDS is not transmitted by just being in contact with others. This is not appropriate teaching.
116. Comprehension, implementation, physiological (b)
    1 The residual amount of feeding should not be over half of the amount being given. In this case 240 ml or less should have been aspirated. The residual amount indicates that the patient is not absorbing the feeding as fast as it is being given. The physician should be notified.
    2 Continuing the feeding could result in distention and aspiration pneumonia.
    3 If the patient has not tolerated 480 ml, it is doubtful that more will be tolerated in one feeding.
    4 Even half of the amount could result in aspiration and should be held.
117. Knowledge, evaluation, physiological (a)
    3 Methocarbamol (Robaxin) is a musculoskeletal relaxant used to relieve spasm and pain.
    1, 2 Although anxiety may be lessened and the patient may sleep better, the primary effect of the medication is decreased muscle spasms.
    4 Pain radiation associated with low back pain is to or down the leg (sciatica).
118. Application, assessment, environment (c)
    3 This question allows the patient to describe the pain experience.
    1, 2, 4 These questions can be answered with a "yes" or "no" and would not provide the information needed about the pain experience.
119. Knowledge, implementation, environment (c)
    1 A myelogram aids in the diagnosis of a herniated intervertebral disk. Medication is injected into the lumbar subarachnoid space.
    2 This describes electromyography (EMG).
    3 This describes an electroencephalogram (EEG).
    4 This describes computerized axial tomography (CAT).

120. Comprehension, planning, physiological (c)
    4 The nurse uses the logrolling technique to keep the body in alignment and to lessen strain on the vertebral column.
    1 The nurse should assist the patient in turning.
    2 To ensure alignment, pillows are used between the legs when the patient is in the side-lying position.
    3 The nurse will encourage, not limit, range-of-motion exercises.

COMPREHENSIVE EXAMINATION ONE: PART 2

121. Knowledge, evaluation, environment (a)
    4 Stereotyping is labeling of persons into common groups.
    1 A mental set is organization of an individual's perceptions in a particular way.
    2 An ideology is a manner of thinking that is characteristic of an individual.
    3 A halo effect is a tendency to be influenced by a personal impression.

122. Comprehension, assessment, physiological (c)
    1 The individual exhibits a mask-like appearance, drooling, and a shuffling gait.
    2 An exaggerated sense of euphoria would not be typical. Although there is increased salivation and defects in judgment and emotional instability may occur, intelligence is *not* impaired.
    3 These are signs and symptoms of a brain tumor.
    4 These are signs and symptoms of a head injury.

123. Application, evaluation, environment (c)
    4 An adverse effect of the medication is urine retention; this is a serious problem and should be reported promptly.
    1, 2, 3 These are not associated with amitriptyline (Elavil) therapy.

124. Knowledge, planning, environment (c)
    4 Unless there are physical or neurologic changes such as a recent memory loss, the functions of habit, judgment, creativity and problem-solving are maintained.
    1, 2 Motor response and visual and auditory acuity all decrease with age.
    3 These are not pertinent to cognitive tasks.

125. Application, planning, health (c)
    2 Blues and greens are not seen clearly by older adults. Avoiding objects on the floor prevents falls, and using higher-intensity light assists in better vision as the size of the pupil decreases and is less responsive to light.
    1 High-energy food is necessary because aging affects taste, digestion and metabolism. Because an elderly person may not be aware of extreme loss of body heat, measures to prevent hypothermia include keeping room temperatures slightly higher than usual and staying indoors as much as possible on windy, wet, and cold days.
    3 Because of changes in visual acuity and problems with color interpretation, light intensity and depth perception is aided by avoiding direct lights and white surfaces that produce glare; exposed bulbs can result in burns because of slower response time and reduced ability to feel pain.
    4 Slightly higher-than-normal room temperature prevents hypothermia; signs should have dark backgrounds and light lettering to be more easily seen; daily contact with another person helps in avoiding isolation.

126. Application, evaluation, psychosocial (c)
    1 This best describes precisely what the patient said.
    2, 3 Technical terms could be misinterpreted.
    4 This is not correct; the situation described is an example of seeing, not hearing, voices.

127. Comprehension, assessment, psychosocial (b)
    3 Denial is an unconscious defense mechanism used to avoid feelings or thoughts that are consciously intolerable. The individual refuses to acknowledge an aspect of reality.
    1 Reaction formation is a conscious behavior; it is completely opposite to the unconscious process.
    2 Displacement is use of more socially acceptable substitutes for expression of feelings.
    4 Rationalization is explanation of unacceptable thoughts by logical construction.

128. Application, evaluation, physiological (b)
    3 Antabuse causes extreme illness (vomiting, headache, flushing) when a patient has *any* alcohol including that found in over-the-counter cough syrups.
    1 Any alcohol will affect a patient receiving Antabuse.
    2 Antabuse has no effect on desire for alcohol, except through negative reinforcement.
    4 Although metabolism of alcohol is affected, Antabuse causes the alcohol to have an exaggerated effect.

129. Comprehension, implementation, physiological (c)
    3 Although these drugs may reach therapeutic plasma levels within a few days, it may take 21 or more days to see therapeutic effects.
    1 This should have been done before administration of the initial dose. The delayed effect is expected.
    2 Although this response recognizes the patient's frustration, it becomes a cliché as it attempts to speak for the entire team.
    4 This response is also a cliché; it does not help the patient because it does not give her needed information.

130. Application, evaluation, psychosocial (c)
    2 Denial is the number one defense mechanism used by substance abusers. If he is not discussing his abuse, he probably has not confronted the problem yet.
    1 Manipulation is also a common coping mechanism used by individuals addicted to alcohol, but this is more an example of avoidance and denial than an attempt to get drugs or rewards through manipulating the nursing staff.
    3 Limit setting is appropriate for acting out and other behaviors, but the nurse cannot limit-set with an individual who uses a psychological defense mechanism.
    4 Verbalization of feelings will only occur after patients have accepted the fact that that the problem exists.

131. Comprehension, assessment, environment (b)
    2 This is common in abused children. Other indicators may include unexplained scars, bruises and injuries; signs of physical neglect, such as malnourishment; and the parents' inconsistent emotional reaction in regard to the extent of the child's injury.
    1 This is not a sign of abuse.
    3 Abused children are often suspicious and shy.
    4 This is not typical in an abusive environment.

132. Comprehension, implementation, environment (b)
    4 The vastus lateralis site would be the best choice because this area is not burned and is usually a large muscle in males.
    1 The deltoid site would not be a good choice for an irritating medication such as hydroxyzine (Vistaril), which should be given Z-track.
    2 The dorsogluteal site would involve burned skin, and absorption of the medication could be hindered.
    3 The ventrogluteal site could be chosen if the skin were not severely burned, but a midaxilla site would probably involve this area.

133. Comprehension, evaluation, health (c)
    2 Health-care professionals reporting suspected child abuse cases are protected from civil action.
    1 Nurses are protected from civil action.
    3 The parents may obtain legal services but not to file a suit against the nurse.
    4 The nurse cannot be discharged from hospital employment for reporting documented, suspected child abuse cases.

134. Comprehension, planning, physiological (c)
    1 This is an appropriate nursing diagnosis related to seizure disorders; anxiety is related to self-concept.
    2 This is the nursing diagnosis for degenerative diseases.
    3 This is the nursing diagnosis for Parkinson's disease.
    4 This is the nursing diagnosis for patients with Alzheimer's disease.

135. Comprehension, implementation, physiological (c)
    4 Carbamazepine (Tegretol) is prescribed mainly for grand mal and psychomotor seizures.
    1 Ethosuximide (Zarontin) is often used in petit mal and akinetic seizure types.
    2 Phenotoin sodium (Dilantin) is often the drug of choice for grand mal or focal seizure activity.
    3 Carbamazepine (Tegretol) is not used in petit mal seizures.

136. Comprehension, planning, environment (b)
    2 With reduced blood flow, sodium and water are retained in the body and contribute to generalized edema and increased cardiac workload. Symptoms are exaggerated when pulmonary edema develops.
    1 Diuretics are administered in the morning to prevent nocturia.
    3 The dietary regime varies with patients; all do not need to reduce food intake.
    4 The diet may be limited in sodium and possibly in fluid.

137. Application, evaluation, psychosocial (c)
    2 Patients with obsessive-compulsive behaviors must first learn to substitute other behaviors for the compulsive ones so they can learn other coping mechanisms.
    1 Not using the behaviors as often in the hospital could merely mean the anxiety has been lessened.
    3 This may be an unrealistic expectation and is beyond the stage of identifying feelings.
    4 This does not express dealing with feelings and issues in a realistic manner.

138. Knowledge, assessment, physiological (b)
    3 Multiple sclerosis (MS) is a common degenerative neurologic disease. The cause is unknown. Because of the wide distribution of areas of degeneration, the variety of signs and symptoms is greater than in other neurologic diseases.
    1 These are signs and symptoms of Parkinson's disease.
    2 These are signs and symptoms of cerebral vascular accident—stroke (CVA).
    4 These are signs and symptoms of leukemia.

139. Comprehension, implementation, physiological (b)
    3 Lanoxin strengthens cardiac force and efficiency.
    1 Inderol is used to control irregular heartbeats and elevated blood pressure.
    2 Aspirin suppresses platelet coagulation; it is used for angina pectoris.
    4 Atropine increases heart rate; it is used for cardiac dysrhythmias.

140. Comprehension, planning, physiological (b)
    2 Patient safety is always a high priority especially when equipment and patients with loose ego boundaries are involved.
    1 This would be the second concern. The patient's desire to participate is a sign of progress; however, the activity would be structured to provide safety.
    3 Unit rules in a milieu are a concern, but safety of milieu community members is a main reason for the rules.
    4 This concern area would be lowest in priority. Each patient would be dealt with individually and would confront his or her own concerns.

141. Comprehension, assessment, psychosocial (b)
    2 Ambivalence and inability to make decisions is a key component of schizophrenia.
    1 Apathy is a lack of concern regarding an idea.
    3 Paranoia is fear or illogical delusions.
    4 Ambivalence in combination with schizophrenia becomes more than a simple defensive mechanism for dealing with stress. It contributes to the misperception of reality.

142. Application, planning, physiological (b)
    4 Because of loose ego boundaries and an inability to realistically express themselves, patients with delusions that manifest as a physical symptom should frequently be assessed. It could be a rash or other skin problem, or the patient could grab, scratch and impair his own skin.
    1, 2, 3 These actions by the nurse are supportive of the patient's delusions and hallucinations.

143. Knowledge, assessment, physiological (a)
    4 Impetigo, caused by streptococcus or staphylococcus bacteria, is a highly contagious inflammatory disorder. Common in children, it can be seen at all ages.
    1 This is an atopic dermatitis that may be the result of an allergic reaction or irritant.
    2 Pediculosis is an infestation of lice.
    3 Hives, which are an allergic reaction on the skin, are a result of an allergy to food or drugs.

144. Knowledge, assessment, physiological (c)
    3 The infant's red blood cells are excessively high at birth, but are soon destroyed naturally by the body.
    1 Physiological jaundice does not indicate mother/baby blood incompatibility.
    2 There is no damage to the liver.
    4 This does not cause physiological jaundice.

145. Comprehension, assessment, physiological (c)
    2 Although reflexes are present, the nervous system is not highly developed at birth.
    1 This is a conducive environment for the infant.
    3 Newborns usually have good muscle tone.
    4 This is not necessarily the cause.

146. Comprehension, assessment, physiological (b)
    4 Red blood cell count in newborns is very high (range 5 to 7 million). Red blood cells are destroyed soon after birth.
    1, 2 These are not the cause for bright-red cells.
    3 This is not common in infants; in anemia, skin is pale.

147. Comprehension, implementation, psychosocial (a)
    1 Seeking clarification is taking a patient's broad statement and working to clarify the statements to get more information.
    2 Encouraging comparison is the process of getting patients to compare this feeling or time to similar instances to gain insight.
    3 Summarizing is restating briefly the overall meaning of the interaction.
    4 Focusing is helping to keep the patient dealing with the subject.

148. Comprehension, evaluation, psychosocial (b)
    3 The nurse offered herself as a therapeutic tool to demonstrate acceptance of the patient.
    1 Open-ended questions are those requiring the patient to give answers that are descriptive and not one word.
    2 Although she may have demonstrated empathy in her acceptance of the patient, offering herself was the primary tool. Empathy is placing oneself in another's position.
    4 Reflection is verbalizing to the patient the feelings expressed so the patient will be encouraged to elaborate.

149. Knowledge, assessment, environment (b)
    3 In this specialty, the nurse assists in the process of assisting an individual after a disabling event has occurred. The rehabilitation nurse focuses on creative problem-solving techniques. The goal is to provide a supportive environment that encourages independence while helping the patient to adapt to a different, yet functional, life-style.
    1 This is a definition of geriatrics, which studies the aging process from physiological, pathological, psychological, sociological and economic points of view.
    2 This is a definition of public health nursing. The LPN/LVN contributes by making observations, reporting, documentating, teaching, and technical care.
    4 This is a general definition of nursing. Rehabilitation nursing is just one area of specialty. Job opportunities for nurses are expanding and extending beyond the hospital and nursing homes. Practical/vocational nursing is an exciting, challenging career that provides an opportunity to care for others and to receive personal satisfaction.

150. Knowledge, assessment, health (a)
    1 AIDS is the acronym for acquired immunodeficiency syndrome. The virus causing AIDS is known as human immunodeficiency virus (HIV). The HIV attacks both the immune and nervous systems.
    2 This is the definition of systemic lupus erythematous, an autoimmune disorder.
    3 This is the definition of multiple myeloma, an immunodeficiency disease.
    4 This defines a condition known as atopic dermatitis.

151. Comprehension, implementation, environment (c)
    3 Regular coffee and some colas are stimulants, which would add to tremors and inhibit adequate rest.
    1 This is not correct. Currently, caffeine is viewed as causing physiological, not psychological, problems.
    2 This is not the reasoning; the substitution has to do with the stimulant effect of caffeine.
    4 This is not the correct reasoning.

152. Application, evaluation, physiological (b)
    4 This is an early side effect of niacin.
    1, 2, 3 These are not associated with adverse reactions of niacin.

153. Application, planning, physiological (c)
    3 Patients who have an order for suicide precautions have strictly limited and highly supervised activities until the immediate danger is over.
    1 Occupational therapy allows tools, strings, and other items that are easily used to harm oneself. All therapies are limited until the immediate danger is over.
    2 The patient's anxiety should initially be treated with therapeutic nursing communication and removal from the anxiety-producing area.
    4 Outdoor activities are a privilege after suicide precautions are removed. There is opportunity for self-harm or for the patient to leave the therapeutic environment.

154. Knowledge, assessment, psychosocial (b)
    3 Thinking that others are looking at or judging them in a harmful or negative way is a common thought disorder of many forms of psychosis.
    1 The thought-about aliens are not connected in any way to anything else.
    2 This is a general term that does not describe the specific symptoms that Joanne is experiencing.
    4 This term describes a physical symptom.

155. Comprehension, implementation, environment (b)
    3 This response validates the feelings of the patient.
    1 This does not address the reality of the patient.
    2 This reinforces the patient's delusional thinking.
    4 This response gives false assurance; the patient has no reason to believe this.

156. Application, planning, health (b)
    2 Young adolescents often seek independence from the family and hold viewpoints that are different from those of the parents.
    1 Seeking assistance from a qualified source does not necessarily mean that the adolescent is becoming disrespectful.
    3 Seeking independence from the family normally begins in early adolescence (ages 11 to 14 for females and ages 13 to 15 for males).
    4 There is no indication that professional therapy is needed. Most adolescents do not need professional therapy at this stage of development.

157. Comprehension, planning, health (a)
    3 Acceptance by peers, as well as peer relationships are important to young adolescents.
    1 Dressing in the same manner as the peer group is normal for this age group.
    2 This is not considered narcissistic but a normal part of development.
    4 There is no evidence of promiscuity.

158. Application, implementation, health (b)
    1 During the first year or so after menarche, periods are often irregular because initial menstrual periods are anovulatory.
    2 Irregular menses during the first year after menarche are considered normal.
    3 This response ignores the adolescent's concern.
    4 The nurse should instruct the adolescent about normal menstrual concerns and should encourage her to communicate with her parents if possible.

159. Application, implementation, health (b)
    2 Tub bathing or showering is a good hygiene practice. Soap and water ensure cleanliness.
    1 Either tub bathing or showering should be encouraged.
    3 This is an old wives' tale.
    4 Fresh water and soap will not contaminte or bring bacteria to the perineal area.

160. Knowledge, assessment, physiological (b)
    3 Increased vaginal discharge is common.
    1 Minor swelling is expected, but reporting excessive swelling of hands, feet, ankles and face is a must.
    2 Early morning vomiting during the first 3 months is normal, but persistent vomiting at any time during pregnancy is serious.
    4 This is abnormal; the nurse must report to the physician.

161. Comprehension, evaluation, physiological (c)
    2 The placenta is located near the cervical os. As the cervix prepares for labor, separation occurs, resulting in painless bleeding.
    1 Abdominal pain is more often noted with abruptio placentae.
    3 Uterine tenderness is more often noted with abruptio placentae.
    4 Tetanic contractions are also common with abruptio placentae.

162. Comprehension, assessment, physiological (c)
    4 Normally, the placenta is located in the upper portion of the posterior or anterior wall of the uterus.
    1 This is called abruptio placentae.
    2 This is correct; however, it does not relate to this situation.
    3 See no. 4, above.

163. Comprehension, implementation, physiological (c)
    3 Sterile water is given as the first oral feeding to the neonate to determine the patency of the esophagus. Baby Zellers may be manifesting signs of esophageal atresia, as evidenced by his moist respirations.
    1, 2 Baby Zellers is demonstrating abnormal symptoms that need to be reported.
    4 Although babies do need to learn to suck and swallow, moist respirations are abnormal.

164. Application, implementation, physiological (b)
    2 With any respiratory distress, clearance and airway patency must be established.
    1 The nurse must stabilize the neonate, then notify the charge nurse.
    3 This nursing action may not be sufficient to establish airway patency.
    4 Oxygen given under pressure increases the likelihood of further obstruction; the mucus should be removed first.

165. Knowledge, implementation, environment (a)
    3 Handwashing is the *most important* barrier against transmission of infection.
    1 Sterilization of all baby linen is impractical and not necessary.
    2 This is an appropriate action, but it is not scientifically proved to decrease the spread of infection.
    4 This is not cost-effective. However, steps are taken to decrease the possibility of infection by cleansing, scrubbing, and use of disinfectants.

166. Comprehension, planning, physiological (b)
    3 Pain is related to loss of skeletal integrity and soft tissue trauma. Impaired physical mobility is related to neuromuscular/skeletal impairment, pain, and discomfort. Altered peripheral tissue perfusion is related to vascular injury or interruption of arterial/venous flow, secondary to edema.
    1 This is a nursing diagnosis for the patient with Meniere's disease.
    2 This is a nursing diagnosis for hypoglycemia.
    4 This is a nursing diagnosis for amputation of the leg, above or below the knee.

167. Knowledge, evaluation, health (b)
    1 Literature documents that the medicine should be held if the heart rate is 60/min or below. A heart rate of 50/min may be acceptable to her physician; orders should be written to cover the nurse.
    2 A heart rate of 50/min is too low to safely assume that the beta blocker should be continued.
    3 Beta blockers should not be abruptly discontinued; 1 week without the medication could cause serious consequences.
    4 Beta blockers should not be abruptly discontinued.

168. Comprehension, evaluation, physiological (a)
    2 The medicine was absorbed systemically to affect the heart (palpitations) and the central nervous system (feeling faint). The nurse should have worn gloves during application.
    1 A local effect would have been manifested on or around the hands in the form of burning, a rash, or irritation to the skin.
    3 An additive effect involves the complimentary effect of one drug given with another drug.
    4 A teratogenic effect involves congenital anomalies when a fetus is exposed to drugs during pregnancy.

169. Application, implementation, physiological (b)
    4 An explanation of the need to prevent decubitus will help the family to understand and cooperate with the plan; it also recognizes their concern for her need to rest.
    1 This option ignores the family's concerns and could evoke anger, especially if the family is fearful of her deteriorating condition.
    2 The nurse could choose to wait another hour if concern was not high for the patient developing a decubitus; however, an explanation to the family would be best.
    3 This is also ignoring the family's concern. The nurse can independently explain the purpose of the treatment.

170. Application, implementation, environment (a)
    2 $\dfrac{0.25 \text{ mg}}{0.125} \times 1 \text{ tab} = 2$
    1 This is an incorrect calculation; dose is too low.
    3, 4 These are incorrect calculations; doses are too high.

171. Application, planning, health (b)
    4 Restraints should be loosened every 2 hours for range of motion and to ensure that circulation is not being hindered. This also allows for repositioning the patient.
    1 There is not enough information to suggest that the restraints could be left off all day.
    2 The patient should be turned more frequently than 6 to 8 hours to prevent decubitus.
    3 As written, this option is too vague to offer safe care. A few hours could be any number.

172. Application, implementation, environment (a)
    2 $8 \text{ oz} = 240 \text{ ml} \quad \dfrac{4340 \text{ ml}}{240 \text{ ml}} = 18$
    1, 3, 4 These are incorrect calculations.

173. Application, implementation, health (c)
    2 Obtaining some history is essential to quickly and safely treat this patient.
    1 This does not address the safety needs of this patient.
    3 Although she is an adult, she may not be competent or legally responsible at this time.
    4 Her confidentiality is not violated by obtaining a health history from her family, because she is incoherent.

174. Knowledge, planning, environment (b)
    2 Anxiety, if not addressed promptly and appropriately, can increase the severity of symptoms and make treatment more difficult.
    1, 4 These are appropriate diagnoses, but they are not the first priority.
    3 There is no evidence to suggest a potential for violence.
175. Knowledge, implementation, environment (b)
    4 These agents are used to treat patients with thought disorders.
    1 These are used to treat depression.
    2 These agents are used to treat depression and enuresis.
    3 These agents are used to help induce sleep.
176. Application, implementation, health (c)
    4 If Joanne is a danger to herself because she is delusional, she can be committed to the hospital even if she does not want to stay there.
    1 Her roommate cannot take responsibility for Joanne's welfare.
    2 Her parents cannot legally sign her out of the hospital if the psychiatrist determines that she needs to stay.
    3 Joanne cannot be detained in the emergency room; she must either be allowed to leave or be committed to the hospital as an inpatient.
177. Comprehension, assessment, health (b)
    4 A 1-month-old infant is usually able to lift his head and turn it from side to side while in a prone position.
    1 Smiling and laughing are expected at 2 to 3 months of age.
    2, 3 Holding a rattle and rolling from his back to his side are characteristics of the infant at around 4 months of age.
178. Comprehension, assessment, health (b)
    3 Usually an infant of 4 months is not able to sit without support.
    1, 2, 4 Usually 4-month-old infants demonstrate these.
179. Comprehension, assessment, health (b)
    4 Usually muscle coordination increases and teeth erupt. The infant is resistant to being held close while feeding.
    1, 2, 3 The infant may also demonstrate other signs, but these are not necessarily signs that he is ready for weaning.
180. Comprehension, assessment, health (b)
    3 Aspirin should never be given with chicken pox because it has been implicated in development of Reye's syndrome. Because the child has a slight fever, only Tylenol should be given.
    1 These are clinical signs and symptoms of rubeola (regular measles).
    2 These are symptoms of German measles (rubella).
    4 These are clinical symptoms of mumps.
181. Knowledge, assessment, environment (a)
    1 In the first trimester, the fetus is developing through a rapid process of cellular growth that allows basic organs and systems to be formed. Because of this process, the fetus is more susceptible to genetic mutation and/or malformation.
    2, 3 During the second trimester, the fetus is already formed; therefore, malformations are less likely to occur.
    4 The last half of pregnancy includes the second and third trimester.
182. Knowledge, implementation, health (a)
    1 The Food and Nutrition Board recommends an increase of 300 calories per day during pregnancy.
    2 500 calories per day is the recommendation for lactating mothers.
    3, 4 These amounts are not usually recommended, because an undesirable weight gain could occur.

183. Comprehension, implementation, psychosocial (a)
    3 This response acknowledges the patient's feelings and allows the patient to express her concerns.
    1, 2 These responses discount the patient's concerns and feelings.
    4 Use of direct questioning is a nontherapeutic response.
184. Comprehension, assessment, physiological (a)
    2 Eating small, frequent, nongreasy foods aids in the digestive process and helps eliminate digestive problems.
    1 Eating one large meal each day promotes delayed digestion and absorption.
    3 Sodium bicarbonate is an alkaline substance that may alter the pH level of the blood.
    4 Antacids should be used with discretion because they may alter the fluid and electrolyte balance.
185. Knowledge, assessment, physiological (a)
    1 Fluids, fresh fruit, vegetables, and fiber increase peristalsis and promote bowel regularity.
    2 Use of a Fleet enema may induce labor.
    3 Good posture promotes well-being, but it does not necessarily aid in bowel elimination.
    4 Suppositories are not recommended unless ordered by a physician.
186. Application, implementation, environment (c)
    3 At age 85, this person is outside the range of the normal adult dose and, with an emaciated appearance, probably does not weigh close to 150 lb. Her dose would probably need to be decreased.
    1 At age 16, this person is outside the age range, but at 200 lb could probably tolerate an adult dose without adverse effects.
    2 Although an individual with liver disease could develop toxicity quicker, he or she is of normal weight and height. This is not the best answer.
    4 This person is also outside the adult range, but his generally good health would allow him to tolerate the adult dose with little or no adverse effects.
187. Comprehension, assessment, physiologic (b)
    1 The barium used could block the intestines and should be passed after the test. If no bowel movement has occurred or if the stool is hard and white, a laxative may be needed.
    2 Bowel sounds are important but can be present even though no bowel movement has occurred. Also, this does not indicate whether the barium has been passed.
    3 The last bowel movement could have been before the test; this information would not assess the bowel activity since the test.
    4 Flatus can be passed even when a blockage occurs; it does not indicate whether the barium has been passed.
188. Application, implementation, physiological (a)
    1 The blue pigtail should be irrigated with air; this does not require disconnection of the sump to the suction apparatus.
    2 Water should never be introduced into the pigtail.
    3 Unless absolutely necessary, the suction does not have to be disconnected for irrigation if the pigtail is used. Disconnecting the suction would require additional time for the pressure to build up once the suction is reconnected.
    4 Saline, not water, is recommended by most physicians for irrigation.
189. Application, implementation, environment (a)
    2 Convert grams to milligrams
    0.2 g = 200 mg
    $$\frac{\text{Desired}}{\text{Have}} \times \text{Quantity}$$
    $$\frac{200 \text{ mg}}{50 \text{ mg}} \times 1 = 4 \text{ capsules daily} = 1 \text{ capsule/dose}$$
    1 This is an incorrect calculation; dose is too low.
    3, 4 These are incorrect calculations; doses are too high.

190. Comprehension, assessment, physiological (a)
     1 Leg pain not associated with activity (intermittent claudication) is typical with Buerger's disease.
     2 This is an indication of phlebitis.
     3 This is an indication of varicose veins.
     4 This is an indication of thrombophlebitis.
191. Knowledge, planning, physiological (c)
     4 This is a noninvasive test that measures the amplitude of the pulsations over an artery.
     1 This makes echoes from sound waves used to study movements and dimensions of the cardiac structure.
     2 This is a test designed to detect cardiac ischemia during exercise or exertion.
     3 This is a tracing of the electrical impulses of the heart.
192. Knowledge, assessment, physiological (a)
     2 The pain is a cramping pain in the legs and is not usually related to activity.
     1 This is pain (cramping in legs) usually associated with exercises.
     3 This is pain on dorsiflexion of the foot that is significant with thromobophlebitis.
     4 This is a term to describe redness of lower extremities when in a dependent position.
193. Comprehension, planning, physiological (a)
     4 Because smoking constricts blood vessels, it should be avoided; cold temperatures aggravate the symptoms.
     1, 2 These do not relate to Buerger's disease.
     3 This would not be sufficient to provide warmth, which is recommended for patients with Buerger's disease.
194. Application, planning, environment (c)
     3 For the safety of the patients, things such as sharp objects or anything that could be used to harm self or others must be removed.
     1 This is an inaccurate answer, and it gives false assurance.
     2 This is an inaccurate answer, and it could frighten the patient.
     4 This is not the reason some of her possessions might be sent home; they might also be kept on the unit for her.
195. Application, implementation, environment (b)
     2 Extrapyramidal symptoms are both the most common and most serious side effects of antipsychotic medications; they are controlled with antiparkinson's drugs.
     1 Weight gain is a common side effect of antipsychotic drugs. Calorie intake should be monitored, not encouraged.
     3 Antipsychotic drugs do not cause or contribute to potassium excess.
     4 Antipsychotic drugs can cause drowsiness and lethargy; usually these patients require extra rest, not exercise.
196. Comprehension, assessment, health (b)
     2 The average incubation period is 10 to 21 days.
     1 This is the incubation period for diphtheria.
     3 This is the incubation period for encephalitis.
     4 This is the incubation period for mumps.
197. Comprehension, assessment, physiological (b)
     2 In addition to the stated signs and symptoms, poor skin turgor also indicates dehydration.
     1 These signs and symptoms are the exact opposite of those in No. 2 and are not symptomatic of dehydration.
     3 These are signs and symptoms of failure to thrive.
     4 These are symptoms of celiac disease.
198. Comprehension, assessment, health (c)
     4 The causes of acute diarrhea may vary; many causes are considered infectious. *Escherichia coli* is an example of a common causative organism.
     1, 2, 3 These may be the causes of *chronic* diarrhea.

199. Comprehension, assessment, health (c)
     1 During the toddler period, growth is slower than in infancy; gross motor coordination increases. Toddlers gain about 5 to 10 lb (2 to 4.5 kg) each year and 3 in (7.5 cm) in height per year.
     2 Expected growth is 5 to 10 lb each year and 3 in in height.
     3 Just the opposite is true.
     4 This is characteristic of a 3 to 5 year old child.
200. Application, implementation, physiological (b)
     2 The patient's head should be turned to the side to prevent aspiration.
     1 This is not the priority measure; it can be done after the patient is in the bed.
     3 He can be safely placed in bed after he stops vomiting.
     4 This is not a priority measure. After he is safely in bed, the ordered medication can be given. If this does not help the patient, the physician may need to be notified.
201. Comprehension, planning, physiological (b)
     1 The ventrogluteal site is a safe and less painful location for an intramuscular injection.
     2 The syringe should be held at a 90-degree angle.
     3 The site should be marked with the use of the nurse's fingers and palm.
     4 A 1½-inch needle is the most common for an average-size adult. A ⅝-inch needle is not likely to reach the muscle.
202. Application, implementation, physiological (a)
     3 The drainage bag should be lower than the level of the bladder to prevent urinary stasis and backflow of urine.
     1 Extra loops of hanging tubing will contribute to urinary stasis.
     2 To prevent bacterial contamination, the drainage system should never be taken apart.
     4 The catheter should be taped to the abdomen for the adult male patient. This prevents pulling of the catheter.
203. Application, assessment, physiological (b)
     4 A 2-cm spot of blood on the dressing is not uncommon after surgery. The spot should be marked and assessed for evidence of further bleeding.
     1 The team leader or physician need only be notified if there is evidence of an abnormal amount of bleeding.
     2 The first surgical dressing is usually removed by the physician unless there is an unusual reason not to do so.
     3 Reinforcing the dressing for a very small spot makes further assessment difficult.
204. Application, evaluation, physiological (b)
     3 The dressing should not be damp with serosanguinous drainage. This may be an indication of wound dehiscence.
     1 This is a good indication of a well-hydrated patient.
     2 This is an expected reaction to incisional pain on the third postoperative day.
     4 This is a normal response for a recovering patient.
205. Application, implementation, physiological (a)
     2 The nurse should check the incision for possible dehiscence.
     1 This gives the patient the notion that he caused the problem or had some control over it.
     3 This response ignores the patient's concerns and provides false assurance.
     4 This is not a priority action in this situation.

206. Comprehension, assessment, health (b)
    1 This is developing and demonstrating autonomy in addition to maintaining a sense of security and control.
    2 These are characteristics of infants 6 to 7 months of age.
    3 These are characteristics of infants 8 to 9 months of age.
    4 These are characteristics of preschoolers (3 to 5 years of age).

207. Comprehension, assessment, health (b)
    4 This is a result of the 2-year-old's inquisitive, assertive behavior that helps him learn by touch, taste, and sight.
    1 These are the most common accidents for infants 7 to 12 months of age.
    2 These are the most common accidents for newborns.
    3 These are the most common accidents for infants 1 to 6 months of age.

208. Application, implementation, physiological (b)
    4 Isolation should be implemented because chicken pox is spread indirectly through articles freshly soiled by discharges from the skin or mucous membrane of infected persons.
    1 This is the nursing intervention for rebeola (regular measles).
    2 This is the nursing intervention for mumps.
    3 This is the nursing intervention for pertussis (whooping cough).

209. Knowledge, assessment, psychological (a)
    3 Separation anxiety is common in children this age and may be exaggerated during times of illness.
    1 Temper tantrums may occur in children this age, but the description given does not suggest an outburst usually seen in tantrums.
    2 Neither the nurse nor the mother did anything that would support loss of self-image in this situation.
    4 Although the child is dependent on his mother for support at this time, a dependent coping mode is usually identified in an older child who refuses to perform independent activities.

210. Comprehension, implementation, physiological (c)
    1 The temperature would be 102.6° F (39.2° C), and the Tylenol should be given as ordered.
    2 The nurse could be held liable for any consequences that may occur if the orders were clear and not followed.
    3 The nurse could have made an error in calculation, but she would be held accountable for the error.
    4 A rectal or axillary temperature is usually preferred in pediatric patients unless the child is old enough to safely follow instructions for an oral temperature.

211. Comprehension, implementation, psychosocial (a)
    1 In this option, the nurse is correcting a misconception and supporting the patient's desire to breast-feed.
    2 This response is not therapeutic; it discourages the patient's choice.
    3 This reply does not address the patient's feelings about breast-feeding.
    4 This is an example of advice-giving, which is nontherapeutic.

212. Knowledge, assessment, physiological (a)
    3 when the urinary bladder is distended, the uterus is displaced to the right side.
    1 Stomach distention will not displace the uterus.
    2 The normal anatomical position of the uterus is midline.
    4 When the uterus fills with blood, it usually becomes relaxed but remains midline.

213. Comprehension, implementation, psychosocial (a)
    4 The use of therapeutic communication techniques help identify the reason for her behavior.
    1 This ignores the patient's needs.
    2 Inappropriate; there is no given data to support any history of mental illness.
    3 This response ignores the patient's needs and is a nontherapeutic nursing action; emotional responses such as this are within nursing's domain for appropriate action.

214. Knowledge, implementation, environment (a)
    2 Examining the perineum would be the initial action to adequately validate the complaint of the patient.
    1 This may be appropriate if ordered, but assessment is imperative for collection of baseline data.
    3 Heat enables healing; however, initial assessment is done first.
    4 Assessment must take place before reporting findings to the nurse in charge.

215. Knowledge, implementation, health (a)
    3 The postpartum follow-up visit takes place at 6 weeks, at which time the physician assesses healing and the process of involution. Sexual intercourse may be resumed when involution and healing are complete.
    1, 2 The healing process may be interrupted and/or an increased risk for infection may occur if sexual relations are resumed too soon.
    4 Healing and involution process is usually complete in 6 weeks; therefore there is no need to wait 12 weeks.

216. Application, assessment, physiological (b)
    1 The nurse should notify the team leader or physician because the patient's potassium level is below the normal range (3.5 to 5 mEq/L) and may affect the administration of anesthesia.
    2 This is not a priority action.
    3 The team leader or physician should be notified.
    4 Although orange juice does contain potassium, the priority is to notify the team leader or physician to get the physician's decision on the correct source of potassium, if any, to be administered.

217. Application, implementation, physiological (b)
    3 The answer is 31 gtt/min. ($125 \times 15 = 1875$; $1875 \div 60 = 31.2$)
    1 15 is the ratio of drops per milliliter.
    2, 4 These are incorrect calculations.

218. Comprehension, evaluation, physiological (b)
    3 Skin that is cool to the touch and even slightly swollen is an indication that the IV is infiltrated.
    1 A backflow of blood when the IV bag is lowered is an indication that the IV is patent.
    2 There are many reasons why the IV is dripping too slowly; for example, the roller clamp may be too tight, or the IV bag is hanging too low.
    4 The connection needs to be tightened, the IV may be patent.

219. Knowledge, implementation, physiological (b)
    2 A Foley catheter, 14- to 16-gauge, with a 5-cc balloon should be used for the average adult woman.
    1 A straight catheter is not a retention catheter.
    3 An 8- to 12-Fr gauge is pediatric size.
    4 A Coude catheter is usually used for elderly men with enlarged prostate glands.

220. Application, implementation, physiological (a)
    4 Because the patient will most likely become drowsy, the nurse should pull up the side rails as a safety measure.
    1 The gown should be changed before the medication is given.
    2 Preoperative teaching should be done before the medication is given.
    3 After the patient is given medication, she is considered no longer able to give legal consent for surgery.

221. Application, implementation, psychosocial (a)
    1 This response allows the nurse to further explore the patient's feelings before deciding on further action.
    2, 3 This response negates the patient's feelings and is nontherapeutic.
    4 This action may be appropriate after the patient further explains her feelings and the nurse determines that medical assistance is needed.
222. Application, implementation, physiological (c)
    3 Acyclovir will help resolve the lesions in 2 to 6 weeks.
    1 There is no known cure for herpes infections. Acyclovir will only treat the symptoms.
    2 Ms. Jones should not decrease her fluid intake. This may lead to a urinary tract infection.
    4 Soaking in warm water may help the patient by easing the discomfort of the lesions.
223. Application, evaluation, health (b)
    2 Patients with active genital herpes (lesions present or developing) should not engage in sexual activity. Sexual relations at this time can easily transmit the virus to the partner.
    1 Condoms should always be worn as a part of safe-sex practice.
    3 The diaphragm does not protect against any type of sexually transmitted disease.
    4 Ms. Jones should have regular Pap smear tests because there is a relationship between genital herpes and an increased risk of cervical cancer.
224. Application, evaluation, physiological (b)
    2 The use of alcohol while taking metronidazole can cause severe gastrointestinal distress.
    1 The medication should be taken as ordered for the best results.
    3 It is recommended that partners be treated.
    4 The use of dairy products should not cause any problems with this medication.
225. Application, planning, physiological (b)
    2 The nurse should ascertain that the patient is not pregnant. These medications are not recommended for women in the first trimester of pregnancy.
    1 These medications do not usually affect the hemoglobin levels, although the white blood cells may be affected.
    3 There is no relationship between eggs and these medications.
    4 There is no relationship between the patient's normal diet and these medications.
226. Knowledge, assessment, physiological (b)
    2 Thrombophlebitis occurs most commonly in the deep veins in the legs.
    1 Thrombophlebitis can occur in superficial peripheral veins, for example after an IV infusion, but this is not the most common incidence.
    3 Exercise during pregnancy is health-promoting and does not normally cause a condition like thrombophlebitis.
    4 Thrombophlebitis does not occur in arteries.
227. Comprehension, implementation, physiological (b)
    3 To avoid bruising, the syringe should not be aspirated.
    1 A ½-inch, 25- to 26-gauge needle is recommended.
    2 The deltoid muscle is used for intramuscular injections.
    4 The site should not be massaged to avoid bruising.

228. Application, implementation, physiological (b)
    3 Aspirin can interfere with her therapy by altering the results of the prothrombin time. The nurse should obtain another order for medication.
    1 Aspirin should not be given when the patient is receiving heparin.
    2 Ibuprofen is in the same family of drugs as aspirin and should not be given when the patient is receiving heparin.
    4 A headache is not normally expected. The patient should be further assessed.
229. Application, planning, physiological (b)
    2 The patient is considered at risk for a pulmonary embolism.
    1 The patient will need to be on bed rest with exercises contraindicated at this time.
    3 Reducing fluid intake will decrease the plasma fluid, increasing the patient's risk of an embolism.
    4 The affected leg should be elevated to promote venous return.
230. Knowledge, assessment, physiological (a)
    3 A "burning" or painful sensation when voiding accompanied by frequency of urination are the most common symptoms of a urinary tract infection, specifically cystitis.
    1 Most patients do not feel faint. Another cause for this symptom should be investigated.
    2 The inability to void is a possible symptom of a urinary tract infection (UTI); however, because this only occurs when she is away from home, the possibility of the "bashful bladder syndrome" should be investigated.
    4 This is not a common symptom. Another cause should be investigated.
231. Application, evaluation, health (a)
    1 Voiding after intercourse helps cleanse the urethra from any invading bacteria.
    2 Nylon underpants even with a cotton crotch keeps moisture against the skin. This can lead to the growth of bacteria. Only all-cotton underpants should be worn.
    3 The perineal area should always be wiped in a front-to-back direction.
    4 Deodorant perineal pads may be an irritant to sensitive tissues, making the area more susceptible to bacterial invasion.
232. Application, planning, physiological (b)
    2 A clean-catch urine specimen is adequate for a routine urine culture.
    1 A bedpan is not considered clean for a urine specimen. The entire amount of urine is not needed.
    3 Catheterization is an invasive procedure not normally required for a urine culture.
    4 A 24-hour specimen is not needed. Only 1 oz of urine is necessary for a culture.
233. Knowledge, assessment, physiological (a)
    2 The use of antibiotics can alter the normal flora of the vaginal area and urethra, leading to the invasion of the fungal organism *Candida.*
    1 Yogurt has no relationship to a fungal infection.
    3 Normal use of deodorant soaps should not cause fungal infection.
    4 The use of scented toilet paper is not recommended for women who have repeated urinary tract infections, but by itself this does not cause a fungal infection.

234. Application, implementation, physiological (a)
    2 Mrs. Smith will need to drink plenty of fluids to flush the bladder after the procedure.
    1 There should not normally be a bloody drainage afterwards, but the urine may be pink-tinged or have small clots. A pad should not be necessary.
    3 Under normal circumstances, Mrs. Smith will not need to take sick leave from work.
    4 A bubble bath is contraindicated because it promotes the development of a urinary tract infection.

235. Application, evaluation, health (c)
    4 Methenamine will make the urine a blue or blue-green color.
    1 Nitrofurantoin, not methenamine, will make the urine a red-orange color.
    2 A patient with an infection or bladder inflammation should increase the amount of fluids taken.
    3 Urine that appears pink or bloody should be reported to the physician because it is not caused by the medication.

236. Application, implementation, physiological (a)
    3 Respiratory distress must be treated immediately as per the physician's orders.
    1 If the chemotherapy is ordered to be resumed, it can be done after her immediate needs are met.
    2 Pain relief should be accomplished after treating the respiratory problems.
    4 Orienting the patient is a normal admission procedure, but it is not a priority in this situation.

237. Application, assessment, psychosocial (a)
    4 The patient in the stage of depression may be nonverbal while realizing she is going to die and feeling a severe sense of loss.
    1 During denial, the patient does not believe the diagnosis is correct. This is not evident in this situation.
    2 During the stage of anger, the patient usually verbalizes anger with a sense of helplessness.
    3 During bargaining, the patient is usually trying to bargain his/her way out of the situation. This is not evident in this situation.

238. Knowledge, assessment, psychosocial (b)
    3 Altered family processes are evident in the family's behavior. Assistance with coping behaviors can be facilitated by the nurse.
    1 When a nursing diagnosis is written, the relational statement should be something that the nurse can change. This is not true in this statement.
    2 The nurse cannot change or cure the patient's illness.
    4 Inappropriate nursing diagnosis; this is not evident.

239. Knowledge, evaluation, environment (c)
    4 A living will allows the patient to decide that extraordinary measures not be taken.
    1 The intent of a living will is to allow the patient, not the family, to decide what measures will be taken.
    2 This is a legal (probated) will; it does not take the place of a living will.
    3 A living will states what should not be done in the event of a terminal illness.

240. Application, implementation, psychosocial (a)
    2 This is the recommended statement by E. Kubler-Ross. It is important for the patient to know that the nurse will try to help the patient. This response does not negate the patient's sense of hope.
    1 This relates a false sense of hope.
    3 This relates a false sense of hope and gives the patient a sense of doubt about the adequateness of her health-care providers.
    4 This does not recognize the patient's concerns or feelings.

COMPREHENSIVE EXAMINATION TWO: PART 1

1. Application, evaluation, physiological (b)
   3 Any difficulty breathing (dyspnea, wheezing, SOB, orthopnea) can be signs of a blood reaction and should be immediately reported. The blood transfusion should be stopped at once.
   1 Blood is often slightly cooler than vascular temperature. If chilling occurs, provide blankets. Blood should be warmed. Significant chilling can be an adverse reaction.
   2 Voiding is a normal occurrence, especially with the IV fluid administration.
   4 Blood is normally given very slowly for the 15 minutes. If the patient is not considered high risk for circulatory overload, the rate can then be increased.

2. Application, implementation, physiological (b)
   3 Nitro-Bid has a vasodilating effect and may cause orthostatic hypotension. For safety, the medication is administered when the patient is in a recumbent position.
   1 Although the dose may be calculated by the patient's weight, the physician orders the amount of medication to be administered.
   2 Nitrate levels are not usually obtained when taking nitroglycerin derivatives.
   4 Nitro-Bid does not effect the ECG pattern.

3. Knowledge, assessment, physiological (a)
   4 An elevated white blood cell count is indicative of an inflammatory process.
   1 Red blood cell elevation is correlated with diseases of the blood-forming organs, such as polycythemia.
   2 An elevated hemoglobin level may indicate dehydration, pulmonary obstructive disease, or congestive heart failure and is not necessarily an inflammatory process.
   3 Serum lipase is usually elevated in biliary disease.

4. Knowledge, planning, physiological (a)
   4 Beverages containing caffeine are avoided by patients with peptic ulcer disease because caffeine stimulates gastric secretions; this increases gastric mucosal irritation.
   1 Caffeine physiologically stimulates the central nervous system; it does not depress it.
   2 Caffeine does not specifically alter the fluid electrolyte balance.
   3 The use of caffeine products actually *increases* rather than delays the production of gastric secretions.

5. Knowledge, assessment, physiological (a)
   3 With a perforation of an ulcer, the abdominal cavity fills with fluid or blood, leading to distention.
   1 Clay-colored stools indicate a lack of bile, which may be associated with gallbladder dysfunction.
   2 Coffee-ground emesis is indicative of an upper gastrointestinal bleed, possibly related to ulcer pathology; this is not a sign of perforation.
   4 Distention after eating is usually related to the type of foods ingested or to decreased peristalsis.

6. Application, implementation, health (c)
   2 Once a person has an episode of major depression, his or her chances of having another one are increased.
   1 This is false assurance, which is nontherapeutic.
   3 This could be true, but it is not necessarily the case.
   4 This is false assurance, which is nontherapeutic. She could become depressed again despite these treatments.

7. Application, implementation, environment (c)
   3 Patients are disoriented after electroconvulsive therapy (ECT) and require orientation as they begin to awaken.
   1 Patients are not alert enough after ECT to take fluids.
   2 Patients should be allowed to rest and sleep as they recover from anesthesia.
   4 Patients are not alert enough after ECT to eat.

8. Knowledge, implementation, health (b)
   3 Both of these foods contain tyramine, which causes hypertension in combination with an monoamine oxidase (MAO) inhibitor.
   1 This is necessary with lithium, not with MAO inhibitors.
   2 This is a side effect of lithium, not of MAO inhibitors.
   4 This is a symptom of lithium toxicity, not of MAO inhibitors.

9. Knowledge, implementation, physiological (a)
   1 Keeping a child in an upright position helps ease the motion of their diaphragm in breathing.
   2 Oxygen may not be needed; also, the child has not been examined by a physician who has given this order.
   3 This child is in respiratory distress and is having difficulty breathing, so this would not be the first thing to do in this situation. The physician has not seen the child to give an order for aerosol treatment.
   4 The nurse should monitor the respiratory rate more frequently, but this would not be the nurse's first intervention.

10. Knowledge, implementation, physiological (a)
    4 The child will most likely be able to sit alone using hands for support by 6½ to 7½ months.
    1 In motor sequence, walking with assistance starts between 11 and 12 months of age.
    2 In motor development, the child can feed herself with a spoon and will have some spills at 15 months of age.
    3 In motor sequence, standing holding onto furniture or pulling self up starts about 9 to 11 months of age.

11. Knowledge, implementation, health (a)
    1 For children under 3 years of age, the ear is drawn down and back; Jeanette is 5 months old.
    2, 3 For older children and adults, the ear is pulled up and back.
    4 For infants the ear is pulled down and back.

12. Knowledge, implementation, physiological (a)
    4 A drainage of purulent fluid accumulates in the middle ear, causing earache and other discomfort.
    1 The ear may be warm as a result of the infectious process caused by swelling and accumulation of infectious fluid.
    2 Cilia are hairlike processess projecting from epithelial cells, which would not be seen by the mother.
    3 There may be a color change, but this would be as a result of the swelling caused by the fluid accumulation.

13. Knowledge, assessment, physiological (a)
    4 Otitis media is a common complication of an upper respiratory tract infection in young children.
    1, 2, 3 These conditions can accompany otitis media, but they are not the most common complications.

14. Knowledge, assessment, physiological (a)
    1 Down syndrome is the most common chromosomal abnormality of a generalized syndrome and is caused by the presence of an extra chromosome 21 in the G group or, in a small percentage of cases, by the translocation of chromosomes 14 or 15 in the D group and chromosomes 21 or 22.
    2 Patau's syndrome (trisomy 13) has an extra chromosome at the number 13 position.
    3 Turner's syndrome (XO) or (45 XO), appearing in females, is characterized by the absence (missing of) one X chromosome.
    4 Klinefelter's syndrome (XXY), a syndrome of gonadal defects appearing in males, is characterized by an extra X chromosome.

15. Application, implementation, psychosocial (b)
    3 This statement reflects the mother's feelings and encourages her to continue and express herself fully.
    1 This gives false assurance; it is a clichéd answer and is nontherapeutic.
    2 This gives unrealistic advice; advice is nontherapeutic.
    4 This assumes the child is ill. Alpha-fetoprotein is a non-diagnostic screening tool.

16. Knowledge, assessment, physiological (b)
    1 Breast changes are a subjective, presumptive sign of pregnancy.
    2 Goodell's sign is a softening of the cervix, an objective probable sign of pregnancy.
    3 Positive urine pregnancy test is an objective probable sign of pregnancy.
    4 Chadwick's sign is an objective probable sign of pregnancy.

17. Comprehension, planning, health (a)
    2 Using Nägele's rule, take the first day of the last menstrual period (October 4), count back 3 months (July 4), and add 7 days (July 11).
    1, 3, 4 These are incorrect calculations.

18. Knowledge, assessment, physiological (a)
    3 When the fundal height is at the umbilicus the pregnancy is half over (20 weeks).
    1 At 10 weeks the fundus is often at the level of symphysis pubus.
    2 At 12 weeks the fundus is half way to the umbilicus.
    4 At 30 weeks the fundus is almost to the rib cage.

19. Comprehension, assessment, physiological (b)
    4 Any unusual vaginal discharge requires immediate evaluation because it may be amniotic fluid.
    1 Quickening may not yet have occurred.
    2 Dependent swelling is not unusual.
    3 Weight gain over 2 lb/week is significant.

20. Comprehension, implementation, physiological (a)
    3 A nursing judgment requires that equipment and additional assessment data be obtained before initiating any other actions.
    1 This action is contraindicated in abdominal surgery patients without the order of the physician.
    2 This action would require additional assessment and is beyond the scope of practice for the licensed practical nurse in this situation.
    4 This action may be taken, but it is not the initial approach in this situation.

21. Comprehension, planning, health (b)
    1 The suggested diet for patients with diverticulitis is low-fat, no fried foods, and moderate fiber intake.
    2 This selection includes foods that are fried and high in fat.
    3 This selection includes foods with high fat content.
    4 Strawberry yogurt may be appropriate if it is low fat, but the chocolate chip cookies are not.

22. Knowledge, assessment, physiological (a)
    3 Appendicitis is the inflammation of the cecum and is not related to hernia formation.
    1 Congenital defects may allow for hernia formation.
    2 Obesity increases muscular weakness with the possibility of herniation.
    4 A weakened muscular wall will increase the likelihood of hernia formation.

23. Application, planning, physiological (b)
    2 Supportive therapy, such as blood transfusion, pain relief, and fluids, is necessary.
    1 This is not treatment for sickle cell crisis or sickle cell anemia.
    3 Fluids are appropriate in this situation.
    4 Passive range-of-motion exercises are performed to promote circulation.

24. Knowledge, implementation, physiological (a)
    1 Tinctures are alcohol or water and alcohol solutions that can produce reactions when mixed with Antabuse.
    2 Oral solutions usually contain only water and the medication particles; they should not interfere with Antabuse.
    3 Enteric-coated tablets are protected by a coating from dissolving in the stomach; they should not interfere with Antabuse.
    4 Sustained-release tablets allow slow distribution over time and will not interact with Antabuse.

25. Application, implementation, environment (c)
    2 $\dfrac{30 \text{ gtt}}{1 \text{ min}} \times \dfrac{1 \text{ ml}}{60 \text{ gtt}} \times \dfrac{1 \text{ g}}{500 \text{ cc}} \times \dfrac{1000 \text{ mg}}{1 \text{ g}} = \dfrac{2}{2} = 1$
    1 This is an incorrect calculation; dose is too low.
    3, 4 These are incorrect calculations, doses are too high.

26. Application, planning, environment (c)
    4 The intervention should state how often and by whom, as well as the characteristics of the sputum to be assessed.
    1 This is within the nurse's realm and does not require a physician's order.
    2 The intervention is appropriate, but it gives little direction for others using the plan.
    3 It is an appropriate but poorly written intervention.

27. Application, planning, psychological (b)
    2 Allowing the patient time to communicate her feelings and ventilate her frustrations will help the nurse to determine appropriate nursing interventions and will let the patient know the nurse cares.
    1 Medical intervention is premature at this time; nursing interventions should be tried before calling the physician.
    3 At age 25, a fresh makeover with her own personal gown may help; however, a depilitary might require handling and rubbing of the leg.
    4 The family could play an important part in the patient's recovery at this time, but she may not respond to them either.

28. Comprehension, implementation, physiological (b)
    4 Massaging the calf could result in dislodging part of the clot and is contraindicated.
    1 A bed bath should not produce any harm to the patient as long as excessive rubbing to the right leg does not occur.
    2 Showering should not be allowed with an order for bed rest.
    3 Turning the patient will not produce any harmful effects, but proper alignment should be maintained on the weak side.

29. Comprehension, planning, environment (b)
    4 This combination would allow for two meals on days, one meal at evening and fluid for medications at night.
    1 Most patients do not need 400 ml of fluid on the night shift.
    2 This does not allow for two meals on 7 to 3 shift or any fluids at night.
    3 This does not equal 1400 ml of fluid for 24 hours.

30. Application, implementation, physiological (b)
    3 The nurse should not give pain medication earlier than ordered unless the physician orders it.
    1 Vital signs may not be the same as during the preoperative period, but they are still within a safe range.
    2 Respirations of 18 are within normal limits; oxygen does not interfere with narcotic administration.
    4 Other measures can be effective and safe in controlling pain, but they do not always work.

31. Application, implementation, environment (b)
    1 $\frac{3}{4} \text{ gr} \times \frac{60 \text{ mg}}{1 \text{ gr}} \times \frac{1 \text{ ml}}{30 \text{ mg}} = \frac{\frac{3}{4} \times 2}{1} = 1.5 \text{ ml per dose}$
    2, 3, 4 These calculations are incorrect; amounts are too high.

32. Application, assessment, physiological (b)
    4 A rebound effect can occur 15 minutes after Narcan is given. Although vital signs should increase immediately after the medicine is given, a drop in respirations to the original rate may occur in 15 to 20 minutes.
    1 An increase in blood pressure can occur with too rapid of a reversal. The antagonist (naloxone) will also antagonize beneficial analgesic effects, and pain will return. Increased blood pressure is an observable sign of acute pain.
    2 The pulse may stay the same or rise slightly after Narcan is given, especially if the pain returns.
    3 An increase in respirations would be expected immediately after giving Narcan.

33. Application, implementation, environment (b)
    2 This allows the nurse and patient to establish a working relationship and gives the patient support and reinforcement.
    1 Ignoring these symptoms could be dangerous and may communicate a lack of caring to the patient.
    3 She is unable to set limits for herself and needs the nurse to do so for her until she is healthier.
    4 This is punitive and nontherapeutic; it does not help the goal of encouraging the patient to participate as much as she is able.

34. Comprehension, planning, environment (b)
    2 Limited fluid intake can lead to serious fluid and electrolyte imbalances and requires careful monitoring.
    1 The patient may or may not be anxious in relation to the environment.
    3 This might be true; but it is not the highest priority.
    4 This is a priority, but it is not the highest.

35. Application, implementation, health (b)
    3 This answers their question and also provides an opening to obtain support and information from the family.
    1 This is an inaccurate answer; the patient cannot get better simply because she wants to or not.
    2 This is a closed answer and does not engage the family.
    4 This may or may not be true, but it gives the family false assurance and is nontherapeutic.

36. Knowledge, assessment, psychosocial (b)
    1 The symptoms described here are the diagnostic criteria for major depression.
    2 There is nothing in this patient's history to indicate a personality disorder.
    3 She could be using substances, but this is not the most likely diagnosis.
    4 There is no evidence of a formal thought disorder.

37. Knowledge, planning, physiological (b)
    3 Excessive coughing exhausts the child, so care must include comfort and rest.
    1 The child is not severely ill, but complications can occur.
    2 This condition does not necessarily require hospitalization.
    4 Careful medical attention is required.

38. Knowledge, implementation, environment (b)
    2 Mumps involves swelling and pain in the parotid glands.
    1 Measles is a communicable disease involving runny eyes and nose, followed by rash.
    3 Scarlet fever does not affect the parotid glands.
    4 Chickenpox involves skin eruptions.

39. Knowledge, assessment, environment (a)
    4 Rubella, German measles, and 3-day measles are the same.
    1 This is not German measles.
    2 Roseola is another communicable disease.
    3 Scarlet fever is another communicable disease that has no immunization.

40. Comprehension, assessment, health (a)
    2 A DPT booster is recommended for children between 4 and 6 years of age.
    1 He should have received them as an infant followed by a booster before starting school.
    3 No chicken pox vaccine is currently available.
    4 Not required.

41. Comprehension, assessment, physiological (c)
    3 The clumping of malformed cells obstructs blood vessels and destroys red blood cells.
    1 No infection is involved.
    2 This is not relative to the situation at this time.
    4 White blood cells are not involved.

42. Application, implementation, environment (b)
    3 With the head lower than the body, the drops will flow by gravity into the swollen nasal passages.
    1 Sitting up does not promote flow by gravity.
    2 The infant's head should remain lower than the body for 2 to 3 minutes.
    4 This is not the preferred position.

43. Application, planning, psychosocial (b)
    3 Women facing possible loss of a child have great amounts of grief (anticipatory) and stress.
    1 With a threatened abortion, care will be aimed at preserving the fetus, not in removal of retained tissue.
    2 If the patient was heavily bleeding, fluid replacement would be a priority. At this time electrolyte replacement may not be necessary.
    4 Oxytocin would only be used in an incomplete abortion.

44. Knowledge, assessment, physiological (a)
    2 Abruptio placentae symptoms include severe pain, tense boardlike abdomen, fetal distress, and often concealed bleeding.
    1 Bleeding would only occur with a partial separation and apparent hemorrhage. It is not the norm for all abruptio placentae patients.
    3 Most often the abdomen is boardlike, and individual contractions are not apparent.
    4 These are symptoms of placentae previa.

45. Application, intervention, physiological (b)
    4 The most common reason for postpartum bleeding is a relaxed fundus. Massage will cause the muscles to tighten and will constrict blood vessels.
    1 This action would be taken second to check the extent of fluid loss. The first action should be to stop the cause.
    2 This is not a primary intervention for a conscious patient.
    3 A patient at risk for blood loss and shock should not be given PO fluids until his status is assessed and found stable.

46. Knowledge, assessment, physiological (b)
    2 The presence of inner epicanthal folds and small ears, sometimes low-set, are characteristics of Down syndrome.
    1 Blue hands and feet (acrocyanosis) and irregular respirations are normal immediately after birth.
    3 The normal head circumference is 2 to 3 cm (1 inch) larger than the chest circumference at birth. If the baby has a considerable amount of molding, the circumferences may be equal for a few days after birth.
    4 This is normal infant posture (the fetal position).

47. Application, assessment, physiological (c)
    1 The nurse should carefully assess the baby's heart sounds because cardiac anomalies are commonly found with Down syndrome.
    2 Cognitive (learning) deficits cannot be assessed immediately after birth.
    3 Visual impairments should be evaluated later by a pediatric ophthalmologist.
    4 Hearing impairments should be evaluated by a pediatric physician specialist.

48. Application, implementation, psychosocial (c)
    4 It is not possible to determine the extent of disability, retardation, or learning ability immediately after birth. Specialists will make this determination over a period of time.
    1 Genetic counseling can normally determine the source of the problem, but it cannot predict the extent of disability.
    2 The nurse should not predict the extent of disability or lead the mother to believe something that may not be true.
    3 The nurse cannot predict the extent of disability.

49. Application, evaluation, health (c)
    4 Because of the characteristically small nose and nasal passages and decreased muscle tone that can inhibit respiratory efforts, the baby will be more inclined to upper respiratory infections (URIs) than will other newborns.
    1 Overfeeding will lead to obesity, a common problem of Down syndrome children.
    2 The baby should be dressed in the same manner as other babies.
    3 The baby should be treated the same as other babies in regard to visitors. Normal socialization should be encouraged.

50. Application, evaluation, environment (c)
    2 Tachycardia is often a side effect of theophylline and may require monitoring and further evaluation. The licensed practical nurse is expected to know the effects of medications administered.
    1, 3 Bronchodilatation and improved breathing patterns are the expected outcomes of theophylline preparations.
    4 Theophylline breaks down to a stimulant in the body; tachycardia is a common side effect.

51. Application, evaluation, health (c)
    1 Asking the mother for feedback is the best way for the nurse to determine if the instructions were understood.
    2 Providing opportunity for feedback fosters communication and will enable the nurse to immediately modify her teaching plan, if appropriate. To instruct the mother to call with any questions blocks communication.
    3 Interpreting all medical terms should have been done in teaching. Feedback from the mother will still be necessary to determine if the medical terms were understood.
    4 Checking for the presence of communication barriers should have been done before teaching in the assessment phase.

52. Application, assessment, environment (c)
    2 This is true. *All 50 states require this to be reported.*
    1 This statement is only partially true. The nurse can report directly to proper authorities as well as to the physician.
    3 This is untrue. Laws *do grant immunity* from civil suits to those who are required to report child abuse.
    4 This is untrue. This is *not* considered legal privileged communication. All states require notification.

53. Comprehension, assessment, environment (b)
    4 This is a common characteristic of parents who abuse children.
    1, 2, 3 These are not factors in abusive families.

54. Knowledge, assessment, physiological (b)
    2 Nursing interventions for this condition include keeping the omphalocele covered with gauze and moistened with normal saline until surgery can be performed.
    1 This is where the upper esophagus ends in a blind pouch.
    3 This is a distention of the lower colon caused by lack of nerve cells in the wall of the colon.
    4 This is a narrowing of the distal end of the stomach.

55. Application, assessment, health (c)
    3 The most important role of the nurse is to assist the patient in regaining his or her psychological balance despite current stressful circumstances.
    1 This may or may not be the case, depending on the individual patient's support system.
    2 This must be done by the patient himself; the nurse can only assist in the process.
    4 Her primary responsibility is to the patient.

56. Application, planning, health (b)
    2 The goal in crisis intervention is to assist the patient to return to at least their precrisis level of function.
    1, 4 The situation does not identify the nature of the situational crisis.
    3 This would occur as a result of a return to her precrisis level of function.

57. Application, planning, health (c)
    4 Giving patients long-acting injectable forms of antipsychotic drugs has been shown to increase compliance because the patient is not responsible for medicating himself and the number of appointments to the outpatient mental health clinic for medications is reduced.
    1 This might increase the chances he would get his medication, but it would not further other important goals such as maintaining or increasing his independence.
    2 This would remove the responsibility from the patient and place it onto his health providers.
    3 This might increase his compliance only if the timing of his medications is the reason for noncompliance.

58. Application, planning, health (c)
    2 This is the least threatening and most structured way for a patient to both obtain social skills and have increased social interaction with those likely to be receptive to him.
    1 This is probably not realistic and may be setting the individual up for failure.
    3 This may be too complex a task for the patient; it would not necessarily provide opportunities for socialization.
    4 This is a potentially helpful means for greater social contact for this patient, but it does not provide assistance for him to develop social skills.

59. Application, implementation, health (b)
    3 It is important that the nurse give him an explanation about why she is not available to date him. This reinforces the limits of their therapeutic relationship.
    1 This is nontherapeutic; it does not provide an opportunity to do patient teaching.
    2 This is a rejection of the patient and is not therapeutic.
    4 It is not appropriate for the nurse to be upset by this question because it is normal for patients to test the limits of the therapeutic relationship.

60. Application, implementation, environment (c)
    1 This offers the presence of the nurse to help the patient feel safe and decreases the potential for violence.
    2 Secluding a patient who is hearing voices serves no therapeutic benefit.
    3, 4 These do not acknowledge what the patient is feeling, nor do they address the potential for violence.

61. Comprehension, planning, physiological (c)
    3 Immediately after surgery, it would be important to assess the patient's respiratory status because of her history of smoking.
    1 Not a priority, as the situation does not identify this as a problem.
    2 Mrs. Flow may have difficulty ambulating the first time because of pain, but this would not be the immediate postoperative concern.
    4 Her weight needs to be addressed in the care plan, but this would not be the immediate concern.

62. Comprehension, assessment, physiological (b)
    4 Excretion may be hindered by the ineffective action of the kidneys, thereby affecting the half-life of a drug. The kidneys are the main organs involved in excretion, thus causing a higher dose of the medication to circulate over a longer period of time.
    1 Absorption is involved with the process from the time the drug enters the body and the bloodstream.
    2 Distribution is involved with the transportation of the drug through the body.
    3 Metabolism is the way the body inactivates the drug; it primarily involves the liver.

63. Comprehension, assessment, physiological (b)
    2 A baseline heart rate is needed to determine any adverse reactions that may occur during administration of the drug. Adverse reactions include palpitations and increased heart rate.
    1 Temperature should not be indicative of any adverse reaction to the drug.
    3 The sputum specimen is not altered by the use of metoproterenol (Alupent).
    4 Blood specimens are not altered by the use of metoproterenol.

64. Application, implementation, environment (b)
    2 $0.5 \text{ gr} \times \dfrac{60 \text{ mg}}{1 \text{ g}} \times \dfrac{7.4 \text{ ml}}{30 \text{ mg}} \times \dfrac{1 \text{ tsp}}{5 \text{ ml}} = \dfrac{7.4}{5} = 1.48 \text{ tsp}$
    1 This is an incorrect calculation; dose is too low.
    3, 4 These are incorrect calculations; doses are too high.

65. Knowledge, evaluation, physiological (b)
    1 Drug tolerance is a condition of cellular adaptation to a substance so that increasingly larger doses are necessary to obtain the desired effect.
    2 An additive effect is the increased effect of combining two drugs with similar actions.
    3 An idiosyncratic reaction is an unusual reaction the first time the drug is taken.
    4 Effects of psychological dependence occur when the user desires the drug during withdrawal.

66. Knowledge, implementation, physiological (a)
    4 Human chorionic gonadotropin stimulates ovulation for women trying to become pregnant.
    1 Rho-gam is given after pregnancy to Rh-negative mothers delivering Rh-positive babies.
    2 Ergot alkaloids are used to treat postpartum hemorrhage.
    3 Androgens are male hormones used for replacement therapy and to relieve postpartum breast engorgement.

67. Knowledge, assessment, physiological (a)
    2 Anorexia, nausea, and vomiting are symptoms of digitalis toxicity.
    1 Back pain is not an adverse reaction to digitalis.
    3 Weight gain should be monitored during digitalis toxicity and may indicate that the medicine is not working well, but weight gain does not imply toxicity.
    4 Although fatigue can be an adverse reaction, signs and symptoms of digitalis toxicity are more prominent.

68. Comprehension, evaluation, physiological (b)
    4 Elevation of the feet will aid in increasing the blood pressure; another dose of nitroglycerin would only lower the blood pressure further.
    1 The priority is to increase the patient's blood pressure and notify the physician.
    2 Although both of these actions should be initiated, the nurse could first try to elevate the blood pressure by measures that do not require a physician's order.
    3 The first part of the answer is correct, but the administration of another dose of nitroglycerin is contraindicated because of the blood pressure reading.

69. Comprehension, implementation, environment (c)
    2 Vital signs are necessary to determine if the nitrate can be given without harmful effects to the patient; sublingual (SL) nitrate is fast-acting.
    1 A transdermal patch is usually not used for chest pain; it is used for prevention of chest pain.
    3 This is unsafe practice. The blood pressure could have been too low before the first dose, and another type of medication may be needed.
    4 Taking a *detailed* history would be unsafe in the presence of chest pain. The nurse can quickly secure enough history about the chest pain to appropriately intervene.

70. Application, implementation, physiological (b)
    3 With decreased protection from the leukocytes, the defense against infection is greatly reduced. Prevention of infections is crucial to the patient's survival.
    1 Bleeding precautions are associated with thrombocytopenia (decreased platelets).
    2 Rest is important but not specific to leukopenia.
    4 Antiemetics are used to manage nausea and vomiting.

71. Comprehension, implementation, environment (c)

    4 Neither the patient nor any of his belongings are radioactive when external radiation therapy is used. Patients should be informed of this information before the therapy commences.

    1 External radiation is directed at a specific target area that is carefully identified and outlined (by purple marks).

    2, 3 The patient is not radioactive at any time during the treatment.

72. Knowledge, implementation, environment (a)

    2 Checking the breast in both the supine and erect positions allows one to examine the breasts and the chest area. In the supine position, the breasts "flatten," making them easier to examine.

    1 The breasts should be examined 7 to 10 days after menses. Breasts have a tendency to become swollen and lumpy before the start of the menstrual period.

    3 The examination should be done monthly, preferably on the same day.

    4 Women should use the flat part of the fingers for the examination.

73. Knowledge, assessment, environment (a)

    1 With biopsy, a small amount of breast tissue is removed for examination under a microscope. Actual malignant cells can be seen and identified.

    2 Ultrasonography is useful in distinguishing between cystic and solid tumor bodies.

    3, 4 These are radiographic examinations. No direct tissue is examined. Mammography, the radiographic examination of the breast, is a useful screening device for detection of breast tumors.

74. Application, implementation, psychosocial (b)

    3 This response allows the patient the opportunity to express her feelings about the surgery.

    1 The patient may not know the answer to this "why" question. Not knowing what to answer may increase her anxiety.

    2 This statement ignores the patient's concerns about surgery and her fear of dying.

    4 This offers false assurance, does not address the patient's concerns, and is nontherapeutic.

75. Comprehension, planning, physiological (b)

    4 Circulation is decreased in the right arm (operative arm) because the axillary lymph nodes have been removed. An invasive procedure (drawing blood) increases risk of infection. Lymphedema may also occur in the operative arm.

    1 Movement is encouraged, not limited. Arm exercises help the patient retain the use of the arm.

    2 Elevation of the right arm will aid in decreasing edema.

    3 The patient should be encouraged to use her right arm.

76. Comprehension, assessment, physiological (c)

    2 The cell-life cycle is disrupted with the use of chemotherapeutic drugs. Cells most vulnerable are those that are actively dividing or about to divide. As a result, both normal and malignant cells are affected/destroyed.

    1 Both single and combination chemotherapeutic agents may cause numerous side effects.

    3 Chemotherapeutic drugs may be given by many routes, all of which produce numerous side effects.

    4 Chemotherapeutic drugs must be given more than once because only a fraction of cells are dividing at one time. Side effects are also related to dose strength. As doses are increased, major toxicities are more likely.

77. Knowledge, assessment, physiological (a)

    4 Clinical findings associated with hypothyroidism include edema of the face and eyelids.

    1,2,3 These symptoms are associated with hyperthyroidism.

78. Knowledge, planning, physiological (a)

    3 Individuals with hypothyroidism have a decreased tolerance to cold. A warm environment should be provided.

    1, 2 These interventions are appropriate for the patient with hyperthyroidism.

    4 If hypoglycemia is evident, serum glucose levels would be the most accurate indicator.

79. Comprehension, assessment, physiological (c)

    1 These are average vital signs for a 2-year-old.

    2 These are average vital signs for a newborn.

    3 These are average vital signs for a 12-year-old.

    4 These are average vital signs for a 6-year-old.

80. Comprehension, planning, health (b)

    4 The juice will disguise the flavor and sucking on a straw will prevent the iron from staining the teeth.

    1 The child may refuse the milk with the iron and even without the iron later on, which could be detrimental to growth and development.

    2 Administered with a dropper is not appropriate, as the iron could come in contact with the teeth.

    3 Even on a cookie, the iron may come in contact with the teeth.

81. Knowledge, assessment, physiological (a)

    1 Cyanosis develops as the child grows and stenosis becomes more severe; the infant is called a "blue baby." The squatting position improves oxygenation.

    2 Pink tetralogy is seen when infundibular stenosis is minimal and no cyanosis develops. Clubbing of fingers is the result of inadequate oxygen supply that causes cyanosis.

    3 Retarded growth is usually seen in patent ductus arteriosus.

    4 These symptoms occur in coarctation of the aorta.

82. Comprehension, planning, psychosocial (c)

    3 This is the most frequent reason patients with schizophrenia are readmitted to the hospital.

    1 This could be a significant stressor, but it is not as likely to cause a relapse if he is taking his medications.

    2 Dietary protein restrictions are not important with antipsychotic medications.

    4 This could be a significant stressor, but it is not as likely a cause for relapse as is medication noncompliance.

83. Application, planning, environment (b)

    3 Many developmentalists have suggested that adolescents have not reached a cognitive level at which they can fully understand what will happen as a result of their actions.

    1 This is not necessarily true.

    2 Not all adolescents need to do this.

    4 Adolescents as a group are more likely to be trusting of health-care providers than of other adults.

84. Comprehension, assessment, psychosocial (b)

    4 Erickson theorized that the greatest challenge of adolescence is the formation of a unique identity.

    1 This is the task of the toddler stage.

    2 This is the task of the preschool stage.

    3 This is the task of young adulthood.

85. Application, implementation, environment (b)

    4 The nurse must let the patient define exactly what she needs the most—when and how.

    1 This is important, but it is not the nurse's first priority.

    2 This may or may not be necessary and is not the highest priority.

    3 This is very important, but she is probably not able to use this information at this time.

86. Knowledge, assessment, psychosocial (b)
    2 This is the most common reaction immediately following an attack, especially rape. Most victims report later that they felt numb and removed from any feelings about the experience immediately afterwards.
    1 This is unlikely because the experience of being raped produces profound shock.
    3 An unfortunate and false assumption sometimes made about women who are raped is that they wanted to have sex with their assailant.
    4 This is possible, but it is not the most likely explanation.

87. Knowledge, assessment, psychosocial (b)
    2 Rape is an act of violence and aggression expressed through sexual means; the object is the expression of violent feelings, not sexual ones.
    1 A common misconception is that the rapist is physically frustrated. This is untrue; many acts of rape are committed by men who are sexually dysfunctional.
    3 This is also untrue; the only dominance involved is that of aggressor/assailant over victim.
    4 This is another misconception, that the rapist is someone who has questions about his or her sexuality and uses the rape to reassure themselves.

88. Knowledge, assessment, psychosocial (b)
    3 Rape is a crime that victimizes persons of all age and ethnic/racial groups; it is committed by the same cross-section of the population.
    1 It is a common misconception that rape is a crime committed by members of the lower class.
    2 It is a common prejudice that blacks commit or are the victims of more rapes than whites.
    4 It is also a common prejudice that persons of color or urban dwellers are more likely to rape or be raped.

89. Comprehension, planning, physiological (a)
    4 Meperidine (Demerol) is relatively safe and 50 mg is an acceptable dose.
    1 The dose is within normal limits.
    2 The infant will not require naloxone (Narcan) if meperidine is given during the active stage of labor.
    3 The oral route is the slowest-acting.

90. Application, implementation, physiological (b)
    4 Fertilization occurs in the outer one third of the fallopian tubes.
    1 The uterus is the site of implantation.
    2 The corpus luteum is a yellowish mass formed in the graafian follicle after the egg has been released from the ovary.
    3 The vagina is the female organ of copulation.

91. Comprehension, implementation, physiological (a)
    1 Any tissue passed vaginally must be examined to determine if products of conception were expelled.
    2 The position of the patient is not a priority unless she is hemorrhaging.
    3 Providing a quiet environment is conducive to well-being; however, it is not the priority in the choice of answers.
    4 Fluids may need to be held in this situation, given the possibility of a dilatation and curettage (D & C) in the future.

92. Comprehension, implementation, physiological (a)
    3 The greatest risk of hemorrhage occurs within a few hours of delivery; the uterus must remain firm to control bleeding.
    1 Keeping the environment comfortable is desired but not essential.
    2 Offering sips of water is appropriate, but the concern for hemorrhage is greater than fluid deficit in the early period.
    4 Taking the temperature is an appropriate measure, but assessing the uterus takes precedence.

93. Knowledge, implementation, physiological (a)
    3 The nurse should remain with the patient until seizure activity has stopped. During this time the nurse can protect the patient from injury as well as observe the seizure activity.
    1 Inserting an object *during* the seizure can cause teeth damage.
    2 The patient should not be left alone.
    4 Resistance against the restraints can cause injury.

94. Comprehension, implementation, physiological (b)
    2 This allows any accumulated secretions to drain from his mouth.
    1 If activity has ceased, this is not an appropriate first action.
    3 If activity has ceased, this is not an appropriate first action. When a patient is on seizure precautions, vital signs should be checked at regular intervals because hyperthermia may bring about seizure activity.
    4 Oxygen may be needed during a seizure if he is hypoxic.

95. Application, implementation, environment (c)
    4 Periocular edema often occurs on the side of the incision. This may cause the eye to be swollen. It will typically subside in a few days.
    1 This is not the most appropriate action. The physician does not need to be notified.
    2 Keeping the head of the bed elevated to 30 degrees and not in a flat position will facilitate drainage of fluid.
    3 This action is not the most appropriate choice. The glasses may be another source of discomfort because the area around the eyes is already swollen. Light, cool compresses over the eyes will help reduce the edema.

96. Comprehension, assessment, physiological (b)
    1 Changes in level of consciousness (e.g., drowsiness) occur because of reduced oxygen supply to the cortex. The level of consciousness is a sensitive indicator of the patient's neurological status.
    2, 3, 4 These signs of increased intracranial pressure often do not appear until the intracranial pressure has been elevated for some time.

97. Comprehension, evaluation, physiological (c)
    4 Pituitary function disturbances in the form of diabetes insipidus (DI) can occur after intracranial surgery. DI is manifested by polyuria and urine that is low in specific gravity.
    1 The increase in temperature may be related to infection or an increase in intracranial pressure.
    2 Sluggish pupils are more likely related to changes in neurological status, such as an increase in intracranial pressure.
    3 Clear drainage on the dressing often indicates the occurrence of a cerebrospinal fluid leak.

98. Application, implementation, physiological (c)
    1 Clear drainage from the nose or ear often indicates the occurrence of a CSF (cerebrospinal fluid) leak. The patient may also complain of a "postnasal drip." The physician should be notified because meningitis could develop.
    2 Because of the danger of meningitis, the physician should be notified.
    3 This type of drainage is not normal mucus drainage. The drainage will be clear to pale-colored and may be seen as a "halo" around sanguineous or serosanguineous drainage.
    4 This is not the appropriate action; reinforcing the dressing and waiting until the physician arrives leaves the patient at risk for infection.

99. Comprehension, assessment, physiological (c)
    3 The Glasgow Coma Scale provides information about the patient's level of consciousness. The areas assessed are the patient's ability to speak, obey commands, or open the eyes.
    1 Emotional reactions are not part of the Coma Scale assessment.
    2 Intellectual functioning is not part of the Coma Scale assessment.
    4 These areas of neurological assessment are important, but the Coma Scale assesses level of consciousness only.

100. Comprehension, implementation, physiological (b)
    2 The patient should sit upright for meals and for 30 minutes after meals to decrease aspiration risk.
    1 Sitting up for meals should be encouraged.
    3 Swallowing with the head slightly flexed facilitates the swallowing process and reduces aspiration risk.
    4 Weakness is on the right side, so the patient should be encouraged to place food in the unaffected (left) side of the mouth.

101. Application, implementation, physiological (c)
    2 A regular voiding schedule helps prevent overdistention of the bladder. The schedule can be started with offering the urinal or toileting the patient every 2 hours and then gradually increasing the time span.
    1 An adequate fluid intake is important to help ensure an ample urine supply. Fluids should be taken at regular intervals during the day and should be limited in the evening hours.
    3 Checking for residual urine is an invasive procedure and places patient at risk for infection.
    4 Adult diapers are not part of a retraining program and do not support the patient psychologically.

102. Comprehension, planning, health (b)
    4 Emptying the breast with each feeding promotes the supply-and-demand principle. By emptying the breast, a supply of milk will be available for the next feeding.
    1 An exercise regime promotes well-being but does not ensure an adequate supply of milk.
    2 Adequate oral fluid intake is important; however, it does not have to be milk. The supply-and-demand principle supersedes the adequate fluid intake.
    3 Protein in itself does not ensure an adequate milk supply.

103. Knowledge, implementation, physiological (a)
    3 Gentle pressure on the infant's chin breaks the suction, decreasing trauma to the nipple.
    1 Pressure to the infant's lips would not comfortably release the suction and could potentially injure the infant or harm the nipple.
    2, 4 The nose and forehand have no anatomical relationship to the lips and the reflex of sucking.

104. Comprehension, evaluation, physiological (c)
    3 With increased blood volume, both become lower: Hgb 12 to 16 g/dl blood; Hct 37% to 47%.
    1, 2, 4 Both decrease; see No. 3 response.

105. Comprehension, evaluation, health (b)
    4 Cigarettes can retard fetal growth. Research indicates that smoking may complicate a pregnancy.
    1, 2 These are true statements.
    3 There is no safe limit of alcohol for a fetus. The patient should eliminate alcohol intake.

106. Knowledge, evaluation, physiological (a)
    3 Buccal tablets are to dissolve next to the cheek.
    1 A troche can dissolve anywhere in the mouth.
    2 Often tablets that dissolve should not be followed with water.
    4 This is sublingual administration.

107. Comprehension, evaluation, health (a)
    3 The pancreas either decreases the amount of insulin production or fails to produce insulin, causing the glucose level to elevate in the blood.
    1 This may cause a temporary increase of blood glucose, but it does not cause diabetes mellitus.
    2 Eating less would cause a decrease of blood glucose. Eating or avoiding certain foods does not cause diabetes mellitus.
    4 This produces insulin shock.

108. Comprehension, evaluation, physiological (c)
    1 Miotic drugs cause constriction of the pupils, which helps to facilitate the drainage of the aqueous humor.
    2 Mydriatic drugs cause dilation of the pupils, which would further hinder the circulation of the aqueous humor.
    3 Diaphoresis is the term for excessive perspiration.
    4 Diuresis is the term for increased urinary output.

109. Application, evaluation, health (b)
    1 Diets high in purines should be restricted because purines break down into uric acid.
    2, 3, 4 These nutrients do not apply to gout.

110. Comprehension, evaluation, physiological (a)
    4 Pernicious anemia results from the lack of the intrinsic factor found in the lining of the stomach. This is a chronic condition and must be treated with injections of vitamin B_{12}.
    1 Whole blood is usually given to patients with hemorrhagic anemia because of the loss of a large quantity of blood.
    2 Packed cells may be given when only the cells of blood need to be replaced, such as in sickle cell anemia.
    3 Injections of Imferon are usually administered to patients with severe iron-deficiency anemia.

111. Comprehension, evaluation, environment (c)
    4 A hemolytic reaction is a result of incompatible blood, which may result in decreased urine output and hematuria.
    1 This is an allergic reaction.
    2 This is a pyogenic reaction as a result of contaminated blood.
    3 This is not a result of a hemolytic reaction. Hypertension makes this statement incorrect. Hypotension occurs.

112. Comprehension, evaluation, environment (b)
   3 When a patient is given incompatible blood, the red blood cells react by clumping, or agglutinating.
   1 Achromia refers to the absence or loss of normal skin pigment.
   2 Agnosia is the total or partial loss of the ability to recognize familiar objects or persons through sensory stimuli as a result of organic brain syndrome.
   4 Anticoagulation refers to the prevention or delaying of coagulation (clotting) of the blood.

113. Comprehension, evaluation, environment (b)
   1 Any pain, dyspnea, change in blood pressure or dysrhythmia that is precipitated by an activity could indicate the patient's inability to tolerate activities.
   2 This does not necessitate stopping rehabilitation, because the patient must be taught to understand risk factors regarding health.
   3 This does not necessitate stopping rehabilitation, because the patient must be taught dietary modifications.
   4 The patient must be instructed about prescribed medications.

114. Knowledge, evaluation, physiological (b)
   2 Nitrates dilate central vessels; this causes an increase in cranial pressure, resulting in headaches.
   1 Nitrates may reduce, not increase, blood pressure.
   3 Nitrates do not directly effect the pulse rate.
   4 Nitrates do not cause drowsiness.

115. Application, evaluation, health (a)
   4 Weighing a patient daily is an accurate measurement for fluid increases and/or decreases.
   1 Daily weighing is only one factor in the assessment of medication change.
   2 Daily weighing is not indicated when weight reduction is the goal.
   3 Inappropriate response; the patient's diagnosis should be discussed with her by her physician.

116. Comprehension, evaluation, physiological (b)
   1 Absorption is decreased when diarrhea occurs. The drug is passed through the intestine too quickly for proper absorption to occur.
   2 Drug elimination involves primarily the kidney.
   3 Drug metabolism involves primarily the liver.
   4 Drug distribution would be altered by blood flow within the vessels.

117. Application, evaluation, environment (b)
   3 It is important for the nurse to always follow facility policy and procedure for reporting errors or omissions. The Quality Assurance committee should be made aware of such incidents to determine if a problem does exist.
   1 The physician is not next in authority on the unit and would probably defer to the supervising nurse.
   2 Confrontation is not the responsibility of the staff nurse; it could result in unpleasant working conditions.
   4 Unnecessary and inappropriate; follow facility policy and procedure.

118. Application, evaluation, environment (b)
   4 This is actual and factual data that does not imply the nurse's opinion or dissatisfaction.
   1 This is labeling the patient instead of describing what was measurable about his behavior.
   2 Although it is important to note in the chart, this is too vague as written.
   3 The first part is an opinion and labels the patient.

119. Knowledge, evaluation, health (a)
   2 A tetanus booster is recommended every 10 years; the patient should make a notation of the date it was received.
   1 Within 3 years, the booster should be sufficient for any major injuries.
   3 A tetanus injection offers active immunity but does not offer protection for life.
   4 If the patient suffers another accident and cannot remember the date, the physician may elect to order another booster.

120. Comprehension, evaluation, physiological (b)
   4 Illness weakens the body's ability to fight infection. An elderly individual may have a lowered defense because of age. Hospitalized patients are also at higher risk of developing nosocomial infections.
   1 Terminal illness can cause an individual to be more susceptible to infection, but the home environment may not be as risky as the hospital.
   2 If a nursing student follows hospital policy and uses proper protocol, the student is at no greater risk of infection than are other health personnel.
   3 Although a laceration can become infected as a result of a break in the skin barrier, proper cleaning at home will allow for healthy recovery.

COMPREHENSIVE EXAMINATION TWO: PART 2

121. Comprehension, planning, environment (b)
   2 In this situation, turning the patient to decrease further breakdown and to aid in increasing circulation does not require a physician's order.
   1 Whirlpool baths require a physician's order.
   3 Penicillin is a medication that requires a physician's order.
   4 Hydrogen peroxide and povidoneiodine (Betadine) are treatments requiring a physician's order.

122. Application, planning, psychological (c)
   1 A psychological problem may be of higher priority than a physical one. Mr. Snell's fear of dying needs to be dealt with to lower his anxiety.
   2 The anxiety is probably a result of the fear of dying. If the fear is causing the problem of anxiety, then fear should be priority.
   3 Although impaired gas exchange is of concern because of his chest trauma, it is not life-threatening at this time.
   4 This choice is not the best because resolving both the fear and anxiety first may subsequently reduce the shortness of breath.

123. Application, implementation, environment (c)
   $$\mathbf{2} \quad \frac{100 \text{ ml} \times 10}{x} = 33$$
   $$33x = 1000$$
   $$x = 30$$
   1, 3, 4 These are incorrect calculations.

124. Application, implementation, environment (b)
   2 A portable chest x-ray examination should be done in the room to prevent disease transmission to others in the hospital.
   1 Because the patient is coughing frequently, the mask is needed; disease transmission during a trip to the radiology department is high.
   3 The infection control nurse could be contacted, but she will probably suggest either notifying the physician or option No. 2.
   4 Although the technicians should be protected, the risk of contamination during a trip to the radiology department is high.

125. Application, implementation, physiological (b)
    2 The wound should be irrigated with the flow of liquid from the least contaminated to the most contaminated area, best facilitated by a dangling position.
    1 Lying flat would soil the linen and possibly cross-contaminate the wound during irrigation.
    3, 4 These positions could result in the liquid flowing from the most contaminated area (ulcer) to the least contaminated area (laceration).

126. Knowledge, implementation, health (a)
    3 Activity eases false labor; it will not affect true labor.
    1 False labor often begins in the lower abdomen.
    2 False labor is characterized by irregular contractions that do not increase in duration or intensity.
    4 Breathing techniques control pain, not contractions.

127. Application, planning, physiological (b)
    2 Vaginal examinations may precipitate acute bleeding. The physician will determine if delivery will be by cesarean section. Labor progression will be determined by monitoring contractions.
    1 Ultrasound is a possibility but requires a physician's order.
    3 This situation does not indicate active bleeding. Also, women in active labor do not wear pads.
    4 There is no information related to blood loss in this situation; type and cross match requires a physician's order.

128. Comprehension, assessment, environment (a)
    3 Following rupture of membranes (ROM), a prolapsed cord may occur, causing fetal distress. Initially the nurse must check fetal well-being.
    4 This will be done routinely q15min.
    1 If the fetus is fully engaged there is less chance of cord pressure occurring, but fetal heart tones are a better indication of fetal well-being.
    2 Labor may accelerate following membrane rupture.

129. Knowledge, assessment, environment (a)
    1 A gush of blood or transient increase in bleeding is a sign of placental separation.
    2 The umbilical cord lengthens with placental separation.
    3 The uterus tightens just before placental separation.
    4 Placental separation decreases cord pulsation.

130. Application, implementation, physiological (b)
    2 Most often hypotension in labor is a result of uterine pressure decreasing venous return.
    1 This position counteracts the normal direction and pressure on the diaphragm.
    3 If there were a continued decline in hemodynamic status this would be appropriate.
    4 This would be appropriate routine monitoring if blood pressure and pulse declined further, but immediately turning the patient will promote placental perfusion and increase venous return. This may be all that is needed.

131. Application, planning, health (c)
    1 The "morning after" pill is the only known therapy currently prescribed to prevent a pregnancy after unprotected intercourse.
    2 This is untrue. If she were ovulating at the time of the rape, she could become pregnant.
    3 This is only true if she elects not to use hormonal therapy.
    4 Spermicidal douche will not prevent pregnancy after unprotected intercourse, especially since several hours have elapsed since the rape.

132. Knowledge, planning, environment (c)
    3 It is mandatory that all cases of suspected or actual child abuse be reported to child protection authorities immediately. The nurse has a legal as well as an ethical obligation to do so.
    1 This is important and should occur as part of treating this family, but it is not first priority.
    2 This should not be done until child protection authorities are contacted.
    4 This should not be done until child protection authorities are notified; it should not be done by the family.

133. Application, planning, psychosocial (b)
    2 Safety of the students is the most important priority. In cases of alleged abuse by teachers, teachers are usually put on leave until the situation is resolved.
    1 This is important, but not as important as ensuring safety and protection from further abuse.
    3 This is important, but it will be easier if she believes that adults around her can protect her from further abuse.
    4 This is not the responsibility of the nurse.

134. Application, assessment, psychosocial (c)
    4 Children who are abused most often feel guilty about what has occurred and responsible for not stopping the abuser.
    1 Many times children are not certain about this, which is one reason the abuse is often not immediately revealed.
    2 This might be true, but rituals are patterns of behavior, not emotions.
    3 This might also be true, but rationalization is not a defense likely to be employed by a child.

135. Application, implementation, health (c)
    4 This acknowledges that the mother feels upset and disappointed in her ability to protect her daughter.
    1 This is a falsely reassuring answer. It does not address the reality of what her mother is feeling.
    2 This gives false reassurance. The nurse cannot know at this time how much of an effect the abuse will have.
    3 This is also not the case. The child will be upset over what has occurred whether or not her mother shows that she is upset.

136. Application, assessment, physiological (a)
    3 If an infection is present, tonsil surgery is postponed until infection subsides.
    1 This is not necessarily needed.
    2 Hemorrhage could occur after, not before, surgery.
    4 This is not accurate information.

137. Knowledge, planning, environment (b)
    2 The nurse should position the patient slightly on the side to facilitate drainage. Flexing knees eliminates use of pillows; it does not hamper breathing.
    1 The prone position increases chance of aspiration.
    3, 4 These positions do not facilitate drainage after a tonsillectomy and adenoidectomy.

138. Knowledge, assessment, physiological (b)
    1 Hemorrhage is the single most common complication because bleeding is concealed.
    2 This is not a complication.
    3 This is not relative to this condition.
    4 It might hurt to talk, but there is no loss of speech.

139. Comprehension, assessment, physiological (c)
    3 Frequent swallowing, restlessness, spitting up bright-red blood, and increased respirations and pulse are indications of excessive bleeding.
    1 Flushed face is not indicative of excessive bleeding. Loss of consciousness may result but would not be an early sign of excessive bleeding.
    2 Tarry stools are indicative of bleeding at this time.
    4 These signs do not indicate bleeding.

140. Application, implementation, physiological (b)
    2 Clear liquids and Gatorade are less irritating than natural juices.
    1 Natural juices are irritating to the throat.
    3 Cool drinks are more soothing to the throat.
    4 Milk products are not used initially because they coat the mouth and throat, causing the child to clear her throat more often. This could initiate bleeding.

141. Comprehension, implementation, psychosocial (b)
    4 Thrombolytic agents dissolve clots, decreasing and preventing extension of the existing clot.
    1 Thrombolytic agents do not "thin" the blood as was once thought.
    2 This is a description of products such as aspirin with anticoagulant properties.
    3 This is a description of the action of an anticoagulant.

142. Application, implementation, environment (c)
    4 $\dfrac{\text{Desired}}{\text{Have}} \times \text{Quantity}$

    $\dfrac{8,000 \text{ U}}{5,000 \text{ U}} \times 1 \text{ ml} = 1.6 \text{ ml}$

    1, 2, 3 Incorrect calculations.

143. Comprehension, implementation, environment (b)
    1 The recommended site for subcutaneous administration of heparin is the abdomen; injection sites should be rotated to avoid bruising.
    2 Rubbing the site after administration of subcutaneous heparin can increase the risk of bleeding and bruising.
    3 The intramuscular route is not recommended due to risk of hematoma.
    4 IV heparin should be on an infusion pump or other volume-controlled unit for accuracy and safety.

144. Application, planning, health (a)
    4 These are signs of inflammation and should be clarified with patients even though many may know the signs already.
    1 Although swelling may be of concern, coolness is not a sign of infection.
    2 Some soreness and bruising is expected around the site; the patient should know the difference between pain and soreness.
    3 This explanation is too vague and assumes that the patient knows what to look for.

145. Knowledge, implementation, environment (a)
    2 Diabetic individuals are prone to infections and heal poorly. Clean footwear assists in preventing infections. The nails should be trimmed carefully to avoid cutting the surrounding skin or producing ingrown nails.
    1 Diabetic individuals should assess the feet daily for cuts and irritations. Vascular changes associated with diabetes contribute to poor healing.
    3 Improper footwear and nail-trimming can lead to serious complications for the diabetic as described in Options Nos. 1 and 2.
    4 Diabetic individuals should assess their feet daily.

146. Comprehension, assessment, physiological (b)
    2 A thrill should be palpated over the shunt if the shunt is patent. The shunt could have clotted off if the thrill is absent.
    1 Blood pressure measurement should not be taken under any circumstances in the arm with the shunt.
    3 Soreness would not be an immediate concern after surgery.
    4 Although concern for HIV infection may need to be addressed, it is not an immediate concern.

147. Knowledge, planning, health (a)
    3 These foods contain high levels of tyramine, which could cause hypertension. Compliance in taking the medication is necessary; it should not be abruptly stopped.
    1 Bananas and yogurt contain moderate amounts of tyramine and should be consumed only occasionally. The medicine is usually not ordered prn.
    2 Seasonings and milk are not on the listed foods containing tyramine and therefore present no harm.
    4 Colas and fruit are not on the listed foods containing tyramine; however, the last part of the answer is correct.

148. Application, assessment, environment (b)
    1 The change in condition could be related to other reasons, but it may be drug related.
    2 Further evaluation by the physician is needed to determine the cause of central nervous system (CNS) changes.
    3 The signs and symptoms are indicative of CNS depression; they would worsen with additional medication.
    4 Close observation would be needed for the next few hours whether or not the medication were administered.

149. Application, implementation, environment (c)
    2 Two cans q4h would equal 12 cans in 24 hours, 2880 calories, and less than 3000 milliliters.
    1 One and a half (1.5) cans would result in 9 cans in 24 hours and only 2160 calories.
    3 This would be over the amount of calories and milliliters ordered by the physician.
    4 There are six 4-hour periods in 24 hours; this could cause confusion in the number of cans needed.

150. Application, assessment, physiological (b)
    3 The complaints suggest a fecal impaction, which should be ruled out before administration of medicine or other treatments.
    1 A laxative could cause severe cramping if a fecal impaction is present.
    2 An antidiarrheal medication could worsen an impaction.
    4 The patient's physical condition should be the priority concern.

151. Comprehension, implementation, physiological (b)
    3 Most physicians will allow showers eventually, but the patient must be able to stand on his own without complications.
    1 The nurse should be with the patient the first time the shower is taken, but the first day is too soon for a shower.
    2 This response allows the patient to freely ambulate on his own, and he may not know when to limit activity.
    4 Most physicians allow showers before suture removal. The nurse can coordinate the time of the dressing change and the shower when ordered.

152. Comprehension, implementation, physiological (b)
    3 Inhalation anesthetic drugs are eliminated by the lungs; proper aeration of the alveoli aids in the elimination of these gases after surgery.
    1 Age may determine the use of a triflow, but the triflow is not standard for all patients. The condition of the lungs, length of the surgery, and anticipated recovery also determine the use of a triflow.
    2 Although partially correct, this is not the best explanation for the patient who does not feel he needs the treatment.
    4 Secretions will not necessarily be loosened by a triflow.

153. Application, implementation, environment (b)
    3 $\dfrac{\text{Desired}}{\text{Have}} \times \text{Quantity} =$
    $\dfrac{1200 \text{ mg}}{100 \text{ mg}} \times 1 \text{ tab} =$
    $12 \times 1 \text{ tab} = 12 \text{ tablets} =$
    4 tablets three times a day (tid)
    1, 2 These are incorrect calculations; doses are too low.
    4 This is an incorrect calculation; dose is too high.

154. Comprehension, implementation, environment (b)
    1 Drowsiness and dizziness may occur and should decrease after a few weeks. If the side effects do not subside, the physician may need to adjust the medication. Driving is contraindicated in the presence of these side effects.
    2 Absorption is enhanced by administration with meals.
    3 Abrupt withdrawal of medication can precipitate seizures.
    4 Photosensitivity may occur; the patient requires protection with sunscreen and proper clothing.

155. Application, implementation, physiological (b)
    4 Further footdrop can be prevented by proper positioning of the feet. A foot board is helpful in maintaining this proper alignment.
    1 This should be done regardless of footdrop, but it will not guarantee that the footdrop will not worsen.
    2 This may help and is an appropriate choice, but it should not limit the nurse in independent measures as explained in the correct response.
    3 This option may help, but the footdrop will worsen if the foot is not properly positioned between exercises.

156. Comprehension, implementation, environment (a)
    2 A 24-hour specimen begins with the patient emptying his bladder and then discarding that specimen. The nurse notes the time the bladder was emptied and instructs the patient to save each urine specimen. The urine collection procedure is ended 24 hours after the patient first emptied his bladder. The patient voids at this time, and this last urine collection is added to the sample.
    1, 3, 4 These are not accurate 24-hour urine collection procedures.

157. Comprehension, assessment, environment (b)
    1 The anemia associated with chronic renal failure reflects hypoproliferative activity of the bone marrow. The main cause is decreased production of erythropoietin by the kidney.
    2 Hypertension usually occurs and is probably a result of sodium retention and increased extracellular fluid volume.
    3 Hyperkalemia, not hypokalemia, is one of the most serious electrolyte problems seen in chronic renal failure.
    4 Weight gain as a result of fluid retention frequently occurs.

158. Application, implementation, physiological (c)
    1 The access should be palpated to check and document the presence of adequate blood flow.
    2 There will be some swelling in the extremity after the procedure; it is necessary to keep the extremity elevated.
    3 Blood pressure should not be taken in the arm with the access, nor should blood be withdrawn from that arm.
    4 The only restriction is the avoidance of tight clothing around the access because this may decrease blood flow and cause clotting.

159. Comprehension, assessment, environment (b)
    2 This is descriptive of hemodialysis.
    1 This is descriptive of continuous arteriovenous hemofiltration.
    3 This is descriptive of peritoneal dialysis.
    4 This is descriptive of continuous ambulatory peritoneal dialysis.

160. Comprehension, implementation, physiological (b)
    2 Lowering protein intake decreases metabolic end products such as urea. Sodium is restricted, depending on the degree of edema and hypertension. Potassium is usually restricted because of the problems with hyperkalemia.
    1 Fluids are usually restricted so that the patient does not have excess weight gain between dialysis treatments.
    3 Protein and sodium are usually decreased.
    4 Sufficient calories are needed from fat to maintain body weight.

161. Knowledge, assessment, physiological (a)
    2 Phenylalanine is found in the blood of infants with phenylketonuria (PKU).
    1 Tyrosine results when phenylalanine is properly digested.
    3 Phenylpyruvic acid is a derivative of phenylalanine and is found in the urine of a child with PKU.
    4 Phenylalanine hydroxylase is an enzyme that converts phenylalanine to tyrosine.

162. Knowledge, assessment, physiological (a)
    3 Interference with proper nervous system development in the child with phenylketonuria (PKU) results in mental retardation in most affected infants. This is a result of phenylalanine accumulating in the blood.
    1, 2 PKU does not affect these organs directly.
    4 PKU does not cause seizures.

163. Knowledge, planning, health (a)
    3 Animal and vegetable proteins should be controlled in the diet. Protein contains phenylalanine.
    1, 2, 4 A low-protein diet is prescribed for a patient with phenlketonuria (PKU); these substances are not modified.

164. Knowledge, assessment, psychosocial (b)
    2 This is absolutely essential. She may be in danger of serious illness or death from her severe weight loss.
    1, 3 These are important, but they are not the nurse's first priority.
    4 This should be done in cooperation with her physician after her physical status is assessed.

165. Knowledge, planning, physiological (b)
    4 Safety and physiological integrity are always the most appropriate short-term goals.
    1 This is a long-term goal.
    2 Alteration of body image is a very long-term goal.
    3 This is important, especially to help reinforce the gains that the patient needs to make in treatment, but it is a long-term goal.

166. Knowledge, assessment, psychosocial (b)
    2 Delirium is characterized by sudden onset of symptoms with no prior deficits.
    1 This is more suggestive of normal aging or dementia.
    3 This reflects a bias about the elderly; people do not necessarily present with delirium just because they get older. There is no indication of the patient's age in this situation.
    4 The symptom of depression is more similar to that of dementia, not delirium.

167. Comprehension, assessment, psychosocial (c)
    2 Diuretic drugs are more likely to cause electrolyte imbalances, which can lead to delirium.
    1 Antibiotics can cause gastrointestinal disturbance, which can disrupt electrolyte balance. No. 2, however, is the more likely problem.
    3 This could have caused disruption at the time, but it is most likely not contributing to the present problem.
    4 This is not an abnormally large weight loss.

168. Comprehension, implementation, environment (b)
    4 Patients with delirium are extremely disoriented and need to be frequently reoriented to help them feel safe.
    1 This is impractical with a patient in delirium.
    2 She is unlikely to be able to read or use them.
    3 She is unlikely to be able to understand or follow verbal instructions.

169. Comprehension, planning, environment (b)
    4 She is definitely at risk for harm if she is not closely supervised.
    1, 2, 3 These are true, but they are not the highest priority.

170. Application, assessment, environment (b)
    1 Orientation to time is an important indicator of the general level of confusion or orientation.
    2 This is more appropriate to assess mood.
    3 This is more appropriate to assess short-term memory.
    4 This is more appropriate to asess judgment.

171. Application, planning, environment (b)
    2 There is the possibility of aspiration of formula and air in stomach.
    1 There is still the possibility of aspiration, a dangerous result of bottle-feeding.
    3 The mother needs rest. Sitting and holding baby allows for rest, enjoyment, and bonding.
    4 Holding the baby provides cuddling and close contact.

172. Knowledge, implementation, psychosocial (a)
    4 Newborns usually need 18 to 20 hours of sleep daily.
    1 Infants need more than brief naps.
    2 Newborns are not likely to stay awake all night.
    3 After 1 month, infants usually sleep 15 to 18 hours a day.

173. Knowledge, implementation, environment (a)
    4 He needs a quiet environment within normal limits.
    1 There is no need for sedation every 4 hours.
    2 A dark room would frighten him and make him anxious.
    3 He needs rest, and so does his mother.

174. Knowledge, assessment, physiological (b)
    2 Croup is spasmodic laryngitis.
    1 It is not an infection of the pharynx.
    3 Croup is characterized by spasms of larynx, not trachea.
    4 Croup does not affect lung tissue.

175. Application, planning, physiological (b)
    4 $\dfrac{\text{Desired}}{\text{Have}} \times \text{Quantity} = \dfrac{250 \text{ mg}}{125 \text{ mg}} \times 5 \text{ ml} =$
    $2 \times 5 \text{ ml} = 10 \text{ ml}$
    1, 2, 3 These are insufficient quantities.

176. Comprehension, assessment, physiological (b)
    1 Elevated serum glucose levels, dehydration, and nausea and vomiting are some of the clinical findings associated with hyperglycemia.
    2, 3, 4 All are clinical findings associated with hypoglycemia.

177. Comprehension, planning, physiological (b)
    3 NPH, an intermediate-acting insulin, is used as part of insulin-maintenance therapy.
    1 Regular insulin (short-acting) is used as part of "sliding scale" coverage; it may be used as supplemental doses when patients are medically unstable.
    2 Acute hypoglycemia is treated with glucose, not with insulin.
    4 Regular (fast-acting) insulin, not an intermediate acting insulin, is needed in treating acute ketoacidosis. Regular insulin is usually given intravenously.

178. Application, implementation, health (c)
    4 The diabetic patient may not feel pressure points from tight-fitting socks/stockings. Feet with arterial insufficiency are prone to necrosis and infection. To avoid pressure points, stockings with seams or mended socks should not be used.
    1 The toenails should be cut straight across because cutting the toenails in a curved fashion could lead to ingrown nails.
    2 Alcohol will dry the skin; it places the skin at risk for damage.
    3 Heating pads should not be used. The diabetic patient may experience burns because discomfort may not be felt.

179. Application, evaluation, health (b)
    4 Regularly scheduled meals are part of the overall treatment plan. The timing of the meals and allowed snacks help prevent problems such as hypoglycemia and hyperglycemia.
    1 Desserts can be included in the diet as part of the daily caloric requirements. Desserts are not restricted to fresh fruit.
    2 Food may need to increased during periods of heavy exercise.
    3 The exchange system allows for substitutions and flexibility in the diet. So-called "dietetic" foods do not have to be used. Often, these foods are high in sodium and can be more costly.

180. Comprehension, assessment, physiological (b)
    2 An Apgar score of 4 to 7 indicates a mild to moderately depressed newborn.
    1 An Apgar score of 8 to 10 indicates vigorous newborn.
    3 An assessment of 0 is given when respiration is initiated or absent. Respiratory efforts are usually affected when the Apgar score is 4.
    4 The respiratory rate of newborn is faster, if there are no problems, it is usually between 30 and 45.

181. Knowledge, implementation, physiological (a)
    3 Moro or startle reflex is elicited by a loud noise or sudden movement.
    1 The grasp reflex is elicited by placing a finger in the ulnar side of the infant's palm.
    2 Babinski's reflex or grasp reflex is elicited by stimulating the outer sole of the foot.
    4 Tonic neck reflex is elicited when the infant's head is quickly turned to one side.

182. Knowledge, assessment, health (a)
    3 Morning sickness is the appropriate term for nausea and vomiting during pregnancy, occurring usually during the first trimester.
    1 Pernicious vomiting is a term used to designate vomiting occasionally occurring in pregnancy that becomes so prolonged and excessive as to threaten the mother's life.
    2 Vomitus marinus refers to seasickness.
    4 Hyperemesis gravadarum is another term for pernicious vomiting.

183. Knowledge, assessment, health (c)
    3 Human chorionic gonadatropin (HCG), originating in chorionic tissue, is excreted in the urine during early stages of pregnancy. It is also secreted by choriocarcinomas.
    1 The adrenocorticotropic hormone is excreted by the pituitary gland and stimulates the cortex of the adrenal gland.
    2 The follicle-stimulating hormone is excreted by the pituitary gland and stimulates the follicle to produce estrogen in the female.
    4 The thyroid-stimulating hormone stimulates the thyroid to produce thyroid hormone.

184. Application, implementation, environment (a)
    4 The patient is lying on her back with legs in stirrups. This enables the physician to examine the genitals and do a pelvic examination.
    1 The patient is lying on her back with legs straight; all body parts are in appropriate alignment; unable to examine genitals and do a pelvic examination in this position.
    2 Supine position is the same as the horizontal recumbent position.
    3 This dorsal recumbent position has the patient lie on her back with knees flexed. Although this position may be used, it is not the preferred position for a pelvic examination.

185. Knowledge, assessment, health (b)
    1 This is a condition occurring in the latter months of pregnancy. It is characterized by acute elevation of blood pressure, edema and proteinuria, but without convulsions or coma as seen in eclampsia.
    2 This is a condition occurring in the second half of pregnancy and sometimes in the puerperium. It is characterized by acute elevation of blood pressure, proteinuria, edema, sodium retention, convulsions and sometimes coma.
    3 This is excessive tension or pressure exerted by body fluids; also known as high blood pressure.
    4 This is a condition of exalted strength or tone of the body.

186. Comprehension, planning, health (b)
    3 The patient has symptoms of preeclampsia. Bed rest and decreased salt intake will help to reduce the symptoms.
    1 Bed rest is appropriate, but decreasing caloric intake would not be therapeutic in preeclampsia.
    2 These would be contraindicated.
    4 Reducing the salt intake is appropriate, but moderate exercise is contraindicated.

187. Comprehension, implementation, health (c)
    2 A person can stop using alcohol and be in recovery, but this does not mean that the underlying illness has disappeared. Alcohol dependence is a chronic illness, even if the person is not currently using the substance.
    1 No, her underlying illness is still present.
    3 This response does not answer the mother's question.
    4 Her illness is present whether or not she has any permanent physical changes.

188. Knowledge, planning, environment (b)
    4 The most important concern of the nurse in this phase is preventing physical harm while the substance is withdrawn from the patient's body.
    1, 2 These are important goals but only after detoxification.
    3 This is important but secondary to physiologic safety factors.

189. Comprehension, assessment, environment (b)
    3 The history she has given indicates a recent onset of symptoms and also identifies possible reasons for the crisis.
    1 She does not have the changes in function that would indicate depression, not is there indication of a prior history of depression.
    2 The situation does not present signs and symptoms of an anxiety neurosis.
    4 There is no indication in the situation that Bernice is a schizophrenic.

190. Application, assessment, psychosocial (c)
    2 Current coping is most strongly determined by how the patient has coped with stress in the past.
    1 This could serve to moderate the immediate crisis, but it will not be the final determination of what the patient will do to get himself to his precrisis level.
    3 This may not be what is necessary to decrease feelings of being overwhelmed or inadequacy.
    4 Therapy promotes long-term change, but it is not a good predictor of how a patient will react to or resolve a crisis.

191. Knowledge, planning, environment (b)
    4 Verbalization of concerns will decrease the need to have somatic and other types of symptoms.
    1 This could be an appropriate long-term goal, but it is not the immediate primary focus.
    2 This will be a consequence of helping the patient to verbalize, which is the priority.
    3 This may not be necessary, and it is not appropriate as an immediate goal.

192. Knowledge, planning, environment (b)
    1 Drugs such as Valium are highly addictive and should be prescribed only when absolutely necessary.
    2 This is true, but it is not the most important reason they are not usually prescribed to treat anxiety symptoms.
    3 This can occur in individuals who are physically and/or psychologically dependent on them.
    4 This is not necessarily true; antianxiety drugs can be very effective in treating symptoms such as muscle tension and gastrointestinal complaints.

193. Knowledge, implementation, environment (a)
    3 To provide a safe distance that does not endanger skin integrity, the heart lamp should be applied at a distance of 1½ to 2 feet.
    1 Heat lamps do not need to be warmed up. The warmth begins as soon as the lamp is turned on.
    2 The strongest wattage to be used for heat applications is 40 watts.
    4 To protect the skin from damage, heat lamps should be used for no more than 20 minutes.

194. Comprehension, implementation, physiological (b)
    2 Fluids will allow softer stools, and exercise promotes peristalsis.
    1 Analgesia often slows peristalsis.
    3 Rest will slow peristalsis. Calories have no effect on stools.
    4 Laxatives will aid with elimination, but they should only be used after nursing measures of increased fiber, fluids, and activity. Laxatives require a physician's order. Sitz baths do not promote elimination.

195. Knowledge, planning, psychosocial (a)

    3 This is factual and supportive, truthful information.

    1 This response ignores patient's question and is non-therapeutic.

    2 This response fails to identify the patient's emotional need.

    4 This response is patronizing, devalues the patient's feeling, and is nontherapeutic.

196. Comprehension, implementation, physiological (b)

    2 Following a cesarean section and general anesthesia, peristalsis is slowed. The nurse acknowledges the patient's request and provides an explanation that is therapeutic.

    1 This reply avoids the patient's emotional need.

    3 This is a nontherapeutic response; it does not acknowledge the patient's emotional need.

    4 This response neither directly answers the question posed by the patient, nor is it factually correct; IV fluids do not quench the thirst drive.

197. Comprehension, implementation, physiological (b)

    2 This response is a prudent nursing measure because the patient will be more cooperative when pain is well-managed.

    1 Although dangling will increase lung expansion, it does not help or eliminate the pain.

    3 Explanations do not necessarily promote patient cooperation.

    4 This does not help the patient to cooperate with the nursing intervention; also, the nurse is ignoring the responsibility to the patient.

198. Knowledge, planning, psychosocial (a)

    3 These are all symptoms characteristic of a personality disorder.

    1 This is not an accepted psychiatric diagnosis.

    2 This does not cover all the symptoms mentioned.

    4 Substance abuse is one of the symptoms in this case; it is not the diagnosis.

199. Application, evaluation, health (c)

    2 This indicates that her sense of reality is intact and that she understands the need for support and reinforcement of the gains she made during hospitalization.

    1 This indicates that she is still not accepting that she has a chronic illness and will need to take medication on a permanent basis.

    3 This indicates that she is still thinking in a manic grandiose way.

    4 This also could indicate that she is not accepting realistic limits.

200. Knowledge, assessment, environment (a)

    4 The clinical findings of hyperthyroid disease result from thyroid hormone excess. Heat intolerance is often a common complaint.

    1, 2, 3 These findings are associated with hypothyroid function (insufficient thyroid hormone).

201. Knowledge, assessment, environment (a)

    2 Bulging or protrusion of the eyeballs and orbit and lid muscle function are altered with hyperthyroidism. The patient also appears to be staring because blinking is reduced. These eye changes are referred to as exophthalmos.

    1, 3, 4 These findings are associated with problems of visual acuity and inflammation.

202. Comprehension, planning, physiological (b)

    2 A low-stimulus, quiet environment should be provided. Fatigue, dyspnea, tachycardia, and constant activity place the patient at risk for congestive heart failure.

    1 The hyperthyroid patient will need a high-calorie diet and between-meal feedings. Most hyperthyroid patients experience weight loss even with an increased appetite.

    3 Skin is usually warm and moist with increased perspiration. Frequent hygiene measures (e.g., baths, change of clothing and bed linens) should be encouraged.

    4 The room is usually kept cool because the patient typically has heat intolerance.

203. Knowledge, assessment, physiological (a)

    4 A potential side effect is agranulocytosis. The occurrence of a sore throat and fever should be reported immediately.

    1 Tachycardia often occurs in the hyperthyroid patient and is not abnormal for this condition.

    2 Body weight should be monitored, but some weight gain may occur as the metabolic rate is adjusted.

    3 A metallic taste is associated with iodine preparations (Lugol's solution, saturated solution of potassium iodide [SSKI]) used in the treatment of hyperthyroidism.

204. Comprehension, assessment, physiological (b)

    4 Bleeding may not be visible on the front of the dressing because it will drain down by gravity to the back of the patient's neck.

    1 Just an inspection of the dressing for dried blood is not thorough enough.

    2 Changes in hemoglobin and hematocrit could reflect more than bleeding.

    3 Checking the wound in this manner places the patient at risk for infection.

205. Comprehension, evaluation, physiological (c)

    2 Postoperative edema, intubation for surgery, and surgical damage to the laryngeal nerves can all cause damage to the laryngeal nerve with resulting vocal changes. The voice should be assessed for tone and quality. Having the patient speak when vital signs are checked in the postoperative period is an important part of nursing care.

    1 Hemorrhage is evaluated through such assessments as vital signs, skin color, and dressing checks.

    3, 4 Assessing the patient's ability to speak after a thyroidectomy is related to concerns about laryngeal edema or damage; it is not a measure of lower airway problems or level of consciousness. Airway obstruction problems would result in such symptoms as stridor and cyanosis.

206. Comprehension, assessment, environment (b)

    2 The first changes usually associated with chronic glaucoma are associated with peripheral visual ability. Patients may complain of bumping into things or stumbling.

    1 Eye pain can be associated with acute closed-angle glaucoma, burns, or corneal injuries.

    3 Tearing and redness after reading may indicate a refraction disorder.

    4 A decreased ability to focus on near objects is indicative of a refraction disorder.

207. Application, implementation, physiological (b)
    3 Medication should be placed in the conjunctival sac, not on the cornea. The eye should not be touched with the dropper or the tip of the tube.
    1 Pressure should not be applied to the eye because corneal damage could occur.
    2 The eye should be gently closed for 2 to 3 minutes to spread the medication.
    4 Excess fluid or encrusted secretions should be cleaned by wiping from inner to outer canthus. Cleaning from outer to inner canthus could spread infection.
208. Application, implementation, psychosocial (c)
    3 The clinical picture of acute spinal injury changes as edema develops or subsides or if complications occur. Telling the parents that at this time "it is too early to know" provides them with feedback and gives an honest answer to their questions.
    1 It is too early after the injury to know the full extent of function impairment.
    2, 4 These responses give false reassurance and are nontherapeutic.
209. Knowledge, planning, environment (a)
    2 Following the fracture, skeletal traction is used to immobilize the cervical region at the level of the injuries. Pain and muscle spasms are reduced, and the injured vertebrae are aligned into position.
    1 Even with cervical tongs in place, the patient will not have *normal* head and neck movement. The patient must be moved as a unit to prevent movement of the spine. The patient may be placed on a special bed (e.g., the Kinetic Rotorest bed) to facilitate turning.
    3 This type of traction is used to support the injured cervical vertebrae.
    4 Traction addresses the fracture, but it is not used to prevent the development of spinal shock. Spinal shock usually occurs with spinal cord injuries and may last from days to months.
210. Comprehension, assessment, environment (c)
    1 Following the acute injury at the cervical level, the patient will have a loss of reflexes below the level of injury.
    2 Deep-tendon reflexes will be absent, not hyperactive, following the acute injury.
    3 Paralysis, not sensory loss, is noted below the injury.
    4 Temperature sensation (sensory) is lost below level of the injury.
211. Knowledge, assessment, physiologic (a)
    2 Bradycardia, or slowing of the heart rate, occurs in spinal shock. Vasoconstrictive responses are blocked, blood pressure drops, and heart rate slows.
    2 Hypotension, not hypertension, is associated with spinal shock.
    3 Muscle flaccidity, not spasticity, is associated with spinal shock.
    4 Seizures do not occur in spinal shock.
212. Comprehension, implementation, physiological (c)
    4 The halo fixation device provides for spinal stabilization and the promotion of further healing without the use of a special bed.
    1 Pins are used to insert the traction apparatus, and pin site care is provided to prevent infection at the pin sites.
    2 The use of the halo apparatus provides for greater mobility, but the patient will still have limited head motion and will need assistance with mobilization.
    3 Traction weights are not used with this type of spinal immobilization.

213. Application, planning, health (c)
    3 Urinary stones frequently develop in spinal cord–injured patients. The need for increasing the intake of fluids should be emphasized.
    1 Fluids are primarily given to combat the formation of calculi.
    2 Because of immobility, the patient is at increased risk for pulmonary problems, but the primary concern is renal calculi.
    4 Spinal shock occurs after the acute injury.
214. Knowledge, assessment, physiological (c)
    3 This is correct; the eustachian tube is shorter, wider, and straighter in an infant.
    1, 4 These are not true. See correct response, above.
    2 This is not relevant to the situation.
215. Knowledge, assessment, physiological (a)
    2 The Croupette is used for smaller patients and provides cool moist air and oxygen to facilitate breathing.
    1 Aerosol therapy is inappropriate for a 16-month-old and does not deliver cool, moist air and oxygen.
    3 This does not provide cool moist air
    4 Air provided should be cool and moist, not warm and moist.
216. Comprehension, implementation, environment (b)
    1 Changing damp gowns and bedding prevents the child from chilling.
    2 This does not directly aid in promoting safety or comfort.
    3 The child needs freedom to move in the crib.
    4 The child should be positioned for maximum lung expansion, for example in high-Fowler's position.
217. Comprehension, assessment, physiological (c)
    4 Air passages are smaller in children and when these passages swell, respiratory distress occurs.
    1 The infant's diet is not necessarily a factor at this time.
    2 This is not true.
    3 Infants can be given antibiotic drugs if necessary.
218. Knowledge, implementation, environment (a)
    4 Cleansing from front to back with an individual wipe and voiding a small amount in the toilet before the sample cleanses the meatus of microorganisms.
    1 The word "void" may not be understood by the patient; in addition, the wipes are not provided for cleansing the hands.
    2 This explanation does not offer enough instruction on the cleansing.
    3 Although this would not violate the technique for collection of the specimen, it is inconvenient for the patient.
219. Knowledge, assessment, environment (a)
    2 The brachial artery is located on the inner aspect of the antecubital fossa.
    1 The radial artery is where the pulse is normally taken.
    3 The correct location is the inner aspect of the antecubital fossa.
    4 This is not an exact location.
220. Application, planning, health (a)
    3 The removal of nits from the hair shaft is essential and may be easier if the comb is fine-toothed and dipped in vinegar.
    1 The shampoo is usually recommended for 8 to 10 minutes.
    2 A repeat of the shampoo is recommended in 7 to 10 days.
    4 All bed linen and clothing should be washed in hot water, using bleach if possible.

221. Application, implementation, environment (b)
  3 Clorox is a caustic agent and should not be vomited. Because of the child's age and the unknown amount of Clorox, a physician should assess the child's condition.
  1, 2 The syrup of ipecac will cause vomiting, which is contraindicated in this situation.
  4 The first part of the answer is correct, but because the child is so young and the amount unknown, a panic-stricken mother cannot adequately assess the child.

222. Application, implementation, environment (b)
  3 $\dfrac{500 \text{ ml}}{50 \text{ ml}} = 10$ hrs.
  1, 2, 3 These are incorrect calculations.

223. Comprehension, implementation, psychological (b)
  2 Acknowledging her concerns will allow the mother to further communicate her fear.
  1 This statement does not offer assurance and would probably hinder further conversation.
  3 The nurse should be sincere and listen carefully to what the patient is saying without belittling.
  4 This action would convey to the patient that either the nurse is not listening or she does not care.

224. Application, planning, health (b)
  4 The expectorant produces coughing to relieve the respiratory fluids and should be given during the daytime "awake" hours; the antitussive suppresses the cough so the child can sleep.
  1 The two agents together will counteract each other and be ineffective.
  2 The expectorant should be taken during working hours to decrease accumulation of respiratory fluids, the antitussive at night to suppress coughing, and the antibiotics q6h as ordered.
  3 Taking the expectorant during the night will keep the child awake, and the antitussive may cause drowsiness during the day.

225. Knowledge, evaluation, physiological (a)
  3 Daily weights reflect water retention (1 kg = 1 L water) and can be used to estimate fluid retention.
  1 Intake and output records are important, but weight is the most accurate indicator.
  2 Blood urea nitrogen (BUN) levels measure the amount of urea nitrogen in the blood. BUN levels and their relationship to serum creatinine concentration are useful in evaluating fluid volume status. Fluid volume deficit would be indicated by a BUN out of proportion to the serum creatinine level.
  4 Skin turgor refers to the elasticity of the skin. A test for skin turgor is not the most accurate method of evaluating fluid status.

226. Comprehension, evaluation, health (b)
  2 Constrictive clothing should be avoided over the area. The skin is more sensitive in the treatment area and is subject to injury.
  1 Creams, lotions, and deodorantss should not be used on the area. After the first 2 weeks of treatment, the skin usually becomes red and dry. Changes in the skin are common during therapy.
  3, 4 The skin is already dry, use of an astringent or alcohol on the area will only make the skin more dry.

227. Knowledge, evaluation, environment (a)
  3 Both food and insulin may need to be adjusted when an exercise program is started. The best way to determine the needs is to have the patient check his blood sugar level before and after excerise.
  1 The effects of insulin may be potentiated by exercise; therefore, exercise may cause the blood sugar to drop.
  2 Fruit or juice may be necessary to prevent hypoglycemia.
  4 Planned exercise is important and should be part of the diabetic individual's treatment program. Insulin-dependent diabetic individuals can participate in an exercise program.

228. Comprehension, evaluation, physiological (b)
  1 Thyroid hormone replacement therapy helps restore a normal metabolic rate but also places stress on the cardiovascular system. The patient should be monitored for signs of heart failure or chest pain. The patient should be taught to take his pulse and to report chest pain or shortness of breath.
  2, 3 Constipation and decreased activity are associated with hypothyroidism.
  4 Sore throat and fever are side effects of certain antithyroid medications.

229. Application, evaluation, physiological (c)
  3 Complaints of tingling or numbness in fingertips are associated with hypocalcemia.
  1, 2, 4 These complaints are not associated with tetany.

230. Knowledge, evaluation, physiological (a)
  3 Pilocarpine is used in the treatment of glaucoma because intraocular pressure is lowered, thus increasing the outflow of aqueous humor.
  1 Pilocarpine creates miosis (constriction) of the pupil.
  2, 4 These are not the actions of the drug.

231. Application, evaluation, health (b)
  4 Gingival hyperplasia often occurs. The nurse should stress oral hygiene on an ongoing basis as part of discharge planning/teaching.
  1 The medication is given on a prescribed basis, and serum blood levels can be done to determine the best dose.
  2 Alcohol should not be taken because it decreases the effect of the medication.
  3 The patient should have an available supply, but it is not necessary to keep it with him at all times. It should be taken only as prescribed by a physician.

232. Application, evaluation, psychosocial (c)
  4 After a stroke, both the individual and the family are at risk for coping problems related to the various physical and mental changes as a result of the stroke. Emotional lability is often a part of the problem.
  1 The data do not support a nursing diagnosis of severe anxiety.
  2 The data do not support the nursing diagnosis of a deficit related to diversional activity.
  3 The data do not support an alteration in terms of sensory-perceptual abilities.

233. Comprehension, evaluation, physiological (c)
  4 Signs of respiratory distress and tachycardia are associated with circulatory overload.
  1 Febrile reactions include chills, fever, and headache. These usually occur 1 to 1½ hours after the start of the transfusion.
  2 Allergic reactions usually occur within the first 30 minutes and are associated with hives, itching, facial edema, and wheezing.
  3 An acute hemolytic reaction usually occurs immediately and is associated with a burning sensation along the vein, chest pain, low back pain, abrupt fever, and chills.

234. Comprehension, evaluation, health (b)
 3 Oral iron preparations may cause constipation and dark-colored (black) stools.
 1 Because side effects include gastrointestinal upset, the medication may be taken with meals.
 2 Liquid iron preparations may stain the teeth.
 4 Vitamin C aids in the absorption of iron.
235. Comprehension, evaluation, physiological (b)
 3 When myocardial cells are injured, intracellular enzymes are released. CK-MB (formerly called CPK) is the most specific enzyme indicating myocardial injury. CK-MB rises within 4 to 8 hours of the infarction.
 1 This is indicative of injury, not infection.
 2 The myocardial infarct location is noted on the ECG.
 4 The CK-MB is specific for the myocardium, not the kidneys.
236. Knowledge, evaluation, physiological (a)
 4 A decreased supply of oxygen to the brain can cause confusion, impaired judgment, and altered levels of consciousness.
 1 Tachycardia, not bradycardia, is associated with hypoxia.
 2 Retention of carbon dioxide can cause a red or ruddy skin color.
 3 Auscultation of breath sounds provides information about airflow through the tracheobronchial tree.
237. Application, evaluation, health (b)
 4 Sublingual nitroglycerin should be taken at the *earliest* sign of chest discomfort. The patient should sit down, place one tablet under his tongue, and allow it to dissolve.
 1 A patient may be taught to dissolve one tablet under the tongue 5 minutes before participating in an activity that the patient knows causes chest discomfort. However, taking the medication at the *earliest* sign of chest discomfort is the most appropriate patient response in the beginning stage of patient teaching.
 2, 3 Sublingual nitroglycerin is for use when chest discomfort occurs.

238. Comprehension, evaluation, physiological (c)
 3 When the lung has reexpanded, no fluctuation of fluid in the long tube of the water-seal bottle will occur. If there is an absence of complications, the lung usually reexpands in 2 to 3 days.
 1 Fluctuation in the water-seal chamber indicates that the lung has not reexpanded.
 2 With a pneumothorax, the chest tube releases air from the pleural cavity.
 4 Continuous bubbling usually indicates an air leak.
239. Application, evaluation, health (b)
 3 The stoma should be cleaned with a clean wash cloth. The use of soaps should be avoided because they irritate the skin around the stoma.
 1 This is a healthful practice that should be done. This statement indicates patient understanding of discharge teachings.
 2 The stoma should be assessed daily for any sign of infection. This statement indicates patient understanding of discharge teachings.
 4 Foreign material (hairs) could lead to inhalation. This statement indicates patient understanding of discharge teachings.
240. Comprehension, evaluation, environment (a)
 4 The normal range for the systolic pressure is 120 to 140; the normal diastolic range is 60 to 90. A diastolic pressure above 90 may be indicative of hypertension.
 1, 2 Both the systolic and diastolic pressure values are within the average range.
 3 Although both the systolic and diastolic pressures are slightly low, this is not considered abnormal.